Genetics and Public Health in the 21st Century

OXFORD MONOGRAPHS ON MEDICAL GENETICS

General Editors

Arno G. Motulsky   Martin Bobrow   Peter S. Harper   Charles Scriver

Former Editors

J.A. Fraser Roberts   C.O. Carter

OXFORD MONOGRAPHS ON MEDICAL GENETICS NO. 40

GENETICS

AND

PUBLIC HEALTH

IN THE

21st CENTURY

Using Genetic Information to Improve Health and Prevent Disease

Edited by

MUIN J. KHOURY, M.D., PH.D
Director, Office of Genetics and Disease Prevention
Centers for Disease Control and Prevention
Atlanta, Georgia

WYLIE BURKE, M.D., PH.D.
Associate Professor of Medicine
Department of Medicine
University of Washington
Seattle, Washington

ELIZABETH J. THOMSON, M.S., R.N., C.G.C.
Director, Ethical, Legal and Social Implications Research Program
National Human Genome Research Institute
National Institutes of Health
Bethesda, Maryland

OXFORD
UNIVERSITY PRESS

2000

OXFORD
UNIVERSITY PRESS

Oxford   New York
Athens Auckland Bangkok Bogotá Buenos Aires Calcutta
Cape Town Chennai Dar es Salaam Delhi Florence Hong Kong Istanbul
Karachi Kuala Lumpur Madrid Melbourne Mexico City Mumbai
Nairobi Paris São Paulo Singapore Taipei Tokyo Toronto Warsaw

and associated companies in
Berlin   Ibadan

Library of Congress Cataloging-in-Publication Data
Genetics and public health in the 21st century:
using genetic information to improve health and prevent disease/
edited by Muin J. Khoury, Wylie Burke, Elizabeth J. Thomson.
p.; cm. Includes bibliographical references and index.
ISBN 0-19-512830-3
1. Genetic screening. 2. Public health. 3. Medical genetics.
I. Khoury, Muin J. II. Burke, Wylie. III. Thomson, Elizabeth J. (Elizabeth Jean), 1950– .
[DNLM: 1. Human Genome Project 2. Public Health. 3. Epidemiology, Molecular. 4. Genetic
Engineering. 5. Genetic Predisposition to Disease—prevention & control. 6. Genetic Screening.
7. Genetics, Biochemical. 8. Health Planning. 9. Preventive Medicine.
WA 105 G328 2000] RB 155.65 .G465 2000 616'.042—dc21 99-049548

9 8 7 6 5 4 3 2 1

Printed in the United States of America
on acid-free paper

Preface

During the next few years, all of the estimated 50,000 to 100,000 human genes will be identified as a result of the Human Genome Project. As genome technology moves from the laboratory to the healthcare setting, a complex array of challenges will face medical and public health professionals in the appropriate use of genetic information to improve health and prevent disease in individuals, families, and communities. Human genetic variation is associated with many, if not all, human diseases and disabilities, including the common chronic diseases of major public health impact. Genetic variation interacts with environmental and sociocultural influences to modify the risk of disease.

Because the broad mission of public health is to fulfill society's interest in assuring conditions in which people can be healthy, there will be an unavoidable integration of new genetic technologies and information into public health programs to target intervention strategies that will prevent morbidity, mortality, and disability from a wide array of conditions. Public health professionals will increasingly use genetic technologies and information in research, policy, and program development. This is not different from the expected integration of genetics into health care in general across the various subspecialties.

In anticipation of the expected growth at the interface of genetics and public health, we have attempted in this book to delineate a framework for the integration of advances in human genetics into public health practice. The book is intended to be a resource to public health students, researchers, and practitioners. Our contributors come from a wide range of disciplines including epidemiology, biostatistics, clinical medicine, health policy and management, health services research, behavioral and social sciences, ethics, law, health economics, and laboratory sciences. Researchers, students, and practitioners in various medical and nursing fields should also benefit from having their perspectives on the emerging and often complex issues of genetic testing as a public health issue.

The book is divided into six parts. Part I presents overarching principles of human genetics in public health. It includes a framework for integrating genetics into public health practice (Chapter 1), historical perspectives (Chapter 2), an update on the impact of the Human Genome Project (Chapter 3), an overview of models of public health policy decisions in genetics (Chapter 4), and a discussion of the multidisciplinary nature of research and training in genetics and public health (Chapter 5).

Part II covers issues related to public health assessment in genetics. It provides an overview of the interface between epidemiology and molecular biology (Chapter 6) and discusses issues of surveillance in birth defects and genetic disorders (Chapter 7), with a focus on hematologic diseases (Chapter 8). This section further deals with public health assessment in the genetics of cancer (Chapter 9), infectious diseases (Chapter 10), and occupational health (Chapter 11).

Part III presents selected examples of public health evaluation of genetic testing. It discusses various strategies to ensure the quality, safety, and effectiveness of genetic testing (Chapter 12) and gives a specific example of newborn quality assurance screening (Chapter 13).

Part IV identifies approaches and gives examples for developing, implementing, and evaluating population interventions that use genetic information to improve health. It contains chapters on population needs assessment and delivery of genetic services (Chapters 14 through 17), the application of prevention effectiveness principles to genetics programs (Chapter 18), and the impact of genetic counseling on public health (Chapter 19). Additional chapters in this section illustrate the process of policy and program development and evaluation in relation to specific disease conditions, such as phenylketonuria (Chapter 20), cystic fibrosis (Chapter 21), sickle cell disease (Chapter 22), hemochromatosis (Chapter 23), and coronary heart disease (Chapter 24).

Part V addresses some but not all of the emerging ethical, legal, and social issues related to the integration of genetics into public health practice. It covers the interface among public health, genetics, and the law (Chapter 25), the informed consent process in traditional public health genetics programs (Chapter 26), and issues surrounding public health surveillance and information systems (Chapter 27).

Finally, Part VI deals with communication, education, and the dissemination of genetic information in public health practice. It presents overall principles of communication science related to genetics and public health (Chapter 28), an overview of efforts to train public health professionals in genetics (Chapter

29), consumer perspectives on genetic testing (Chapter 30), and an account of the use of the Internet as an emerging medium for information dissemination in genetics and public health (Chapter 31).

Although the interface of genetics and public health will continue to evolve over the next few years, we hope this volume will provide a solid foundation for increasing the level of awareness of the emerging role of genetics in public health practice in the 21st century.

Atlanta, Ga.   M.J.K.
Seattle, Wash.   W.B.
Bethesda, Md.   E.T.
September 1999

Acknowledgments

We thank the numerous distinguished contributors to this book. In particular we acknowledge the mark of Dr. Roger Williams, who died tragically in the crash of Swissair Flight 111 in September 1998 before completing Chapter 24. Dr. Williams was the founder and director of the University of Utah Cardiovascular Genetics Research Clinic, and he served on many state, national, and international committees for both public and private organizations. Over a career that spanned almost 25 years, he authored or co-authored more than 200 professional publications, taught at universities throughout the world, and was the recipient of numerous awards for his achievements.

We are grateful to the following individuals for reviewing drafts of selected book chapters: Jean Anderson, Melissa A. Austin, Roy Baron, Barbara Bowman, George C. Cunningham, Paul M. Fernhoff, Nancy Fisher, Norman Fost, Jan Friedman, H. Wayne Giles, W. Harry Hannon, James Hanson, Roy Ing, Ronald La Porte, Arno G. Motulsky, John Mulvihill, Claudia F. Parvanta, Margaret Piper, Nancy Press, Scott Ramsey, Sonja A. Rasmussen, Mark A. Rothstein, Thomas H. Sinks, James R. Sorenson, Suzanne P. Tomlinson, Deborah Tress, Michael S. Watson, Ellen Wright-Clayton, and Elizabeth Gettig, who read and commented on many parts of the manuscript. In addition, we thank Diane Mayes for her skills in compiling the manuscript and her diligence and support in the creation of this project.

Contents

Contributors

MICHAEL AIDOO, PH.D.
Molecular Vaccine Section,
  Immunology Branch
Division of Parasitic Diseases
National Center for Infectious
  Diseases
Centers for Disease Control and
  Prevention
Atlanta, Georgia

MELISSA A. AUSTIN, PH.D.
Department of Epidemiology
Public Health Genetics Program
Public Health and Community
  Medicine
University of Washington
Seattle, Washington

DIANE L. BAKER, M.S., C.G.C.
Department of Human Genetics
University of Michigan Medical School
Ann Arbor, Michigan

CAROL J. BELL B.S.,
  MT (ASCP)
Newborn Screening Quality Assurance
  Program
Division of Laboratory Sciences
National Center for Environmental
  Health
Centers for Disease Control and
  Prevention
Atlanta, Georgia

JUDITH L. BENKENDORF, M.S.,
  C.G.C.
Division of Genetics
Department of Obstetrics and
  Gynecology
Georgetown University Medical
  Center
Washington, DC

LORENZO D. BOTTO, M.D.
Birth Defects and Genetic Diseases
  Branch
National Center for Environmental
  Health
Centers for Disease Control and
  Prevention
Atlanta, Georgia

WYLIE BURKE, M.D., PH.D.
Department of Medicine
University of Washington
Seattle, Washington

SCOTT BURRIS, J.D.
James E. Beasley School of Law
Temple University
Philadelphia, Pennsylvania

SUSAN M. CAUMARTIN, PH.D.
Department of Epidemiology
School of Public Health
University of Michigan
Ann Arbor, Michigan

MARY E. COGSWELL, DR. P.H.
Division of Nutrition and Physical
 Activity
National Center for Chronic Disease
 Prevention and Health Promotion
Centers for Disease Control and
 Prevention
Atlanta, Georgia

DEBRA L. COLLINS, M.S.
University of Kansas Medical Center
Kansas City, Kansas

FRANCIS S. COLLINS, M.D.,
 PH.D.
National Human Genome Research
 Institute
National Institutes of Health
Bethesda, Maryland

CELESTE M. CONDIT, PH.D.
Department of Speech Communication
University of Georgia
Athens, Georgia

STEVEN S. COUGHLIN, PH.D.
Division of Cancer Prevention and
 Control
Centers for Disease Control and
 Prevention
Atlanta, Georgia

KAREY DAVID, B.A.
Alliance of Genetic Support Groups
Washington, DC

MARY E. DAVIDSON, M.S.W.
Genetic Alliance
Washington, DC

D. GAYLE DeBORD, PH.D.
Molecular and Genetic Monitoring
 Section
Biomonitoring and Health Assessment
 Branch
Division of Applied Research and
 Technology
National Institute for Occupational
 Safety and Health
Centers for Disease Control and
 Prevention
Cincinnati, Ohio

JANICE S. DORMAN, PH.D.
Department of Epidemiology
Graduate School of Public Health
University of Pittsburgh
Pittsburgh, Pennsylvania

MARIE V. DOWNER, M.D.,
 M.P.H.
Immunogenetics Section
Immunology Branch
Division of AIDS, STD and TB
 Laboratory Research
National Center for Infectious
 Diseases
Centers for Disease Control and
 Prevention
Atlanta, Georgia

DEBRA LOCHNER DOYLE,
 M.S., C.G.C.
Genetic Services Section
Washington State Department of
 Health
Seattle, Washington

BRUCE L. EVATT, M.D.
Hematologic Diseases Branch
Division of AIDS, STD, and TB
 Laboratory Research
National Center for Infectious Diseases
Centers for Disease Control and
 Prevention
Atlanta, Georgia

PHILIP M. FARRELL, M.D.,
 PH.D.
University of Wisconsin Medical
 School
Madison, Wisconsin

ROBERT M. FINEMAN, M.D.,
 PH.D.
Office of Maternal and Child Health
Washington State Department of
 Health
Seattle, Washington

LESLIE FINK, B.S.
Office of Communications and Public
  Liaison
National Institute of Allergy and
  Infectious Diseases
National Institutes of Health
Bethesda, Maryland

ADELE FRANKS, M.D.
Prudential Center for Healthcare
  Research
Atlanta, Georgia

LAWRENCE O. GOSTIN, J.D.,
  L.L.D.
Georgetown/Johns Hopkins University
Washington, DC

SCOTT D. GROSSE, PH.D.
Office of Program Evaluation and
  Legislation
National Center for Environmental
  Health
Centers for Disease Control and
  Prevention
Atlanta, Georgia

W. HARRY HANNON, PH.D.
Newborn Screening Quality Assurance
  Program
Division of Laboratory Sciences
National Center for Environmental
  Health
Centers for Disease Control and
  Prevention
Atlanta, Georgia

L. OMAR HENDERSON, PH.D.
Newborn Screening Quality Assurance
  Program
Division of Laboratory Sciences
National Center for Environmental
  Health
Centers for Disease Control and
  Prevention
Atlanta, Georgia

THOMAS HODGE, PH.D.
Immunogenetics Section
Immunology Branch
Division of AIDS, STD and TB
  Laboratory Research
National Center for Infectious
  Diseases
Centers for Disease Control and
  Prevention
Atlanta, Georgia

GARY HOFFMAN
Newborn Screening
State Laboratory of Hygiene
Madison, Wisconsin

PAUL N. HOPKINS, M.D.
  M.S.P.H.
Cardiovascular Genetics Research
  Clinic
University of Utah School of Medicine
Salt Lake City, Utah

NANCY HSU, B.A.
University of Wisconsin Medical
  School
Madison, Wisconsin

STEVEN C. HUNT, PH.D.
Cardiovascular Genetics Research
  Clinic
University of Utah School of Medicine
Salt Lake City, Utah

MUIN J. KHOURY, M.D., PH.D.
Office of Genetics and Disease
  Prevention
Centers for Disease Control and
  Prevention
Atlanta, Georgia

MICHAEL R. KOSOROK, PH.D.
Department of Biostatistics and
  Medical Informatics
University of Wisconsin Medical
  School
Madison, Wisconsin

RONALD H. LAESSIG, PH.D.
Department of Preventive Medicine
University of Wisconsin Medical
   School
State Laboratory of Hygiene
Madison, Wisconsin

ANITA LAXOVA, B.S.
Department of Pediatrics
University of Wisconsin Medical
   School
Madison, Wisconsin

CARYN LERMAN, PH.D.
Department of Oncology
Georgetown University Medical
   Center
Lombardi Cancer Center
Washington, DC

JANE S. LIN-FU, M.D.
Genetic Services Branch
Maternal and Child Health Bureau
Health Resources and Services
   Administration
U.S. Department of Health and Human
   Services
Potomac, Maryland

MICHELE LLOYD-PURYEAR,
   M.D, PH.D.
Genetic Services Branch
Maternal and Child Health Bureau
Health Resources and Services
   Administration
U.S. Department of Health and Human
   Services
Rockville, Maryland

CARL F. MARRS, PH.D.
Department of Epidemiology
University of Michigan
Ann Arbor, Michigan

PIERPAOLO MASTROIACOVO,
   M.D.
Institute of Pediatrics
Catholic University
International Center for Birth Defects
Rome, Italy

DONALD R. MATTISON, M.D.
March of Dimes Birth Defects
   Foundation
White Plains, New York

SHARON M. MCDONNELL,
   M.D., M.P.H.
Division of Nutrition and Physical
   Activity
National Center for Chronic Disease
   Prevention and Health Promotion
Centers for Disease Control and
   Prevention
Atlanta, Georgia

JANET M. MCNICHOLL, M.D.,
   M.S.
Immunogenetics Section
Immunology Branch
Division of AIDS, STD and TB
   Laboratory Research
National Center for Infectious
   Diseases
Centers for Disease Control and
   Prevention
Atlanta, Georgia

BETH O'GRADY, B.S.
Department of Speech Communication
University of Georgia
Athens, Georgia

LESLIE A. O'LEARY, PH.D.
Office of Genetics and Disease
   Prevention
Centers for Disease Control and
   Prevention
Atlanta, Georgia

RICHARD S. OLNEY, M.D.
   M.P.H.
Division of Birth Defects and Pediatric
   Genetics
National Center for Environmental
   Health
Centers for Disease Control and
   Prevention
Atlanta, Georgia

GILBERT S. OMENN, M.D., PH.D.
Departments of Medicine, Genetics, and Public Health
University of Michigan
Ann Arbor, Michigan

ROXANNE L. PARROTT, PH.D.
Department of Speech Communication
University of Georgia
Athens, Georgia

KENNETH A. PASS, PH.D.
Newborn Screening and Genetic Services
Wadsworth Center
State of New York Department of Health
Albany, New York

VICTOR B. PENCHASZADEH, M.D., M.S.P.H.
Albert Einstein College of Medicine
Division of Medical Genetics
Beth Israel Medical Center
New York, New York

BETH N. PESHKIN, M.S., C.G.C.
Department of Oncology
Georgetown University Medical Center
Lombardi Cancer Center
Washington, DC

PATRICIA A. PEYSER, PH.D.
Department of Epidemiology
Public Health Genetics Interdepartmental Concentration
School of Public Health
University of Michigan
Ann Arbor, Michigan

TONI I. POLLIN, M.S.
University of Maryland School of Medicine
Division of Diabetes, Obesity, and Nutrition
Baltimore, MD

NANCY PRESS, PH.D.
Department of Public Health and Preventive Medicine
Oregon Health Sciences University
Portland, Oregon

FREDERICK R. RICKLES, M.D.
George Washington University Medical Center
Washington, DC

MICHAEL J. ROCK, M.D.
Department of Pediatrics
University of Wisconsin
Madison, Wisconsin

PAUL A. SCHULTE, PH.D.
Education and Information Division
National Institute for Occupational Safety and Health
Centers for Disease Control and Prevention
Department of Health and Human Services
Cincinnati, Ohio

J. MICHAEL SOUCIE, PH.D.
Hematologic Diseases Branch
Division of AIDS, STD and TB Laboratory Research
National Center for Infectious Diseases
Centers for Disease Control and Prevention
Atlanta, Georgia

MARK L. SPLAINGARD, M.D.
Pulmonary Department
Children's Hospital of Wisconsin
Milwaukee, Wisconsin

LEO P. TEN KATE, M.D., PH.D.
Vrije Universiteit
Amsterdam, The Netherlands

STEVEN M. TEUTSCH, M.D.,
M.P.H.
Outcomes Research & Management
Merck & Co., Inc.
West Point, Pennsylvania

ELIZABETH J. THOMSON, M.S.,
R.N., C.G.C.
National Human Genome Research
Institute
National Institutes of Health
Bethesda, Maryland

DEBORAH TRESS, J.D.
Office of the General Counsel
Centers for Disease Control and
Prevention
Atlanta, Georgia

VENKATACHALAM
UDHAYAKUMAR, PH.D.
Molecular Vaccine Section,
Immunology Branch
Division of Parasitic Diseases
National Center for Infectious
Diseases
Centers for Disease Control and
Prevention
Atlanta, Georgia

MICHAEL S. WATSON, PH.D.
Washington University School of
Medicine
Washington University Medical
Center
St. Louis Children's Hospital
St. Louis, Missouri

JOAN O. WEISS, M.S.W.
Alliance of Genetic Support Groups
Chevy Chase, Maryland

BENJAMIN S. WILFOND, M.D.
National Human Genome Research
Institute
Department of Clinical Bioethics
National Institutes of Health
Bethesda, Maryland

NACHAMA WILKER
Alliance of Genetic Support Groups
Washington, DC

ROGER R. WILLIAMS, M.D.[†]
Cardiovascular Genetics Research
Clinic
University of Utah School of Medicine
Salt Lake City, Utah

MARY ANN WILSON
Alliance of Genetic Support Groups
Washington, DC

ELLEN WRIGHT CLAYTON, M.D.,
J.D.
Department of Pediatrics
Vanderbilt University
Nashville, Tennessee

LILY WU, PH.D.
Cardiovascular Genetics Research
Clinic
University of Utah School of
Medicine
Salt Lake City, Utah

LAN ZENG, M.S.
Department of Pediatrics
University of Wisconsin Medical
School
Madison, Wisconsin

[†] Deceased.

I

GENETICS AND PUBLIC HEALTH: AN OVERVIEW

1

Genetics and public health: A framework for the integration of human genetics into public health practice

Muin J. Khoury, Wylie Burke, Elizabeth J. Thomson

As we enter the 21st century, health care is undergoing phenomenal changes driven, in part, by the Human Genome Project and accompanying advances in human genetics (1). All of the 50,000 to 100,000 human genes will be identified in the next few years (2). As of 1999, more than 10,000 genes have been discovered and catalogued (3). Tests for more than 600 gene variants are already available in medical practice (4). Gene variants found thus far include not only those associated with rare diseases, but those that increase susceptibility to common chronic diseases, such as cancer and heart disease (5) (Table 1.1). Risks for almost all human diseases result from the interactions between inherited gene variants and environmental factors, including chemical, physical, and infectious agents and behavioral or nutritional factors, which raises the possibility of targeting disease prevention and health promotion efforts to individuals at high risk because of their genetic makeup (6).

Need for Public Health Leadership in Genetics

How to use knowledge from genetics research to promote health and prevent disease—the fundamental mission of public health—is now being explored. However, we lack population-based information about the distribution of genotypes in different populations, the benefits and risks of genetic testing, and the efficacy of early interventions. Moreover, the complex issues that have emerged (e.g., rapid commercialization of genetic tests, quality of laboratory

Portions of this chapter are based on the Centers for Disease Control and Prevention "Translating Advances in Human Genetics into Public Health Action: A Strategic Plan" (1997) (11).

Table 1.1 Number of Genes Reported to Increase
Susceptibility to Selected Conditions

Condition	Number of Genes*
Mental retardation	872
Congenital abnormalities	594
Cancer	554
Heart disease	408
Anemia	331
Infection	318
Diabetes	292
Thyroid	242
Dementia	137
Arthritis	111
Asthma	55

* Includes identified or mapped genes.
Source: Online Mendelian Inheritance in Man [database] (1999) (3).

testing, availability of and access to interventions, and potential discrimination against and stigmatization of individuals and groups) call for public health leadership.

Almost daily, gene discoveries are reported for human diseases (7). Unfortunately, what happens after a new gene discovery is announced is often a haphazard mixture of scientific excitement, heightened public awareness, and commercial interest in developing and marketing genetic tests. This problem is exemplified by events following the 1997 publication of an association between familial colorectal cancer in Ashkhenazi Jews and the presence of a common genetic variant in the adenomatosis polyposis coli (APC) gene (8). In one example of the accompanying news coverage, a 1998 article titled "Genetic Defect Doubles Colon Cancer Risk" (9) stated:

> Researchers have found a new genetic defect present in one of every 17 American Jews that doubles a person's colon cancer risk. This mutation is now the most common cancer-associated gene defect identified in any ethnic population. Rarely present in non-Jews, the mutation appears to be responsible for about one in four cases of inherited colon cancer in Askhenazi Jews—those of Eastern European ancestry who constitute more than 95% of America's six million Jewish people. The good news is that scientists have developed a blood test, available for $200, that can detect this genetic defect. The test is advisable for everyone in the Ashkhenazim population, whether they have a family history of colon cancer or not.

Although this study needed further confirmation, and its implications for medical practice still remain far from clear, the response illustrates the mounting pressures for a rapid transition from gene discovery to integration in clinical practice, which could result in the premature development and offering of genetic tests.

Over the last 5 years, public health agencies have begun examining how advances in human genetics can be used to prevent disease and improve the health of the population (10). As the Centers for Disease Control (CDC) developed a strategic plan (11) to address both the opportunities and challenges posed by advances in human genetics on public health practice, for example, it became clear that much of public health training, infrastructure, policy and program development has not taken genetics into consideration. Notable exceptions are newborn screening programs for metabolic diseases, birth defects surveillance systems, and programs for children with special health care needs. Yet, as the science of gene discovery matures, there will be an increasing role for public health in closing the gap between gene discovery and applications to prevent human diseases, especially adult-onset chronic diseases.

The Institute of Medicine (IOM) report on the future of public health (12) can be used as a starting point for developing a long-term strategic plan to integrate genetics into public health practice. The IOM report defined three core functions for public health agencies: assessment, policy development, and assurance. Although genetics was not mentioned specifically in the IOM document, the substantial recommendations of this report apply to all emerging areas in public health, including genetics.

The Interface of Genetics and Public Health

In recent years, a new hybrid subspecialty of genetics and public health has emerged. *Public health genetics* (a term mostly used in the United States [13,14]) has been defined as the application of advances in genetics and molecular biotechnology to improve public health and prevent disease (14). *Community genetics* (a term mostly used in Europe [15]) has been defined as "a branch of genetics that has service and science components." The service component seeks to integrate genetic services into community interventions. The science component encompasses the research needed to develop and evaluate services (15). Public health genetics and community genetics could be viewed as one and the same. Nevertheless, as we think about the broader mission of public health, namely "to fulfill society's interest in assuring conditions in which people can be healthy" (12), there will be unavoidable integration of new genetic information into all public health programs and across all diseases, whether or not the diseases are labeled "genetic diseases" or the services are termed "genetic services." All public health professionals, therefore, will need an increasing appreciation for integrating genetic research, policy, and program development into their daily work. This is not different from the expected integration of genetics into health care in general and across the various medical subspecialties (16,17). Although recognizing the need for a cadre of public health researchers and practitioners fully trained in genetics, we also believe that all public health professionals will be using advances in human genetics in research and practice. We do not particularly endorse the creation of a new public health subspecialty in genetics; rather, we encourage and emphasize the smooth integration of genetics into public health practice. Some of the distinctions between these views are shown in Table 1.2. Nevertheless, the reader will see various terminologies and definitions used by contributing authors to address the interface between genetics and public health (18).

One might wonder, What is the meaning of prevention in the context of genetics and public health? Juengst (19) used the terms "genotypic prevention"—the interruption of genetic trait transmission from one generation to the next through reproductive counseling, carrier testing, prenatal diagnosis, and pregnancy termination—and "phenotypic prevention"—the prevention of disease and death among people with specific genotypes (19). In its strategic plan (11), the CDC clearly endorses the concept of phenotypic prevention as the strategy for public health-driven programs. Phenotypic prevention can be achieved by interrupting harmful interaction of environmental cofactors with human genetic variation or by using gene therapy to correct deficiencies in gene products.

Although public health-driven prevention may be clear-cut for adult-onset multifactorial conditions such as cancer and heart disease, its role is more problematic for early-onset, lethal single-gene conditions such as Tay-Sachs disease and other severe conditions affecting children. It has been argued that an important role still exists for public health activities in prenatal diagnosis and genotypic prevention of severe or lethal conditions (20). Assurance of individuals' and couples' access to reproductive-risk information could improve their own well-being, a goal that could be encompassed within a broad definition of health. For many couples, the availability of prenatal diagnosis provides a level of reassurance that permits them to proceed with childbearing they would otherwise forgo. Assuring the availability and voluntary access to prenatal services and evaluating the impact of these services would fall within the purview of public health practice; nevertheless, although the

Table 1.2 Genetics in Medicine and Public Health: Emphasis of Different Terminologies

Emphasis	Medicine	Public Health
Specialization	Medical genetics	Public health genetics and Community Genetics
Integration	Genetics in medicine	Genetics in public health

public heath community should take an active role in promoting the use of genetic tests and services when there are proven and cost-effective interventions to prevent disease, death, or disability (e.g., phenylketonuria or PKU), public health agencies cannot play a role in promoting the use of genotypic prevention as a method to improve the public's health.

Another philosophical issue in the integration of genetics into public health is what defines a genetic condition. Geneticists often make a distinction between single-gene disorders and susceptibility genes that are disease risk factors along with other genes and environmental exposures involved in disease development. This distinction is embodied in the concept of *genotype penetrance*. The distinction tends to fade when one realizes that all human disease is the result of interactions between genetic variation and the environment (broadly defined to include dietary, infectious, chemical, physical, and social factors). Even many of the classical single-gene metabolic disorders are the result of a deficiency in a nutritional enzyme combined with dietary exposure to one or more chemicals (e.g., phenylalanine and phenylalanine hydroxylase deficiency in PKU; and iron intake and mutations in the HFE gene in hereditary hemochromatosis (17). As Rothman stated: "It is easy to show that 100% of any disease is environmentally determined and 100% is genetically determined as well. Any other view is based on a naive understanding of causation" (21). Perhaps the wide range of penetrance with respect to clinical disease could be due, in part, to variations in the prevalence of interacting cofactors (e.g., other genes and modifiable risk factors). Universal exposure of newborn infants to phenylalanine through their diets leads to a high incidence of mental retardation among those who inherit a deficiency in phenylalanine hydroxylase.

If we accept the fundamental premise that genetic variation is associated with all human disease, there is no compelling reason to label a disease as genetic or not. For example, one can label hereditary hemochromatosis as an iron overload disorder resulting from the interaction between an inherited variation in iron transport, iron intake, and iron loss. Similarly, breast cancer in some individuals could result from the interaction between an inherited mutation in the BRCA1 gene and yet-to-be-described cofactor(s), including other genes and modifiable risk factors. When the authors of this volume refer to "genetic disorders," they are usually referring to conditions in which a single gene, with either high penetrance or a chromosomal abnormality, has been implicated. It is implicit, however, that genetic factors do play a role in the etiology of virtually all human diseases, even those that are traditionally not thought of as "genetic" (e.g., infectious and occupational diseases).

Thus, an important theme of this book is the need to identify the modifiable risk factors for disease that interact with the genetic variation and that may be used to help target preventive interventions. Recognition of the need to apply knowledge about the interaction between environment and genetics to health care has been described in the popular press (22).

Finally, an inherent assumption in our discussion of the future of genetics in public health is that much of the delivery of genetic tests and services for disease prevention and health promotion, including adequate family history assessment and genetic counseling, will be done within the context of the broader health-care system. Managed-care organizations will play an important role in integrating genetic services into disease prevention and health promotion activities.

Framework for Integrating Genetic Discoveries into Public Health Functions

A framework for applying essential public health functions in evaluating the relevance of gene discoveries to disease prevention and health promotion was developed as part of the CDC's strategic plan for genetics and public health (11). This framework encompasses four essential public health functions and three critical issues that affect each function (Table 1.3). The rest of this book is largely organized according to these public health functions and related critical issues. The following provides a brief overview.

THE FRAMEWORK

The Role of Public Health Assessment in Genetics

Public health assessment in genetics relies on scientific approaches to assess the impact of discovered genes on the health of communities. The traditional forms of applied research in public health include surveillance and epidemiology, which are explored in more detail in Part II (Chapters 6 through 11).

Table 1.3 Genetics, Public Health Functions, and Critical Issues

---

Public Health Functions
 Public health assessment
 Evaluation of genetic testing
 Development, implementation, and evaluation of population
  interventions
 Communication and information dissemination

Critical Issues
 Partnerships and coordination
 Ethical, legal, and social issues
 Education and training

Source: Adapted from CDC (1997) (11).

Surveillance

In general, surveillance—the systematic gathering, analysis, and dissemination of population data (23)—is needed to determine the population frequency of genetic variants that predispose people to specific diseases, both common and rare; the population frequency of morbidity and mortality associated with such diseases; and the prevalence and effects of environmental factors known to interact with given genotypes in producing disease. Information could be gathered also through broader surveillance of the economic costs of the genetic component of various diseases (e.g., expressed by health care costs, hospitalization rates, years of potential life lost, and other measures); genetic testing issues (e.g., access to services, quality of tests, usage by providers and potential discrimination); and issues related to interventions (e.g., availability, safety, and effectiveness). Examples of existing surveillance and health information systems include the National Health and Nutrition Examination Survey (24), population-based birth defects surveillance systems (25), and cancer surveillance systems (26).

Epidemiology

Epidemiology is often viewed as the scientific core of public health. A widely used definition is "the study of the distribution and determinants of health-related states or events in populations, and the application of this study to control health problems" (27). Epidemiologists not only investigate outbreaks of disease in different populations but also conduct studies to determine risk factors for various diseases, identify high-risk subpopulations to which to target prevention and intervention actions, and evaluate the effectiveness of health programs and services in improving the population's health (28).

Over the last two decades, epidemiologic methods and approaches have been increasingly integrated with those of genetics through the discipline of *genetic epidemiology*, which seeks to identify the role of genetic factors in disease occurrence in populations and families (29). In addition, a new brand of epidemiology has emerged—*molecular epidemiology*—that seeks to study disease occurrence using biological markers of exposure, susceptibility, and effects (30).

Most discoveries for gene variants are based on studies of high-risk families or selected groups. To translate the results of this genetic research into opportunities for treating and preventing disease and promoting health, population-based epidemiologic studies are increasingly needed to quantify the impact of gene variants on the risk of disease, death, and disability, and to identify and quantify the impact of modifiable risk factors that interact with gene variants. The results of such studies will help health professionals to better target medical, behavioral, and environmental interventions. Epidemiologic studies are also required for clinically validating new genetic tests, monitoring a population's use of genetic tests, and determining the safety, effectiveness, and impact of genetic tests and services in different populations.

To accomplish translation of genetic discoveries into public health practice, epidemiologists must collaborate with practitioners of other disciplines such as clinical genetics, laboratory sciences, behavioral and social sciences, communication sciences, ethics, and law. A combined genetic–epidemiologic approach is essential for better understanding disease etiology and developing molecular diagnostics. Data generated from such collaborations are urgently needed in developing medical and public health policy. For example, issues have been debated regarding population-based genetic testing for breast cancer in relation to the BRCA1 gene (31); Alzheimer's disease in relation to the Apolipoprotein E-E4 allele (32); and iron overload in relation to the hemochromatosis gene (33). Given the paucity of population-based epidemiologic data regarding the frequency of and disease risks and environmental interactions for many newly discovered human gene variants, there is concern that appropriate health policy on the use of genetic tests may not be possible.

Human Genome Epidemiology

The term "human genome epidemiology" (HuGE) denotes an evolving field of inquiry that systematically applies epidemiologic methods and approaches in population-based studies of the impact of human genetic variation on health and disease. The HuGE can be viewed as the intersection between genetic epidemiology and molecular epidemiology (34). Whereas genetic epidemiology has traditionally focused on techniques to find disease genes using linkage and segregation analysis, molecular epidemiology focuses on using biological markers in epidemiologic studies.

The wide spectrum of topics addressed by investigators working on human genome epidemiology and selected examples are shown in Table 1.4 (35). The spectrum ranges from population-based epidemiologic research on gene variants to evaluation of genetic tests and services. Ultimately, HuGE represents the application of clinical and molecular research to a population setting and involves the collaboration and contribution of numerous specialties.

In 1998, a collaboration of individuals and organizations launched the Human Genome Epidemiology Network (HuGE Net [36]). This global effort seeks to (1) promote collaboration in developing and disseminating of peer-reviewed epidemiologic information on human genes, (2) to develop an updated and accessible knowledge base on the World Wide Web, and (3) to promote use of this knowledge base by health care providers, researchers, industry, government, and the public for making decisions involving the use of genetic tests and services for disease prevention and health promotion (34,35).

Table 1.4 Categories and Examples of Human Genome Epidemiology Studies

Category	Example
Assess the prevalence of gene variants in different populations.	Using the National Health and Nutrition Examination Survey III, a nationally representative sample of the U.S. population, to assess the prevalence of gene variants in population subgroups (24).
Assess the magnitude of disease risk associated with gene variants in different populations.	Using population-based, case-control studies of neural tube defects to assess the etiologic role of an allelic variant in the methylene tetrahydrofolate reductase enzyme (37).
Assess the contribution of gene variants to the occurrence of a disease in different populations.	Using population-based cancer registries to assess the contribution of BRCA1 mutations to the risk of breast cancer in the general population (38).
Assess the magnitude of disease risk associated with gene-gene and gene-environment interactions in different populations.	Using case-control studies to assess the interaction between the factor V Leiden and the use of oral contraceptives in relation to the risk of venous thrombosis (39).
Assess the clinical validity and utility of genetic tests in different populations.	Using a randomized clinical trial to assess the impact of newborn screening for cystic fibrosis in Wisconsin on height and weight in the first 10 years of life (40).
Evaluate the determinants and impact of using genetic tests and services in different populations.	Using newborn screening programs for sickle cell disease in three states to evaluate gaps in utilization of health care (e.g., penicillin prophylaxis) and the determinants of morbidity and mortality (41).

Evaluation of Genetic Testing

The book focuses on two main types of evaluation-related activities: (1) the assessment of how and when genetic tests can be or are used to promote health and to diagnose and prevent human disease; and (2) the development of standards and guidelines for assuring quality genetic testing. As defined by the Task Force on Genetic Testing, genetic tests include the analysis of human DNA, RNA, chromosomes, proteins, and certain metabolites to detect a person's genotype for clinical purposes, including predicting risk of disease, identifying carriers, and establishing prenatal and clinical diagnosis or prognosis (42).

The Task Force on Genetic Testing recognized the need to evaluate several types of data parameters (analytic validity, clinical validity, and clinical utility, as defined in Table 1.5) for each genetic test before transitioning the test from research to clinical practice. Because evaluation of genetic tests used in the prediction of adult-onset diseases may require years of follow-up, the Task

Table 1.5 Parameters for Evaluating the Population Use of Genetic Tests

Data Parameter	Definition
Analytic validity	How good is the test in predicting underlying genotype (i.e., sensitivity, specificity, and predictive values with respect to genotype)?
Clinical validity	How good is the test in diagnosing or predicting phenotype or disease (i.e., sensitivity, specificity, and predictive values with respect to phenotype or disease)?
Clinical utility	What are the benefits and risks that accrue from genetic tests and ensuing interventions?

Source: Holtzman and Watson (1997) (42).

Force also outlined the need for postmarket reevaluation of the same three parameters for genetic tests in the context of "real-world" use and to reevaluate policies and recommendations on the use of genetic tests. These and other parameters of the preanalytic and postanalytic testing process need to be continuously evaluated in population-based settings.

The second main area of evaluation concerns the development of standards, regulations, and guidelines to ensure the accuracy, validity, and precision of laboratory procedures and to ensure that other quality assurance issues are also addressed.

All clinical laboratories in the United States that provide information to referring physicians are certified under the Clinical Laboratory Improvement Act (CLIA) Amendments of 1988 (43). The CLIA standards for quality control, proficiency testing, personnel, and other quality assurance practices apply to all genetic tests; CLIA regulations, which are jointly developed and administered by the Health Care Financing Administration and CDC, include additional specific requirements for cytogenetic testing. A genetics subcommittee of the CLIA Advisory Committee has considered more specific requirements for molecular genetic testing.

Another role for public health could be development of model quality assurance programs, including proficiency testing programs for genetic testing in public health programs such as the Newborn Screening Quality Assurance Program (Chapter 13). These model programs would set standards for testing, monitor the quality of testing, and recommend improvements for laboratory quality assurance.

The need for quality assurance programs in molecular genetic testing is highlighted in the results of a mail survey of 245 molecular genetic testing laboratory directors conducted by McGovern et al. (44). Researchers collected and analyzed data regarding availability of clinical molecular genetic testing, including data on personnel standards and laboratory practices. They found a wide range of mean quality assurance (QA) scores, with 15% of the laboratories scoring lower than 70%, suggesting that both personnel qualification and laboratory practice standards are in need of improvement to ensure quality in clinical molecular genetic testing laboratories. Evaluation of genetic testing is explored in more detail in Part III (Chapters 12 and 13).

Development, Implementation, and Evaluation of Population Interventions

The translation of advances in human genetics into actual disease prevention opportunities requires strong public health leadership in developing, implementing, and evaluating disease intervention strategies. Burgeoning genetic knowledge is accompanied by high expectations that identification of genetically susceptible people will permit tailoring of prevention efforts to improve their effectiveness; yet, the clinical use of genetic information poses risks as well. Social scientists have postulated an adverse effect of genetic testing on psychological well-being and family functioning (45,46). The potential for loss of health, life or disability insurance or other discrimination as a result of genetic testing has also been raised (47). Of equal concern is that genetic tests will be used to identify persons at increased risk of disease before effective measures to reduce their risk are available. To formulate sound policy decisions regarding the appropriate use of genetic information in population-based testing programs, a systematic, evidence-based approach should be used to assess the potential benefits and risks of genetic testing.

Since 1968, principles for population-based screening programs have been developed (48) and modified by various groups (e.g., the American College of Medical Genetics [49], and the National Academy of Sciences, [50]) with respect to genetic screening. More recently, Coughlin et al. (51) have synthesized from the literature emerging elements of a set of principles on the use of genetic information in population-based, adult-onset chronic disease prevention programs. These principles include (1) assessment of scientific evidence on the relationship among genotype, disease, and genetic test parameters (shown in Table 1.5); (2) systematic review of the benefits, risks, and costs of screening to the target population; (3) a policy development process using consensus conferences, workshops, or other approaches to evaluate the appropriateness of population testing; and (4) an evaluation process that should include various measures of access to the testing program as well as impact and effectiveness, including need for revision of testing recommendations based on new scientific evidence.

Thus, an important role of public health will be to develop intervention strategies for diseases with a genetic component, implement pilot demonstration programs, and evaluate the impact of interventions on reducing morbidity and mortality in the population. Part IV of this book discusses needs assessment and delivery of genetic services (Chapters 14 through 17), application of prevention effectiveness principles to genetics programs (Chapter 18), and impact of genetic counseling on public health (Chapter 19). Additional chapters in Part IV illustrate the process of policy and program development and evaluation in relation to specific disease conditions, including PKU (Chapter 20), cystic fibrosis (Chapter 21), sickle cell disease (Chapter 22), hemochromatosis (Chapter 23), and coronary heart disease (Chapter 24). Although much of the discussion of genetic services still focuses on traditional genetic programs related to reproductive genetics and child health, an increasing emphasis in the next few years will be on the utility of genetic testing for preventing adult-onset diseases.

Communication and Information Dissemination

The fourth public health function in genetics is developing and applying communication principles and strategies related to advances in human genetics, the use of genetic tests and services, interventions, and the ethical, legal, and social issues related to these topics. The relevance of advances in human genetics to disease prevention and health promotion needs to be communicated to a large number of audiences, including policymakers, health care providers, researchers, and the general public (11). Public health agencies can play a crucial role in translating the ever-growing amount of complex information related to genetics and disease prevention to health care providers and communities alike. Early on, the public health community needs to develop a baseline understanding of both professional and consumer perceptions of and attitudes toward the recent developments in and future expectations for human genetics.

Because the subject of human genetics can be sensitive, effective communication will be key to the success of public health programs involving genetic research results. Effective communication could be achieved by coalition building among federal agencies, professional organizations, consumers, private industry, and state and local health departments to develop and evaluate communication strategies for genetics and public health. Communication effectiveness will hinge on many factors, including coordinating communication strategies among various groups; targeting appropriate audiences with messages that result in health promotion and disease prevention; and providing messages that are accurate and appropriate on technical and cultural levels. Particular attention must be given to primary-care physicians, nurses, and other health professionals who will often serve as a conduit for information and who can help shape widespread attitudes and behaviors. Finally, an appropriate mix of mechanisms should be used for disseminating information, including distance-based interactive meetings, information centers and means of electronic communication (e.g., the Internet). Chapter 28 discusses overall principles of communication science related to genetics and public health and focuses on the Internet as an emerging medium for information dissemination (Chapter 31).

Critical Issues in Genetics and Public Health

To integrate genetics into the four public health functions discussed (public health assessment, genetic testing evaluation, public health intervention, and communication), three critical issues must be addressed for each: partnerships and coordination; ethical, legal, and social implications (or issues); and education and training. Details on these critical issues are provided in the CDC strategic plan on genetics and public health (11). Part V of this book (Chapters 25 through 27) addresses some of the emerging ethical and legal issues related to the integrating of genetics into public health practice. Part VI deals with other critical issues such as training public health professionals in genetics (Chapter 29), and consumer and public perspectives on genetic testing (Chapter 30). The following are highlights of these topics.

Partnerships and Coordination

For all of the public health functions in genetics discussed earlier to be carried out, strong partnerships and coordination of efforts among various groups need to occur (11), including partnerships and coordinated efforts among various agencies of the federal government; federal, state, and local agencies; the public and private sectors; and the public health, medicine, and academic sectors, with various community and consumer involvement.

One example of such partnership is annual national meetings on genetics and public health. The CDC, the Health Resources and Services Administration (HRSA), the National Human Genome Research Institute, and the Association of State and Territorial Health Officials (ASTHO) and affiliates held the First Annual Conference on Genetics and Public Health in Atlanta, Georgia, in May 1998 (52). This first meeting addressed the public health opportunities and challenges presented by advances in human genetics research. The conference sought to establish awareness about the scope of and process for integrating advances in human genetics into public health programs and strengthening partnerships for disease prevention and health promotion efforts. The conference was attended by nearly 400 people from federal, state, academic, consumer, community, and industry organizations, representing 41 states and several European countries. The second annual meeting was held (December 1999), sponsored jointly by ASTHO in collaboration with the Maryland Department of Health and the Johns Hopkins University School of Hygiene and Public Health. These meetings will provide crucial gatherings for exchanging information and building partnerships among various groups.

Ethical, Legal, and Social Issues

As the Human Genome Project was being planned, there was widespread recognition that the information gained from sequencing the human genome would have profound implications for individuals, families, and society. A number of complex ethical, legal, and social issues can arise around the integration of genetic technologies in practice, and the use and interpretation of genetic information. To address these issues, the Ethical, Legal and Social Implications (ELSI) Program was established as an integral part of the Human Genome Project (53,54). The program has provided leadership in scientific research by identifying, analyzing, and addressing the ethical, legal, and social implications of human genetics research as basic scientific discoveries were made. The overarching aims of the ELSI Program have been to assure that: (a) genetic research is conducted in an ethically sound manner; (b) genetic technologies and information are appropriated integrated into clinical and nonclinical settings; (c) genetic information is interpreted accurately and used appropriately; and (d) professionals and the public become more "genetically literate."

Over the past decade, emphasis has been placed on privacy and fairness in the use and interpretation of genetic information. Privacy and fairness issues include (a) privacy and confidentiality of genetic information, including issues of ownership and control of genetic information and consent to disclosure and use of genetic information; (b) fair use of genetic information (e.g., related to insurance and employment); (c) individual, family, and group psychological interactions and stigmatization related to genetic information; (d) cultural differences in the uses of genetic information; and (e) the impact of genetic information on the concept of disability (53).

Another ELSI research emphasis has been addressing issues related to genetic research, particularly research in which the risks and benefits to participants are not fully known. Specific topics in this area have included the elements of informed consent for individuals participating in genetics research; the role of institutional review boards in genetics research; policies related to effectively maintaining privacy and confidentiality of genetic information about individuals and families participating in genetics research; and issues raised by commercialization of the products from human genetics research (e.g., ownership of tissue and products, patents, and so forth).

Although much of ELSI research has been driven by concerns about the human rights of individuals and their families in the context of genetic testing for single-gene disorders with relatively high penetrance (e.g., mutations conferring cancer predisposition), the interface between ELSI and public health practice (or PHELSI) leads to concerns that are somewhat different from the traditional clinical practice involving genetic testing and counseling of high-risk families (Table 1.6). Part V addresses some but not all of these issues, including the interface between public health and the law (Chapter 25), the informed consent process in traditional public health genetics programs (Chapter 26), and issues surrounding public health surveillance

Table 1.6 Examples of Public Health Ethical, Legal, and Social Issues

---

I. Informed consent in public health genetic research

How can truly informed consent for genetic testing be obtained in public health practice (versus clinical practice, in which personal contact and the opportunity for one-on-one interaction is greater)?

How does informed consent for genetic testing in public health practice differ from informed consent for other public health services?

Should genetic counseling services be provided as part of public health practice even when risks associated with different genetic polymorphisms and mutations vary widely? And how can such services be provided?

How can stored samples on large-scale populations (e.g., newborn screening blood spots) be used for epidemiologic research?

Under what circumstances is new consent for archived specimens needed for public health investigations?

Under what circumstances, if any, is it appropriate to make specimens anonymous? Do situations occur in public health when genetic testing could be done on identifiable specimens without informed consent?

II. Legal issues for public health genetics programs

Should genetic programs in the public health setting be mandated by law? What legal protections can be used to ensure confidentiality to persons participating in screening programs?

What laws and regulations are needed to ensure the safety and effectiveness of genetic tests?

III. Population access to clinical and preventive services

How can population access to genetic tests and services be ensured?

IV. Privacy concerns in population-based surveillance programs

How can privacy and confidentiality be maintained in the public health setting?

How should population-based disease registries be handled? What are their immediate and long-term benefits? What are their immediate and long-term risks?

How can public health agencies maximize benefits and minimize the risks associated with such registries?

V. Group stigmatization

How can concerns about potential stigmatization of population groups resulting from research or testing programs be addressed?

Source: CDC (1997) (11).

and information systems (Chapter 27). At this time, many of these issues are unresolved. Public health leadership is needed to ensure discussion of sensitive issues and consensus building that balances individual rights with societal concerns, and they highlight an urgent need for population-based epidemiologic research.

One issue that has received a lot of attention over the past decade is the informed consent process for using stored genetic research tissue samples (55–58). In a public health setting, stored samples from large-scale national surveys or newborn blood spots could be used to conduct human genome epidemiologic studies for evaluating the impact of genetic variation on the burden of disease in the population. Although universal agreement exists on the need to obtain informed consent from subjects participating in genetic research, opinions differ regarding the use of stored samples from population surveys for which there is no or inadequate informed consent. There has been debate about the practicality of recontacting subjects from population studies; whether or not genetic studies pose more than "minimal risks" to subjects; the definitions and desirability of "anonymization" of existing samples; and whether or not coded but "linked" or "linkable" samples can be used (e.g., Clayton et al.,) (Table 1.6).

In these discussions, a distinction has been made between allelic variants that have high penetrance or risk for disease and the more common genetic variants (e.g., blood groups, HLA antigens, variants in drug metabolizing enzymes) that are neither necessary nor sufficient for disease development (58–60). The latter group of genetic variants are risk factors that act in combination with other genes and environmental factors and are often associated with low relative risks for disease; however, in most existing recommendations and guidelines put out by various groups, the distinction between the two types of genetic variation has not been considered, perhaps implying that all genetic testing should be treated the same with respect to potential harm to individuals. Currently, the National Bioethics Advisory Commission, appointed by the President of the United States, has deliberated on genetic research on stored tissue samples (61). As recommendations on informed consent issues are developed by various groups, it is obvious that public health officials and researchers need to work with clinicians, ethicists, social scientists, lawyers, consumers and other groups, and to participate through individual action and through professional organizations, in defining and resolving these issues for public health practice.

Education and Training

The rapid expansion of the field of human genetics strains the ability of public health researchers, health practitioners, policymakers, and consumers to keep abreast of new information and its potential ramifications for policy, research, and practice; therefore, concerted efforts are needed to provide various audiences, especially public health professionals, with the knowledge and skills they need to integrate genetics into public health activities. This emphasis on educating public health professionals is exemplified by ongoing CDC training activities (62) as well as the development of several genetics training programs in various U.S. schools of public health. An overview of such efforts appears in Chapter 29.

There have been other national efforts to address education of professionals in various health disciplines other than public health in genetics. In 1996, the American Medical Association, the American Nurses Association, and the National Human Genome Research Institute formed the National Coalition for Health Professional Education in Genetics (NCHPEG) to promote health professional education and access to information about advances in human genetics (1). The NCHPEG is a multidisciplinary group of leaders from more than a hundred diverse health professional organizations, consumer and voluntary groups, government agencies, private industry, managed-care organizations, and genetics professional societies.

To accelerate training in genetics for public health professionals, the content of existing courses will have to be supplemented by revised curricula or course work. For example, training for laboratory personnel will need to cover new genetic tests and reagents and may result in recertification of these professionals. Training modules that address each component of the proposed framework (public health assessment, genetic testing evaluation, intervention, and communication) will need to be incorporated into the training of professionals in various public health disciplines (e.g., epidemiology, biostatistics, behavioral and social sciences, health services research, economics, health policy and management, and environmental health). A minimum level of competence needs to be achieved not only in genetics and disease prevention but also in the ethical, legal, and social issues related to it.

Members of the general public will need to be similarly educated to become informed consumers of medical and genetic services and to be aware of potential misuse of genetic information. In addition, incorporating information on genetics into the life science curricula of elementary and secondary schools will help prepare the next generation to be responsive to the challenges and opportunities of genetic technology.

Concluding Remarks

With acceleration of the discovery of human genetic variation and associated diseases in the next few years, public health professionals will not only be confronted with but will help develop, analyze, and disseminate a large body of scientific information that will guide public health action. The potential for inappropriate or premature use of genetic information without adequate protections for privacy and confidentiality will demand public health leadership in evaluating and resolving the many ethical, legal, and social issues associated with genetic information. In the not too distant future, however, disease prevention and health promotion programs will routinely consider whether or not to use genetic information to help target intervention activities so as to maximize benefit and minimize costs and harm to individuals. For this to occur, however, genetics needs to be incorporated into training programs for numerous fields (e.g., epidemiology, laboratory sciences, legislation and policy, medicine, nursing, behavioral and social sciences, and communication sciences). This will require changes in professional training programs and the retraining of many public health professionals. Only then can we achieve a true integration of human genetics into public health practice in the 21st century.

References

1. Collins FS. Preparing health professionals for the genetic revolution. JAMA 1997;278:1285–1286.

2. Collins FS, Patrinos A, Jordan E, et al. New goals for the U.S. Human Genome Project: 1998–2003. Science 1998;282:682–689.

3. Center for Medical Genetics, Johns Hopkins University and National Center for Biotechnology Information, National Library of Medicine. Online Mendelian Inheritance in Man, OMIM™ [database]. 1999; World Wide Web URL:http://www.ncbi.nlm.nih.gov/omim.

4. Pagon RA, Covington M, Tarczy-Hornoch P. Helix: a directory of medical genetics laboratories. World Wide Web URL:http://www.hslib.washington.edu/helix/.

5. Coughlin SS. The intersection of genetics, public health, and preventive medicine. Am J Prev Med 1999;16:89–90.

6. Khoury MJ. Genetic epidemiology and the future of disease prevention and public health. Epidemiol Rev 1997;19:175–180.

7. Centers for Disease Control and Prevention, Office of Genetics and Disease Prevention. Genetics in the news. Available from URL:http://www.cdc.gov/genetics/News.htm.

8. Laken SJ, Petersen GM, Gruber SB, et al. Familial colorectal cancer in Ashkhenazim due to hypermutable tract in APC. Nat Genet 1997;17:79–83.

9. Cancer Research Foundation of America. Cancer Research Foundation of America web site. 1998; http://www.preventcancer.org/.

10. Khoury MJ, and the CDC Genetics Working Group. From genes to public health: applications of genetics in disease prevention. Am J Public Health 1996;86:1717–1722.

11. Centers for Disease Control and Prevention. Translating advances in human genetics into public health action: a strategic plan (1997). Available from URL:http://www.cdc.gov/genetics/Strategic.html.

12. Institute of Medicine. The future of public health. Washington, DC: National Academy Press, 1988.

13. University of Washington, School of Public Health and Community Medicine. Multidisciplinary program in public health genetics in the context of law, ethics and policy. Available from URL:*http://weber.u.washington.edu/~phgen/*.

14. University of Michigan. Public health genetics. Internet URL:*http://www.sph. umich.edu/genetics/*.

15. Ten Kate L. Editorial. Community Genetics 1998;1:1–2.

16. King RA. Genetics and the practice of medicine: the future is here. Genet Med 1998;1:1.

17. Collins FS. Genetics: not just somewhere but at the very center of medicine. Genet Med 1998;1:3.

18. Khoury MJ. The interface between medical genetics and public health: changing the paradigm of disease prevention and the definition of a genetic disease. Am J Med Genet 1997;71:289–291.

19. Juengst ET. "Prevention" and the goals of genetic medicine. Hum Gene Ther 1995;6:1595–1605.

20. Clayton EW. What should be the role of public health in newborn screening and prenatal diagnosis? Am J Prev Med 1999;16:111–115.

21. Rothman KJ. Modern epidemiology. Boston: Little, Brown, 1986, p. 14.

22. Jaroff L. Keys to the kingdom. Time 1996;148:24–29.

23. Teutsch SM, Churchill RE (eds). Principles and practice of public health surveillance. New York: Oxford University Press, 1994.

24. Steinberg KK, Sanderlin KC, Ou CY, et al. DNA banking in epidemiologic studies. Epidemiol Rev 1997;19:156–162.

25. International Center for Birth Defects. World atlas of birth defects (1st ed). Geneva: World Health Organization, 1998.

26. National Cancer Institute. Surveillance, epidemiology and end results (SEER) program. Internet URL:*http://www-seer.ims.nci.nih.gov/*.

27. Last JM. A dictionary of epidemiology (3rd ed). New York: Oxford University Press, 1995.

28. Terris M. The Society of Epidemiologic Research and the future of epidemiology. Am J Epidemiol 1992;136:909–915.

29. Khoury MJ, Beaty TH, Cohen BH. Fundamentals of genetic epidemiology. New York: Oxford University Press, 1993.

30. Schulte PA, Perera FP (eds). Molecular epidemiology: principles and practice. New York: Academic Press, 1993.

31. American Society of Human Genetics. Statement on genetic testing for breast and ovarian cancer predisposition. Am J Genet 1994;55:i–iv.

32. American College of Medical Genetics/American Society of Human Genetics Working Group. Statement on use of Apolipoprotein E testing for Alzheimer disease. JAMA 1995;274:1627–1629.

33. Burke W, Thomson E, Khoury MJ, et al. Hereditary hemochromatosis: gene discovery and its implications for population-based screening. JAMA 1998;280:172–178.

34. Khoury MJ, Dorman JS. The human genome epidemiology network (HuGE Net). Am J Epidemiol 1998;148:1–3.

35. Khoury MJ. Human Genome Epidemiology (HuGE): translating advances in human genetics into population-based data for medicine and public health. Genet Med 1999;1:71–73.

36. Centers for Disease Control and Prevention. The Human Genome Epidemiology Network. Internet URL:http://www.cdc.gov/genetics/huge.htm.

37. Shaw GM, Rozen R, Finnell RH, et al. Genetic variation in infant methylene

tetrahydrofolate reductase and risk of spina bifida: effect of maternal vitamin use. Am J Epidemiol 1998;148:30–37.

38. Malone KE, Daling JR, Thompson JD, et al. BRCA1 mutations and breast cancer in the general population: analyses of women before age 25 years and in women before age 45 years with first-degree family history. JAMA 1998;279:922–929.

39. Vandenbroucke JP, van der Meer FJ, Helmerhorst FM, Rosendaal FR. Factor V Leiden: should we screen oral contraceptive users and pregnant women? BMJ 1996;313:1127–1130.

40. Farrell PM, Kosorok MR, Laxova A, et al. Nutritional benefits of neonatal screening for cystic fibrosis. N Engl J Med 1997;337:963–969.

41. Centers for Disease Control and Prevention. Morbidity and mortality among children with sickle cell disease identified by newborn screening during 1990–1994—study protocol at http://www.cdc.gov/genetics/publications/sickle.htm#Morbidity and Mortality.

42. Holtzman NA, Watson MS (eds). Promoting safe and effective genetic testing in the United States: final report of the Task Force on Genetic Testing 1997. Internet URL:*http://www.nhgri.nih.gov/ELSI/TFGT_final/*.

43. Centers for Disease Control and Prevention. Regulations for implementing clinical laboratory improvement amendments of 1988: a summary. MMWR 1992;41(RR-2):1–17.

44. McGovern MM, Benach MO, Wallenstein S, et al. Quality assurance in molecular genetic testing laboratories. JAMA 1999;281:835–840.

45. Marteau TM. Psychological implications of genetic screening. Birth Defects Original Articles Series 1992;28:185–190.

46. Lerman C, Croyle R. Psychological issues in genetic testing for breast cancer susceptibility. Arch Intern Med 1994;154:609–616.

47. Hudson K, Rothenberg KH, Andrews LB, et al. Genetic discrimination and health insurance: an urgent need for reform. Science 1995;270:391–393.

48. Wilson JMG, Jungner F. Principles and practice of screening for disease (Public Health Papers No. 34). Geneva: World Health Organization, 1968.

49. American College of Medical Genetics. Principles of screening: report of the Subcommittee on Screening of the American College of Medical Genetics Clinical Practice Committee, 1997. http://www.faseb.org/genetics/acmg/pol-26.htm.

50. Committee for the Study of Inborn Errors of Metabolism. Genetic screening: programs, principles, and research. Washington, DC: National Academy of Sciences, 1975.

51. Coughlin SS, Burke W, Lee NC, et al. Toward principles of population screening for genetic susceptibility to adult-onset chronic disease. Am J Public Health (in press).

52. Khoury MJ, Puryear M, Thomson E, Bryan J. First annual conference on genetics and public health: translating advances in human genetics into disease prevention and health promotion. Community Genetics 1998;1:93–108. Also available at URL:http://www.cdc.gov/genetics/publications/abstracts.htm.

53. National Human Genome Research Institute. Ethical, legal, and social implications of human genetics research. Internet URL:*http://www.nhgri.nih.gov/elsi/*.

54. U.S. Department of Energy. Ethical, legal, and social issues (ELSI). Internet URL: http://www.ornl.gov/TechResources/Human_Genome/resource/elsi.html.

55. Clayton EW, Steinberg KK, Khoury MJ, et al. Informed consent for genetic research on stored tissue samples. JAMA 1995;274:1786–1792.

56. American Society of Human Genetics. Statement on informed consent for genetic research. Am J Hum Genet 1996;59:471–474.

57. American College of Medical Genetics (ACMG) Storage of Genetics Materials Committee. Statement on storage and use of genetic materials. Internet URL:*http://www.faseb.org/genetics/acmg/pol-17.htm.*

58. Hunter D, Caporaso N. Informed consent in epidemiologic studies involving genetic markers. Epidemiology 1997;8:596–599.

59. Schulte PA, Hunter D, Rothman N. Ethical and social issues in the use of bio-markers in epidemiologic research. IARC Sci Publ 1997;142:313–318.

60. Steinberg KK. Informed consent for stored tissue samples: the NHANES III experience. 1997 USPHS workshop proceedings: determining the role of environmental exposures as risk factors for B-cell chronic lymphoproliferative disorders. Internet URL:http://www.cdc.gov/nceh/programs/lab/flowcyto/pub/1997/html/doc25.htm.

61. National Bioethics Advisory Commission. National Bioethics Advisory Commission homepage. Internet URL:*http://bioethics.gov/cgi-bin/bioeth_counter.pl.*

62. Centers for Disease Control and Prevention, Office of Genetics and Disease Prevention. Training opportunities. Internet URL:http://www.cdc.gov/genetics/Training.htm.

2

Genetics and public health: Historical perspectives and current challenges and opportunities

Gilbert S. Omenn

Genetics and public health share a focus on populations in practice, research, and policy-making. Cultural, social, ethnic, and racial dimensions are recognized by both fields as crucial for clinical preventive services and for investigation and reduction of environmental and behavioral risk factors.

The marriage of genetics and public health is certain to usher in a golden age for the public health sciences. The concepts and methods of biostatistics and bioinformatics, epidemiology and population-based prevention trials, environmental and occupational health, health services research, health behavior, health education, and health policy are essential for interpreting the coming avalanche of data about the human genome and about genetic variations among people. To understand the functions of genes and the significance of variation in specific genes, researchers will need to learn how those genes and their gene products interact with metabolic, nutritional, and behavioral factors and with exposures to various environmental chemical, physical, and infectious agents. In addition, gene expression is influenced by the effects of many other genes. Cause-and-effect hypotheses from epidemiology and from clinical observations will need to be tested with pharmacologic, dietary, and behavioral interventions in randomized clinical prevention trials. Similarly, we will need to demonstrate the significance of environmental exposures on health risks by showing—through properly conducted population studies of the impact of various regulatory, technological, and behavioral innovations— that a reduction in levels of exposure will lead to a reduction in disease incidence (see Table 2.1).

This chapter traces the historical paths that have led to the emergence of *public health genetics*. The importance of anticipating and addressing the social, ethical, and legal ramifications of scientific advances and of medical and

Table 2.1 The Postgenomic Era Will Depend Upon the Public Health Sciences

---

Epidemiology
  All the factors that play upon/determine the expression of genetic variation identified in
  sequences; role of biomarkers

Biostatistics and bioinformatics
  Platforms and methods for designing studies and for analyzing the avalanche of data

Environmental health sciences/"ecogenetics"
  Understanding the host variation in host/agent interactions; risk assessment/risk management

Pathobiology/infectious disease
  Host–pathogen genomic interactions
  Host–pathogen–environmental interactions

Behavioral sciences
  Genetic predispositions to aspects of smoking behavior and other unhealthful behaviors

Health services research fields
  Designing and assessing well-targeted, cost-effective genetic clinical and preventive services
  that improve quality of life

---

public health applications of genetics is also discussed. It is essential to be sensitive to the legacy of the eugenics movement of several decades ago, and to recognize the problems associated with making medical diagnoses (including prenatal diagnoses) when no treatment or preventive intervention is known. We must learn from the grade-school-based sickle cell trait screening programs and from the neonatal phenylketonuria screening programs how to make future screening less stigmatizing and more specific. Research can help show how to present and explain the purposes and results of such screening for specific families. Especially in a country lacking universal health insurance, such as the United States, we must guard against discriminatory use of genetic information by insurers and employers. And more knowledge is needed about the heterogeneity of genetic predispositions, environmental exposures, and disease risks. In short, a scientifically-sound, cost-effective strategy must be developed for using genetics to improve health and prevent disease, the overarching mission of public health.

Historical Perspectives: Human Genetics

Philosophers, early scientists, and laypeople have observed similarities and dissimilarities among individuals, family members, tribes, and communities from the beginning of time. Curiosity about the biological basis for different male and female anatomy, physiology, reproductive roles, and social roles and about the basis for different characteristics of offspring led to explanatory speculations ascribed to Hippocrates, Anaxagoras, and Aristotle (1). In the *Statesman* and later in the *Republic*, Plato proposed that mates be selected with similar personality traits, though he worried about the consequences of such selective mating over many generations because of a lack of balancing traits. In contrast, Democritus claimed that more people become able by exercise than by their natural predisposition (1). Here we see the forerunner of debates about nature versus nurture, genetics versus environment. It is important that the emergence of public health genetics reinforce the modern conclusion that genetic and environmental factors interact in so many ways that disputes about which is primary are inappropriate (2,3).

About 2000 years elapsed without much attention to human genetics, at least in Western countries. Breeding of animals was progressing empirically throughout the planet, but few connections were made between agriculture or biology and prescientific medicine. In the 17th century, Anton van Leeuwenhoek, the inventor of the microscope, discovered sperm in the semen, and in the next century medical reports began to appear about the pattern of inheritance of specific clinical conditions, such as polydactyly and hemophilia. Deductions from pedigrees led a British physician, Joseph Adams, to remarkable insights for genetic counseling in a book published in 1814, *A Treatise on the Supposed Hereditary Properties of Diseases* (see ref. 4). Adams differentiated between familial congenital disorders and later-manifesting hereditary conditions, recognized that the parents of children with (recessive) familial conditions manifest at birth were often near-relatives, and emphasized that hereditary conditions can become clinically apparent at various ages. He noted that disease predispositions may lead to manifest disease only under the additional influence of environmental factors and that the risk can be transmitted to the next generation even when the parent does not manifest the condition. Adams also realized that clinically identical diseases can have heterogeneous genetic bases. He noted a higher frequency of familial disease in isolated populations with inbreeding, and he concluded that many hereditary diseases are associated with reduced reproduction, thus reducing the long-term incidence of the disease unless the effect of reduced reproduction is matched by what we would call new mutations.

The year 1865 was a watershed for the development of human genetics. First, Francis Galton, the pioneer of the biometrics approach to traits with continuous variation—like height, skin color, blood pressure, and behaviors—published papers on *Hereditary Talent and Character* (5). In this approach, one measures performance, intelligence, stature, or other quantifiable traits as accurately as possible and then compares the results among individuals of known degree of relationship (siblings, twins, parent/child, and so forth) with statistical tests. Galton collected biographies of prominent individuals, from which he analyzed pedigrees for familial relationships among such people. He found similar high percentages of close relatives reaching eminence in science, literature, and the law, as well as in political, economic, and military spheres, where family connections were expected to be more influential. Though he had modern caveats about ascertainment bias and about social and economic advantages for those in prominent families, he went on to recommend various eugenic policies.

Meanwhile, in Brno (now in the Czech Republic) in 1865 Gregor Mendel published his findings from experiments with peas, which had been stimulated by his earlier observations on color variants in ornamental plants. He deduced three laws of heredity: the law of uniformity, which states that offspring of parents homozygous for different alleles of a gene are identical and heterozygous at that gene locus in the first generation; the law of segregation, which describes the ratios of homozygotes and heterozygotes in the intercrosses of heterozygotes and backcrosses of heterozygotes with homozygotes; and the law of independence, which states that different segregating genes are transmitted independently. These results were rediscovered independently in 1900 by several investigators, at the same time that Karl Landsteiner reported the ABO blood groups on red blood cells (1).

Also around the turn of the 20th century, Sir Archibald Garrod proposed that genes were linked causally to familial clinical disorders through enzymes and body chemistry. His description of inherited disorders as inborn errors of metabolism began with his 1902 paper, *The Incidence of Alkaptonuria: A Study in Chemical Individuality* (6). Garrod made the first explicit application of Mendel's laws to human diseases. He recognized that there was no graded response: Siblings would be either normal or excrete large quantities of the abnormal metabolic product, homogentisic acid, in urine. He noted the crucial features of autosomal recessive inheritance: siblings affected, parents normal, and affected children often resulting from the intermarriage of first cousins. He explicitly tied his deductions to a 1902 report of the Evolution Committee of the Royal Society. He suggested several other recessive disorders that would be inborn errors of metabolism, as well as the likelihood of differential responses among individuals to drugs and infectious agents. Unfortunately, even though Garrod became Sir William Osler's successor in the leading chair of medicine at Oxford, his contributions to human genetics were little appreciated during his lifetime. Biologists in the early part of the 20th century were uninterested in human studies, and physicians were not scientifically inclined (1).

Cytogenetics has a history parallel to that of biochemical genetics, with seminal work on chromosomes about 1900; a long period of stagnation; clarification in 1956 that normal diploid human cells contain 46 chromosomes, not 48, as had been believed for decades; then rapid expansion of knowledge about disorders of chromosome number or structure, which often lead to fetal or congenital abnormalities. Banding techniques introduced in 1969 by Torbjorn Caspersson made it feasible to identify each human chromosome, which in turn facilitated the mapping of individual genes to chromosomes in combination with in vitro culturing of somatic cells and of mouse/human hybrid cells.

The two paradigms of biometrical or statistical analysis of traits and of biologically based deduction of genes (on chromosomes; transmitted by germ cells, the eggs and sperm) were given a common basis in 1918 by the distinguished biostatistician R.A. Fisher, who emphasized that the actions of several specific genes could be the basis for correlations between relatives demonstrated by biometric analysis (7). Nevertheless, the two paradigms developed separately for many decades, with the Galtonian biometric approach dominating, especially with regard to predispositions to common diseases and in behavioral genetics. Mendelian analysis seemed to be useful only for quite rare hereditary diseases. Most human traits could not be classified as alternatives, like round versus shrunken peas. Moreover, the phenotypes depended upon exogenous, environmental influences, as well as genetics. For such important traits as intelligence and personality, and for common diseases and mental retardation, the only feasible research at the time was based on Galton's statistical correlations.

The emergence of an understanding of genes and gene action took decades. In 1924, Felix Bernstein established that three alleles of one gene accounted for the ABO blood groups. In 1944, Alfred Day Hershey and Martha Chase proved that the hereditary material is DNA (not proteins). In 1949, Linus Pauling and colleagues demonstrated that sickle cell disease was due to a specific homozygous mutation in hemoglobin beta-chains. In 1953, James Watson and Francis Crick proposed the double-helix model for DNA structure and function. Meanwhile, genetic research in fruit flies, viruses, and bacteria progressively revealed a universal molecular basis for human genetics and for evolution.

Historical Perspectives: Public Health

Organized efforts to improve the health of the public can be identified in every society from antiquity. Isolation of individuals with contagious illnesses, sanitation to manage wastes and control pests and infections, and various community-level nutritional, shaman, and medical interventions addressed the overwhelming problems of infection and of malnutrition.

The earliest public health organizations in the United States were established in the rapidly growing port cities of the eastern seaboard. The primary focus was on protecting the population from the introduction of epidemic diseases, such as the yellow fever epidemic that crippled Philadelphia in 1793 and later the cholera pandemics. There emerged a struggle between those who relied on the police function of quarantines and those who believed that the diseases could be prevented by cleaning up filthy conditions of workplaces, food and water, docks, alleys, and streets that made local residents vulnerable. The "accepted" epidemic conditions of that time—typhoid, typhus, measles, diphtheria, influenza, tuberculosis, and malaria—were "met with a stolid indifference born of familiarity and a sense of helplessness" (8). There is an apparent analogy in today's indifference or ineffectiveness in the face of drug abuse, violence, teen pregnancy, sexually transmitted diseases, and alcoholism.

The late 19th century was marked by social-reform movements and the emergence of such organizations as the American Public Health Association (1872), the American Red Cross (1882), and the American Tuberculosis Association (1904). The Committee of One Hundred on National Health (including Jane Addams, Andrew Carnegie, William H. Welch, and Booker T. Washington) campaigned for federal regulation of public health. One government response was the establishment just before World War I of the U.S. Public Health Service, built upon the long-standing Marine Hospital Service (1798). In 1920, William H. Welch of Johns Hopkins would proclaim to an audience of philanthropists, "Merely from a mercenary and commercial point of view it is for the interest of the community to take care of the health of the poor. Philanthrophy assumes a totally different aspect in the eyes of the world when it is able to demonstrate that it pays to keep people healthy" (8).

There arose a demand for individuals trained in public health to direct local, state, and national programs on a full-time professional basis. The Rockefeller Foundation was instrumental in stimulating and funding the development of schools of public health at leading universities in the United States (Johns Hopkins, Harvard, Yale, Columbia) and elsewhere (London, Toronto, São Paulo). From the beginning, however, there was a dilemma: Few young physicians chose to take public health training after earning their medical degree, largely owing to the higher remuneration in clinical practice. The public health students were either older physicians who had worked in public health positions without specialist qualifications or young scientists interested in the new fields of bacteriology, epidemiology, and statistics.

Public health—then, as now—was defined by its goals: to prevent disease and to maintain the health of the population. Public health was not defined by any specific body of knowledge, by a particular type of discipline, or by personnel. Physicians, sanitary engineers, epidemiologists, vital statisticians, lawyers, public health nurses, inspectors, and administrators were all needed and recognized for their roles in the community. Meanwhile, scientists in the laboratory, especially bacteriologists following the work of Louis Pasteur and Robert Koch, became powerful figures. Their disease-specific and agent-specific approach to control of infectious diseases caused a collision with the practice of medicine and drew public health away from the multifactorial conditions of the external environment. Nevertheless, several heroes of the early 20th century did pursue nonbacteriologic pathways, including Charles-Edward Winslow in sanitation and health education, Joseph Goldberger in the epidemiology of pellagra, Alice Hamilton in industrial hygiene, and E.V. McCollum in nutrition.

Origins of Public Health Genetics

In the 1940s and 1950s, several scientists established pioneering programs of epidemiological research of genetic diseases, notably T. Kemp in Copenhagen, James Neel at the University of Michigan, and A. C. Stevenson in Northern Ireland and later at Oxford. They investigated prevalence, modes of inheritance, heterogeneity, mutation rates, and attributable risk for common diagnoses (1). Genetic epidemiology became more statistical and less clinical, with models aimed at distinguishing the major effects of single unidentified genes from the effects of multiple factors, while mainstream research in medical genetics and population screening for specific genetic diseases focused more on biochemical studies of specific genes and gene products in the laboratory. Only now are molecular epidemiology research initiatives seeking to combine these complementary statistical and clinical approaches. Certain practical clinical applications were approached on a population basis with public health goals. The biochemical genetics path led to neonatal screening for inborn errors of metabolism and later screening of children or adults for sickle cell trait or Tay-Sachs carrier status. In the late 1960s, prenatal genetic diagnosis for chromosomal and biochemical disorders emerged. Most of these applications were devised and conducted by clinicians, rather than by public health professionals, with the exception of the statewide mandatory neonatal screening programs.

Meanwhile, population genetics was advanced through comparative multination studies of clinical findings (9). An important advance in public health sciences was the discovery of the selective influence that common infectious diseases had on the prevalence of disease genes. For example, the probability that infected children would survive falciparum malaria was greater in those carrying genes for sickle cell hemoglobin, beta-thalassemia, or glucose-6-phosphate dehydrogenase deficiency; these abnormal genes, in single dose, make red blood cells less sensitive to malaria infestation, thereby slowing the growth cycle of the parasite and increasing the survival chances of infected children. Other infectious diseases likely to be responsive to natural selection can be grouped as epidemic diseases, such as plague, cholera, and smallpox; chronic infections, such as tuberculosis and syphilis; intestinal infections in children; and tropical diseases of children and young adults.

Unfortunately, most public health researchers studying infectious diseases and environmental chemicals paid little attention to inherited variation in susceptibility to these agents; instead, they focused only on identifying and controlling the agents. Both medical and epidemiological researchers have often neglected the crucial principle of heterogeneity in human population studies in an effort to generate sufficient numbers of subjects and disease endpoints to justify the analysis statistically. In epidemiological studies of risk factors for common chronic diseases, such as elevated total or LDL cholesterol as a risk factor for coronary heart disease, and in clinical trials of pharmaceuticals for common diseases, researchers neither sought information on genetic variation nor used such information to create more homogeneous subgroups for more specific analyses. Today, genetics is at the core of research on cancers, coronary heart disease, high blood pressure, neurological and psychiatric disorders, and a host of other common clinical conditions (10–12).

CURRENT OPPORTUNITIES

Genetic approaches should become pervasive throughout all the disciplines that make up the public health sciences and all the subfields that make up public health practice. The biological substrate for interactions with environmental, metabolic, nutritional, and behavioral variables will no longer be a black box. Researchers' capacity to identify biologically significant and clinically important variation in the biological substrate will grow. Meanwhile, their ability to interpret the significance of genetic variation will depend upon the application of epidemiology, biostatistics, environmental health sciences, health behavior, and health education all in cultural, ethical, and public policy contexts. Here I highlight a few special opportunities to bring together genetics and public health.

Ecogenetics and Environmental Health

The field of environmental and occupational health has been developing rapidly under the impetus of regulatory requirements with a strong public health intent. For example, the Occupational Safety and Health Act of 1970 requires the regulatory agency in the Department of Labor to set health standards so that no worker shall suffer adverse effects even if exposed to potential toxins at the maximum permissible exposure level for a full working lifetime (13). Section 109 of the Clean Air Act of 1970, amended in 1977 and 1990, requires the Environmental Protection Agency to set national ambient air quality standards for air pollutants to which all of us are exposed (particles, sulfur oxide, carbon monoxide, ozone and related photooxidants, nitrogen dioxide, hydrocarbons, and lead), such that even the most susceptible subgroups (not defined) would be protected with an "adequate margin of safety." Children with cystic fibrosis might be a relevant subgroup. Section 112 of the Clean Air Act, covering life-threatening hazardous air pollutants, requires a similar process to identify population subgroups especially suscep- tible to these carcinogens and neurotoxins, to ensure that people are protected with the prescribed "ample margin of safety."

The Presidential/Congressional Commission on Risk Assessment and Risk Management (14) and numerous National Research Council and specialty scientific society panels have recommended that interindividual variation be more carefully investigated and be used in standard-setting and in risk man- agement to protect subgroups in the population. Understanding the mecha- nisms of action of known carcinogenic, teratogenic, or neurotoxic agents should empower us to anticipate and predict which other exogenous chemi- cal agents would be biotransformed similarly or attack similar receptors or other targets. Better mechanistic and empirical data would enable scientists and regulators to insert real data (instead of automatic factors of 10) for inter- species, intraspecies, and dose-extrapolation variables when they calculate safety factors for exposures to agents shown to be hazardous at high doses in animals (15). Recognition of specific relevant subgroups, especially subgroups at high risk for adverse health effects from particular exposures, can help in proving that an environmental exposure is, indeed, hazardous. Thus, when the difference in disease incidence between exposed and nonexposed people in a broad population may not be sufficient to show a statistically significant asso- ciation between the exposure and the disease risk, the difference in disease incidence between exposed and nonexposed members of a specific subgroup might be much larger. In addition to genetic predispositions, genetic variation can be the result, the dependent variable, when exogenous agents cause mutations in the DNA or other effects on gene expression; we call this area *genetic toxicology*, a prominent component of the required testing of new chemicals.

The Risk Commission proposed a new way of thinking about environmen- tal health protection, "putting each environmental problem into public health context" and trying to estimate the attributable risk, not just the relative risk, that a given type of exposure poses for asthma, lung cancer, birth defects, or other adverse health outcomes (16). Furthermore, the commission urged that stakeholders be actively engaged in the formulation of the problem, the risk assessment, the decision process, and the much-needed evaluation later of what was actually accomplished (14).

In 1996 Congress enacted the Food Quality Protection Act, which updated the pesticide control laws of the United States. A specific provision, recom- mended by the Risk Commission and other groups, was the requirement to address explicitly the hazards incurred by vulnerable or unusually exposed subgroups in the population. A salient example involves infants and children who might be highly exposed to pesticide residues in fruit juices at a time of rapid organ growth (17). The U.S. Environmental Protection Agency (EPA) used this law as impetus to create a Child Health Initiative, which has drawn the attention of many schools of public health and public health agencies. Geneticists should be actively engaged in this process of identifying predisposing factors and mechanisms for protection of children.

The National Institute for Environmental Health Sciences, under the leadership of Kenneth Olden, has mounted an Environmental Genome Initiative, aimed at using emerging knowledge of genes and genetic variation from the National Human Genome Program and powerful new methods of microchip technology to study gene-environment interactions and health risks. To evaluate variation in numerous biologically related genes, researchers will need to analyze multiple interacting factors with new bioinformatics methods for handling the data.

Nutrition and Genetics

Despite the importance of our diets to good health and the management of disease and disease risks, nutritional sciences have lagged behind other fields in biomedical and behavioral research. Genetics may help modernize nutrition research through its emphasis on metabolic and biochemical mechanisms and its recognition of the marked variation in responses of people to the variable nutrients and contaminants in their diverse diets.

Cholesterol fractions, trans-fatty acids, Lp(a), apolipoprotein variants, lipoprotein lipase, and other lipid components are important risk factors for coronary heart disease and stroke, and possibly for several major cancers and Alzheimer's disease. Nevertheless, individuals with similarly elevated cholesterol levels have a variety of underlying conditions for which different dietary and pharmacologic approaches are needed (18). With recent evidence that "statin" drugs can reduce mortality risks for coronary patients with serum total cholesterol levels in the normal range (19), the use of these drugs is certain to be expanded; careful pharmacogenetic and dietary studies of the variation in human responses to these drugs and of their cost-effectiveness in specific subgroups will be essential guides for public health strategies.

Another important risk factor for coronary heart disease, stroke, and peripheral vascular disease is a high concentration of serum homocysteine. Homocysteine levels are greatly influenced by a person's dietary intake of the vitamins folic acid, B12, and B6 (20). In turn, genetic variation in the enzymes in the metabolic pathways of folate, B12, and B6 influence the levels of these circulating vitamins. The clue that homocysteine might be important in cardiovascular disease was deduced 30 years ago from descriptions of the arterial and venous thromboses in patients with the inborn error of metabolism, homocystinuria (21). Mild hyperhomocysteinemia occurs in about 5% of the general population. Homocysteine acts on the arterial endothelial lining cells, on platelets, and on blood-clotting mechanisms to increase the risk of athero-sclerosis and thrombosis in the coronary, cerebral, and peripheral vasculature (22). Boushey et al. (20) estimated that 10% of the risk of coronary artery disease in the general population can be attributed to hyperhomocysteinemia. They projected that an increase of 5 μmol homocysteine per liter plasma raises the risk of coronary artery disease by as much as an increase of 20 mg cho-lesterol/dL (0.52 mmol/L). Studies of folic acid intake (by diet, fortification of foods, or vitamin supplements) indicate that increases of 200 μg/day could reduce plasma homocysteine concentrations by about 4 μmol/L, a reduction that could save tens of thousands of lives annually in the United States. Randomized clinical trials are being planned to test the clinical utility of this strategy. A special subset of patients on kidney dialysis for end-stage renal disease deserves clinical trials with folic acid (and B12 and B6); these patients have extraordinarily high levels of circulating homocysteine and high cardio-vascular mortality.

Randomized clinical preventive trials have proved that increased supple-mental intake of 4 μg/day folic acid is protective against the occurrence of neural tube birth defects, through mechanisms and genetic predispositions that have not yet been elucidated (23). Setting the right levels will surely require accommodation of response variation in women and fetuses. Nevertheless, the Centers for Disease Control and Prevention, the Food and Drug Administration, the March of Dimes, the Robert Wood Johnson Foundation, and numerous state and local organizations have mobilized to increase folic acid intakes through fortification of wheat grains, through increased use of folic acid-containing vitamin supplements, and through greater consumption of fruits and vegetables in people's diets. My colleagues and I believe it is important to include B12 in folic acid-fortified foods and folic acid-containing vitamin supplements in order to be confident that no adverse effects will be induced in individuals with markedly deficient absorption of B12 (20). Health behavior research is at the heart of efforts needed to significantly increase the folic acid levels of women before they become pregnant; because the neural tube of a fetus should close by the 23rd day of gestation, it is too late to recommend supplementation or diet changes after the pregnancy has been recognized.

Iron is required in our diets to avoid iron-deficiency anemia, a prevalent and debilitating condition worldwide, especially in children and women; iron is needed for hemoglobin and also for many tissue proteins, such as cytochrome P450 enzymes. Carriers of the common gene for excessive iron absorption (called HFE; *H* for HLA-H, *Fe* for iron) are at risk of developing iron over-load in the liver, pancreas, heart, testes, and skin; this condition, known as hemochromatosis, affects an estimated 1 million Americans (24). Ironically, in

1996 the CDC, the College of American Pathologists, and other groups seemed prepared to launch a much-needed hemochromatosis screening program based on serum iron, iron-binding capacity, and transferrin saturation tests. However, when the HFE gene was discovered, questions arose about using genotypic diagnosis instead of or in addition to iron status tests. Early detection is crucial, because all the complications of diabetes, cardiomyopathy, hepatic cirrhosis, liver cancer, and hypogonadism can be prevented—or reversed if detected in time—by reducing a person's iron simply via periodic phlebotomy. Meanwhile, the assurance that hemochromatosis gene carriers can be detected and protected from excessive iron might put to rest the criticisms of those who fear that carriers might suffer adverse consequences if society-wide fortification of foods with iron is implemented to prevent iron-deficiency states. It is likely that a combination of genotypic and phenotypic tests can be devised to achieve screening and confirmation (25).

The demonstration more than 40 years ago that the inborn error of metabolism phenylketonuria (PKU) could be diagnosed at birth and that children treated with a phenylalanine-limited diet would avoid developing mental retardation exploded two myths about genetics: first, that genetic effects are immutable, and, second, that nature and nurture are competing explanations, rather than interacting factors, in health and disease. However, scientists and physicians were slow to recognize that high levels of phenylalanine in newborn blood could arise from multiple different mutations; only about half of the infants who tested positive on the screening test actually had PKU, and some, fortunately rare, infants had a mutation that made them need more phenylalanine in the diet to develop normally.

This failure to recognize the multiple genetic mutations associated with PKU occurred because researchers ignored an important epidemiologic clue: The incidence rate of PKU appeared to double when the newborn screening was introduced. Other inborn errors of metabolism, such as histidinemia, were associated with risk for mental retardation only because of ascertainment bias: Early studies were done on specimens from children in homes for the developmentally disabled. Meanwhile, in the case of galactosemia, diagnosis must lead to immediate treatment in order to gain the preventive benefits of a galactose-restricted diet. These disorders illustrate the importance of detailed knowledge about genetic heterogeneity, metabolism, nutrition, and clinical epidemiology in organizing and providing public health services.

Infectious Disease Genetics

As noted at the outset of this chapter, infectious diseases have been powerful forces of natural selection in human populations because of genetic differences in susceptibility to specific infectious agents. The survival advantage of children and young adults with hemoglobin variants S, C, D, and E, the thalassemias, or glucose-6-phosphate dehydrogenase deficiency in the face of infection with falciparum malaria, is a classic example (1,26). An extensive compilation of host/pathogen interactions is available (27).

Tuberculosis (TB) remains a major public health problem throughout the world. It has reemerged in the United States during the past 15 years because the number of immune-compromised people has grown and poor treatment practices have permitted drug-resistant strains of the TB organism to become prominent. Research on TB was neglected for about 30 years; no new drugs were developed to treat TB, and no new methods were developed to diagnose the disease. During the past decade, as a result of public health needs, such research has been resumed, and diagnostic gene probes have made it feasible to detect TB in hours rather than weeks, including multiple-drug-resistant strains whose detection is so important to a patient's choice of treatment and to efforts to control the spread of the disease among health care personnel and in the larger community. Such DNA diagnostic techniques are transforming infectious disease practice and surveillance. Interactions between genetic and multiple environmental factors can be illustrated by the report that iron overload predisposes people to TB (28).

No disease has been more dramatic in its presentation and ramifications over the past two decades than HIV infection and AIDS. Variation in susceptibility to infection and to development of clinical manifestations should have been expected based on general principles. However, evidence was lacking for quite a long time. Now polymorphic host genes important in HIV pathogenesis can be grouped into those involved in HIV entry into cells (chemokine receptors), those involved in general immune function (such as HLA, tumor necrosis factor, and complement), and genes that may indirectly affect pathogen entry or clearance, such as Lewis blood group antigens (27). Chemokine-receptor polymorphisms have been recognized in several countries; they are responsible for resistance to HIV infection even in individuals with extensive exposure to the virus. A specific deletion mutation of a 32 base-pair segment in the CCR5 gene coding for a transmembrane-receptor protein results in a nonfunctional receptor (29). The HIV strains that enter via this receptor are unable to do so in people homozygous for the deletion, so these individuals remain HIV-negative. Heterozygotes seem to have partial protection, including delay in progression to clinical manifestations of AIDS. The CCR5 mutations so far explain only a minority of HIV-negative/uninfected or HIV-positive/nonprogressor people among those who have been highly exposed to HIV. Such genetic variation reveals possibilities for entirely new routes of clinical and public health intervention, both for treatment and for prevention.

Genetics of Unhealthful Behaviors

We could use the tabulation by McGinnis and Foege (30) of the lifestyle factors that contribute to about half of the 2 million deaths annually in the United States as a framework for examining the interplay among genetic predispositions and environmental and behavioral risk factors in various diseases (see Table 2.2). This table is a call to action for public health.

Behavioral genetics has been a particularly controversial area of human genetics because of difficulties in measuring such traits as personality and intelligence and because of racial and educational biases in many such measures. However, emerging findings related to tobacco use and addiction and alcohol use and addiction may now be more readily tied to underlying pharmacology and toxicology and to preventive strategies related to these overwhelming public health problems. Similar approaches are being applied to common psychiatric conditions, notably depression, which frequently complicates other medical conditions and thus markedly increases the complexity of clinical care and the attendant costs.

Smoking and Genetics. A recent review (31) concluded that knowledge

Table 2.2 Leading Medical Causes of Death in the United States

	LISTED CAUSES
Heart Disease	720,000
Cancers	505,000
Cerebrovascular disease	144,000
Unintentional injuries	92,000
Chronic lung disease	87,000
Pneumonia and influenza	80,000
Diabetes mellitus	48,000
Suicide	31,000
Cirrhosis/liver disease	26,000
HIV infection	25,500
TOTAL U.S. DEATHS (all causes)	2,148,000
	"REAL CAUSES"
Tobacco	400,000
Diet/activity patterns	300,000
Alcohol	100,000
Microbial agents	90,000
Toxic agents	60,000
Firearms	35,000
Sexual behavior	30,000
Motor vehicles	25,000
Illicit use of drugs	20,000
TOTAL	1,060,000

about the specific genes involved in the initiation, maintenance, cessation, and recurrence of smoking behavior is extremely limited, although twin studies consistently indicate that genetic factors play an important role in the initiation of smoking. Much attention is now focused on dopaminergic neurons and receptors and the related pharmacology. Habit-forming actions of nicotine may be triggered at nicotinic receptors on the cell bodies of dopaminergic neurons in the mesolimbic system of the brain, a system tied to rewarding behavioral responses. The same system is thought to be involved in addictions to cocaine, opiates, and alcohol and in schizophrenias. The extent of genetic variation is being investigated for each step in dopamine synthesis, dopamine release by presynaptic neurons, receptor activation of postsynaptic neurons, dopamine reuptake by presynaptic neurons, and metabolism of released dopamine. Analogous studies are underway in relation to smoking cessation and particularly smoking cessation facilitated by pharmacologic aids; the purpose of these studies is to identify subgroups most likely to respond (32).

Likewise, there is variation in susceptibility to the organ-system-specific consequences of smoking, including lung cancer, other cancers, coronary heart disease, emphysema and ulcer disease, as well as in risks to the fetus. Cigarette smoke is loaded with known chemical carcinogens, which themselves are subject to genetically polymorphic enymatic biotransformation through cytochrome P450s, glutathione-S-transferases, and N-acetyltransferases (33).

Alcoholism and Genetics. Polymorphisms of dopamine-receptor alleles are being investigated for influence on alcohol behavior and chronic alcoholism risk. For example, the Addiction Research Foundation in Toronto conducted a study of the D4 dopamine-receptor genotype in 72 severely affected chronic alcoholics and reported a higher prevalence of D4(3) and D4(6) among alcoholics than among nonalcoholic controls (34). Frequency of other drug abuse was higher in the D4(3,3) and D4(4,7) subgroups, and family history of alcoholism was strikingly positive in the D4(2,4) group. These results are quite preliminary. Related studies, especially with broad categories of substance-abuse patients, seem to show no obvious associations (35).

Genetic dissection of dopamine receptors is progressing rapidly, revealing a family of receptor genes, as has been found for serotonin and other neurotransmitter systems. As with smoking, chronic alcohol exposure leads to organ-specific damage, including cirrhosis of the liver, pancreatitis, cerebellar degeneration, and cardiomyopathy; for all these effects, people show striking variability in susceptibility, partly on an inherited basis (36). In addition, alcohol-drinking behavior, smoking behavior, clinical depression, mood and affect have been shown to be highly interrelated (37).

Educational Initiatives in Public Health Genetics

In 1997 the University of Washington in Seattle launched a university-wide initiative from the President's Initiatives Fund under the broad banner of Public Health Genetics in Legal, Ethical, and Policy Context. The core members of the group carrying out this initiative represent the full array of public health science disciplines within the University's School of Public Health. The school has a long tradition in environmental health and ecogenetics, with numerous links with experts in biostatistics, epidemiology, molecular biotechnology, and health policy. The new program across the university, the Cancer Center, and the Washington State Department of Health also has expertise in law, public policy, anthropology, philosophy, ethics, biotechnology, and population-oriented clinical genetic services. This approach is highly complementary to the Public Health Genetics program started earlier at the University of Michigan, which is more oriented toward policy development and the provision of clinical genetic services. Both programs are described by Austin et al. (34); see Chapter 5, this book.

CHALLENGES

Wise choices in public health and medicine depend upon excellent science, compassionate values, effective communication, appreciation of diverse cultures and preferences, openness to new knowledge and alternative views, commitment to disease prevention and health promotion, and progress in closing the gaps between diagnosis and treatment and between diagnosis and prevention.

Priorities

There is a perpetual tension in public health between applying more broadly what we know or think we know about health promotion and disease prevention and doing more research to build the knowledge about causes and effective interventions. Too often the lack of an experimental basis for successful interventions is neglected. Intervening in heterogeneous populations often has limited effectiveness. Many citizens ignore the advice of public health experts; the expert's approach is ineffective in either the justification or the communication of the advice. I believe that about 20% to 30% of the $1.2 trillion spent on health care annually in the United States is used to try to detect and control symptoms as well as one can for common diseases (cancers, psychoses, degenerative neurological diseases, gastrointestinal disorders, arthritis, and others) for which too little is known about the underlying causes and processes to prevent or reverse those processes. We should beware of hubris about our current knowledge and capabilities. The nation should enhance its huge expenditure in providing the American people access to current medical care and public health services with a substantial investment in research designed to make certain that such care and services are more effective and also more cost-effective in the not-too-distant future.

Training

Few public health professionals, including physicians, have received the education necessary to use complex genetic information in preventive medicine and public health. The subject matter comprises a formidable array of molecular and cell biology, clinical medicine, statistical genetics, epidemiology, ecogenetics, evaluation of screening and testing methods, ethics, and public policy (39,40). The Josiah Macy Jr. Foundation has embarked upon an initiative to stimulate educational initiatives for current professionals and for students in various stages of training (41). Federal and state investment in such training will be needed. It is important that genetics become one of the core integrating fields for public health training.

The National Human Genome Research Institute of the National Institutes of Health has established a National Coalition for Health Professions Education in Genetics (NCHPEG). This clearinghouse is a boon for genetic counselors and an important link to the Program on Ethical, Legal, and Social Implications (ELSI) of the Genome Institute. The ELSI program supports studies and conferences on clinical integration of genetic technologies, privacy and fair use of genetic information, implications of cataloguing genetic variation, and conduct of genetic research.

Ethics

The development of the Human Genome Project by the National Institutes of Health (NIH) and the Department of Energy in the United States and similar initiatives in France, the Nordic countries, and elsewhere have brought great public attention to the technologies, potential applications, and ethical issues involved in sequencing the human genome and applying that knowledge. From the outset, questions were asked about whose genome would be sequenced and whether there might be proprietary implications. In addition, these projects reignited fears of the misguided eugenics movement of the early decades of the 20th century. Thus, it was wise of James Watson to respond to a reporter's inquiry with the impromptu announcement that, as the initial Director of the Human Genome Project in 1988, he would earmark a portion of the funding for consideration of the ethical, legal, and social implications (ELSI) of the project (40). The result has been a generally admirable effort to define genetic issues; to engage ethicists, social scientists, philosophers, and historians to anticipate the implications of genetic discoveries; and to reach out through highly interdisciplinary conferences to representatives of employers, insurers, workers, community groups, and policymakers. Science in general and genetics in particular should not be conducted as if they were isolated from the larger society.

There is particular public angst about physicians being able to diagnose a genetically determined disease, such as Huntington disease, or a genetic predisposition to disease, such as specific breast cancer (BRCA1) gene mutations, if they have no effective preventive or therapeutic intervention to offer. In the case of untreatable Tay-Sachs disease, it was possible to offer community-based counseling and specific carrier testing for this autosomal recessive condition among Ashkenazi Jews. In the case of cystic fibrosis, no specific population subgroup could be targeted for community-based counseling and screening; furthermore, multiple mutations were associated with the disease, and the disease is not as severe or untreatable as is Tay-Sachs disease. Thus, cystic fibrosis carrier-detection programs were deferred after both the American Society for Human Genetics and the NIH ELSI program published social impact assessments and recommended against general-population screening programs.

The decision to use genetic testing involves very complex questions about informed consent, confidentiality, privacy, and duty to warn (2,3,42). The risk of discrimination in insurance and in employment is substantial; in fact, genetic counselors commonly advise new patients to first be sure they are adequately insured before undergoing genetic assessments and tests. An admirable state-level process has generated well-balanced recommendations to the governor and legislature in Michigan (43), reflecting the legacy of James Neel (44).

One can predict with confidence that genetics will continue to grow in importance in public health as more effective strategies are developed for treatment and especially for prevention, the special province of public health, and as the public becomes more knowledgeable about genetic services. Therefore, establishing a credible process for public discourse and for respectful consideration of diverse views will be critical to the development and application of public health genetics.

References

1. Vogel F, Motulsky AG. Human genetics: problems and approaches (3rd ed). Berlin, Heidelberg, New York: Springer-Verlag, 1997.
2. Khoury MJ and the Genetics Working Group. From genes to public health: the

applications of genetic technology in disease prevention. Am J Public Health 1996;86:1717–1722.

3. Omenn GS. Genetics and public health. Am J Public Health 1996;86:1701–1703.

4. Motulsky AG. Joseph Adams (1756–1818). Arch Intern Med 1959;104:490–496.

5. Galton F. Hereditary talent and character. Macmillan's Magazine 1865; 12:157–166.

6. Garrod AE. The incidence of alkaptonuria: a study in chemical individuality. Lancet 1902;ii:1616–1620.

7. Fisher RA. The correlation between relatives on the supposition of mendelian inheritance. Trans R Soc Edinburgh 1918;52:399–433.

8. Fee E. The origins and development of public health in the United States. In: Holland WW, Detels R, Knox G (eds). Oxford textbook of public health (2nd ed). New York: Oxford University Press, 1991, pp. 3–22.

9. Allison AC, Blumberg BS. Polymorphism in man. Boston: Little, Brown, 1965.

10. Lander ES, Schork NJ. Genetic dissection of complex traits. Science 1994;265:2037–2048.

11. Sing C, Haviland MB, Reilly SL. Genetic architecture of common multifactorial diseases. In: Ciba Foundation Symposium 197: Variation in the human genome. Chichester, UK: Wiley, 1996, pp. 211–232.

12. Gelehrter TD, Collins FS, Ginsburg D. Principles of medical genetics (2nd ed). Baltimore: Williams & Wilkins, 1998.

13. Omenn GS, Motulsky AG. Ecogenetics: genetic variation in susceptibility to environmental agents. In: Cohen BH, Lilienfeld AM, Huang PC (eds). Genetic issues in public health and medicine. Springfield, IL: Thomas, 1978, pp. 83–111.

14. "Risk Commission", The Presidential/Congressional Commission on Risk Assessment and Risk Management. Risk assessment and risk management in regulatory decision-making. Final report, Volume 2, 1997. Washington, DC: Government Printing Office; *www.riskworld.com*.

15. Omenn GS, Faustman EM. Risk assessment and risk management. In: Detels R, McEwen J, Beaglehole R, Tanaka H (eds). Oxford textbook of public health (4th ed). New York: Oxford University Press, 2000 (in press).

16. Omenn GS. Putting environmental risks in a public health context. Public Health Rep 1996;111:514–516.

17. Goldman LR. Linking research and policy to ensure children's environmental health. Environ Health Perspect 1998;106:857–862.

18. LIPID, The Long-Term Intervention with Pravastatin in Ischaemic Disease, Study Group. Prevention of cardiovascular events and death with pravastatin in patients with coronary heart disease and a broad range of initial cholesterol levels. New Engl J Med 1998;339:1349–1357.

19. Motulsky AG, Brunzell JD. The genetics of coronary atherosclerosis. In: King RA, Rotter JI, Motulsky AG (eds). The genetic basis of common diseases. New York: Oxford University Press, 1992, pp. 150–169.

20. Boushey C, Beresford SAA, Omenn GS, Motulsky AG. A quantitative assessment of plasma homocysteine as a risk factor for vascular disease: probable benefits of increasing folic acid intakes. JAMA 1995;274:1049–1057.

21. McCully K. Vascular pathology of homocysteinemia. Am J Pathol 1969; 56:111–128.

22. Welch GN, Loscalzo J. Homocysteine and atherosclerosis. N Engl J Med 1998;338:1042–1050.

23. Institute of Medicine. Dietary reference intakes: thiamin, riboflavin, niacin,

vitamin B6, folate, vitamin B12, pantothenic acid, biotin, and choline. Washington, DC: National Academy Press, 1998, Chapter 8.

24. Cogswell ME, Burke W, McDonnell SM, Franks AL. Prevention of iron overload disease due to hemochromatosis. Am J Prev Med 1999;16:134–140.

25. Motulsky AG, Beutler E. Population screening in hereditary hemochromatosis. Annu Rev Public Health 2000; 21 (in press).

26. Miller LH. Impact of malaria on genetic polymorphism and genetic diseases in Africans and African-Americans. Proc Natl Acad Sci U S A 1997;91:2415–2419.

27. McNicholl JM, Cuenco KT. Host genes and infectious diseases: HIV, other pathogens, and a public health perspective. Am J Prev Med 1999;16:141–154.

28. Gordeuk VR, McLaren CE, MacPhail AP, Deichsel G, Bothwell TH. Associations of iron overload in Africa with hepatocellular carcinoma and tuberculosis: Strachan's 1929 thesis revisited. Blood 1996;87:3470–3476.

29. Samson M, Libert F, Doranz BJ, et al. Resistance to HIV-1 infection in Caucasian individuals bearing mutant alleles of the CCR-5 chemokine receptor gene. Nature 1996;382:722–725.

30. McGinnis JM, Foege WH. Actual causes of death in the United States. JAMA 1993;2207–2212.

31. Rossing MA. Genetic influences on smoking: candidate genes. Environ Health Perspect 1998;106:231–238.

32. Pomerleau OF. Individual differences in sensitivity to nicotine: implications for genetic research on nicotine dependence. Behav Genet 1995;25:161–177.

33. Eaton DL, Farin F, Omiecinski CJ, Omenn GS. Genetic susceptibility. In: Rom WN (ed). Environmental and occupational medicine (3rd ed). Philadelphia: Lippincott-Raven, 1998, pp. 209–221.

34. Gross SR, Cheng R, Nguyen T, Israel Y, O'Dowd BF. Polymorphisms of the D4 dopamine receptor alleles in chronic alcoholism. Biochem Biophys Res Commun 1993;196:107–114.

35. Gelernter J, Kranzler H, Coccaro E, Siever L, New A, Mulgrew CL. D4 dopamine-receptor (DRD4) alleles and novelty seeking in substance-dependent, personality-disorder, and control subjects. Am J Hum Genet 1997;61:1144–1152.

36. Omenn GS. Genetic investigations of alcohol metabolism and of alcoholism. Am J Human Genet 1988;43:579–581.

37. Barondes SL. Mood and genes. San Francisco: W.H. Freeman, 1998.

38. Austin MA, Peyser PA, Khoury MJ. The interface of genetics and public health: research and educational challenges. Annu Rev Public Health 2000; 21 (in press).

39. Vogel F, Motulsky AG. Human and medical genetics. In: Detels R, Holland W, McEwen J, Omenn GS (eds). Oxford textbook of public health (3rd ed). New York: Oxford University Press, 1997.

40. Juengst ET. Self-critical federal science? The ethics experiment within the U.S. human genome project. Soc Philos Policy 1996;13:63–95.

41. Hager M (ed). Education for more synergistic practice of medicine and public health. New York: Josiah Macy, Jr., Foundation, 1999.

42. Rothstein MA. Genetic secrets: protecting privacy and confidentiality in the genetic era. New Haven, CT: Yale University Press, 1997.

43. Michigan Commission on Genetic Privacy and Progress. Final report and recommendations. Michigan Department of Community Health, Lansing, February 1999.

44. Neel JV. Physician to the Gene Pool: Genetic Lessons and Other Stories. New York: John Wiley, 1994.

3

The human genome project: evolving status and emerging opportunities for disease prevention

Leslie Fink and Francis S. Collins

The history of biology was forever altered a decade ago by the bold decision to begin a directed research program to characterize in ultimate detail the complete set of genetic instructions for human beings. The idea captured the public imagination, perhaps not so much like America's targeted health wars on cancer or AIDS, but rather like the great expeditions—those of Lewis and Clark, Sir Edmund Hillary, and even Neil Armstrong. Scientists wanted to map the human genetic terrain, knowing it would lead them to previously unimaginable insights and from there to the common good. That good would include a new understanding of genetic contributions to human disease and the development of rational strategies for minimizing or preventing disease phenotypes altogether.

History and Accomplishments of the Human Genome Project

The endeavor undertaken was both awesome and chancy. The instruction book—the human genome—was vastly larger than any genetic endowment tackled so far; and in 1990, the tools were not yet powerful enough to perform the task. Critical social questions, such as whether the new technologies for reading our genetic constitution would challenge our identities, our fundamental right to privacy, or our freedom from discrimination, loomed without answers.

Portions of this chapter have been previously published in Collins FS. Medical and Societal Consequences of the Human Genome Project. New England Journal of Medicine 1999;341: 28–37.

Yet a public science initiative focused so sharply on the molecular essence of humankind was too intriguing and too promising to forgo. Since the 1970s, nearly all biomedical research avenues increasingly led to the gene, for genes contain the basic information about how a human body carries out its duties from conception until death. In between, of course, our bodies struggle to survive in a challenging environment. We fare better or worse largely, but not entirely, on the basis of our genetic makeup.

Not surprisingly, disease researchers wanted to identify their leading gene suspects as soon as possible and at the least expense. This was no small order— the 80,000 or so human genes are scattered throughout the genome like stars in the galaxy, with genomic light-years of noncoding DNA in between. The "billions and billions" of uncharted DNA units (approximately 3 billion base pairs in human beings) have frustrated searches regularly, often at great health and financial cost. If gene hunters were to mine miracles from the human genome, they needed more powerful tools and more ambitious strategies.

In 1988, the U.S. Congress appropriated funds to the Department of Energy (DOE) and the National Institutes of Health (NIH) to begin planning the Human Genome Project. Planners set a 15-year time frame, estimated a $3 billion price tag, and laid out formal goals to get the job done (1). On October 1, 1990, the Human Genome Project officially began (2). According to early plans, the human race would witness its own blueprint in fine detail in the year 2005.

In the fall of 1998, though, improvements in technology, success in achiev-ing early mapping goals (see below), emerging research opportunities, and accelerating demand for the human DNA sequence prompted project leaders in the United States and abroad to promise the blueprint—the complete DNA sequence of the human genome—two years ahead of schedule, in 2003 (3). The technology to accomplish such a task is at hand.

The NIH and DOE genome programs in the United States expect to con-tribute 60% to 70% of that sequence. Scientists funded by the Wellcome Trust at the Sanger Centre in Cambridge, England, along with other international partners, will produce the remainder. In March 1999, 15% of the sequence was in finished or nearly finished form. The largest centers participating in the Human Genome Project received new grants to begin full-scale sequencing and the timetable was moved up yet again. Pilot sequence projects had been so suc-cessful that the planners of the Human Genome Project now felt confident that at least 90% of the human sequence could be completed in "working draft" form by the spring of 2000. The sequencing centers achieved two milestones in late 1999. First, in November, project scientists celebrated completion and deposi-tion into the public database, Genbank, of 1 billion base pairs of human genome DNA sequence. Shortly thereafter, Human Genome Project scientists announced they had completed the sequence of human chromosome 22 (3a).

Though the "working draft" sequence will be of lower accuracy and contiguity, it will nevertheless be very useful, especially for finding genes, exons, and other genomic features. But because the working draft will contain gaps, it will not be as useful as a finished sequence for studying DNA features that span large regions or require high sequence accuracy over long stretches.

The final product must have four characteristics—the "4 A's" of the Human Genome Project: (*1*) the sequence must be *accurate*, that is, the DNA spellings must have an accuracy of 99.99% or better; (*2*) because large-scale sequencing relies on the accurate assembly of smaller lengths of sequenced DNA into longer, genomic-scale pieces, the human sequence must be *assembled* into long pieces that reflect the original genomic DNA; (*3*) because human DNA sequence must also be *affordable*, technology development must aim to reduce cost as much as possible; (*4*) finally, human DNA sequence should be *accessible* within 24 hours through public databases.

As plans for the period between 1998 and 2003 were being developed, two corporate ventures announced initiatives to sequence a major fraction of the human genome, using strategies that differ fundamentally from the publicly funded approach. The stated intention of one of those ventures to release its data publicly creates the possibility of synergy with the effort by the federal government. If the corporate data and the public data can be merged, the depth of sequence coverage will be greater, allowing a broader range of polymorphisms to be captured. And, because the public sequence will be obtained from mapped DNA, it will provide critically needed anchoring to sequence data generated by private-sector efforts.

Prior to the 1998–2003 plan, the scientific goals of the Human Genome Project addressed mostly genome mapping, technology development, and work to characterize the genomes of certain laboratory organisms. One type of map, known as a *genetic map*, is particularly helpful for following the inheritance of a disorder through several generations of a family. Genetic maps consist of a series of sequence-based markers that can be used to pinpoint the likely neighborhood of an altered gene responsible for a disease phenotype or other trait. Such maps have been invaluable in identifying and isolating highly penetrant gene mutations with mendelian inheritance patterns. The goal was to establish markers close enough to give a gene hunter a high likelihood of placing a gene in a reasonably searchable interval. A year ahead of schedule, an international consortium with major players in France and the United States published a genetic map containing almost 6000 markers, spaced less than 1 million bases apart (*4*). Such detail was four to six times greater than called for in the 1990 goals.

A second type of map, known as a *physical map*, provides cloned and ordered sets of contiguous DNA that represent regions of a chromosome, or even a whole chromosome. Once genetic markers define the region containing the sought-after gene, cloned pieces from the physical map provide a resource from which investigators can then isolate the gene. A copied replica of 98% of the human genome, consisting of thousands of linked pieces of DNA, is complete and meets the genome project's goal for physical mapping (5). This map contains over 41,000 DNA markers, known as "sequence-tagged sites," or STSs, that properly align the pieces. At that marker density, any gene in the human genome should lie within fewer than 100,000 bases of an STS.

The Human Genome Project recognized from its inception its responsibility not only to develop gene-finding and analysis technologies, but also to address the broader societal implications of these newfound abilities to decipher genetic information. To fulfill this responsibility, the project commits 5% of its annual research budget to study the "ethical, legal, and social implications (ELSI)" of genome research. Historically, the ELSI program has focused on four high-priority areas: (1) the use and interpretation of genetic information; (2) clinical integration of genetic technologies; (3) issues surrounding genetics research; and (4) public and professional education and training about these issues.

The plan covering the years 1993 to 1998 expanded the mapping goals and explicitly included new objectives for identifying and mapping not just systems of anonymous markers, but the genes themselves (6). Scientists at the National Library of Medicine, at genome research centers, and in private industry later began a program to position expressed DNA from gene regions (also called "expressed sequence tags" or ESTs) on the physical map. After two editions, this gene map represents the most extensive effort so far to locate and identify the 80,000 genes in the human genome. Over 30,000 gene tags now give disease-gene hunters a ready list of candidate genes residing in the chromosomal neighborhood they know is involved in a disease (5).

Before 1996, goals for DNA sequencing were largely targeted toward genomes of model organisms. From those efforts, scientists have sequenced the genomes of *Saccharomyces cerevisiae,* a species of yeast valuable to biologists and commonly used by bakers and brewers (7) and *Escherichia coli,* a mainstay of basic biology and the biotechnology industry (8). The first complete genome sequence of a multicellular organism, the round worm *Caenorhabditis elegans*, was completed in late 1998 (39) and, through a public—private collaboration, the sequence of the fruitfly *Drosophila melanogaster* was completed in March 2000.

The yeast genome contains 12,057,500 base pairs in its nuclear DNA. Containing some 6000 genes arranged on 16 chromosomes, yeast has already provided biologists with a valuable resource for determining the function of individual human genes involved in medical problems such as cancer.

The 97-million base-pair *C. elegans* genome is distributed among six chromosomes and contains over 19,000 genes. Although barely visible with the naked eye, the tiny round worm has become an invaluable tool for studying biological processes such as development, neurobiology, and aging. The worm project began in 1990, as a collaboration between researchers at Washington University in St. Louis, Missouri, and at the Sanger Centre in Cambridge, England. Computer comparisons between the worm sequence and those of other organisms have shown that about 40% of the *C. elegans* genes found so far are novel. A major fraction of the genes is likely to be similar to those of humans and other more advanced organisms.

Now the complete sourcebook for these organisms will allow scientists to piece together for the first time a comprehensive look at how all the genes in a eukaryotic cell and a multicellular viganism function as an integrated system.

The 1998–2003 plan also contains goals for new areas of study, including how variations in human DNA sequence among different populations relate to the development of, or protection from, disease; new technologies and strategies for studying genetic function on a whole-genome scale; and new areas of ELSI research, such as identifying and addressing issues that link genetics to personal identity and racial or ethnic background, and the implications of these issues for philosophical and religious traditions.

Implications of Gene Discovery for Understanding Human Genetic Illness

Maps and other genome technologies provide the tools for a gene-isolation technique known as *positional cloning* (9). This technique allows a researcher to confirm the genetic basis of a disease and locate the gene, even when little is known about the gene's function. So far, over 100 disease-linked genes have been isolated using the positional cloning technique. Whereas gene discovery once took years to decades, an investigator using these powerful tools can now sometimes map and isolate a gene in a matter of weeks. Increasingly, gene hunters are combining positional cloning techniques with information in EST databases to narrow their gene searches to rational candidates. This method, called "positional candidate cloning" (10), has been used to isolate many altered genes associated with human disease.

Gene isolation provides the best hope for understanding human disease at its most fundamental level. Knowledge about genetic control of cellular functions will underpin future strategies to prevent or treat disease phenotypes. The recent isolation of mutations associated with Parkinson disease (PD) (11–14), for example, has dramatically pushed molecular research forward on that baffling disorder. In one study, gene hunters mapped a suspect gene to a region of chromosome 4 (11). Although the region contained approximately 100 genes, one was already known to encode the protein alpha-synuclein.

Earlier research had shown that alpha-synuclein builds up in brain cells of people with Alzheimer disease (15), and people with PD have similar deposits. In just a few months, the researchers showed conclusively that a missense mutation in the alpha-synuclein gene caused PD in the study families. Further research has shown that a mutation in a gene encoding a protein critical to the breakdown of alpha-synuclein and other proteins also results in the PD phenotype (14). Understanding the genetic control of the proteolytic processes of brain proteins may provide new targets for interventions in a number of related neurodegenerative disorders characterized by the accumulation of protein deposits, including Alzheimer disease, Huntington disease, and spinocerebellar ataxia.

Even before a gene's role in disease is fully understood, diagnostic applications can be useful in minimizing or preventing the development of health consequences. The DNA tests that look for the presence of disease-linked mutations, for example, are proving to be the most immediate commercial application of gene discovery and the one now encountered most frequently by clinicians. These tests may assist in the correct diagnosis of a genetic disease, foreshadow the development of disease later in life, or identify healthy heterozygote carriers of recessive diseases. Genetic tests can be performed at any stage of the human life cycle, with increasingly less-invasive sampling procedures. Whereas genetic testing was once sought almost exclusively by couples with a family history of early-onset disease for the purpose of family planning, information about genetic status is increasingly sought by individuals who wish to learn their own predisposition to later-onset illness.

In a growing number of instances, strategies can be implemented to reduce or prevent illness when a genetic etiology or predisposition is known. Successes in reducing disease through treatment have been achieved for the hereditary disorders hemochromatosis, phenylketonuria, and familial hypercholesterolemia, among others. Risk reduction through early detection and lifestyle changes may be available for disorders associated with predisposing mutations, such as some cancers. As therapies build on knowledge gained about the molecular basis of disease, increasing numbers of illnesses, now refractory to treatment, may in the future yield to molecular medicine (Fig.3.1A,B).

The recent discovery of an altered gene (HFE) that leads to hereditary hemochromatosis (HH) (16), a common disorder of iron metabolism, provides an interesting example of the potential for using mutation information to prevent an adult-onset disease phenotype. A recessive condition, HH affects about 1 in 300 people of northern European descent and is easily treatable if diagnosed early. Its major symptoms—liver cirrhosis, heart failure, diabetes, arthritis, and other organ damage—do not occur until midlife and are easily misdiagnosed. Untreated, the disease causes early death, but treatment by phlebotomy to remove excess iron allows people with HH to live a normal life

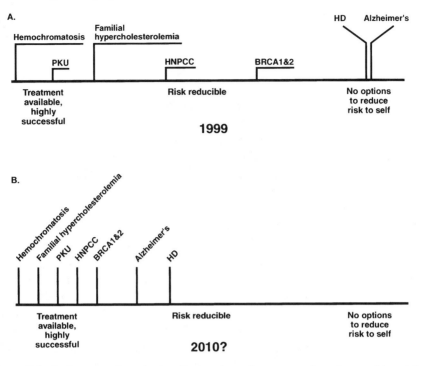

Figure 3.1. **A.** *Successes in reducing disease through treatment have been achieved for the hereditary disorders hemochromatosis, phenylketonuria (PKU), and familial hyper-cholesterolemia, among others. Risk reduction through early detection and lifestyle changes may be available for disorders associated with predisposing mutations, such as some cancers.* **B.** *As therapies build on knowledge gained about the molecular basis of disease, increasing numbers of illnesses, now refractory to treatment, may in the future yield to strategies of molecular medicine.*

span. A single substitution of the amino acid cysteine by tyrosine at codon 282 accounts for the majority of cases (17).

At first glance, HH seems like an ideal target for public health approaches to hereditary disease prevention: The disorder is common, the number of disease-linked mutations in the gene are few, and effective treatment can minimize or eliminate the effects of the disease. But closer examination reveals a number of complexities that have so far mitigated against rapid introduction of this genetic test as a tool for disease prevention (16). Two HFE mutations, C282Y and H63D, have been identified. The C282Y/C282Y genotype accounts for most cases of hemochromatosis, but it has also been observed in healthy elderly persons (Ref. 16; see also Chapter 20 in this volume). The C282Y/H63D and H63D/H63D genotypes appear to confer a much lower risk of disease than the C282Y/C282Y genotype, but the penetrance of these genotypes is not yet established. (16) At the moment, simple detection of HFE mutations does not predict the most likely clinical course. Before population testing for HFE mutations is considered, further research is needed to explain the variations in phenotype among mutation carriers and to correlate genotype more closely with health outcomes.

Implications for the Study of Complex Disorders

The rather straightforward mendelian rules that govern inheritance of disease traits have been worked out for many rare disorders resulting from highly penetrant changes in a single gene. But teasing out the genetic components of the so-called complex disorders—diabetes, heart disease, most common cancers, autoimmune disorders, and psychiatric disorders, which result from the interplay of environment, lifestyle, and small effects of many genes—remains a formidable task. Most successes in identifying genes associated with common diseases have focused on highly heritable subsets, including BRCA1 (18) and BRCA2 (19) for breast cancer, HNF-4 α for maturity-onset diabetes of the young (MODY) 1 (20), GCK for MODY 2 (21), HNF-1 α for MODY 3 (22), hMSH2 (23,24), and hMSH1 (25) for hereditary nonpolyposis colon cancer, and α-synuclein for Parkinson disease (11). Linkage analysis and positional cloning techniques are well suited to discovering genes with such strong influence. But strategies for finding the multiple, low-penetrance variants, which in the aggregate account for a larger percentage of illnesses, are not currently as well developed. Identification of weakly penetrant alleles contributing to common disorders will require new approaches.

To assist in those efforts, the Human Genome Project is initiating new studies on genetic variation in the human population to provide a dense map of common DNA variants. The DNA sequence variations include insertions and deletions of nucleotides, differences in the copy number of repeated sequences, and single-nucleotide polymorphisms, or SNPs (pronounced "snips"), which occur most frequently throughout the human genome. About 1 in every 300 to 500 bases in human DNA may be a SNP.

The SNPs can be used as markers in whole-genome linkage analyses of families with affected members, as well as in association studies of individuals in a population. Association studies might directly test a potential functionally important variant or may take advantage of the phenomenon of linkage disequilibrium—in which a marker and a gene are inherited together—to map gene variants associated with disease. Because the human species consists of relatively few generations, recombination events have not disrupted linkage disequilibrium over distances of 10,000 to 100,000 bases in most populations. Consequently, association studies view large human populations as evolutionary families and do not rely on nuclear family studies for gene mapping (26,27).

Some SNPs may contribute directly to a trait or disease phenotype by altering function. Though most SNPs are located outside of protein-coding sequences, those within coding sequences, called cSNPs, are of particular interest because they are more likely to affect cell function. A large, well-characterized collection of SNPs will become increasingly important to the discovery of DNA sequence variations that affect biological function.

New Technologies for Genetic Analysis and Risk Assessment

The transition from genetics to "genomics" marks the evolution from understanding single genes and their individual functions to understanding the actions of multiple genes and their control of biological systems. Whereas Human Genome Project tools initially advanced research on single genes, they are now forming the basis for genomic-scale analysis of the human organism.

The so-called DNA chip currently provides one promising approach to genome-scale studies of genetic variation (28), detection of heterogeneous gene mutations (29), and gene expression (30). A next-generation adaptation of filter blot hybridization techniques, DNA chips, also called "microarrays," generally consist of a thin slice of glass or silicon about the size of a postage stamp upon which threads of synthetic nucleic acids are arrayed. Sample probes are added to the chip, and matches are read by an electronic scanner. As with semiconductors, the capacity of DNA arrays has doubled about every two years. Thus, chips that held a few hundred arrays not so long ago now hold hundreds of thousands.

Microarray technology has been used to detect DNA variations and to detect the expression of mRNA in individual cells and tissues. Microarrays are used clinically to monitor HIV sequence variation, to detect p53 gene mutations in breast tissue, and to assess expression of cytochrome P450 genes. In the laboratory, microarray technology has also been applied to genomic comparisons across species (31), genetic recombination (32), and large-scale analysis of gene copy number and expression, as well as protein expression in cancerous tissues (33).

Application of microarrays to the detection of DNA variation holds promise, along with family histories and data from large population studies, for establishing an individual's risk of developing common, adult-onset disorders. A baseline genome scan could provide helpful information about an individual's disease risk profile and point to which prevention strategies—when available—should be put into place.

Genetic Knowledge and Personalized Medicine

Identifying human genetic variations will eventually allow clinicians to sub-classify diseases and adapt therapies to the individual. Large differences in the effectiveness of medicines may exist from one individual to the next. Toxic reactions can also occur and are likely in many instances to be a consequence of genetically encoded host factors. That basic principle has spawned the burgeoning new field of *pharmacogenomics*, which aims to use information about genetic variation to predict responses to drug therapies.

For example, researchers discovered that Alzheimer's patients with the gene subtype ApoE4, which affects cholinergic function in the brain, are less likely to benefit from the cholinomimetic drug tacrine (34). Such a finding will help data analysis of clinical trials of Alzheimer's therapies and will promote targeting of new therapies specifically to ApoE4 carriers.

In another example, the formation of venous blood clots in the brain or legs is a rare but serious side effect of taking birth control pills. One study has shown a dramatically increased risk for cerebral vein thrombosis among women taking oral contraceptives who also carry the blood-clotting variant factor V Leiden (35). Foreknowledge of the presence of that variant, and consideration of alternate forms of birth control, might be useful in minimizing the risk for thrombosis among these women.

Pharmacogenomics may also present new possibilities for refinements in breast cancer treatment. A recent study found that the estrogen-receptor blocker tamoxifen reduced the incidence of breast cancer by 45% among women at high risk for the disease (36). Women whose breast cancer risk was reduced with tamoxifen treatment may represent a subset of individuals with a certain genetic makeup; as one approach to this possibility, studies are now underway to determine whether the responder phenotype correlates with BRCA1/2 mutation status.

More generally, genetic approaches to disease prevention and treatment will include an expanding array of gene products developed into drug therapies. Ever since the Food and Drug Administration's (FDA) approval of recombinant human insulin in 1982, over 50 additional gene-based drugs have come on-line. These include drugs for the treatment of cancer, heart attack, stroke, and diabetes, as well as many vaccines (37).

Not all therapeutic advances for gene discovery will be genes or gene products. In other instances, molecular insights into the disorder, derived from gene discovery, will suggest a new treatment. Phenylbutyrate, for example, which is approved for the regulation of blood ammonia, is being tested in clinical trials for the treatment of cystic fibrosis (CF) (38). The main clinical phenotype in people with CF results from a mutation in the cystic fibrosis transmembrane conductance regulator (CFTR) gene, which prevents normal amounts of CFTR protein from crossing the cell membrane, thus diminishing the ability of chloride and water to enter and exit the cell. Phenylbutyrate apparently stimulates expression of the CFTR protein, allowing more of it to reach its correct location.

The Ethical, Legal, and Social Implications of Genetic Knowledge

One of the most active ELSI areas has been policy development related to the privacy and fair use of genetic information, particularly in health insurance, employment, and medical research. Debates in this area focus largely on the potential of genetic information to predict an increased likelihood that a currently healthy individual will later develop a disease phenotype.

Although many states have attempted to address "genetic discrimination" in health insurance and the workplace, federal legislation would provide the most comprehensive protections. In research, fears about the privacy of genetic information and the loss of a job or insurance coverage may make people hesitant to use medical advances or to volunteer for studies of disease-linked gene mutations for fear the results could be used against them.

Largely on the basis of recommendations from workshops held by the Human Genome Project and the National Action Plan on Breast Cancer (NAPBC), the Clinton Administration endorsed the need for congressional action to protect against genetic discrimination in health insurance and employment. In 1996, Congress enacted the Health Insurance Portability and Accountability Act (HIPAA), which took a significant step toward protecting access to health insurance in the group market but left several serious gaps in the individual market that still must be closed.

In the area of workplace discrimination, the Equal Employment Opportunity Commission (EEOC) has interpreted the Americans with Disabilities Act (ADA) to cover on-the-job discrimination based on "genetic information relating to illness, disease or other disorders." But there have been no genetic discrimination complaints filed with the EEOC, and the guidance has yet to be tested in court. Thus, the amount of protection actually provided by the ADA remains uncertain. In February 2000, President Clinton signed an Executive Order prohibiting genetic discrimination in the federal workplace and legislation to extend these protections to the private sector is pending in the U.S. Congress.

In the area of privacy, as part of the NAPBC–Human Genome Project partnership, medical researchers, policymakers, and representatives of law, government, the insurance industry, and public health have recently assessed current policies and practices to protect confidentiality in genetics research and have identified areas where new or modified policies or practices might enhance privacy protections and promote the conduct of research. The group developed a set of principles for researchers, research institutions, state and federal agencies, and policymakers to consider in formulating privacy protections for research information.

Other significant steps have been taken to ensure the responsible integration of genetic tests into clinical practice. For the most part, genetic testing in the United States has developed successfully, and people tested have been provided options for avoiding, preventing, and treating inherited disorders. But the rapid pace of test development combined with the rush to market these developments may create an environment in which genetic tests are available to health care consumers before they have been adequately validated. Upon the recommendation of the Task Force on Genetic Testing (39), created by the Human Genome Project's NIH-DOE ELSI Working Group, the Secretary of the Department of Health and Human Services has created an advisory panel to ensure safe delivery of genetic tests into clinical practice.

The completion of the first human genome sequence and the expansion of human genetics research to include studies of genetic variation among human subpopulations have raised new ELSI questions. The 1998–2003 plan includes goals for examining those issues as well as for integrating genetic technologies and information into health care and public health activities; for integrating knowledge about genomics and gene-environment interactions into nonclinical settings; for example, how new genetic knowledge may interact with a variety of philosophical, theological, and ethical perspectives; and for examining how racial, ethnic, and socioeconomic factors affect the use, understanding, and interpretation of genetic information, the use of genetic services, and the development of policy (3).

Conclusions

Ever since the Human Genome Project's inception, the increasing detail and quality of genome maps have reduced the time it takes to locate a gene from years, to months, to weeks. We have learned the location of approximately half of the 80,000 or so genes packaged on human chromosomes. Genome researchers are at the forefront of cross-disciplinary technology development for the identification and analysis of not just single genes, but whole genomes.

Most recently, we have begun to get the first glimpses of the human genome at its most detailed level: as of March 2000, More than 2 billion of the 3 billion bits of DNA code that spell out instructions for every function a human body carries out is now available in public databases. In the years ahead, the full DNA sequence of humans will give us unprecedented opportunities to observe and understand the "Book of Life".

As genome technologies move from the laboratory into the health care setting, new methods will make it possible to read the instructions contained in an individual's DNA. Such knowledge may foretell of future disease and alert patients and their health care providers to begin better prevention strategies. In the wrong hands, however, that same information could be used to discriminate against or stigmatize an individual. The Human Genome Project has catalyzed the development of policy options for lawmakers to consider in their efforts to prohibit genetic discrimination and to protect the privacy of genetic information.

As hoped, genome maps, sequence, and analytical tools are providing a robust technological infrastructure for biomedical research well into the 21st century. The project's commitment to make these powerful tools freely available means any scientist with an Internet connection can already apply genomic approaches to individual research problems. High-technology research tools developed by the Human Genome Project will offer researchers unprecedented opportunities to study human biology and disease in entirely new ways.

References

1. Committee on Mapping and Sequencing the Human Genome. Mapping and sequencing the human genome. Washington, DC: National Academy Press, 1988.

2. U.S. Department of Health and Human Services, U.S. Department of Energy. Understanding our genetic inheritance: the U.S. human genome project. The first five years: FY 1991–1995. NIH publication No. 90-1590, 1990.

3. Collins FS, Patrinos A, Jordan E, et al. New goals for the U.S. human genome project: 1998–2003. Science 1998;282:682–689.

3a. Dunham I, Shimizu N, Roe BA, et al. The DNA sequence of human chromosome 22. Nature 1999;402:489–495.

4. Murray JC, Buetow KH, Weber JL, et al. A comprehensive human linkage map with centimorgan density. Science 1994;265:2049–2054.

5. Deloukas P, Schuler GD, Gyapay G, et al. A physical map of 30,000 human genes. Science 1998;282:744–746.

6. Collins FS, Galas D. A new five-year plan for the U.S. human genome project. Science 1993;262:43–46.

7. The yeast genome directory. Nature 1997;387(6632 Suppl):5–••.

8. Blattner FR, Plunkett G III, Bloch CA, et al. The complete genome sequence of *Escherichia coli* K-12. Science 1997;277:1453–1462.

9. C. elegans Sequacing Consortium. Genome sequence of the nematode C. elegans: a platform for investigating biology. Science 1998;282:2012–2018.

10. Collins FS. Positional cloning: let's not call it reverse genetics anymore. Nat Genet 1992;1:3–6.

11. Collins FS. Positional cloning moves from perditional to traditional. Nat Genet 1995;9:347–350.

12. Polymeropoulos MH, Lavedan C, Leroy E, et al. Mutation in the alpha-synuclein gene identified in families with Parkinson's disease. Science 1997;276:2045–2047.

13. Glasser T, Muller-Myhsok B, Wszolek ZK, et al. A susceptibility locus for Parkinson's disease maps to chromosome 2p13. Nat Genet 1998;18:262–265.

14. Jones AC, Yamamura Y, Almasy L, et al. Autosomal recessive juvenile parkinsonism maps to 6q25.2–q27 in four ethnic groups: detailed genetic mapping of the linked region. Am J Hum Genet 1998;63:80–87.

15. Leroy E, Boyer R, Auberger G, et al. The ubiquitin pathway in Parkinson's disease. Nature 1998;395:451–452.

16. Ueda K, Fukushima H, Masliah E, et al. Molecular cloning of cDNA encoding an unrecognized component of amyloid in Alzheimer disease. Proc Natl Acad Sci U S A 1993;90:11282–11286.

17. Burke W, Thomson E, Khoury MJ, et al. Hereditary hemochromatosis: gene discovery and its implications for population-based screening. JAMA 1998;280:172–178.

18. Feder JN, Gnirke A, Thomas W, et al. A novel MHC class I-like gene is mutated in patients with hereditary haemochromatosis. Nat Genet 1996;13:399–408.

19. Miki Y, Swensen J, Shattuck-Eidens D, et al. A strong candidate for the breast and ovarian cancer susceptibility gene BRCA1. Science 1994;266:66–71.

20. Wooster R, Bignell G, Lancaster J, et al. Identification of the breast cancer susceptibility gene BRCA2. Nature 1995;378:789–792.

21. Yamagata K, Futura H, Oda O, et al. Mutations in the hepatocyte nuclear factor 4 alpha gene in maturity-onset diabetes of the young (MODY 1). Nature 1996; 384:458–460.

22. Froguel P, Zouali H, Vionnet N, et al. Familial hyperglycemia due to mutations in glucokinase: definition of a subtype of diabetes mellitus. N Engl J Med, 1993;328:697–702.

23. Yamagata K, Oda N, Kaisaki PJ, et al. Mutations in the hepatocyte nuclear factor 1 alpha gene in maturity-onset diabetes of the young (MODY3). Nature 1996;385:455–458.

24. Fishel R, Lescoe MK, Rao MR, et al. The human mutator gene homolog MSH2 and its association with hereditary nonpolyposis colon cancer. Cell 1993;75:1027–1038.

25. Leach FS, Nicolaides NC, Papadopoulos N, et al. Mutations of a mutS homolog in hereditary nonpolyposis colorectal cancer. Cell 1993;75:1215–1225.

26. Papadopoulos N, Nicolaides NC, Wei YF, et al. Mutation of a mutL homolog in hereditary colon cancer. Science 1994;263:1625–1629.

27. Schafer AJ, Hawkins JR. DNA variation and the future of human genetics. Nature Biotechnol, 1998;16:33–39.

28. Collins FS, Guyer MS, Charkravarti A. Variations on a theme: cataloging human DNA sequence variation. Science 1997;278:1580–1581.

29. Wang DG, Fan J-B, Siao C-J, et al. Large-scale identification, mapping and genotyping of single-nucleotide polymorphisms in the human genome. Science 1998;280:1077–1082.

30. Hacia JG, Brody LC, Chee MS, et al. Detection of heterozygous mutations in BRCA1 using high-density oligonucleotide arrays and two-color fluorescence analysis. Nat Genet 1996;14:441–447.

31. DeRisi J, Penland L, Brown PO, et al. Use of cDNA microarray to analyse gene expression patterns. Nat Genet 1996;14:457–460.

32. Hacia JG, Makalowski W, Edgemon K, et al. Evolutionary sequence comparisons using high-density oligonucleotide arrays. Nat Genet 1998;18:155–158.

33. Winzeler EA, Richards DR, Conway AR, et al. Direct allelic variation scanning of the yeast genome. Science 1998;281:1194–1197.

34. Kononen J, Bubendorf L, Kallioniemi A, et al. Tissue microarrays for high-throughput molecular profiling of tumor specimens. Nat Med 1998;4:844–847.

35. Poirer J, Delisle M-C, Quirion R, et al. Apolipoprotein E4 allele as a predictor of cholingergic deficits and treatment outcome in Alzheimer disease. Proc Natl Acad Sci U S A 1995;92:12260–12264.

36. Martinelli I, Sacchi E, Landi G, et al. High risk of cerebral-vein thrombosis in carriers of a prothrombin-gene mutation and in users of oral contraceptives. N Engl J Med 1998;338:1793–1797.

37. Fisher B, Costantino JP, Wickerham DL, et al. Tamoxifen for prevention of breast cancer: report of the National Surgical Adjuvant Breast and Bowel Project P-1 study. J Natl Cancer Inst 1998;90:1371–1388.

38. New Medicines in Development. Biotechnology 1998. Pharm Res Manufac Am 1998: 35.

39. Rubenstein RC, Zeitlin PL. A pilot clinical trial of oral sodium 4-phenylbutyrate (Buphenyl) in deltaF508-homozygous cystic fibrosis patients: partial restoration of nasal epithelial CFTR function. Am J Respir Crit Care Med 1998;157:484–490.

40. Task Force on Genetic Testing. Holtzman NA, Watson MS (eds). Promoting safe and effective genetic testing in the United States. Baltimore: Johns Hopkins University Press, 1998.

41. Adams MD, Celniker SE, Holt RA, et al. The genome sequence of drosophila melanogaster. Science 2000;287:2185–2195.

4

Models of public health genetic policy development

Benjamin S. Wilfond and Elizabeth J. Thomson

As more genes associated with diseases are identified, it will become increasingly necessary for public health agencies, professional organizations, and consumer organizations to make policy decisions about genetic testing programs designed to promote health or prevent disease. Thus, it is important to have a framework for policymakers to utilize in making such decisions. This framework should include both substantive criteria and procedural approaches to these issues.

This chapter begins with a history of policy development for genetic services in the United States. It includes a discussion of early genetic screening programs, a review of part policy statements about genetic screening, and a more detailed discussion of the consistent substantive criteria for genetic diagnostic services that have been recommended by various policy-making bodies. The chapter also presents two conceptual models for the development of public policy, the extemporaneous and the evidentiary models. The development of policy for cystic fibrosis newborn screening is used to illustrate both the value and the limitations of these models.

The analysis presented here is based on four main assumptions. The first is that society will ultimately benefit from advances in genetic knowledge and further development of genetic technologies. This does not mean that there are no concerns about the potential (mis)use of genetic information, but that on balance, these advances will be a benefit. The second assumption is that the potential psychosocial harms associated with learning genetic information about individuals, families, and groups must be taken very seriously. The third assumption is that the potential benefits and harms must be assessed empirically in observational studies and clinical trials, just as is done with new pharmaceutical interventions prior to clinical implementation. The final assumption is that the decisions to develop public health genetic programs are not exclusively medical decisions but are also societal decisions. Determining whether information may be of value to individuals, families, and society is a decision that ought to be made by society as a whole and not solely by medical or public health professionals and organizations. Thus, regardless of what public health genetic policy-making process is utilized, substantial public input is highly desirable. These fundamental assumptions are derived, in part, from an examination of the previous experiences in the United States with genetic screening programs. They are articulated to a large extent in policy-making statements that have been developed over the last 20 years concerning the integration of genetic services into health care.

History of Screening Programs

Definitions

It is important to note that certain terms are used inconsistently and lack clear definitions in policy analyses. First, the term *genetic* commonly has been used to connote "single gene" disorders (e.g., cystic fibrosis, Huntington disease, muscular dystrophy). More recently, however, the term has come to include diseases with more complex genetic and environmental interactions (e.g., cardiovascular disease, diabetes, and asthma). Additionally, genetic *tests* have often narrowly referred only to DNA-based tests, although a broader view of genetic tests might include gene products (e.g., protein levels) or manifestations of a disease secondary to abnormal protein structure or function (e.g., measurement of sweat chloride in cystic fibrosis). A family history itself can provide limited information to individuals, family members, health care providers, or others about the risk of a person developing symptoms of a genetic disease. Thus, although the issues surrounding the dilemmas posed by genetic advances may not be new (e.g., family history), given the technological advances, they will be raised more and more frequently.

Various distinctions have been proposed between the terms genetic "screening" and genetic "testing." Generally, *screening* refers to a preliminary form of testing, requiring diagnostic confirmation through subsequent testing. The assessment of asymptomatic populations also has been called "screening." This remains the case even though some of the tests now used in such population assessments are diagnostic in nature. Sometimes certain demographic characteristics, such as age or ethnicity, are utilized to target "screening" in asymptomatic individuals (e.g., women over 35 years of age, or Ashkenazi Jews). The term "screening" is sometimes used to signify interventions that occur outside the context of the usual physician/patient interaction. The distinctions between "screening" and "testing" are often blurred. This issue will not be resolved in this chapter, and the term "genetic screening" will be used interchangeably with "genetic testing."

Newborn Screening

One of the first genetic screening programs to be developed in the United States was newborn screening for phenylketonuria (PKU) (see Chapter 20). Currently, newborn screening for PKU is considered one of the hallmark successes of a public health genetic screening program. However, at the time the program was developed and implemented in the 1960s, many questions still remained unanswered (e.g., how frequent the disorder was; whether there were variations in this disorder; and how best to implement such testing, interpret the test results, and treat children diagnosed with PKU) (1). In a rapid and unprecedented fashion, PKU screening was mandated in almost all of the states within the space of a few years; despite the objections of the American Academy of Pediatrics (2). In fact, it took more than a decade after mandatory PKU screening had been adopted to develop adequate information about the optimal diagnosis and management of PKU and to organize treatment programs, which resulted in the screening programs' ultimate success. Further, it took several decades to learn about some of the long-term consequences of newborn screening for PKU such as the length of time that dietary adherence is desirable and the potential implications for women with PKU who have children (i.e., mental retardation). Meanwhile, numerous children were incorrectly labeled as affected with PKU, and some children were inappropriately treated; still others were correctly identified as affected with PKU, but lacked access to appropriate therapy. This situation was never well documented because controlled clinical trials were never carried out (3).

Although there were a number of unanticipated consequences of the early PKU screening programs, the most significant is the legacy of state-run "mandatory newborn screening programs," which have become the gold standard for newborn screening throughout the United States. Testing is done, in all but one state, without the informed permission of the parents. The ability of parents to "opt out" of this testing for their child is generally allowed, particularly for religious objections. While each state "mandates" its own list of required tests, three tests are almost universally provided: PKU, hypothyroidism, and sickle cell anemia (4). This mandatory testing is today an anomaly, in contrast to most other aspects of pediatric care, in which a physician has a conversation with one or both parents, recommends a course of action, and obtains permission for a particular intervention. Recently, it has been suggested that newborn screening should move away from "mandatory" screening toward mandatory "offering" of newborn screening (5,6). Many reasons exist for suggesting this change. Perhaps the most compelling arguments relate to the availability of new DNA diagnostic capabilities, which allow for testing of newborns for literally hundreds of disorders (including ones that are not treatable; ones that become symptomatic far later in life; ones for which interventions are as yet unproven; and ones that identify not only affected individuals, but also individuals who are healthy, but carriers of single gene disorders) (7).

Opponents of voluntary testing with informed consent argue that testing will often not get done and that many babies will be harmed as a result (8). Proponents of voluntary testing argue that parents, who are the most likely to have their child's best interests in mind, should have a role in determining what testing is done on their newborn (5). Thus, while newborn screening represents the potential promise of genetic testing exemplified by the prevention of mental retardation in PKU, it also raises a number of ethical and health policy issues, including those of informed permission for genetic testing, privacy, and the potential for unanticipated consequences of such testing.

Reproductive Testing

A number of other early genetic screening programs met with mixed results. Perhaps two of the most classic examples were those of *sickle cell anemia carrier screening in the African American population* and *Tay-Sachs carrier screening in the Ashkenazi Jewish population.* The development of sickle cell anemia carrier testing in the 1970s began with what appeared to be well-intended and sincere enthusiasm to identify those who were carriers of the gene for this disorder. For many reasons, this screening program has become the example of the potential problems that can be associated with genetic screening efforts. The community targeted for sickle cell screening was African American, and few African Americans were engaged in the policy discussions about whether and how to implement such a screening program. There was limited evidence that the African American community was interested in this screening. In addition, there was a great deal of confusion about the meaning and interpretation of test results. In particular, confusion existed about the distinction between actually having the disease and the carrier state (often referred to as the "trait"), which resulted in stigmatization of and discrimination against healthy carriers (9). Finally, there was also a perception by some in the African American community that any recommendation about carrier testing, prenatal diagnosis, and possible abortion had racist and eugenic overtones.

Contemporaneous with development of sickle cell screening programs was the development and implementation of screening programs for Tay-Sachs disease in the Ashkenazi Jewish population (10). Several differences existed in the development and implementation of this screening program. A number of the researchers and health care providers involved in setting up the screening programs were members of the Jewish community. In addition, extensive consultation with Jewish leaders and education of community members resulted in a widespread acceptance of the program within the community as well as acceptance of the concept of carrier detection, prenatal diagnosis, and possible abortion, especially since Tay-Sachs disease is inevitably fatal in early childhood. Thus, Tay-Sachs screening is often heralded as one of the successes of genetic screening of the 1970s. However, even the Tay-Sachs screening programs have not been without critics. Some have suggested that the brochures used were factually misleading and overstepped the bounds of nondirectiveness to achieve their own goals (11). Others have suggested the program had eugenic overtones, even though individual couples made their own choices concerning testing and abortion.

Testing for Adult-Onset Diseases

More recently, genetic testing for cancer risks (12,13) and hereditary hemochromatosis (14) has been debated. When one of the first major genes predisposing to the development of breast cancer was discovered, discussion ensued about who might benefit from this testing. In the test for breast cancer, unlike that for Tay-Sachs, a mutation in the BRCA1 gene did not predict with certainty who would get the disease, when the disease would occur, or how severe the disease would be. Additionally, it was not clear at the time whether effective interventions existed to reduce risk. Despite these uncertainties, rapid commercialization and marketing of BRCA testing has occurred, even though such testing is still considered to be experimental by some.

Hemochromatosis (*hh*) is another important example of a late-onset disorder for which genetic screening is now possible. Although this disorder does appear to have an effective intervention, the fact that many unanswered questions remain has dampened the enthusiasm for such testing. While a gene for *hh* has been identified, the prevalence, penetrance, and genotype-phenotype correlations for the known mutations remain to be clarified (14). Furthermore, issues such as whether and when to intervene so as to reduce health risks for individuals with identified genetic changes, but no other evidence of disease, are not clear. Thus, one very important question is whether screening for *hh* by a phenotypic test (e.g., abnormal transferrin saturation) may be clinically more useful (and potentially less stigmatizing) than DNA or genotypic screening. Studies are underway to answer some of these questions in a deliberative manner. When available, these answers will provide important information regarding decisions on whether to test, when to test, who to test, and how to begin to offer such screening (see Chapter 23 for further discussion about these issues).

Policy Statements Regarding Genetic Testing

The experiences with genetic testing, from PKU screening in the 1960s to the present day, have resulted in a number of multidisciplinary policy statements that have attempted to articulate principles by which proposed new genetic screening and testing programs should be assessed. These statements include ones from the Hastings Center in 1972 (15), the National

Academy of Sciences in 1975 (3), the President's Commission on Ethical Issues in Medicine Biomedical and Behavioral Research in 1983 (16), the Institute of Medicine in 1993 (6), and the NIH-DOE Task Force in Genetic Testing in 1997 (17).

These reports considered various aspects of genetic testing and genetic screening programs, and they articulated a surprisingly congruent set of principles (Table 4.1). One of the most important principles, uniformly recommended from the 1970s to the present day, is the need for empirical research about the benefits and risks of genetic testing prior to the implementation of any mass screening programs. In the section that follows, some of the recommended criteria will be discussed.

NIH-DOE Task Force Criteria

The recent report of the Task Force on Genetic Testing identified three broad criteria that are necessary before using a new genetic test: analytical validity, clinical validity, and clinical utility. *Analytical validity* refers to assuring that the laboratory performance of a genetic test is accurate and precise. A genetic test that may be used should have been proven to be highly analytically sensitive and specific before it is introduced into clinical practice. *Clinical validity* refers to several measures of clinical performance including clinical sensitivity and clinical specificity, and positive predictive value. Before a genetic test is used, it should be established that the results of the test are likely to predict the presence or absence of a clinical disease or the likelihood to develop a disease. Clinical validity involves consideration of broad issues of genotype–phenotype correlations, penetrance of genes, individual and group variations, allelic heterogeneity, and numerous other factors.

The third criteria to be considered is *clinical utility*. This refers to how information from the test can be used in a clinical context to improve people's health. In general, tests should not be used unless the benefits of using the test outweigh the risks. Thus, the determination of clinical utility involves assessments of both safety and effectiveness.

The *safety* of genetic tests does not generally refer to the physical risk of obtaining a DNA sample, but rather to the potential impact that the genetic information may have on the individual and on family members. This is information that can be misinterpreted and misused. It may cause anxiety and alter family relationships. Stigmatization and discrimination of individuals and family members could result should the information become known by others. These are important issues to consider when a genetic test is being considered for widespread use.

Effectiveness is another measure that needs to be considered: A program's success should be measured in terms of its effectiveness in achieving its articulated goals. For example, if the goal of a genetic testing program is to reduce morbidity and mortality, the efficacy must be measured against those

Table 4.1 Principles for Genetic Screening: Areas of Consensus

Principles	Hastings Center*	National Academy of Sciences†	President's Commission‡	Institute of Medicine**	ELSI Task Force Genetic Testing§
Goals of Screening	Improved health in patients with genetic disease; Informed reproductive decisions; Alleviating anxiety of family at risk	Improved health in patients with genetic disease; Informed reproductive decisions; Enumeration of genetic disease	Informed reproductive and personal decisions	Improved health in patients with genetic disease; Informed reproductive decisions	Improved health in patients with genetic disease; Informed reproductive decisions
Attainability of Goals	Define goals; Goals attainable based on pilot studies	Define goals; Goals attainable based on pilot studies; Standardization of projects	Goals attainable based on pilot studies		
Public Involvement in Screening	Supports community participation in education	Supports public participation; Supports involvement of medical community	Supports involvement of medical community	Supports more genetics education for public and medical community	Supports public involvement in nontechnical policy decisions
Access to Screening Services	Information and screening available for all; Priority for high-risk groups	Priority for high-risk groups	Priority for high-risk groups	Priority for high-risk groups	
Necessary Test Characteristics	Precise information to minimize misinterpretation	Acceptable accuracy, validity, sensitivity, and specificity	Acceptable accuracy, validity, sensitivity, and specificity	Acceptable accuracy, validity, sensitivity, and specificity	Acceptable accuracy validity, sensitivity, and specific CLIA approval for labs
Absence of Coercion in Obtaining Services	Voluntary testing only; No constraints on childbearing	Voluntary testing only	Voluntary testing only—newborn screening mandatory only if: (a) Substantial harm, (b) Voluntary program fails	Voluntary testing only	Voluntary testing only newborn screening w/o informed consent if: (a) clinical validity/utility (b) parents understand reason

(continued)

Table 4.1 (*Cont.*)

Principles	Hastings Center*	National Academy of Sciences†	President's Commission‡	Institute of Medicine**	ELSI Task Force Genetic Testing§
Informed Consent	Explicit consent is necessary Prior to testing: Clients need to know risks and benefits Ongoing assessment of effectiveness of consent procedure	Explicit consent is necessary Prior to testing: Clients need to know risks and benefits	Explicit consent is necessary	Explicit consent is necessary Prior to testing: Clients need to know risks and benefits	Explicit consent is necessary Prior to testing: Clients need to know risks and benefits
Protection of Subjects	Screening is a form of human experimentation	Screening is a form of human experimentation	Pilot studies are necessary	Screening is a form of human experimentation until benefits and risks of screening are defined	Screening is a form of human experimentation
Disclosure of Results	Full disclosure	Full disclosure	Full disclosure	Full disclosure	Full disclosure in understandable language
Provision of Counseling	Nondirective Define qualifications Ongoing assessment of: (a) Clients' understanding of information (b) Effect of information on clients' lives	Define qualifications Ongoing assessment of: (a) Clients' understanding of information (b) Effect of information on clients' lives	Nondirective Define qualifications Ongoing assessment of: (a) Clients' understanding of information (b) Effect of information on clients' lives	Nondirective Define qualifications Tailor counseling to cultural perspective of client	Nondirective Define qualifications
Privacy	Information restricted to individual screened	Information restricted to individual screened	Information restricted to individual screened	Information given only to those for whom individual signs release	Information given only to those for whom individual signs release
Laboratory Provisions		Regional Facilities Quality Control	Regional Facilities Quality Control	Regional Facilities Quality Control	Regional Facilities Compliance with (CLIA)

* As reported in reference 15.
† As reported in reference 3.
‡ From the 1983 report of the President's Commission (16).
** As reported in reference 6.
§ As reported in reference 17.

outcomes. If, however, the goal of the program is informed reproductive decision making, the outcomes should be measured in terms of whether women/couples received the information they need to make informed decisions satisfactorily. Such a program should not be measured in terms of the reduction in the number of individuals born with a disease or in reduced health care costs.

The validity, safety, and effectiveness of a genetic test, however, are just some of the important aspects to be considered before developing or implementing a genetic screening program. Other important features to consider are the assessment of community interest; the development and clear statement of program goals; assurance of laboratory quality; the availability of education and optimal informed-consent procedures; assurance of privacy and confidentiality; and the availability of follow-up services for test results including genetic counseling and clinical management. All these issues must be assessed in the context of limited health care resources and the need to prioritize between health programs (18).

Assessment of Community Interest

Before beginning any genetic screening program, it is important to assess community interest in such a program: not only the readiness of health care professionals to provide the services, but also the public's interest in receiving the services. This assessment is particularly critical if there is a group that will be "targeted" for genetic screening. Before any public health screening program is developed, it is important to get input from the community to be screened (19,20). The community should agree that the goals of the screening program are worthwhile, that the test is an acceptable test, and that any risks to the community are outweighed by the potential benefits of such testing. In addition to such "community consultation," it is critical to determine whether health care providers are sufficiently educated about the genetic test itself, including how to interpret and use the test results.

Development of Program Goals

Before undertaking a public health genetic screening program, policymakers must determine and articulate the goals of the proposed program. The effectiveness of a program can be evaluated only if the programmatic goals have been determined. The goals of such a program may depend upon many things, but the most important and overarching goal of any public health genetic screening program should be related to promotion of health and prevention of disease, through phenotypic prevention (see introduction in Chapter 1). It is the authors' view that the goal of *public health* genetic screening programs should not be genotypic prevention, because the decision to undergo prenatal screening, diagnosis, and to consider pregnancy termination is intensely personal and should not be influenced by public health goals, professionals, agencies, or organizations. Although some geneticists have assessed prenatal testing programs on this basis (21), such goals can have eugenic implications.

Assurance of Laboratory Quality

Once it has been decided that a genetic test is analytically sound and Assurance of Laboratory Quality clinically valid, there are various laboratory issues requiring attention. Genetic tests are often developed in research laboratories. Once they move from research into the clinical arena, they need to be performed in a clinical laboratory that adheres to CLIA regulations (22). In addition, those in charge must assure that adequate proficiency testing and quality assurance mechanisms are in place (see Chapter 12), and that staff members are able to provide information about the meaning and interpretation of the genetic test result.

Education and Informed Consent

For a genetic screening program to be effective, issues of education and informed consent must be addressed. Health care providers need to be sufficiently knowledgeable to offer the genetic tests (23). Strategies to educate large numbers of people so that they understand the genetic screening program to be implemented may be challenging (24,25). Issues surrounding informed consent and permission are covered in Chapter 26 and are (and will continue to be) some of the most difficult challenges public health professionals will have to face (26). In general, policy statements have recommended that genetic testing not be done without informed consent. However, as was previously mentioned in this chapter, newborn screening has routinely occurred without informed consent. As public health genetic programs develop, public health professionals will have to determine how to achieve informed consent for genetic testing in public health settings. Further, when a large segment of the population is to be tested and resources to provide such education and counseling are limited, new and innovative approaches to education and consent may be needed. Thus, additional deliberations about balancing the public interest in promoting health with individual interests in medical decision making will be needed to address the role of consent in the public health genetics context. However, these are not necessarily conflicting values: Most people have an interest in promoting their own health, and informed consent (and education) may be important mechanisms to improve health.

Privacy and Confidentiality

These issues are of particular concern in the public health context. Numerous public health registries and databases already exist, to which genetic information could now be added. Given the potential adverse consequences of breaches of confidentiality and possible genetic stigmatization and discrimination, these issues will require even more attention than in the past. There have been numerous state and federal legislative efforts designed to limit the harm that might occur should genetic information about a person become known by third parties. Further, state and federal groups are attempting to improve safeguards for the privacy of medical records, including genetic information, more generally (27). One of the most challenging issues in the future will be determining who should have access to genetic information—individuals, family members, and/or society. State or federal governments may have an interest in this information to further public health goals; however, allowing access to this information may come at the expense of personal liberties and individual risks. This is an issue for which there is as yet no consensus.

Availability of Follow-up Services
Another consideration in the decision to implement a genetic screening program is the availability of adequate follow-up services. These services should include the ability of health professionals to interpret the test results, to provide genetic counseling, and to plan and provide optimal follow-up medical management and treatment or prevention interventions. For example, colon cancer screening may not be effective unless the appropriate intervention follow-up is also available. Programs should probably not be undertaken if no treatment or prevention services are available or if access to them is limited.

Cost and Prioritization of Genetic Health Care Services
In the coming years, genetic tests will abound. The question will inevitably have to be posed, "Because a genetic test becomes available, does it mean that the test should be used?" There will need to be a careful assessment of whether the cost of such screening programs is worth the potential benefit to individuals and society, and whether a particular program has a sufficient priority in an era of limited financial and health care resources.

The Evidentiary and Extemporary Models of Policy Development

The substantive criteria involving the collection of empirical evidence regarding the analytic validity, clinical validity, clinical utility, and programmatic issues have been articulated in various forms for the last 25 years. However, these criteria have not always been utilized in the development of the screening programs. Health policy decisions made in the past have often followed one of two complementary models: either the extemporaneous or the evidentiary model of health policy development (28). Each model describes a mechanism by which new clinical interventions become accepted as standard of care. While many health policy decisions reflect some features of both models, examining the implications of each model can be useful in understanding the basis of health policy decisions about new interventions for the future (see Fig. 4.1).

The Extemporaneous Model

The extemporaneous model is descriptive and acknowledges the role of various stakeholders advocating for their interests. Patient advocacy groups may be enthusiastic about the potential value of screening for "their disorder" based on their own perceptions about how screening might favorably influence their own personal lives. However, extrapolating one's own personal experience to entire populations may be insufficient, because there may be a much wider variability of experiences and impact when a whole population is considered. Industry representatives, with obligations to stockholders, and perhaps, with their own self-interest, might promote financially advantageous technologies that may or may not be beneficial to an individual's health. Physicians and public health departments might be supportive of new tests and treatments because they are enthusiastic about the possible use of new technologies to benefit society. Some physicians might use technologies largely

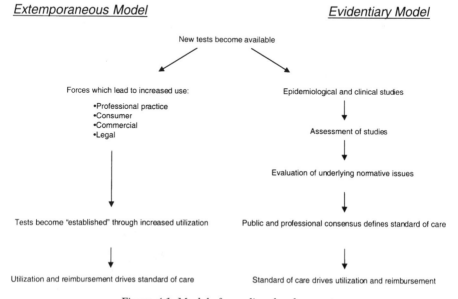

Figure 4.1 Models for policy development.

because of concerns about the legal implications of not providing them to their patients. Private and public insurers might deny adding coverage for new technologies (even when beneficial interventions exist) owing to concerns about limited fiscal resources.

In the extemporaneous model, any one of these groups can influence utilization, reimbursement, and even standard of care, depending on who can most effectively advocate for a particular position. Thus, it is possible that a standard of care will emerge regardless of the effectiveness of the program, the cost, or public consensus about the value of the program. One example of the extemporaneous model of health policy development was the decision to begin newborn screening for PKU in the early 1960s. The decision was based upon the enthusiasm of a few physicians and active consumer groups about the possibility of preventing mental retardation, even though there was no clear evidence of such a benefit at the time.

The Evidentiary Model

The evidentiary model is prescriptive and refers to an explicit approach to policy decisions. This model has three features. The first feature is understanding that empirical data are necessary prior to the development of any health policy decision. There is a growing realization about the importance of such empirical information for all areas of clinical services. However, the model also attempts to articulate the process by which that empirical information is developed into a health policy decision.

The second feature of this model is the acknowledgement that translation into health policy involves a normative assessment. Normative assessments refer to decisions about the value of an intervention. For example, empirical data may describe potential benefits and risks of the proposed intervention. However, the decision that the benefits are sufficiently great to recommend going forward with a program, or that the risks are sufficiently great to recommend against a program, is, in a large part, a value decision. Thus, the evidentiary model is meant to acknowledge that policy decisions should explicitly deal with normative components of the options under consideration. Examples of what may count as normative aspects of such a decision would be whether a particular disease is sufficiently common or severe to warrant a genetic testing program, or whether the benefits are justified by the costs.

The third feature is that the normative assessment must be made not only by scientific professionals, but also by the public. The reason for this need for public imput is that such decisions are not purely scientific or professional decisions, but are value decisions that concern society as a whole. Thus, the evidentiary model also has a place for public participation, including that of advocacy groups and commercial organizations. This model argues for the subsequent evaluation of the normative issues to reflect the concerns of each of those groups rather than the more explicitly political process of trying to accommodate the views of these advocacy groups. In this model, the deliberatively chosen standard of care would determine utilization and reimbursement rather than extemporaneous utilization and reimbursement driving standard of care.

One of the policy recommendations related to genetic testing (made repeatedly over this last decade) (6,28,29) has been the need for a broad-based policy-making group with public representation to make decisions regarding future genetic testing policies. In 1998, the Secretary of Health and Human Services chartered an Advisory Committee on Genetic Testing to potentially fulfill this role (http://www.nih.gov/od/orda/sacgtdocs.htm). This committee will have the opportunity to adopt an evidentiary model that includes explicit attention to the normative dimensions in its deliberations. An examination of a case study of genetic policy—newborn screening for cystic fibrosis—will yield a greater understanding of features of these models.

Cystic Fibrosis Newborn Screening

Clinical Description
Although cystic fibrosis (CF) is discussed in great detail in Chapter 21, in brief, CF is a complex multisystem disease that affects primarily the respiratory, digestive, and reproductive systems (30). In the United States, CF occurs in approximately 1 in 4000 births. It is an autosomal recessive condition, and although it occurs in diverse populations, it is more common in Caucasians, where the carrier incidence is approximately 1 in 30. The presenting symptoms are usually recurring pneumonia and failure to thrive. Not all children are affected the same way. The majority of children are identified during the first year of life, but some individuals with milder symptoms may not be diagnosed until adulthood. Pancreatic insufficiency is treated with pancreatic enzyme supplements and high-fat nutritional supplements. The lung disease is primarily treated with antibiotics and techniques to clear airway mucus. Over time, the lung disease is progressive and is the cause of death in most people. Currently, the median age of survival is 31 years. The usual approach to diagnosing cystic fibrosis is the use of quantitative pilocarpine iontophersis to determine the concentration of chloride in sweat (sweat test). Newborn screening for CF became possible in 1979 after the development of the immunoreactive trypsinogen assay (IRT), which utilizes dried blood spots. DNA diagnosis and carrier detection became feasible in 1989 with the cloning of the cystic fibrosis transmembrane conductance regulator (CFTR) gene.

History of CF Newborn Screening
The advent of the IRT assay led to the initial development of newborn screening programs in some parts of the world, primarily in Europe and Australia in

the early 1980s (31,32). The rationale for newborn screening for CF was a belief that early identification would change the overall prognosis of children by improving their long-term nutritional status and their pulmonary function. There was also the potential benefit of avoiding psychological distress on the part of the family owing to delay in the correct diagnosis of a child with unexplained symptoms, as well as a potential value of the information for future reproductive planning. However, none of these benefits had clearly been established empirically. At the time there were also speculative concerns about the adverse effects on children identified with CF via newborn screening because of a possible impact on the parent–child relationship. In addition, there were concerns about the possible unknown adverse effects from early treatment and about potential psychosocial harms to individuals who, because of elevated IRT levels, had tested "positive" but who were subsequently found not to have CF (false positives). For these reasons, in 1983, the American Academy of Pediatrics recommended against screening newborn for cystic fibrosis unless sufficient evidence of benefit became available, and a determination was made that the risks of screening were not significant (33).

Empirical Research

Because of these concerns, a randomized controlled clinical trial was begun in Wisconsin in 1985 to gather empirical data about newborn screening for CF. As discussed in Chapter 21, the parents of infants in the study group who had an IRT level over the 99.8th percentile were contacted and told that their infant had "screened positive" for CF and were asked to have a diagnostic sweat test performed at one of two control conters. This screening approach was used from 1985 to 1991. The positive predictive value of this approach was approximately 16%, that is, 1 in 7 infants who screened positive actually turned out to have CF (34). The study did show some evidence of transient anxiety, but rarely showed long-term persistent anxiety or confusion among families in which a false-positive test had occurred (35).

By 1997, the study began to show some evidence of nutritional benefits of early diagnosis with improved height and weights that persisted for the first 5 years after birth (35). Although not enough data had been accumulated by 1997 to determine the presence or absence of pulmonary benefit in this population, various observational studies suggested that, in fact, there might be some pulmonary benefit (36,37).

In 1991, because of concerns about the persistent anxiety in a small number of families whose infants were falsely identified as having CF, a new protocol was undertaken that involved a two-tiered approach to screening (34). This new protocol involved a DNA assay that would be performed for the most common CF mutation, ΔF508, after a positive IRT analysis. By doing a DNA assay on any newborn with an IRT greater than the 99th centile, the sensitivity could be maintained while doubling the positive predictive value. In other words, there were half as many newborns falsely identified as having CF for each newborn who truly had the disease. However, because each of the newborns who falsely tested positive was subsequently found to be carriers of CF mutations, parents were provided with genetic counseling and were offered the opportunity for further genetic testing (38).

Because of the unique concerns of presenting complex genetic information to the families of the infants who falsely tested positive, the understanding of the false-positive IRT/DNA group was compared to that of the group testing positive by IRT testing alone (38). A follow-up assessment, at 1 year after the negative sweat test, showed that 7% of the IRT group and 10% of the IRT/DNA families still thought about the results often or constantly. Four percent of the IRT-positive families and 17% of the IRT/DNA positive families believed that their experience of screening affected their feelings about having more children. Perhaps more importantly, at the time of follow-up, approximately half of the families in the IRT/DNA group, including those families who chose to have further genetic testing and genetic counseling, did not understand that they were still at an increased risk of having a child with cystic fibrosis.

Policy Development

The experience of newborn screening policy in Wisconsin illustrates features of both the extemporaneous and evidentiary models. First, the decision to conduct such a randomized controlled trial for a public health genetics program was unprecedented. It remains, to this day, an example of the potential to gather empirical evidence prior to making policy decisions. However, the subsequent policy decisions made on the basis of this data also illustrates that gathering empirical evidence may be insufficient to make sound public policy. Further attention to the normative aspects of policy decisions may have been needed.

The clinical trial in Wisconsin ended in 1994 (39). At that point, even though there was no long-term evidence of nutritional or pulmonary benefits, the state laboratory that had provided laboratory support for the study was in favor of beginning CF screening on a routine basis because the laboratory infrastructure for this program was developed. While the Wisconsin study results were still being analyzed, there appeared to be mounting evidence of pulmonary benefits from observational studies in Europe. In addition, few adverse effects of screening had been reported. As a result, with input from a public advisory group, the State of Wisconsin decided to move forward with implementing a statewide newborn screening program for CF. It is interesting that the decision to implement routine screening in Wisconsin appeared to be based more on the presence of the study rather than the results of the study at that time.

When the routine public health program was implemented in Wisconsin in 1994, several aspects of the screening strategy were changed from the research study, which may have altered the balance of benefits and burdens of such a program. One change resulted in an increase in the number of infants falsely testing positive for CF. The threshold level for the IRT value for DNA testing was decreased (from the 99th percentile to the 96th percentile), resulting in a fourfold increase in the number of newborns requiring DNA testing for ΔF508. This change lowered the positive predictive value to one below that of the early research protocol IRT test alone. Furthermore, the test results of any newborn with an IRT of greater than the 99.8th percentile were still reported to the physician, even if the DNA test was negative, further obviating the advantage of the two-tiered DNA approach in reducing false positives.

A second change in the program was related to the performance conduct of the sweat tests. During the research, sweat tests were performed in only two centers in the state (each had been approved by the Cystic Fibrosis Foundation by meeting its standards for laboratory quality control). When the state program began, community hospitals that did not necessarily adhere to the same laboratory standards began to do sweat tests. A third change that accompanied the decentralization of sweat tests was that genetic counseling, which had been offered as a part of the research protocol, was no longer automatically available through the state program. This lack of counseling created concerns about possible confusion regarding test results and their interpretation. Thus, the routine program adopted strategies that created more false-positive infants and abandoned strategies to minimize risks (genetic counseling).

Finally, at the time of the implementation of the state program, there was no careful tracking of newborns who tested positive, so it was difficult to examine the impact of these results on the families, especially those with false-positive screening results. Thus, it has been extremely difficult to assess whether these differences in approach have had a positive or negative impact on the program and how well these families have fared.

The decision to offer routine newborn screening for cystic fibrosis in Wisconsin exhibited some features of the evidentiary model, but not others. Although there had been a collection of empirical evidence and a public decision to go forward with newborn screening, the decision to go forward did not appear to be very tightly based on the benefits screening identified by the study at that time. Further, the state program made significant modifications to the approach to newborn screening that had been demonstrated through empirical research to be reasonably safe. Unfortunately, no publicly available materials are available that describe the process or reasons that these decisions were make and about how certain normative issues were considered and addressed.

Normative Issues for Newborn Screening

The first normative issue is what sort of informed consent is necessary for the addition of a test in which the potential benefits and harms are unknown or at least qualitatively different from the usual models of newborn screening (5). The State of Wisconsin does provide an educational pamphlet to all parents of newborns, but there is no explicit consent for such testing. The standard model for newborn screening, in which an immediate newborn diagnosis and the implementation of a therapy are necessary to cause irreversible profound harm, does not apply to cystic fibrosis. Informed consent is discussed in much greater detail in Chapter 26.

A second normative issue that needs to be considered is that the benefits of newborn screening for CF may occur in one group (those who are successfully diagnosed and treated), while the possible harms of newborn screening may occur in another group of newborns (those who falsely test positive). Although the potential harms of early identification of newborns with cystic fibrosis have not been observed, misunderstanding and worry in those parent whose infants falsely test positive have been described. The alterations from the research protocol to the routine program represent decisions that apparently did not highly value the importance of minimizing harms to those who falsely test positive. This included the decision to reduce the threshold level to maximize sensitivity and increase the number of false-positive infants, without the benefit of easy access to genetic counseling. The point is not to explicitly suggest that this was inappropriate, but rather that such a decision is not merely technical but is based on underlying normative assumptions about the relative importance of harm to some families from screening in contrast to missed "benefits" of early diagnosis (given the controversial nature of value of the benefits of newborn screening for CF, it is suprising that such a high priority was placed on maximizing sensitivity). However, these normative issues were not explicitly discussed in a public forum where they could be deliberated. This concern may be even further confounded by the fact that it is not likely that there would be any sort of organized representation of the voices of people who may have been harmed by an experience with a false-positive screening test in the same way that there may be support groups for parents of newborns with cystic fibrosis.

A final normative issue is how newborn screening ought to be given priority among other potential services for people with cystic fibrosis. If there is a fixed number of health care dollars available for cystic fibrosis care, there may need to be trade-offs between various approaches to the care that could be provided. Individuals with cystic fibrosis benefit from having access to a wide range of services, including primary care, hospital-based resources as needed, and multidisciplinary out-patient support including nursing, dietary, social work, respiratory therapy, home health care, vocational training, and pulmonary rehabilitation. These services are not always available to all patients with cystic fibrosis. Thus, a decision may need to be made concerning whether greater benefits can be provided to people with cystic fibrosis by improving these services than by implementing a newborn screening program. It is not clear whether such an assessment was made in Wisconsin, but it is likely that different states would come to different conclusions about the value of newborn screening, given the variation in access and availability of routine CF care.

Although there may be increasing enthusiasm for newborn screening for CF and other disorders as further molecular and other diagnostic technologies (40) become available, one should not lose sight of the questions raised by the implementation of CF newborn screening in the State of Wisconsin, an experiment that illustrates some of the challenges of using a robust evidentiary model of health policy development, even when empirical evidence is available. The value of benefits and harms may be weighed differently by different people. Different degrees of importance may be placed on measures to minimize harms or measures to detect problems within the system, in contrast to assessing the program on the basis of the number of missed children with CF. Furthermore, the impact of benefits and harms on different populations needs to be carefully considered as do the prioritization of health resources. Finally, greater attention may need to be given to the role of parents and primary-care physicians in the newborn screening process, thus providing a better mechanism for broader public input into these normative issues.

Conclusions

The experience with CF newborn screening illustrates the need for an evidentiary model for health policy development that can be used for the many anticipated genetic services of the future. It is critical that, in developing health policies, approaches similar to those outlined above must be utilized. The collection of empirical data in research settings is important as is the identification and explicit discussion of normative issues. Public involvement in final health policy decisions is crucial for solid public health policies to be developed and successfully implemented.

References

1. Bessman PS, Swazey IP. PKU: a study of biomedical legislation. Cambridge, MA: Harvard University Press, 1977.

2. American Academy of Pediatrics. Statement on compulsory testing of newborn infants for hereditary metabolic disorders. J Pediatr 1967;39:623.

3. Committee on Inborn Errors of Metabolism. Genetic screening: programs, principles, and research. Washington, DC: National Academy of Sciences, 1975.

4. Stoddard JJ, Farrell PM. State-to-state variations in newborn screening policies. Arch Pediatr Adolesc Med 1997;151:561–564.

5. Clayton EW. Issues in state newborn screening programs. Pediatrics 1992; 90:641–646.

6. Andrews LB, Fullerton JE, Hotzman NA, Motolsky AG. Assessing genetic risks: implications for health and social policy. Washington, DC: National Academy Press, 1994.

7. American Society of Human Genetics Board of Directors and the American College of Medical Genetics Board of Directors. ASHG/ACMG report points to consider: ethical, legal and psychosocial implications of genetic testing in children and adolescents. Am J Hum Genet 1995;57:1233–1241.

8. Laberge CM, Knoppers BM. Newborn genetic screeing: ethical and social considerations for the nineties. Int J Bioeth 1991;2:5–12.

9. Whitten CF. Sickle-cell programming—an imperiled promise. N Engl J Med 1973;288:316–319.

10. Kaback M, Zeiger R. The John F Kennedy Institute Tay–Sachs program: practical and ethical issues in an adult genetic screening program. New York: Plenum Press, 1973, pp. 131–145.

11. Goodman M, Goodman L. The overselling of genetic anxiety. Hastings Cent Rep 1982;12:20–27.

12. American Society of Human genetics. Statement of the American Society of Human Genetics on genetic testing for breast and ovarian cancer predisposition. Am J Hum Genet 1994;55:i–iv.

13. National Action Plan on Breast Cancer. Commentary on the ASCO statement on genetic testing for cancer susceptibility. J Clin Oncol 1996;14:1738–1740.

14. Burke W, Thomson E, Khoury MJ, et al. Hereditary hemochromatosis: gene discovery and its implications for population-based screening. JAMA 1998;280:172–178.

15. Lappe M, Gustafson J, Roblin R. Ethical and social issues in screening for genetic disease. N Engl J Med 1972;286:1129–1132.

16. President's Commission for the Study of Ethical Problems in Medicine and Biomedical and Behavioral Research. Screening and counseling for genetic conditions: the ethical, social, and legal implications of genetic screening, counseling, and education. Washington, DC: U.S. Government Printing Office, 1983.

17. Holtzman NA, Watson MS. Promoting safe and effective genetic testing in the United States: final report of the task force on genetic testing. Bethesda, MD: National Human Genome Research Institute, 1997.

18. Wilfond BS, Rothenberg KH, Thomson EJ, Lerman C. Cancer susceptiblity testing: ethical and policy implications for future research and clinical practice. J Law Med and Ethics 1997; 25:243–342.

19. Foster MW, Sharp RR, Freeman WL, Chino M, Bernsten D, Carter TH. The role of community review in evaluating the risks of human genetic variation research. Am J Hum Genet 1999;64:1719–1727.

20. Juengst ET. Group identity and human diversity: keeping biology straight from culture. Am J Hum Genet 1998;63:673–677.

21. Rowley PT, Loader S, Kaplan RM. Prenatal screening for cystic fibrosis carriers: an economic evaluation. Am J Hum Genet 1998;63:1160–1174.

22. Biesecker LG. Orphan tests. Camb Q Healthc Ethics 1996;5:300–306.

23. Geller G, Tambor ES, Chase GA, Hofman KJ, Faden RR, Holtzman NA. Incorporation of genetics in primary care practice: will physicians do the counseling and will they be directive? Arch Fam Med 1993;2:1119–1125.

24. Wilfond BS, Fost N. The cystic fibrosis gene: medical and social implications for heterozygote detection. JAMA 1990;263:2777–2783.

25. Faden RR, Tambor ES, Chase GA, Geller G, Hofman KJ, Holtzman NA. Attitudes of physicians and genetics professionals toward cystic fibrosis carrier screening. Am J Med Genet 1994;50:1–11.

26. Geller G, Botkin JR, Green MJ, et al. Genetic testing for susceptibility to adult-onset cancer: the process and content of informed consent. JAMA 1997;277:1467–1474.

27. Rothstein MA. Genetic secrets: protecting privacy and confidentiality in the genetic era. New Haven, CT: Yale Univerisity Press, 1997.

28. Wilfond BS, Nolan K. National policy development for the clinical application of genetic diagnostic technologies: lessons from cystic fibrosis. JAMA 1993;270:2948–2954.

29. Rothstein MA, Spence MA, Buffler PA, et al. Report of the Joint NIH/DOE committee to evaluate the ethical, legal, and social implications program of the human genome project. Bethesda, MD: National Institutes of Health/Department of Energy, 1996.

30. Wilfond B, Taussig LM. Cystic fibrosis: clinical overview. In: Taussig LM, Landau LI (eds). Pediatric pulmonary medicine. St Louis, MO: Mosby-YearBook, 1998.

31. Farrell PM. Cystic fibrosis neonatal screening: a continuing dilemma, especially in North America. Screening 1993;2:63–67.

32. Wilcken B. Newborn screening for cystic fibrosis: its evolution and a review of the current situation. Screening 1993;2:43–62.

33. Farrell PM. Early diagnosis of cystic fibrosis: to screen or not to screen—an important question [letter]. Pediatrics 1984;73:115–117.

34. Gregg RG, Wilfond BS, Farrell PM, Laxova A, Hassemer D, Mischler EH. Application of DNA analysis in a population-screening program for neonatal diagnosis of cystic fibrosis (CF): comparison of screening protocols. Am J Hum Genet 1993;52:616–626.

35. Tluczek A, Mischler EH, Farrell PM, et al. Parents' knowledge of neonatal screening and response to false-positive cystic fibrosis testing. J Dev Behav Pediatr 1992;13:181–186.

36. Dankert-Roelse JE, te Meerman GJ. Long-term prognosis of patients with cystic fibrosis in relation to early detection by neonatal screening and treatment in a cystic fibrosis centre. Thorax 1995;50:712–718.

37. Centers for Disease Control and Prevention. Newborn screening for cystic fibrosis: a paradigm for public health genetics policy development—proceedings of a 1997 workshop. MMWR 1997;46:1–24.

38. Mischler EH, Wilfond BS, Fost N, et al. Cystic fibrosis newborn screening: impact on reproductive behavior and implications for genetic counseling. Pediatrics 1998;102:44–52.

39. Farrell PM, Aronson RA, Hoffman G, Laessig RH. Newborn screening for cystic fibrosis in Wisconsin: first application of population-based molecular genetics testing. Wis Med J 1994;93:415–421.

40. Sweetman L. Newborn screening by tandem mass spectrometry. Cin Chem 1996;42:345–346.

5

The multidisciplinary nature of public health genetics in research and education

Melissa A. Austin and Patricia A. Peyser

As the target date of 2003 for the sequencing of the human genome approaches (1), there is growing recognition that public health practice, research, and education will be affected by new genetic technologies and information (1–3). This chapter focuses on the effects of this new genetic knowledge on research and education in public health. Clearly, a multidisciplinary approach is required.

In recent years a new specialty has emerged at the interface of genetics and public health. *Public health genetics* (see Chapter 1 of this text) has been defined as the application of advances in genetics and molecular biotechnology to improving public health and preventing disease. The equivalent term of *community genetics* is used in Europe (4) (see Chapter 16). Because the mission of public health is to fulfill society's interest in assuring conditions in which people can be healthy, there will be unavoidable integration of genetics into public health programs (Chapter 1). Public health professionals, therefore, will see an increasing integration of genetics into public health research, policy, and program development (Chapter 1). Public health practitioners will also have a role in using genetic information and technologies to facilitate both the prevention and treatment of disease (see Chapter 1 for further details)—for example, using genetic screening to identify people with a genetically influenced disease that can be prevented or treated.

What follows is an overview, with illustrative examples, of areas of research that provide information important to genetics in public health (note that several of the research areas are also reviewed in other chapters). This overview should help the reader understand why public health genetics education programs are needed and what their scope should include. Education in public health genetics is also discussed. In-depth descriptions of two emerging graduate programs at the universities of Michigan and Washington are presented. Other educational opportunities are also described. The chapter concludes with a summary of future needs for research and education in public health genetics.

Research

The explosion of genetic knowledge and technology that began in the 1990s has created a growing need for multidisciplinary (or interdisciplinary or cross-disciplinary) research related to public health genetics. It is often difficult to implement multidisciplinary research when traditional, institutional emphases are on focused, disciplinary research (5). This problem is not unique. In fact, research in public health genetics might be characterized as "interdependent research," in which work initially performed completely within one well-defined discipline (genetics) provides the basis for advances in other disciplines. The next section contains brief descriptions of areas of research that are identifying knowledge relevant to education in public health genetics. They are also paving the foundation for research and future applications (see Chapter 1).

Genetic Epidemiology and Molecular Epidemiology

Genetic epidemiology seeks to identify genetic characteristics, and their interactions with environmental exposures, that influence the distribution of disease among relatives and within diverse human populations (6,7). The goal is to understand the genetic etiology of disease better. This knowledge will facilitate early identification of high-risk individuals and families, and the design of more effective interventions. For example, using tools of genetic epidemiology, a susceptibility gene for non–insulin-dependent (type 2) diabetes mellitus was identified on chromosome 2 in a study of 330 Mexican-American sibling pairs (8). Recently, genes on chromosomes 2 and 15 have been shown to interact to increase susceptibility to diabetes in these Mexican-Americans (9). Genetic influences on risk factors, such as lipoproteins associated with risk of heart disease, can also be identified based on studies of relatives, including twins and extended families (10,11).

Rapid advances in molecular biology provide new tools for molecular epidemiology as well as genetic epidemiology. *Molecular epidemiology* is broadly defined as the use of techniques of molecular biology in epidemiologic studies. Molecular epidemiology has increased the understanding of the transmission and pathogenesis of infectious diseases. For example, a comparison of the genetic profile of *Escherichia coli* shared between sex partners allows the identification of genes associated with transmission of uropathogens (12). Chapter 9 in this volume, "Public Health Assessment of

Genetic Predispositions to Cancer," and Chapter 6, "Epidemiology, Molecular Biology, and Public Health," provide additional examples. The impact of genetics and molecular biology on epidemiology is reflected in the issue of *Epidemiologic Reviews* devoted to the methods of genetic epidemiology and applications to specific diseases (13) and in *Molecular Epidemiology: Principles and Practices* (14).

Furthermore, the field of human genome epidemiology (HuGE) has recently emerged, referring to the application of epidemiologic methods and approaches in population-based studies investigating the impact of human genetic variation on health and disease. The spectrum of topics addressed by investigators working on human genome epidemiology ranges from population-based epidemiologic research on gene variants to the evaluation of genetic tests and services in different populations (15). In fact, human genome epidemiology can be viewed as the intersection between genetic epidemiology and molecular epidemiology. To further these efforts, a collaboration of individuals and organizations recently launched the Human Genome Epidemiology Network (HuGE Net). This global effort seeks to (*1*) promote collaboration in developing and disseminating peer-reviewed epidemiologic information on human genes; (*2*) develop an updated and accessible knowledge base on the World Wide Web; and (*3*) promote use of this knowledge base by health care providers, researchers, industry, government, and the public for making decisions involving the use of genetic tests and services for disease prevention and health promotion (16).

Pathobiology and Infectious Diseases

When the focus is infectious disease, molecular epidemiology and pathobiology often overlap. Advances in genotyping technology and sequence analysis hold remarkable potential for better understanding susceptibility and resistance to infectious diseases. For example, a recent report based on five AIDS cohorts revealed a significant association between HLA class I heterozygosity and slower disease progression to AIDS among both Caucasians and African Americans (17). Furthermore, the results suggested that each of the tightly linked HLA class I loci contributed to this protective effect and that specific alleles, B*35 and Cw*04, were associated with disease progression. These findings demonstrate that host susceptibility and resistance to infectious diseases can be genetically mediated.

Concurrently, microbial genome sequencing is advancing rapidly, facilitating the identification of microbial gene products implicated in the infectious process, the screening for "pathogenicity islands" that influence virulence, and the identification of molecular targets for new therapeutic agents (18). Even more important, the combination of identifying genetically influenced host susceptibility and relevant genetic variation in pathogen genomes raises the possibility of characterizing the diversity of host–pathogen genomes, their interactions, and their role in infectious diseases. (See Chapter 10 in this volume, "Public Health Assessment of Genetic Susceptibility to Infectious Diseases," for more on this topic.)

Statistical Genetics

The development of new methods for statistical analysis of genetic data is advancing rapidly, and this will be essential for understanding the data emerging from the Human Genome Project. These methods include gene mapping and positional cloning based on family studies and linkage analysis. They also include methods based on linkage disequilibrium using unrelated cases and controls (19,20). *Statistical genetics* contributes to optimal sampling designs, to the development of better methods of statistical genetic analysis, and the application of these methods to specific diseases. For example, recent developments in statistical genetics have focused on the use of sibling pairs for both linkage and association studies (21,22). An international meeting, the "Genetic Analysis Workshop," is held bi-annually to facilitate advancement of analytical methods, using both simulated data sets and data from large-scale studies. In 1996, for example, the workshop focused on the important problem of detecting genes for complex traits and assessment of the performance of different analytical methods for diseases and their risk factors (23). Statistical issues related to consideration of many genes and environmental exposures simultaneously, as well as the incorporation of all the genetic diversity at a single genetic locus, will pose further statistical challenges (24,25).

Bioinformatics

As the volume of data generated by the Human Genome Project and numerous other genetic research projects accelerates, the organization, rigor, and accessibility of these resources will be essential to translate genetic information into meaningful data that can be used in public health settings. Although the forthcoming sequence of the human genome has been compared to the Rosetta Stone, Gelbart notes that it more closely resembles the undeciphered Phaestos Disk from Crete (1600 B.C.) in terms of our ability to make sense of the information (26). It will likely be through developments in "bioinformatics" that the genome sequences will become truly deciphered.

Bioinformatics is an emerging field combining molecular biology and computer science. Molecular biology is furnishing the extensive knowledge about genes; computer science is furnishing the new hardware and efficient algorithms for symbolic analysis, scientific computation, graphical interpretation, and data management. The establishment and testing of efficient algorithms for extracting and analyzing information is at the heart of bioinformatics. Bioinformatics will provide the tools and approaches for translating all the information available from genomic sequences of thousands of genes so as to understand the risk of many different diseases as well as possible intervention strategies. (See Chapter 3, "The Human Genome Project: Evolving Status and Emerging Opportunities for Disease Prevention.")

Ecogenetics and Pharmacogenetics

In the context of environmental health sciences, *ecogenetics* focuses on the role of gene–environment interactions in relation to health and disease. A recent and intriguing example in this field is the relationship of polymorphisms of the CYP2A6 gene in relation to smoking behavior and risk of cancer. Building on previous work demonstrating potential genetic influences on smoking (27,28), Pianezza and colleagues showed that individual carriers of CYP2A6 null alleles, who are less able to metabolize nicotine, were less likely to be tobacco-dependent (29). Further, those who were already tobacco-dependent were likely to smoke fewer cigarettes. Although this result has not been confirmed by other investigators (30), it does raise the possibility for more effective disease-prevention strategies targeted to individuals with specific genetic susceptibilities. Ecogenetics is discussed in Chapters 2 and 11.

A recent focus in *pharmacogenetics* has been on the interaction between a specific mutation, factor V Leiden, which corresponds to the anticoagulant effect of activated protein C, and use of oral contraceptives. Interestingly, the relative frequency of this mutation varies among ethnic groups (31). The consequences of this mutation and the metabolic changes in the clotting cascade due to oral contraceptives appear to interact to increase the risk of thrombosis in women (32). Currently, the consensus is that screening for this mutation is probably not indicated for women using oral contraceptives because effective contraception would be denied to about 5% of Caucasian women while preventing only a small number of fatal pulmonary emboli. Screening for the mutation is also not indicated for family members of patients with the mutation and venous thrombosis or pregnant women because the risk of severe bleeding associated with prophylaxis exceeds the benefits (33–35).

Nutrition

Similar to the concepts of ecogenetics, gene–environment interactions may involve dietary intake and its relationship to disease susceptibility. For example, there appear to be genetic influences on sensitivity to sweet and bitter tastes (36). These effects may, in turn, influence food preferences and dietary habits, and could modify risk for a variety of chronic diseases.

Health Services

As genetic testing for disease becomes more and more available, a fundamental issue is selecting a screening strategy that balances reduction of morbidity and mortality with the direct and indirect costs of screening on a population basis. For example, genetic testing for hereditary nonpolyposis colon cancer (HNPCC) is currently available. Although a recent report demonstrated that a relatively small proportion of HNPCC family members are likely to use genetic testing (37), the potential for widespread use of such costly genetic tests could consume a tremendous amount of societal resources (38). Thus, prevention-effectiveness analysis, a technique that seeks to identify the strategy that produces the most health benefit per dollar spent from a set of options producing a common health effect, will gain increasing importance in the context of public health genetics (see Chapter 18 for details).

Public Policy

Population-based genetic testing for disease presence and susceptibility is one of the most important potential applications of the advances in molecular biotechnology to public health. Such testing raises some of the most difficult policy decisions for translational research. For example, an expert panel convened at the Centers for Disease Control and Prevention in 1997 concluded that genetic testing for hereditary hemochromatosis, using the candidate gene HFE, should not be endorsed (39). This policy recommendation was based on "uncertainties about prevalence, and penetrance of HFE mutations, and the optimal care of asympotomatic people carrying the HFE mutation" as well as the potential for stigmatization and discrimination. A similar recommendation against screening for the ApoE4 allele as a diagnostic test for Alzheimer disease was recently presented by the Stanford Program in Genomics, Ethics, and Society (40). These recommendations will need to be reevaluated if new information becomes available indicating a health outcome benefit to screening, and as consensus develops regarding the criteria for undertaking genetic testing in a population setting (41).

As the number of genetic tests for disease susceptibility increases exponentially, issues of access to genetic services, including the availability of genetic counseling, will continue to increase. For example, the "duty to recontact" for genetic service providers (i.e., the obligation to recontact former patients about relevant advances in research) takes on new dimensions. A recent survey of physician geneticists, doctoral geneticists, and genetic counselors did not reflect a consensus about the benefits and burdens of such a practice. Although respondents indicated that it was desirable to recontact patients, they did not perceive it as a practical goal within the current health care system (42).

Cultural Anthropology

Genetics research in public health is, by nature, conducted in the context of communities and populations. Perhaps one of the most controversial issues in this area has been the concept of community or group consent for genomic research (43). In a recent publication, interviews with two Native American tribes were used to develop case studies evaluating genetic research and genetic testing (44). The investigators concluded that community review is useful to identify and minimize risks from genetic studies, and that it facilitates the development of partnerships between researchers and communities, thereby enhancing participant recruitment and retention in studies.

Bioethics

The basic ethical principles of biomedical research, respect for persons, beneficence and nonmaleficence, and justice, were established in the Belmont Report in 1979 (45). These principles are applied through the process of informed consent, risk-benefit analysis, and appropriate selection and recruitment of study subjects, respectively. These principles remain applicable to genetic research today. Unlike most medical information, genotypes provide information not only about the patient or study subject, but also about his or her relatives. As a result, considerable controversy has arisen about the use of DNA samples, especially those collected and stored without specific informed consent for genetic research (46,47). Therefore, it has been proposed that informed consent needs to evolve into a process in which study subjects become "limited partners" in research, rather than "subjects" (48). Concerns about privacy and confidentiality are reflected in recent analyses of the publication of pedigrees in biomedical journals (49) and in the creation of a genetic database for the entire country of Iceland (50). These issues demonstrate that ethics "is not just an abstract intellectual discipline. It is about the conflicts that arise in trying to meet real human needs and values" (51), and is of central importance in public health genetics.

Law

Hand in hand with debates on biomedical ethics are questions of tort liability (e.g., medical malpractice, product liability, invasion of privacy, damage to business relationships, and so forth), regulation of genetic technologies and products, and legal enforcement of "rights" to genetic information and services. For example, given that genotypes provide information about relatives of the patient or research subject, do third parties have a right to know this important information? Does this right gain legal vitality when the third party might be able to prevent morbidity or mortality by having the critical information? What are the ethical and legal duties of the patient and/or health provider to warn the third party (52)? Other legal issues include the applicability of antidiscrimination laws (Americans with Disabilities Act, Fair Housing Act, Individual with Disabilities Education Act), civil rights laws (Title VII of the Civil Rights Act), and common law (divorce and custody laws) to alleged genetic discrimination (53).

The commercialization of body tissue, including DNA, as a resource to be "mined or harvested," and the patenting of DNA also create legal issues

(54,55). These questions are not merely ethical and legal in nature. They frequently collide with well-developed cultural mores. For example, the recent implementation of a genetic database composed of samples from the entire Icelandic population would be an anathema to Native Americans, who strongly oppose such invasion of their genome (see Chapter 25, "Genetics, Public Health, and the Law").

Health Behavior and Health Education

There is little doubt that testing for genetic diseases can have profound psychological effects that alter health behavior (56). A striking example is the recent report based on a worldwide assessment of the frequency of "catastrophic events" (suicide, suicide attempt, or psychiatric disorder requiring hospital admission) among those receiving information, based on genetic testing, indicating an increased risk for Huntington disease (57). Two percent of this group experienced such catastrophic events within 2 years of testing, indicating that predictive testing can have serious consequences. It is clear that both the public and health professionals dealing with the public need further education regarding the role of genetics in health and disease.

Education

For many years, schools of public health have offered courses with genetic content or courses that address ethical, legal, and social issues related to genetics. These courses, however, are often independent of each other, and many students are not routinely exposed to genetic concepts and issues. The recent expansion in genetic knowledge and technology is broadly impacting the field of public health, making it necessary for more, if not all, public health students to be exposed to the fundamentals of public health genetics (2). Education in public health genetics needs to address a variety of audiences, including traditional public health graduate students, students from related disciplines, and health professionals. As in research, a multidisciplinary approach is required (see Chapter 29 for additional information).

Genetics in Public Health Training Collaboration

The need to develop more comprehensive public health genetics education programs is now recognized by the academic community. For this reason, six universities formed the Genetics in Public Health Training Collaboration, with liaisons to the Washington State Department of Health, the Centers for Disease Control and Prevention, and the Health Resources and Services Administration. The collaboration included the University of Washington, University of Michigan, University of Minnesota, University of North Carolina, University of Pittsburgh, and Johns Hopkins University.

The first task undertaken by this group was to develop a description of the scope of public health genetics education and training. The collaboration identified a broad set of competencies to reflect the scope of training, beyond the traditional areas of public health, for graduates who want to concentrate in public health genetics. These competencies are applicable to traditional graduate programs and to continuing education programs for public health professionals. The competencies identified are:

1. Apply knowledge of inheritance, including basic cellular and molecular mechanisms, to understanding a variety of rare and common health conditions;
2. Apply epidemiological and statistical approaches to the study of risk factors and diseases with a genetic component;
3. Identify interactions among genes, environmental factors, and behavior;
4. Understand how genetic principles/technologies apply to diagnosis, screening, and interventions for disease prevention and health promotion programs;
5. Incorporate genetic information into assessment, policy development, and assurance activities; and
6. Apply methods to address ethical, legal, social, and financial implications of the use of genetic principles/technologies in public health, including protecting privacy and autonomy, and preventing discrimination.

The collaboration completed its work with a survey of potential employers to more fully identify current and future needs for employees, as well as the competencies desired. The initial results support the competencies identified and establish the availability of employment opportunities.

New Academic Programs
In addition to the long-standing degree programs in Human Genetics and Genetic Counseling at the School of Public Health of the University of Pittsburgh, new programs focusing specifically on the application of the advances in human genetic and molecular biotechnology have recently been implemented at the Schools of Public Health at the University of Michigan and at the University of Washington. These programs differ from past efforts in that they deliberately link courses to develop a multidisciplinary approach to genetics in public health. Although the two programs share common goals and objectives, the approaches differ. The University of Michigan program is an Interdepartmental Concentration that is taken by students who will receive their degree (MPH, MS, or PhD) from one of the five departments of the School of Public Health. The University of Washington program currently grants an MPH degree in Public Health Genetics and a certificate with other

degree programs planned. Descriptions of the two programs are presented below.

UNIVERSITY OF MICHIGAN: PUBLIC HEALTH GENETICS INTERDEPARTMENTAL CONCENTRATION (PHGIC)

The PHGIC was developed because advances in genetics are occurring at a rapid pace, challenging academic institutions to respond to the many social, legal, ethical, and public health policy implications of this information. Twenty-four students have completed the program since 1997. Students in PHGIC obtain MPH, MS, or PhD degrees in one of the five departments while pursuing a concentration in Public Health Genetics. The PHGIC faculty is drawn from all departments in the School of Public Health and relevant departments of other schools and colleges of the university.

The curriculum consists of 13 credit hours of course work: three core courses, a seminar, and one elective. Because many students have not had biochemistry or molecular biology, the first core course was designed to accommodate students without a biology background. This course, "Introduction to Genetics in Public Health," provides the basic scientific understanding of human genetics as well as its applications, including current research and anticipated scientific advances. The objectives are to learn the language of human genetics, to engage in genetic critical thinking, and to be able to define the interface between genetics and public health.

The second core course, "Genetics in Epidemiology," relates genetics to the core public health discipline of epidemiology, emphasizing the use of genetics to help describe disease frequency and distribution and to gain insight into biological etiologies. The third core course, "Issues in Public Health Genetics," focuses on ethical, legal, and social issues and analysis arising from the increasing application of genetic technology to the health of individuals and populations. The course is designed to provide students with a background of the current molecular era, ground them in the principles of genetic screening programs, and demonstrate how various quantitative and humanistic, ethical-legal perspectives bear on policy formation. Guests from the Medical School, the Law School, Michigan State University, the Michigan Department of Community Health, and the National Institutes of Heath participate in the teaching this course. Syllabi for the three core courses are on the PHGIC website (www.sph.umich.edu/genetics/). Interestingly, all core courses have been taken as electives by students not enrolled in PHGIC, including students from other schools (e.g., Law and Medicine). This is believed to reflect the growing awareness of the importance of genetics to the field of public health.

The seminar provides an introduction to public health genetics with a focus on current applications and current controversies. It introduces students to professionals working in public health genetics. Currently, there are 23 courses in the various schools at the University of Michigan identified as electives. These courses have significant content related to public health genetics.

In addition to formal courses, internships and independent studies are directed toward areas related to public health genetics for PHGIC students. Internships are considered an important element of the PHGIC academic program. Since 1997, a total of 20 students have participated in internships with international, national, and state agencies, as well as research laboratories, to gain practical experience in the applications of genetics to public health issues and problems. For example, students analyzed insurance-related genetics issues for Michigan Blue Cross/Blue Shield; worked with the Genome Policy Project, which researches the public's values and perceptions of genetic testing and reproductive technology so that values can be translated into policies for practitioners, government policymakers, and professionals; developed a book and an accompanying interactive CD-ROM for health care providers to educate patients about cancer and genetics; discovered an *E. coli* gene that mediates its attachment to the host in women with urinary tract infections; contacted families identified through the International Fanconi Anemia Registry for family cancer history and blood samples to test carrier status; identified a candidate gene for X-linked retinoschisis and sequenced the putative coding region in affected and normal males; researched and evaluated birth defects surveillance systems; developed a study design to evaluate the efficacy of prophylactic surgery in women who carry a mutation that predisposes them to a higher risk of breast and/or ovarian cancer; evaluated the use and impact of a computer-assisted instruction module on DNA; surveyed families with a child with thalassemia to assess the impact of the disease on families in India; conducted a survey of adolescents with genetic conditions to assess services provided by state agencies; and investigated the association between parental consanguinity and deafness for the World Health Organization (WHO).

The PHGIC curriculum is evolving. The areas of ethical, legal, social, and policy issues are being expanded to meet the student demand for more exposure to these perspectives. New electives are being identified and developed. In the future, students outside the School of Public Health will have the opportunity to earn a certificate in Public Health Genetics. Strong collaboration is being developed with the Michigan Department of Community Health. Graduates of the PHGIC are currently enrolled in doctoral programs in areas related to public health genetics and in medical school. Graduates are working in health departments, in cancer centers, in medical centers, in consulting firms, and in academic departments of schools of public health. Interest in the program continues to be strong with many new School of Public Health students enrolling in PHGIC.

UNIVERSITY OF WASHINGTON: MULTIDISCIPLINARY PROGRAM FOR PUBLIC HEALTH GENETICS IN THE CONTEXT OF LAW, ETHICS, AND POLICY

The academic component of the Public Health Genetics (PHG) program at the University of Washington (web page: http://depts.washington.edu/phgen) consists of a 2-year graduate program leading to a Master of Public Health (MPH) degree in Public Health Genetics and a graduate certificate program. The program is supported by the University Initiatives Fund (UIF) at the University of Washington, and involves seven different schools and colleges: School of Public Health and Community Medicine; School of Law; School of Medicine; College of Arts and Sciences; School of Pharmacy; School of Nursing; and Daniel J. Evans School of Public Affairs. In addition, active collaborative relationships have been established with the Washington State Department of Health (DOH) and the Fred Hutchinson Cancer Research Center, both of which have been instrumental in developing the program to date.

The MPH degree track in Public Health Genetics is the only such degree program in the United States. In addition to course requirements in all the public health disciplines, and a practicum experience, the core curriculum for the PHG track consists of a series of courses intended to introduce students to each of the disciplines integral to PHG. Many of the courses are team-taught by faculty from two or three relevant departments, and the courses are jointly listed in other departments and schools as appropriate. Core Series 1 includes courses on "Genetic Epidemiology," "Legal, Ethical and Social Issues in Public Health," and "Biotechnology, Bioinformatics and Ecogenetics." Core Series 2 provides more in-depth study of the ethical, legal, and social issues, and includes courses on "Sociocultural Perspectives on Public Health Genetics," "Ethical Frameworks of Public Health Genetics," and "Genetics and the Law." Importantly, many of these courses, especially those in Core Series 2, are designed with limited prerequisites so as to be accessible to students from a variety of graduate degree programs.

An interactive seminar series takes place throughout the academic year, highlighting speakers from the numerous fields represented by the program. Because PHG students are drawn from diverse academic backgrounds, ranging from molecular biology to social science, the opportunity to exchange opinions and perspectives in the seminar setting is a defining element of the program. The PHG students can select electives from numerous departments at the University of Washington, and electives developed specifically by the PHG program to date include "Computer Applications in Genetic Epidemiology," and "Animal Models: Genetics and Human Diseases."

The graduate certificate program is designed primarily for students in other graduate degree programs. Students who take PHG Core 1 courses and the seminar series receive a certificate upon graduation and acknowledgment of this training on their transcript. To date, students from graduate programs in Environmental Health, Pharmacy, and Public Policy have earned the PHG certificate.

In addition to academic training, the PHG program is also seeking to facilitate research broadly related to public health genetics. At this writing, the two major aspects of the research program have been initiated.

First, the PHG program funds research pilot projects that are broadly related to genetics in public health. Ten proposals were submitted to the program during this first year, representing a diverse range of projects. Based on evaluations from outside reviewers and a subcommittee of the Internal Advisory Board for the program, two projects were funded: "Genetic Testing in the Workplace: Implications for Public Policy," and "Social Construction of Genetic Knowledge: Interviews with Japanese Americans and U.S. Pacific Islanders." The overall goal of the first project is to explore ethical, legal, social, and economic implications of advances in human genetics and molecular biotechnology for occupational health. The investigators will examine how this information is used in the workplace and what public policies promote the use of genetic information to appropriately balance the interests of employers, workers, and the general public. The overall goal of the second project is to increase understanding of salient cultural features relevant to conducting genetic research with diverse populations. The investigators will develop and test a tool to assess cultural variation in selected domains of meaning that may influence individual and family attitudes about participating in research. This analysis will be based on interviews with individuals from the local Japanese American community and the Pacific Islander community.

Second, the PHG program has a multifaceted, ongoing collaboration with the Center for Ecogenetics and Environmental Health (CEEH), funded as a Center of Excellence from the National Institute of Environmental Health Sciences. The focus of research in the CEEH is on understanding "gene–environment interactions" that lead to chronic diseases of public health importance. Thus, the goals of the CEEH are highly complementary to those of the PHG program. The competitive renewal grant proposal for the CEEH currently includes a new core for research into the "Ethical, Legal and Social Implications" (ELSI) of ecogenetics research. When funded, this core will develop a series of case studies, working closely with researchers from the CEEH.

Training for Public Health Professionals

Although many health-promotion and disease-prevention activities that use genetic information have been ongoing for some time (e.g., newborn screening programs), the field of human genetics continues to expand rapidly. This expansion strains the ability of the public health work force, including officials, researchers, laboratory workers, policymakers, and consumers to keep abreast of new information and its potential implications on public health practice. Therefore, systematic and ongoing education is needed to provide the varied public health audiences with the knowledge and skills necessary to use genetics information in public health programs aimed at preventing disease and improving health. The Centers for Disease Control and Prevention (CDC) offers a number of training programs (58), including short introductory and advanced training courses in genetics and disease prevention, online training materials, lectures, and newsletters. The CDC also offers 12-week internship rotations for students in schools of public health to work in different CDC programs, and 2-year applied epidemiology training in genetics (epidemic intelligence service program). Finally, the CDC offers a special 1–3-year career development opportunity for public health professionals in genetics. The program is multidisciplinary and focuses on the practical application of genetics in public health practice. Areas of concentration include genetic and molecular epidemiology; laboratory sciences; public health policy; health communication; and ethical, legal, and social issues. The emphasis of the program is on (*1*) public health assessment of the impact of genetic variation and disease prevention opportunities through environmental and behavioral modification; (*2*) evaluation of the quality and impact of genetic testing; (*3*) development, implementation, and evaluation of intervention strategies; and (*4*) communication and information dissemination activities.

In recognition of the increasing need for continuing education programs in genetics for current public health professionals, faculty of the University of Michigan, the University of Washington, and the Johns Hopkins University are also developing a multi-institution effort to plan, develop, and implement continuing education courses in public health genetics.

Summary

Research in the emerging field of public health genetics encompasses a broad range of disciplines, and will increasingly involve the interactions among investigators in these fields. The new technologies and information will accelerate scientific advances, but these will need to be evaluated in the context of the societies in which they occur. For example, Breslow has proposed that "disease prevention" should be disentangled from "health promotion," and that health should be viewed as "physical, mental and social well-being, not merely the absence of disease and infirmity" as defined by the World Health Organization (59). Breslow proposes that genetic research should include efforts to identify "genetic indicators of longer and better lives," not just markers of disease susceptibility. Such efforts will necessitate collaboration among scientists, ethicists, social scientists, and legal and policy experts in order to be successful.

Finally, education in public health genetics must also be multidisciplinary and interactive. Students being trained to be the future public health professionals need to understand the role of genetic information in public health and how it relates to their own discipline. Further, the education of public health professionals must be ongoing, so that the potential of genetic technology and information can be appropriately used to benefit the health of all. One of the biggest challenges for society and for public health professionals will be to develop policies and procedures that maximize health benefits derived from genetic advances while ensuring that genetic information is not misused.

Acknowledgments

The authors thank Patricia Kuszler, MD, JD, and Scott Ramsey, MD, PhD, for their assistance in the preparation of this chapter. Portions of this work were derived from a manuscript entitled "Education in Public Health Genetics," prepared for the Josiah Macy Jr. Foundation Conference, "The Implications of Genetics of Health Professional Education," October 1998. This work was performed during Dr. Austin's tenure as an Established Investigator of the American Heart Association. The authors would like to thank Kay Collins for her assistance in preparation of the manuscript.

References

1. Collins FS, Patrinos A, Jordon E, Chakravarti A, Gesteland R, Walters L. New goals for the U.S. Human Genome Project: 1998–2003. Science 1998;282:682–689.

2. Omenn GS. Genetics and public health. Am J Public Health 1996;86:1701–1704.

3. Khoury MJ, and the Genetics Working Group. From gene to public health: the application of genetic technology in disease prevention. Am J Public Health 1996;86:1717–1722.

4. ten Kate L. Editorial. Community Genet 1998;1:1–2.

5. Metzger N, Zare RN. Interdisciplinary research: from belief to reality. Science 1999;283:642–643.

6. Ellsworth DL, Hallman DM, Boerwinkle E. Impact of the Human Genome Project on epidemiologic research. Epidemiol Rev 1997;19:3–13.

7. Khoury MJ, Beaty TH, Cohen BH. Fundamentals of genetic epidemiology. New York: Oxford University Press, 1993.

8. Hanis CL, Boerwinkle E, Chakraborty R, et al. A genome-wide search for human non–insulin-dependent (type 2) diabetes genes reveals a major susceptibility locus on chromosome 2. Nat Genet 1996;13:161–166.

9. Cox NJ, Frigge M, Nicolae DL, et al. Loci on chromosomes 2 (NIDDM1) and 15 interact to increase susceptibility to diabetes in Mexican Americans. Nat Genet 1999;21:213–215.

10. Austin MA, King MC, Vranizan KM, Krauss RM. Atherogenic lipoprotein phenotype: a proposed genetic marker for coronary heart disease risk. Circulation 1990;82:495–506.

11. Austin MA, Talmud PJ, Luong LA, et al. Candidate-gene studies of the atherogenic lipoprotein phenotype: a sib–pair linkage analysis of DZ women twins. Am J Hum Genet 1998;62:406–419.

12. Foxman B, Zhang L, Tallman P, et al. Transmission of uropathogens between sex partners. J Infect Dis 1997;175:989–992.

13. Khoury MJ, Risch N, Kelsey JL. Genetic epidemiology. Epidemiol Rev 1997;19:1–181.

14. Schulte PA, Perera P. Molecular epidemology: principles and practices. San Diego: Academic Press, 1993.

15. Khoury MJ. Human Genome Epidemiology (HuGE): translating advances in human genetics into population-based data for medicine and public health. Genet Med 1999;1:71–74.

16. Khoury MJ, Dorman JS. The Human Genome Epidemiology Network (HuGE Net). Am J Epidemiol 1998;148:1–3.

17. Carrington M, Nelson GW, Martin MP, et al. HLA and HIV-1: heterozygote advantage and B*35–Cw*04 disadvantage. Science 1999;283:1748–1752.

18. Jenks PJ. Microbial genome sequencing-beyond the double helix. BMJ 1998;317:1568–1571.

19. Haines JL, Pericak-Vance MA. Approaches to gene mapping in complex human diseases. New York: Wiley-Liss, 1998.

20. Ott J. Analysis of human genetic linkage. Baltimore: The Johns Hopkins University Press, 1999.

21. Hauser ER, Boehnke M. Genetic linkage analysis of complex genetic traits by using affected sibling pairs. Biometrics 1998;54:1238–1246.

22. Boehnke M, Langfeld CD. Genetic association mapping based on discordant sib pairs: the discordant-alleles test. Am J Hum Genet 1998;62:950–961.

23. Goldin LR, Bailey-Wilson JE, Borecki IB, et al. Genetic analysis workshop 10. Genet Epidemiol 1996;14:549–1142.

24. Kardia SLR, Nelson MR, Ferrell RE, Sing CF. New approaches for identifying multilocus genotypes influencing levels of quantitative risk factors. Am J Hum Genet 1997;61:1167.

25. Nickerson DA, Taylor SL, Weiss KM, et al. DNA sequence diversity in a 9.7-kb region of the human lipoprotein lipase gene. Nat Genet 1998;19:233–240.

26. Gelbart WM. Databases in genomic research. Science 1998;282:659–661.

27. Carmelli D, Swan GE, Robinette D, Fabstiz R. Genetic influence on smoking—a study of male twins. N Engl J Med 1992;327:829–833.

28. Edwards KL, Austin MA, Jarvik GP. Evidence for genetic influences on smoking in adult women twins. Clin Genet 1995;47:236–244.

29. Pianezza ML, Sellers EM, Tyndale RF. Nicotine metabolism defect reduces smoking. Nature 1998;393:750.

30. London SJ, Idle JR, Daly AK, Coetzee GA. Genetic variation of CYP2A6, smoking, and risk of cancer. Lancet 1999;353:898–899.

31. Ridker PM, Miletich JP, Hennekens CH, Buring JE. Ethnic distribution of factor V Leiden in 4047 men and women: implications for venous thromboembolism screening. JAMA 1997;277:1305–1307.

32. Vandenbroucke JP, Koster T, Briet E, et al. Increased risk of venous thrombosis in oral-contraceptive users who are carriers of factor V Leiden mutation. Lancet 1994;344:1453–1457.

33. Middeldorp S, Henkens CM, Koopman MM, et al. The incidence of venous thromboembolism in family members of patients with factor V Leiden mutation and venous thrombosis. Ann Intern Med 1998;128:15–20.

34. McColl MD, Ramsay JE, Tait RC, et al. Risk factors for pregnancy-associated venous thromboembolism. Thromb Haemost 1997;78:1183–1188.

35. Vandenbroucke JP, van der Meer FJ, Helmerhorst FM, Rosendaal FR. Factor V Leiden: should we screen oral contraceptive users and pregnant women? BMJ 1996;313:1127–1130.

36. Drewnoski A, Rock C. The influence of genetic taste markers on food acceptance. Am J Clin Nutr 1995;62:506–511.

37. Lerman C, Hughes C, Trock BJ, et al. Genetic testing in families with hereditary nonpolyposis colon cancer. JAMA 1999;281:1618–1622.

38. Ramsey SD. Economic implications of genetic screening for cancer susceptibility: the case of hereditary nonpolyposis colorectal cancer. First Annual Conference on Genetics and Public Health, Atlanta, GA, 1998.

39. Burke W, Thomson E, Khoury MJ, et al. Hereditary hemochromatosis: gene discovery and its implications for population-based screening. JAMA 1998;280:172–178.

40. McConnell LM, Koenig BA, Greely HT, Raffin TA, and the Working Group of the Stanford Program in Genomics, Ethics, and Society. Genetic testing and Alzheimer disease: has the time come? Nat Med 1998;4:757–759.

41. Andrews LB, Fullarton JE, Holtzman NA, Motulsky AG. Assessing genetic risks: implications for health and social policy. Washington, DC: National Academy Press, 1994.

42. Fitzpatrick JL, Hahn C, Costa T, Huggins MJ. The duty to recontact: attitudes of genetics service providers. Am J Hum Genet 1999;64:852–860.

43. Juengst ET. Groups as gatekeepers to genomic research: conceptually confusing, morally hazardous, and practically useless. Kennedy Inst Ethics J 1998;8:183–200.

44. Foster MW, Sharp RR, Freeman WL, Chino M, Bernsten D, Carter TH. The role of community review in evaluating risk of human genetic variation in research. Am J Hum Genet 1999;64:1719–1727.

45. National Commission for the Protection of Human Subjects of Biomedical and Behavior Research. The Belmont Report. Washington, DC: GPO, 8pp., 1979.

46. Reilly PR, Page DC. We're off to see the genome. Nat Genet 1998;20:15–17.

47. Clayton EW, Steinberg KK, Khoury MJ, et al. Informed consent for genetic research on stored tissue samples. JAMA 1995;274:1786–1792.

48. Greely HT. Genomics research and human subjects. Science 1998;282:625.

49. Botkin JR, McMahon WM, Smith KR, Nash JE. Privacy and confidentiality in the publication of pedigrees: a survey of investigators and biomedical journals. JAMA 1998;279:1808–1812.

50. Specter M. Decoding Iceland. The New Yorker, January 18, 1999, pp. 40–51.

51. Ziman J. Why must scientists become more ethically sensitive than they used to be? Science 1998;282:1813–1814.

52. Safer v. Estate of Pack. (291 N.J. Super. 619), 1996.

53. Miller PS. Genetic discrimination in the workplace. J Law Med Ethics 1998;26:189–197.

54. Nelkin D, Andrews L. Homo economicus: commercialization of body tissue in the age of biotechnology. Hastings Cent Rep September–October 1998:30–39.

55. Hanson MJ. Religious voices in biotechnology: the case of gene patenting. Hastings Cent Rep 1997;November–December:1–21.

56. Koenig BA, Greely HT, McConnell LM, Silverberg AB, Raffin TA, and members of the Breast Cancer Working Group of the Stanford Program in Genomics, Ethics,

and Society. Genetic testing for BRCA1 and BRCA2: recommendations of the Stanford Program in Genomics, Ethics, and Society. J Womens Health 1998;7:531–545.

57. Almqvist EW, Bloch M, Brinkman R, Craufurd D, Hayden MR, on behalf of an international Huntingon disease collaborative group. A worldwide assessment of the frequency of suicide, suicide attempts, or psychiatric hospitalization after predictive testing for Huntington disease. Am J Hum Genet 1999;63:1293–1304.

58. Office of Genetics and Disease Prevention Home Page. http://www.cdc.gov/genetics.

59. Breslow L. From disease prevention to health promotion. JAMA 1999;281:1030–1033.

II
PUBLIC HEALTH
ASSESSMENT

6

Epidemiology, molecular biology, and public health

Janice S. Dorman and Donald R. Mattison

Progress with the Human Genome Project has led, and will continue to lead, to the identification of genes known to contribute to the occurrence of human disease. This knowledge is changing the practice of medicine and public health through the development of molecular diagnostics, targeted interventions for susceptible individuals, and gene therapy. It is also having an enormous impact on society as we address the ethical, legal, and social issues that are becoming apparent as these important discoveries are introduced into practice. Thus, there is an urgent need for the accurate translation of this new genetic information from the laboratory to the community. Molecular epidemiology is at the foundation of this important link, and represents the scientific basis of public health for the 21st century.

Molecular epidemiology has been defined as "a science that focuses on the contribution of potential genetic and environmental risk factors, identified at the molecular and biochemical level, to the etiology, distribution and prevention of disease within families and across populations" (1). Molecular epidemiology creates an interface among epidemiology, basic science, medicine, and statistics, and is, therefore, a collaborative discipline, as is true for many areas of public health. While this collaboration represents the major strength of molecular epidemiology, it also poses its primary challenge. Epidemiologists, biomedical scientists, health professionals, and biostatisticians have different backgrounds, training, experience, and goals. Indeed, they have discipline-specific scientific views and speak different languages. These differences tend to inhibit collaboration. However, with sufficient attention to the development of a common vocabulary and perspective, successful partnerships can be achieved among individuals committed to molecular epidemiology (2,3). Consider the evolution of epidemiology over the past two decades.

During the 1970s and 1980s, rapid advances in computer technology completely revolutionized approaches for database management. Although these developments were initially applied to defense, business, and industry, their usefulness in public health was quickly realized. Keypunch machines using paper cards to contain both the computer program and the data for analyses were replaced with monitors, magnetic storage devices, and computer software that separates the procedures involved in data entry and storage from those utilized for statistical analyses. These advances in computer hardware and software facilitated data collection and processing for large epidemiological studies. At the same time, the availability of computer technology led to the evolution of new statistical methods that were applicable to the more complex analytical issues encountered in epidemiologic research. Initially, these programs were not available on statistical software packages. They were obtained by direct collaboration with the individuals who developed the programs. Thus, partnerships among epidemiologists, statisticians, and computer scientists began to emerge.

Initially, these collaborations were awkward because the individuals involved had a limited understanding of their colleagues' area of research. A "transition period" was required, during which time epidemiologists expanded their knowledge of biostatistics and computer programming, and statisticians and computer scientists became more familiar with the basic tenets of epidemiology and public health. By sharing information, the partners involved established a common knowledge base, which led to an appreciation of the contribution of each respective discipline to the ultimate goals of the partnership. This knowledge-sharing also generated a change in focus for graduate-level training programs in epidemiology and biostatistics. Epidemiology departments began to emphasize biostatistics, data analyses, and study methodology in their curricula. Similarly, many graduate programs in biostatistics accentuated applications to epidemiology and public health. With expanded educational opportunities that stressed the importance of both fields of research, the epidemiologists and biostatisticians of the next generation were better able to collaborate.

At the present time, another revolution in epidemiology is occurring because of recent advances in genetics, molecular biology, and biotechnology (4–6). These developments have facilitated the discovery of new biomarkers of susceptibility, exposure, and effect, which are now being evaluated as part of molecular epidemiological research (7). The magnitude of the potential impact of biomarkers in science and health was well-described by the 1987 report of the Committee on Biological Markers of the National Research Council. In particular, the report noted the dynamic nature of the various types of biomarkers, and stressed their interrelationships on a continuum from health to disease (Fig. 6.1). Thus, rather than studying surrogates to assess risk factor and disease outcomes, precise measures of potential etiologic determi-

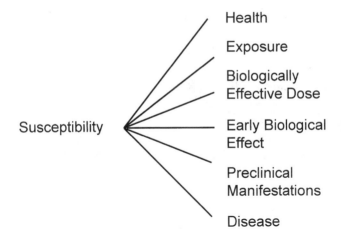

Figure 6.1 Biological markers along the continuum from health to disease.

nants and phenotypes became available for epidemiologic research. However, the report also emphasized the importance of maintaining a global perspective of disease etiology, despite the need to focus on specific types of biomarkers.

Advances in molecular biology and biotechnology have also provided inexpensive and rapid laboratory methods that are required to conduct large population-based studies. As a result, collaborative epidemiological networks have expanded in recent years, and they now include human geneticists and other biomedical scientists. One current challenge for molecular epidemiology is, therefore, to actively sustain these new partnerships. To ensure their development and continuation, collaborators with diverse backgrounds, training, and experience must first acquire a common understanding of the objectives, methods, nomenclature, and results of their colleagues' areas of expertise. New opportunities for training in human genetics and molecular biology for epidemiologists and health practitioners (and in epidemiology and public health for basic scientists and human geneticists) are required to provide the necessary framework for the development of molecular epidemiology.

A second major challenge for molecular epidemiology reflects the need to foster stronger community links among epidemiologists, health practitioners, policymakers, and members of the general population (1,4). An ongoing dialogue across these different groups is essential if all members of society are also to have access to the information necessary to make appropriate decisions regarding genetic testing. This dialogue will initially include formal and informal opportunities for health professionals, policymakers, administrators, industry representatives, and members of the general public to understand the basic concepts of human genetics, molecular biology, and the Human Genome

Project. This will provide a framework for an appreciation of the implications of current research, which will become increasingly important as molecular approaches for predicting and preventing diseases are developed and implemented into practice.

To meet the demands of the 21st century, we must change the language and expertise of public health to include a stronger focus on molecular epidemiology and its applications for disease prevention. In addition, we need to actively promote continuing education in human genetics, epidemiology, and public health for scientists, practitioners, educators, and individuals in the private sector. It is the authors' opinion that leadership from graduate schools of public health is required to meet these challenges. Strategies for addressing this timely issue are discussed in this chapter.

Molecular Epidemiology and Public Health

Although epidemiology has been defined as "the basic science and most fundamental practice of public health and preventive medicine" (8), it has generally not been viewed with such importance by the medical profession or the general public. Indeed, many misconceptions abound concerning the nature of epidemiology, as well as its role in disease prevention. One reason for this confusion is that the discipline focuses on populations rather than individuals. The former is typically not of major concern to health practitioners or members of the general population. An exception is, perhaps, during outbreaks or epidemics, when the need for epidemiologic research to stop the transmission of infectious agents in a community has generally been well-recognized.

We are now experiencing "epidemics" of noncommunicable diseases in populations from both developing and developed countries, yet interest in the epidemiology of these important public health problems has not kept pace with our focus on the molecular aspects of disease. The impression held by many health professionals is that the distribution and risk factors for the major chronic disorders have been well-established, and thus do not require further investigation. Population-based epidemiology is no longer considered a research priority. This perspective is reflected by the recent decline in the resources available for such investigations. Many individuals believe that people will be healthier and live longer in the 21st century because of rapid advances in biotechnology, not epidemiology. Biotechnology will, no doubt, have an enormous influence on our health and well-being in the near future. However, these new developments are unlikely to reduce the risk of disease for an individual or in a population without continuing contributions from molecular epidemiology. Consider the following example.

Breast cancer is one of the leading causes of morbidity and mortality among women in the United States, and incidence rates are increasing worldwide (9,10). The cumulative lifetime risk for Caucasian women in North America and Europe has been estimated at approximately 10%. Population-based epidemiologic research has revealed that age at menarche, diet, reproductive history, and a positive family history of breast cancer are among the major risk factors for the disease. Accurate epidemiologic data regarding the magnitude of these associations were of great importance during the recent controversy concerning mammography and breast cancer screening for the general population (11). Thus, one significant contribution of epidemiology is to provide population-based information for the development of practice guidelines and public health policy for noncommunicable diseases, such as breast cancer.

There has also been enormous interest in the genetics of breast cancer during the past decade. Recent advances from the Human Genome Project led to the identification of several susceptibility genes, including BRCA1 on chromosome 17q21, which is linked to early-onset breast and ovarian cancer (12). Ever since this initial discovery, more than 200 distinct BRCA1 mutations have been identified, none of which appear to be very common (13–15). Therefore, a mutation segregating in one family with early-onset breast cancer is likely to be different from that found in another affected family. Despite the genetic heterogeneity of BRCA1, unaffected relatives who carry the same mutation as do family members with breast cancer appear to be at very high risk for developing the disease (i.e., ≈80%) (16,17).

These statistics received considerable attention in both the literature and the press, and obviously caused great concern among women with a positive family history for breast cancer. However, the estimates quoted were generated from linkage studies, which require large extended families with many affected individuals. The families selected for such analyses were chosen specifically because of their unusually high prevalence of breast and/or ovarian cancer. By definition, they were not representative of most families with early-onset breast cancer. As a result, risk estimates from these cohorts were not applicable to the general population. However, this point is often not recognized by practitioners or the general public.

Only recently have population-based molecular epidemiologic data for BRCA1 and breast cancer become available (18–22) These data are based on studies of women with breast cancer who were not selected on the basis of a family history of the disease, and are, therefore, more representative of the general population. However, the heterogeneous nature of BRCA1 has complicated the technical aspects of genetic screening, and current molecular tests are still limited because of the possibility of false negatives. Despite these difficulties, recent molecular epidemiologic studies of BRCA1 have revealed that a very small proportion of women with early-onset breast cancer from the general population carry known BRCA1 mutations (i.e., ≈3%). Most women with the disease are negative for BRCA1 mutations. Obviously, the implications of these results are considerably different from the findings from the linkage studies. Still, positive test results must be interpreted cautiously because the disease penetrance for BRCA1 has not yet been accurately established. In addition, genetic counseling for BRCA1 carriers is currently limited to risk-factor modification, which is difficult because many of the potential disease determinants relate to reproductive history (e.g., age at menarche, parity). Dietary intervention may also be an option, particularly if molecular epidemiologic studies reveal that gene–environment interactions are significant. More invasive procedures such as hormone therapy and prophylactic mastectomy have also recently been considered.

As a result, the American Society for Human Genetics (ASHG) has discouraged the use of genetic testing for BRCA1 (23). The rationale for this decision was based on the low prevalence of BRCA1 carriers in the general population, and the potential inaccuracies of current molecular tests. Despite the limited usefulness of genetic screening for BRCA1, the health service industry has not followed the recommendation of the ASHG because the potential profits are great. Thus, BRCA1 testing is now available for any woman in the United States who wishes to be tested.

The breast cancer story illustrates the critical need for population-based molecular epidemiologic research to obtain accurate risk estimates for genetic carriers. In addition, the translation of these data to practitioners, health administrators, industry representatives, educators, and members of the general public is essential. This must be an active, not passive, process. After research projects have been conducted, molecular epidemiologists must not only emphasize the importance of population-based data but also promote their use for decision making from an individual, clinical, and public health perspective. This information should be made readily available and carefully interpreted by the above-mentioned groups before genetic screening tests are introduced or utilized, disease interventions are established, or public health policy is developed. Considerable progress has already been made in the area of type 1 diabetes.

Molecular Epidemiology of Type 1 Diabetes

Type 1 diabetes is one of the most common chronic diseases of childhood, with prevalence rates for Caucasians in the United States approximating 2 cases per 1000 population. Moreover, incidence rates appear to be increasing worldwide (24). Significant temporal trends have recently been reported in the United States, Europe, and Asia, the reasons for which are not known. Although it has been established that type 1 diabetes is an autoimmune disease, the etiology of the disorder remains unclear. Following disease onset, individuals with type 1 diabetes often experience acute complications, such as hypoglycemia, ketoaci-dosis, and cerebral edema; and after a decade with the disease, their risk of developing long-term diabetes complications becomes significant (25). These conditions contribute to the high rates of morbidity, mortality, and disability that are commonly observed in type 1 diabetes populations.

Because of the seriousness of type 1 diabetes, the World Health Organi-zation (WHO) recently supported the Multinational Project for Child-hood Diabetes (also known as the WHO DiaMond Project), which is based on the establishment of standardized incidence registries for type 1 diabetes in more than 70 countries worldwide (26). This project began in 1990 and has attracted considerable attention to the epidemiology of the disease. Indeed, the WHO DiaMond Project is the largest known international collaborative study of a noncommunicable disease. Analyses of the vast amount of data generated by this project revealed dramatic geographic differences in the incidence of type 1 diabetes (27,28). Rates are extremely high in Finland, Sardinia, and the Scandinavian countries (>20 cases per 100,000 population per year), but extraordinarily low in Asian and Native American populations (<3 cases per 100,000 population per year). Although the reasons for the worldwide patterns of type 1 diabetes have not been established, the avail-ability of standardized incidence registries facilitated the development of a collaborative population-based study of the molecular epidemiology of type 1 diabetes (29).

Associations between genes in the HLA region of chromosome 6 and type 1 diabetes began to be documented in the mid 1970s, when it was observed that individuals with type 1 diabetes were significantly more likely to be posi-tive for HLA-B8 and -B15 than were individuals without diabetes. With rapid changes in HLA serologic methods and the discovery of class II molecules, stronger associations between the antigens at the DR locus and type 1 dia-betes became apparent (30). Both HLA-DR3 and -DR4, which are in linkage disequilibrium with B8 and B15, respectively, were found in approximately 95% of individuals with type 1 diabetes. Furthermore, those individuals who were heterozygous for DR3 and DR4 were confirmed to be at higher risk for developing the disease than either DR3 or DR4 homozygotes.

With the development of molecular technology, immunogenetic studies from a variety of populations revealed that of the various DQB1 alleles (which code for the HLA-DQβ chain), those that contain DNA sequences for an amino acid other than aspartic acid in the 57th position of the molecule (non-Asp-57; ND) were highly associated with disease susceptibility (31,32). In some populations, relative risk estimates greater than 100 were reported. These relationships were even more striking among individuals who also carried DQA1 alleles (which code for the HLA-DQ chain) containing DNA sequences for arginine in position 52 (non-Arg-52; R) (33). The HLA-DQ and -DR loci are tightly linked, with linkage disequilibrium between the DQA1*R and DQB1*ND alleles, and both DR3 and DR4. Thus, the contributions of HLA-DQ to type 1 diabetes appear to reflect, in part, those documented for DR.

The identification of the extraordinary associations between diabetes and the HLA-DQ alleles, as well as the availability of reliable, valid, and inexpensive molecular tests, and the documentation of worldwide patterns of type 1 diabetes incidence from standardized registries provided the rationale for the WHO DiaMond Molecular Epidemiology Project (34). This multinational study, which began in 1994, was designed to test the hypothesis that the geographic differences in type 1 diabetes risk reflect population variation in the frequencies of DQA1*R-DQB1*ND haplotypes. In areas of high incidence, one would expect a large proportion of the general population to carry HLA-DQ susceptibility alleles. In contrast, areas where the disease is quite rare would likely have few genetically susceptible individuals.

Prior to initiating this project, epidemiologists and immunogeneticists had numerous discussions about the methods required to test this hypothesis. However, epidemiologists had considerable difficulty explaining to their colleagues the importance of a large sample size and the need to develop standard inclusion/exclusion criteria for selecting cases and controls. At the same time, immunogeneticists found it hard to convince epidemiologists that their large studies would place a burden on research laboratories in terms of staff time and available equipment. Thus, considerable effort was required to develop a common understanding of the basic principles and methods of these diverse scientific fields. Epidemiologists learned about the laboratory methods required for HLA molecular typing and also observed the intricacies of processing biological specimens in a small research laboratory. Similarly, immunogeneticists acquired an appreciation for the precise eligibility criteria needed to reduce selection bias in case-control studies, as well as an understanding of the importance of population-based molecular epidemiology data for public health. This "transition" occurred during a period of approximately a year, and was necessary before active collaboration could begin.

After the study design and methods were established, it was necessary to develop standards and quality-control procedures for this large international study. Epidemiologic standards were required for both the selection of cases and controls and for procedures for data collection. Standards for processing and transferring biological specimens to the coordinating center laboratory were also established. Additional discussions focused on issues such as data sharing, analyses, and publication. Finally, a "Method of Operations Manual" for the WHO DiaMond Molecular Epidemiology Project was developed and distributed to all collaborators at a NATO Advanced Research Workshop entitled "Standardization of Epidemiological Studies of Host Susceptibility." The workshop was held in 1994 at the WHO Coordinating Center for Diabetes

Registries and Training, Graduate School of Public Health at the University of Pittsburgh (34).

At present, more than 20 WHO DiaMond Participating Centers from around the globe have contributed to this collaborative effort to study the molecular epidemiology of type 1 diabetes worldwide. All type 1 diabetes cases included in the study were (*1*) diagnosed by a physician as diabetic, (*2*) placed on daily insulin injections before the case's 15th birthday, and (*3*) confirmed as a resident in the area of registration at the time of the first insulin administration. Nondiabetic controls, older than 15 years of age, were identified from the area defined by the registry and group-matched for age, race, and sex. Target sample sizes were based on 100 type 1 diabetic cases and 100 nondiabetic controls for each racial group in the participating registries.

Table 6.1 presents some of the initial results from nine populations representing areas with high, moderate, and low type 1 diabetes incidence rates (35). These data revealed that relative to individuals who carried zero DQA1*R-DQB1*ND haplotypes, those homozygous for DQA1*R-DQB1*ND had a significantly higher risk of developing type 1 diabetes risks in all countries except Japan (Table 6.1). In general, the magnitude of these associations was greater in the moderate-high than in the low-incidence populations. Individuals heterozygous for DQA1*R-DQB1*ND haplotypes were at a moderately increased risk for developing the disease.

Because the descriptive epidemiology of type 1 diabetes was established by each local Participating Center, it was possible to estimate genotype-specific incidence rates for HLA-DQA1*R-DQB1*ND homozygotes, for heterozygotes, and for individuals with no high-risk haplotypes. One of the major advantages of population-based case-control studies, such as those conducted

Table 6.1 Type 1 Diabetes: Estimated Relative and Cumulative Incidence Rates Through Age 40 Years for Individuals with Two Susceptible (S) Haplotypes

Population	Relative Risk for SS	Cumulative Risk (%) for SS
Moderate–High Incidence		
Helsinki, Finland	32.7*	7.1
Allegheny County, PA—Whites	15.4*	2.5
Jefferson County, AL—Whites	14.0*	3.2
Allegheny County, PA—Blacks	>201*	16.5
Jefferson County, AL—Blacks	15.6*	1.7
Auckland, New Zealand	47.1*	2.6
Low Incidence		
Hokkaido, Japan	15.6	0.3
Mexico City, Mexico	50.9*	1.1
Tiajin, China	>79.3*	0.5

*$p < 0.05$.
S = DQA1*R-DQB1*ND.

for the WHO DiaMond Project, is that genotype-specific incidence rates can be determined for an area, where the overall incidence has been established by a registry. Genotype-specific incidence rates can be determined by expressing the overall incidence rate (R) established from the registry as an average of the genotype-specific rates (R_i). The genotype-specific rates are weighted by the proportion of the general population who carry genetically susceptible haplotypes (P_i). Thus, $R = R_2P_2 + R_1P_1 + R_0P_0$, where P_2, P_1, and P_0 are the proportions of the general population who carry two, one, and zero DQA1*R-DQB1*ND haplotypes, respectively. Similarly, R_2, R_1, and R_0 represent the absolute risks of developing type 1 diabetes for individuals in the general population with two, one, and zero DQA1*R and DQB1*ND haplotypes, respectively. The genotype-specific rates R_2, R_1, and R_0 can be determined by using the relative risk estimates established from the case-control analyses to represent the ratios of these rates (i.e., R_2/R_0 and R_1/R_0).

The genotype-specific incidence rates for individuals with two DQA1*R-DQB1*ND haplotypes from the WHO DiaMond Molecular Epidemiology Project are illustrated in Table 6.1. In some of the moderate-high incidence areas, these risk estimates were markedly increased and approximated those typically observed for first-degree relatives of type 1 diabetics (3%–6% through age 35 years) (35). Similar results were apparent in the low-incidence areas. However, the magnitude of these risk estimates was lower than that seen in the moderate-high incidence areas.

Our original hypothesis was that the population distribution of these high-risk haplotypes was responsible for the observed geographic differences in type 1 diabetes incidence. If true, one would expect the genotype-specific rates to be similar across populations, and the variation in the overall incidence rates attributable to differences in the prevalence of susceptible individuals. Although this pattern was apparent for the North American and European populations, it was not observed for those in Asia or Latin America. Thus, data from the WHO DiaMond Molecular Epidemiology Project suggest that other genetic and environmental factors must also be important determinants of the worldwide variation in incidence.

The WHO DiaMond Molecular Epidemiology Project illustrates the need for population-based data for testing hypotheses in molecular epidemiology research. However, it also emphasizes the importance of these estimates for developing primary and secondary prevention strategies. At the present time, it is not possible to stop the onset of type 1 diabetes once beta-cell destruction has occurred, except with the continuous use of immunosuppressives, an intervention that obviously is not appropriate for young children. However, there are currently three major clinical trials focusing on more acceptable, less dangerous, and less effective intervention strategies (36). One of these trials is based on first-degree relatives at high genetic risk. The "Cow's Milk Avoidance Trial" tests the hypothesis that avoidance of cow's milk protein for at least the first 6 months of life will reduce the incidence of type 1 diabetes

(37). Previous epidemiological studies have shown that children exposed to cow's milk protein early in life are more likely to develop type 1 diabetes than those who were exclusively breast-fed. Because of gene–environmental interactions, early cow's milk exposure may be particularly problematic for those at high genetic risk (38). Thus, this trial screens eligible newborns at birth using molecular HLA typing. Those with susceptible genotypes are then randomized to receive either a standard cow's milk baby formula or one containing a nonantigenic protein hydrolyzate at weaning. Infants with moderate or low-risk haplotypes are not eligible for the trial.

In addition, several ongoing prospective population-based studies of the natural history of autoimmunity utilize genetic screening (39–41). For these investigations, newborns are tested at birth for susceptible HLA-DQ haplotypes. Those who are at high genetic risk are eligible for follow-up. The endpoints of interest in the prevention trials and natural history studies include the presence of high titres of islet cell antibodies (i.e., biomarkers of effect), as well as the development of type 1 diabetes.

However, a major concern of limiting prospective studies and clinical trials to susceptible newborns is that children at high genetic risk represent only a fraction of those who eventually develop the disease. Data from the WHO DiaMond Molecular Epidemiology Project revealed that only half of the type 1 diabetics in most areas carry two susceptible haplotypes. Moreover these cases are more likely to be female, to have a young age at diagnosis, and to have a positive family history of type 1 diabetes, compared to those cases with one or zero DQA1*R-DQB1*ND haplotypes. Therefore, the exclusion of moderate and low-risk infants seriously limits the generalizability of data generated from these expensive and labor-intensive clinical trials. It also provides a false assumption that children at moderate or low genetic risk will not develop type 1 diabetes. This impression could have important clinical implications, as parents of these children may be less likely to detect early symptoms, assuming their child is unlikely to develop type 1 diabetes. However, after more extensive beta cell damage has occurred, children are at much greater risk for the serious acute complications of type 1 diabetes, such as ketoacidosis, coma, and death at diabetes onset than are those who are diagnosed early. Thus, genetic screening for the general population, even in high-incidence countries, is unlikely to be a reasonable approach for the primary prevention of type 1 diabetes.

Collaboration Among Basic Scientists and Public Health Professionals

Collaboration among biomedical scientists, clinicians, and public health professionals is required for the evolution of molecular epidemiology. These new partnerships can be facilitated by expanding the availability of training opportunities in human genetics and molecular epidemiology. From the epidemiological perspective, the relevant question is: "How much training in human genetics and molecular biology is necessary to become involved with molecular epidemiology research?" The appropriate response to this inquiry will obviously be personal in nature, depending on the individual's academic interests, position, and responsibilities. However, epidemiology faculty at many institutions in the United States are now receiving requests for training in molecular epidemiology from established epidemiologists, physicians, and other public health professionals who want to update their knowledge of human genetics and molecular biology. Because of the recent interest in molecular epidemiology, workshops were held at the 1998 annual meetings of the Society for Epidemiologic Research (SER) and the American College of Epidemiology (ACE). Attendance was standing-room only at the SER workshops. Thus, these programs will be repeated in 1999 with an expanded format.

Students are also extremely excited by the field. Formal training programs will prepare students and junior-level faculty for exciting new career opportunities in molecular epidemiology. Informal opportunities made available as part of annual professional meetings may be more appropriate for senior-level faculty and other health professionals. Thus, a variety of symposia, workshops, courses, and training programs in molecular epidemiology are now being developed to meet these diverse continuing educational needs. Many such programs are available at graduate schools of public health. These institutions have typically been responsible for training individuals from a variety of backgrounds in disciplines related to the science and practice of public health. They are natural leaders for facilitating training in molecular epidemiology.

As a result of these efforts, basic concepts in human genetics and molecular biology are now being integrated into the core curricula of many epidemiology departments at graduate schools of public health. Terms such as *chromosomes, DNA, genes, loci, alleles, polymorphisms, mutations*, and others that comprise the nomenclature for human genetics and molecular biology are also becoming part of the working vocabulary of epidemiology. The processes of cell division (i.e., mitosis vs. meiosis), transcription, translation, and modes of inheritance, which represent the foundation of human genetics and molecular biology, also have both practical and theoretical implications for molecular epidemiology. Epidemiologists need a clear understanding of the nature of restriction enzymes, cloning, and genomic and cDNA libraries. Other procedures, such as hybridization, Southern and Northern blots, DNA sequencing, and the polymerase chain reaction (PCR), should also be taught. The performance of biomarkers of susceptibility, exposure, and effect in terms of reproducibility, validity, sensitivity and specificity are relevant issues; and the distinction between analytical validity (i.e., the ability of the molecular test to detect the biomarker) and clinical validity (i.e., the ability of the marker to predict disease) should also be emphasized. Approaches for defining "host susceptibility" in molecular epidemiology research require considerable discussion. This topic may be particularly problematic in studies of chronic disease where associations with relevant polymorphisms are seldom absolute.

Biomedical scientists and human geneticists must also acquire an understanding of epidemiology and public health. Training should include discussions of the basics of descriptive and analytical epidemiology, the history of molecular epidemiology, and distinctions between genetic and molecular epidemiology. In addition, the role of molecular epidemiologic research for translating information from the Human Genome Project for medical and public health applications must be the subject of considerable discussion, with an emphasis on population-based research and the importance of considering potential problems such as bias, validity, reproducibility, and generalizability in designing molecular epidemiology studies. Estimating and interpreting genotype-specific morbidity rates from prospective and retrospective investigations should also be described. Finally, ethical, legal, and social issues regarding the use of genetic screening tests in a research study or as part of a public health intervention are important aspects of epidemiology and public health.

Molecular Epidemiology and Public Health Policy

Molecular epidemiology collaborations will provide the foundation for the development of public health policy in the 21st century. An excellent example of how this process is likely to be achieved relates to current discussions regarding population-based screening for hereditary hemochromatosis (HH), which affects iron metabolism, and is the most prevalent autosomal recessive disorder known. Approximately 1 in 200 individuals is homozygous, and 1 in 8 may be genetic carriers (42–47). Individuals with this disease have abnormally high levels of iron absorption, resulting in iron stores exceeding 50 g. Symptoms generally develop after 20 g of iron have accumulated; the condition often occurs during middle age in men and after menopause in women (48,49).

The diagnosis of HH depends upon documenting excessive iron storage. By measuring serum iron and iron-binding capacity, researchers can determine whether the saturation of serum transferrin has been persistently elevated. Levels that exceed 60% among men or 50% among women are diagnostic of HH. Excessive iron deposits affect many organ systems and lead to serious and irreversible complications, such as cirrhosis of the liver, cardiomyopathy, diabetes, polyarthropathy, abnormal pigmentation, hypogonadism, and premature death. Environmental risk factors (i.e., iron and alcohol intake) appear to affect the development of these conditions (50). Many individuals are not diagnosed with HH until they present with complications (51–53). Both a lack of public awareness and misperceptions regarding the rarity of the disease have contributed to the large number of undiagnosed and untreated individuals in many communities.

Early detection could be facilitated if health care providers and the general population were educated about the descriptive epidemiology of the disease. Preventing the complications of HH is simple, low-risk, inexpensive, and extremely effective; it involves repeated therapeutic phlebotomy to remove excess iron and adherence to a diet low in iron. These treatments have dramatically increased the life spans of people with HH, allowing them to survive into their adult years.

The gene for HH has recently been identified. It is linked to the HLA region of chromosome 6, approximately 4 megabases telomeric to HLA-A (54–57). The gene has been assigned the name HFE, and codes for a 343 amino acid protein that is similar in structure to HLA class I antigens. The most prevalent point mutation results in the substitution of tyrosine for cysteine (C282Y). Approximately 80% of affected individuals are homozygous for this mutation. However, another variant has also been identified (H63D). This mutation causes the replacement of histidine with aspartic acid, and occurs with a much lower frequency among affected individuals (i.e., <10%). It has also been observed in the general population. Thus, the contribution of the H63D mutation to the occurrence of HH is unclear. Molecular screening tests are now available for these variants, which are found in approximately 10% in European Caucasian populations. The test appears to be rapid, simple, reproducible, and inexpensive, and could easily be utilized for large-scale population screening.

In 1996, the Centers for Disease Control (CDC) began to develop national guidelines and programs to detect, prevent, and treat iron-overload diseases, such as HH. Because affordable and reliable genetic screening tests are now available, it is possible to prevent the serious complications of HH before they occur by identifying and treating individuals with the relevant HFE mutations at an early age. These individuals would benefit from prophylactic phlebotomy and nutritional counseling to reduce their levels of dietary iron. After much deliberation, a Consensus Statement was recently published, concluding that population-based genetic screening for HH was not appropriate at the present time owing to uncertainties about the prevalence and penetrance of HFE mutations (58). Because of these voids in the literature, the CDC has assigned high priority to population-based HH research.

Molecular epidemiological studies will be required to determine the true incidence of HH, as well as the frequency of mutant alleles among affected and unaffected individuals. Such studies will provide the data necessary to establish accurate risk estimates associated with the presence of these (and possibly other) mutations. In addition, factors that characterize the phenotypic expression of HH, including the age at onset, must be determined. The accept-ability of molecular screening tests to the population, as well as the potential risks in terms of confidentiality, genetic anxiety, and so forth, must be assessed. Finally, cost-effectiveness and efficiency in reducing the burden of the disease should be evaluated. Of particular interest is the cost-efficiency of screening for HH using genetic tests compared to the cost of using transferrin satura-tion testing, which is currently the standard used to detect HH. Results of these molecular epidemiology studies will then be made available to policymakers to aid in making decisions about population genetic screening.

Molecular Epidemiology and the General Public

In 1994, the Committee on Assessing Genetic Risks published a comprehen-sive report outlining the ethical, legal, and social implications of the develop-ment and use of genetic tests. Its major findings noted "both a need and the opportunity to increase public literacy about genetics and genetic testing" (59). The committee advocated that formal genetic education, which should begin in elementary school and continue through college, be considered a national priority. The rationale for this recommendation was that a population literate in genetics would be able to respond appropriately to the introduction of new genetic technologies in our society, and would have a better appreciation of human genetic variation and its personal and social implications. Genetics will affect our society in health care delivery, in the workplace, in insurance appli-cations, and in the ways we think about the issue of privacy. These matters are already becoming more prominent in the media and are receiving greater scrutiny by the government. Knowledge of the genetics and environmental determinants of disease risk is, therefore, important to consumers and practi-tioners; and this is essential for developing prevention strategies and estab-lishing appropriate public health policy.

The importance of educating the public about genetics was echoed through-out the Centers for Disease Control's strategic plan "Translating Advances in Human Genetics into Public Health Action," which was adopted in 1997 (60). Recently, an Ad Hoc Task Force recommended a conceptual framework for the plan that included three critical issues: (*1*) partnerships and coordination; (*2*) ethical, legal, and social issues; and (*3*) education and training. Thus, the CDC is emphasizing the importance of molecular epidemiology for translat-ing genetic information for medicine and public health. This emphasis is clearly reflected by the recent developments at the CDC's Office of Genetics and Disease Prevention, including the establishment of the Human Genome Epidemiology (HuGE) Network (61).

The mission of the HuGE Net is to: (*1*) establish an information exchange network that promotes global collaboration in the development and dissemination of epidemiologic data on human genes; (*2*) develop a knowl-edge base on the World Wide Web (www.cdc.gov/genetics); and (*3*) promote the use of this knowledge base by health care providers, researchers, industry, government, and the public for decision making involving the use of genetic tests and services. The HuGE Net represents the collaboration of individuals, organizations, and academic institutions committed to the development and worldwide dissemination of population-based molecular epidemiology infor-mation on the human genome.

Active formal partnerships between graduate schools of public health and the CDC, such as those created through the HuGE Net, will facilitate the development and implementation of approaches for education in genetics and public health. Schools of public health can contribute by assessing the atti-tudes toward and awareness of genetic testing and environmental risk factors for chronic diseases among different sectors of the population, including groups of practitioners, educators, and the general public. Such opinions are likely to vary by occupation, geography, ethnic group, religion, and gender, and to require careful consideration. Involving members of the community in the initial development of these assessments could ensure that newly developed formal and informal training programs will reflect the needs, ethnic diversity, level of education, socioeconomic background, and religious orientation of the target population.

Approaches to achieving a genetically literate public could also incorporate some of the opportunities for genetic education that have recently become available on the Internet. Since the Committee on Assessing Genetic Risk originally convened, the Ethical, Legal, and Social Issues (ELSI) program of the Human Genome Project has been actively developing on-line genetic edu-cation programs for different subgroups of the population. These educational opportunities could also emphasize the potential environmental determin-ants of noncommunicable disease because they are generally modifiable. Interventions on smoking, nutrition, and physical activity for genetically sus-ceptible individuals, for example, may be even more effective in reducing mor-bidity and mortality than prevention programs targeted for the general population as a whole.

Finally, for these approaches to be successful, greater cooperation among basic scientists, epidemiologists, health professionals, biostatisticians, and members of the general community will be required. Leadership in public health in the 21st century will be central to achieving these goals.

References

1. Dorman JS. Molecular epidemiology and DNA technology transfer: a program for developing countries. In: Dorman JS (ed). Standardization of epidemiologic studies of host susceptibility. New York: Plenum Press, 1994, pp. 241–251.

2. Dorman JS, Siulc ES. Postgraduate programs in molecular epidemiology. Gac Med Mex 1997;133:83–86.

3. Ambrosone CB, Kadlubar FF. Toward an integrated approach to molecular epidemiology. Am J Epidemiol 1997;146:912–918.

4. Khoury, MJ. Genetic epidemiology and the future of disease prevention and public health. Epidemiol Rev 1997;19:1–2.

5. Schulte PA. A conceptual and historical framework for molecular epidemiology. In: Schulte PA, Perera FP (eds). Molecular epidemiology principles and practices. San Diego: Academic Press, 1993, pp. 3–44.

6. Hulka BS. Overview of biological markers. In: Hulka BS, Wilcosky TC, Griffith JD (eds). Biological markers in epidemiology, New York: Oxford University Press, 1990, pp. 3–15.

7. Biological markers in reproductive toxicology. Washington, DC: National Research Council, National Academy Press, 1989, pp. 15–35.

8. Tyler CW, Last JM. Epidemiology. In: Wallace RB, Doebbeling BW, Last JM (eds). Public health and preventive medicine. Stamford, Connecticut: Appleton & Lange, 1998, p. 5.

9. Kuller, LH. The etiology of breast cancer: from epidemiology to prevention. Public Health Rev 1995;23:157–213.

10. Kelsey, JL, Horn-Ross PL. Breast cancer: magnitude of the problem and descriptive epidemiology. Epidemiol Rev 1993;15:7–16.

11. National Institutes of Health Consensus Statement. Breast cancer screening for women age 40–49. January 21–23, 1997. Bethesda, MD: National Cancer Institute, 1997.

12. Hall JM, Lee MK, Newman B, et al. Linkage of early-onset familial breast cancer to chromosome 17q21. Science 1990;250:1684–1689.

13. Xu CF, Chambers JA, Nicolai H, et al. Mutations and alternative splicing of the BRCA1 gene in UK breast/ovarian cancer families. Genes Chromosomes Cancer 1997;18:102–110.

14. Stoppa-Lyonnet D, Laurent Puig P, Essioux L, et al., and the Institut Curie Breast Cancer Group. BRCA1 sequence variations in 160 individuals referred to a breast/ovarian family cancer clinic. Am J Hum Genet 1997;60:1021–1030.

15. Shattuck-Eidens D, Oliphant A, McCllure M, et al. BRCA1 sequence analysis in women at high risk for susceptibility mutations; risk factor analysis and implications for genetic testing. JAMA 1997;278:1242–1250.

16. Szabo CI, King MC. Population genetics of BRCA1 and BRCA2. Am J Hum Genet 1997;60:1013–1020.

17. Ithier G, Girard M, Stoppa-Lyonnet D. Breast Cancer and BRCA1 mutations. N Engl J Med 1996;334:1198–1199.

18. Fitzgerald MG, MacDonald DJ, Krainer M, et al. Breast cancer and BRCA1 mutations in Jewish and non-Jewish women with early-onset breast cancer. N Engl J Med 1996;334:143–149.

19. Couch FJ, DeShano ML, Blackwood MA, et al. BRCA1 mutations in women attending clinics that evaluate the risk of breast cancer. N Engl J Med 1997;336:1409–1415.

20. Krainer M, Silva-Arrieeta S, Fitzgerald MG, et al. Differential Contributions of BRCA1 and BRCA2 to early onset breast cancer. N Engl J Med 1997;336:1416–1421.

21. Newman B, Mu H, Butler LM, et al. Frequency of breast cancer attributable to BRCA1 in a population-based series of American women. JAMA 1998;279:922–929.

22. Malone KE, Daling JR, Thompson JD, et al. BRCA1 mutations and breast cancer in the general population: analyses in women before age 35 years and in women before age 45 years with first-degree family history. JAMA 1998;279:922–929.

23. Statement of the American Society for Human Genetics on Genetic Testing for Breast and Ovarian Cancer Predisposition. Am J Hum Genet 1994;55:i–iv.

24. LaPorte RE, Matsushima M, Chang YF. Prevalence and incidence of insulin-dependent diabetes. In: National Diabetes Data Group. Diabetes in America (2nd ed). Bethesda, MD: National Institutes of Health, National Institute of Diabetes and Digestive and Kidney Diseases, 1995 (NIH Publication No. 95–1468), pp. 37–46.

25. Orchard TJ, Dorman JS, Maser RE, et al. Prevalence of complications in IDDM by sex and duration. Pittsburgh Epidemiology of Diabetes Complications Study II. Diabetes 1990;39:1116–1124.

26. WHO DiaMond Project Group. WHO Multinational Project for Childhood Diabetes. Diabetes Care 1990;13:1062–1068.

27. Karvonen M, Tuomilehto J, Libman I, et al. A review of the recent epidemiological data on the worldwide incidence of type 1 (insulin-dependent) diabetes mellitus. World Health Organization DiaMond Group. Diabetologia 1993;36:883–892.

28. Green A, Gale EAM, Patterson CC. Incidence of childhood-onset insulin-dependent diabetes mellitus: the EURODIAB ACE study. Lancet 1992;339:905–909.

29. Dorman JS, LaPorte RE, Stone RA, et al. Worldwide differences in the incidence of type 1 diabetes are associated with amino acid variation at position 57 of the HLA-DQ β chain. Proc Natl Acad Sci U S A 1990;87:7370–7374.

30. Bertram J, Baur M. Insulin-dependent diabetes mellitus. In: Albert AD, Baur MP, Mayr WR (eds). Histocompatibility testing. Heidelberg: Springer-Verlag, 1984, pp. 348–368.

31. Todd JA, Bell JL, McDevitt HO. HLA-DQ beta gene contributes to susceptibility and resistance to insulin-dependent diabetes mellitus. Nature 1987;329:559–604.

32. Morel PA, Dorman JS, Todd JA, et al. Aspartic acid at position 57 of the HLA-DQ beta chain protects against type 1 diabetes. Proc Natl Acad Sci U S A 1989; 85:8111–8115.

33. Khalil I, Deschamps I, Lepage V, et al. Dose effect of cis- and trans-encoded HLA-DQαβ heterodimers in IDDM susceptibility. Diabetes 1992;41:378–384.

34. Dorman JS, Kocova M, O'Leary LA, et al. Case-control molecular epidemiology studies: standards for the WHO DiaMond Project. In: Dorman JS (ed). Standardization of epidemiological studies of host susceptibility. New York: Plenum Press, 1994, pp. 89–99.

35. Dorman JS, McCarthy B, McCanlies E, et al. Molecular IDDM epidemiology: international studies. Diabetes Res Clin Pract 1996;34(Suppl):S107–116.

36. Schatz DA, Rogers DG, Brouhard BH. Prevention of insulin-dependent diabetes: an overview of three trials. Clev Clin Med 1996;63:270–274.

37. Akerblom HK, Savilahti E, Saukkonen TT, et al. The case for elimination of cow's milk in early infancy in the prevention of type I diabetes: the Finnish experience. Diabetes Metab Rev 1993;9:269–278.

38. Kostraba JN, Cruickshanks KJ, Lawler-Heavner J, et al. Early exposure to cow's milk and solid foods in infancy, genetic predisposition, and risk of IDDM. Diabetes 1993;42:288–295.

39. Rewers M, Bugawan TL, Norris JM, et al. Newborn screening for HLA markers associated with IDDM: Diabetes Autoimmunity Study in the Young (DAISY). Diabetologia 1996;39:807–812.

40. Rønningen, K. S. Genetics in the prediction of insulin-dependent diabetes mellitus: From theory to practice. Ann Med 1997;29:387–392.

41. Roll U, Christie MR, Füchtenbusch M, et al. Perinatal autoimmunity in offspring of diabetic parents. Diabetes 1996;45:967–973.

42. Barton JC, Bertoli LF. Hemochromatosis: the genetic disorder of the twenty-first century. Nat Med 1996;4:394–395.

43. Centers for Disease Control and Prevention. At-a-glance hereditary hemochromatosis—1997. http://www.cdc.gov/genetics/publish/hemoch.htm.

44. Edwards CQ, Griffen LM, Goldgar D, et al. Prevalence of hemochromatosis among 11,065 presumably healthy blood donors. N Engl J Med 1988;318:1355–1362.

45. Hallberg L, Björn-Rasmussen E, Jungner I. Prevalence of hereditary haemochromatosis in two Swedish urban areas. J Intern Med 1989;225:249–255.

46. McLaren CE, Gordeuk VR, Looker AC, et al. Prevalence of heterozygotes for hemochromatosis in the white population of the United States. Blood 1995;86: 2021–2027.

47. Wiggers P, Dalhøj J, Kiær H. Screening for haemochromatosis: prevalence among Danish blood donors. J Intern Med 1991;230:265–270.

48. Witte DL, Crosby WH, Edwards CQ, et al. Hereditary hemochromatosis. Clin Chim Acta 1995;245:139–200.

49. Bothwell TH, Charlton RW, Motulsky AG. Hemochromatosis. In: Scriver CR, Beaudet AL, Sly WS, Valle D (eds). The metabolic basis of inherited disease (Vol. 11). New York: McGraw Hill, 1995, pp. 2237–2269.

50. LeSage GD, Baldus WP, Fairbanks VF et al. Hemochromatosis: genetic or alcohol-induced? Gastroenterology 1983;84:1471–1477.

51. Milman N. Iron status markers in hereditary haemochromatosis: distinction between individuals being homozygous and heterozygous for the haemochromatosis allele. Eur J Haematol 1991;47:292–298.

52. Powell LW, Summers KM, Board PG, et al. Expression of hemochromatosis in homozygous subjects. Gastroenterology 1990;98:1625–1632.

53. Niederau C, Fischer R, Pürschel A, et al. Long-term survival in patients with hereditary hemochromatosis. Gastroenterology 1996;110:1107–1119.

54. Feder JN, Gnirke A, Thomas W, et al. A novel MHC class I-like gene is mutated in patients with hereditary haemochromatosis. Nat Genet 1996;13:399–408.

55. Mercier B, Mura C, Ferec C. Putting a hold on 'HLA-H'. Nat Genet 1997; 15:234.

56. Borot N, Roth M-P, Malfroy L, et al. Mutations in the MHC class I-like candidate gene for hemochromatosis in French patients. Immunogenetics 1997;45:320–324.

57. Carella M, D'Ambrosio L, Totaro A, et al. Mutation analysis of the HLA-H gene in Italian hemochromatosis patients. Am J Hum Genet 1997;60:828–832.

58. Burke W, Thomson E, Khoury MJ, et al. Hereditary hemochromatosis: gene discovery and its implications for population-based screening. JAMA 1998;280:172–178.

59. Committee on Assessing Genetic risks. Assessing genetic risks: implications for health and social policy. Washington, DC: National Academy Press, 1994, pp. 185–201.

60. Center for Disease Control and Prevention. Translating advances in human genetics into public health action: a strategic plan. Atlanta, GA: Task Force on Genetion and Disease Prevention 1997.

61. Khoury MJ, Dorman JS. The Human Genome Epidemiology Network. Am J Epidemiol 1998;148:1–5.

7

Surveillance for birth defects and genetic diseases

Lorenzo D. Botto and Pierpaolo Mastroiacovo

About one in 20 live-born infants is expected to have a single-gene disorder or a condition with an important genetic component by age 25 years (1,2), about 1 in 33 will have a major birth defect (3,4), and a similar proportion will have a significant developmental disability (5). These infants will account for a disproportionate fraction of premature deaths (6,7), pediatric hospitalizations (8–11), and health care costs (12,13). Many of these conditions or their complications can be reduced by timely and effective primary prevention practices, and public health surveillance has the potential to contribute significantly to this goal.

Birth defects surveillance was born in part as a public health response to an international tragedy, the thalidomide epidemic of the late 1950s and early 1960s. Thalidomide, an antinausea drug then widely prescribed during pregnancy, caused thousands of infants to be affected by severe birth defects between 1958 and 1962 (14). Within a few years, monitoring programs for birth defects were created in Europe (e.g., in Norway, Sweden, and Hungary between 1964 and 1967), the Americas (e.g., in Atlanta, Georgia, 1968; in Latin America [ECLAMC], 1968), and elsewhere in the world (15). Since then, public health surveillance for birth defects, while maintaining its original mandate to provide an early warning system for birth defect epidemics, has expanded its scope to include other public health functions such as assessing disease impact on morbidity and mortality, identifying causes, and evaluating policies. At the same time, because of the diverse and changing social, political, and economic environment, birth-defects surveillance has continued to face new challenges, such as the increasing impact of prenatal diagnosis and pregnancy termination, and the changes in the way health care is managed in many countries.

The role of genetics in public health dates back to the same years that witnessed the initial growth of birth-defects surveillance. The public health mandate of such surveillance was driven, at least initially, by the development in 1962 of an easy and inexpensive test to identify infants at risk for phenylketonuria (the "Guthrie" assay). This test provided the health care community with a way to prevent the sequelae of a metabolic disorder through newborn screening. Newborn screening was expanded over the years to more conditions, and its success provided a powerful example of effective integration of genetics into public health practice. Newborn screening also exemplifies a major objective of such integration, namely preventing the disease phenotype by identifying those at risk for the disease and providing them with prevention opportunities (16).

Although very different at the surface, public health genetic programs and birth-defects surveillance share common ground. They often serve similar populations (e.g., stillborn infants, newborns, children), use similar data sources (e.g., birthing hospitals, pediatric wards, cytogenetic laboratories, vital statistics offices), enlist the contribution of similar groups of medical and public health professionals (e.g., geneticists, pediatricians, perinatal and pediatric epidemiologists), and face similar though not identical legal and social issues (e.g., the sharing of confidential and private data, and the risk for discrimination and stigmatization). At the same time, however, each activity confronts specific challenges. Birth-defects surveillance must confront the increasing impact of prenatal diagnosis and pregnancy termination. Public health genetic programs must navigate the complexities of genetic testing, as new tests move from the research laboratory to the clinical world, and they must be particularly sensitive to the ongoing debate on the ethical, social, and legal issues associated specifically with the use and potential misuse of genetic information.

In this chapter we describe some surveillance issues that will likely be increasingly relevant as birth-defects surveillance moves into the future, and that provide instructive similarities and contrasts with the emerging field of genetic disease surveillance. A more general discussion of birth-defects surveillance can be found elsewhere (17–20). Moreover, in our comments on genetic-disease surveillance we shall place a major, though not exclusive, emphasis on high-penetrance, single-gene conditions that usually manifest in the pediatric age group.

Public Health Surveillance and Birth Defects

Public health surveillance has been described as the collection, analysis, and dissemination of outcome-specific data to describe and monitor health events, with the explicit provision that these activities be ongoing, systematic, and timely, and, most importantly, that they be linked to public health practices such as intervention and prevention programs (21,22). In birth-defects surveillance, data can be used to study the prevalence of birth defects, their morbidity, disability, and associated mortality, and their distribution (e.g., geographic and ethnic variation) and evolution in a population. Surveillance must also be timely, ongoing, and linked to public health practice if surveillance data are to help meet public health needs. Such needs include, for example, detecting epidemics, defining and monitoring problems, generating hypotheses, stimulating research, evaluating measures of disease control and prevention, detecting changes in health practices, and facilitating planning.

Uses of Birth-Defect Surveillance

Monitoring prevalence and trends has been traditionally a major focus of birth-defect surveillance. The data gathered through surveillance can also be used to evaluate the significance of apparent birth-defect clusters. For example, following a report of a suspected cluster of limb deficiencies in a coastal area of the United Kingdom, surveillance systems in other countries were able to quickly show that no such cluster had occurred at other coastal sites (23–25), thus providing cost-effective and timely reassurance to the general public and public health professionals.

Surveillance data can also be used to independently verify trends reported by other programs or to suggest potential etiologic studies. For instance, a long-term increase of hypospadias was reported by two monitoring systems in the United States (26). The cause of this increase is still unknown, but it parallels similar increases reported in Europe and Japan in the last decades and which leveled off in the mid-1980s (27). Such trends are of particular interest in light of the current debate on potential endocrine effects of environmental pollutants (28–30). Although the study of trends alone is not sufficient to establish a cause–effect relationship, such studies may provide suggestive evidence, serve as a starting point for etiologic studies, and, if a causal relationship is established, monitor the global impact of the exposure.

Similarly, international differences in the prevalence of neural-tube defects and in their time trends (31,32), integrated with population data on genetic variation (e.g., the frequency of polymorphisms of folate-related genes) and dietary intake (e.g., micronutrient consumption) may provide insight on the role of gene–environment interactions in the etiology of neural-tube defects.

In addition to evaluating the occurrence of birth defects, surveillance systems can be used to assess and monitor the impact of birth defects on mortality, morbidity, and disability (7,11). The addition of geographic information can identify areas where prevention efforts should be intensified. For example, in one study of children with Down syndrome, mortality correlated more strongly with the region of residence than with the occurrence of low birth weight or a heart defect, suggesting that variations in health care practices may account for some of the preventable mortality associated with the syndrome (33).

Birth-defect surveillance systems, when integrated into disease registries, offer a convenient mechanism for enrolling patients in etiologic studies. For example, the Atlanta birth defect case-control study, which was conducted by the Centers for Disease Control and Prevention in the early 1980s and which formed the basis of many etiologic studies (34), was based on an existing population-based monitoring program. The discovery of valproic acid as a cause of spina bifida in humans further underscores the usefulness of monitoring programs in etiologic research. Following the first report of an excess of valproic acid exposures among mothers of infants with spina bifida (35,36), an international study of birth-defect registries quickly confirmed the association (37). In an analogous sequence, the report of a cluster of limb anomalies among a small clinical case-series of infants whose mothers had undergone chorionic villus sampling at one clinic (38) was soon followed by case-control studies based on birth-defects monitoring systems that confirmed the association (39,40). Later studies further added to the evidence (41).

Data from surveillance systems can be used for methodologic studies. For example, surveillance data were used to evaluate the ability of birth-defects monitoring systems to identify new teratogens under different circumstances of exposure frequency, teratogen potency, and etiologic heterogeneity (18). These methods were then applied to known teratogens such as thalidomide (42) and retinoic acid (43). The findings underscored the strengths and limitations of surveillance under realistic scenarios, highlighting, for example, how classification and coding can influence significantly a system's ability to detect birth-defect epidemics.

Data for Surveillance: Approaches and Challenges
Data for birth-defect surveillance can be collected from many different sources, including some that were not developed originally for surveillance. In many countries, the main data sources are birth-defect registries, vital records, and administrative data systems, sometimes supplemented by provider surveys, sentinel networks, and other information systems. Data collection itself occurs through a variety of channels and under different sets of regulations.

In some instances, data collection is mandated by statute or regulation, and the information is reported to public health authorities. In other cases, surveillance is promoted and coordinated by academic or research institutions, often on a voluntary basis. Different systems may coexist in the same country or region. In England and Wales, for example, the monitoring system coordinated by the governmental Office of National Statistics, which is based on notifications from physicians or midwives, coexists with other, smaller registries (e.g., the North Thames registry) that use additional sources of ascertainment (44).

Population-Based and Hospital-Based Systems: Beyond the Labels. Population size, population coverage, and data quality influence considerably the overall usefulness of a surveillance system. Much has been made of the importance of population coverage, and traditionally population-based systems have been contrasted with hospital-based systems. In birth-defect surveillance, population-based systems record data on all births to mothers who reside within a defined area, regardless of where the birth takes place. Hospital-based systems record data on births occurring in certain hospitals, regardless of where the mother lives. In an ideal region where all births occur in hospitals, where all hospitals are part of the system, and where people do not move, such distinctions are meaningless. Most hospital-based systems, however, include only a fraction of the hospitals that serve the resident population. The birth population that is monitored is therefore relatively undefined, making hospital-based systems prone to unrecognized bias. For example, a system that includes few tertiary-care hospitals may record an inflated occurrence of birth defects if such hospitals attract high-risk pregnancies.

Population-based registries, ideally, cover a well-defined population; however, they also have limitations. In particular, they require vast resources to cover a population completely, and, even so, the goal of complete coverage of resident births may not be achieved in practice. Cost usually ensures that current population-based registries are small, unless sustained by a national mandate as in some Scandinavian countries and the United Kingdom.

Because of resource constraints, the size of the population that is monitored within a country is often limited. In practice, a choice has to be made: whether to cover a relatively undefined sample of the population throughout the country using a hospital-based system, or to cover completely a defined population from a smaller geographic area, using a population-based system.

Data quality may vary in both hospital-based and population-based systems. Diagnostic detail, timeliness, and length of follow-up are not necessarily better in population-based than in hospital-based systems. Hospital-based systems can and often do provide high-quality data, as hospitals are often self-selected on the basis of the interest and commitment of staff and management. In either setting, data quality can be improved by using multiple sources of ascertainment and employing registry staff for active case-ascertainment and quality control.

On a more fundamental level, the traditional distinctions between hospital-based and population-based systems must be reevaluated in light of the impact of pregnancy termination on birth-defect prevalence. In this setting, population-based systems should monitor pregnancy terminations in addition to stillbirths and live births, and these data should be collected on all resident women, regardless of where the pregnancy termination takes place. Under these more stringent criteria, few, if any birth defect surveillance systems are truly population-based. The practical challenge for current birth defects surveillance systems, regardless of their label, is to incorporate data on pregnancy terminations, and to do so ethically and lawfully.

Expanding and Integrating Data Sources for Surveillance

Data sources other than disease registries are commonly used to collect information on birth defects, and their strengths and limitations have been discussed in detail elsewhere (20). Morbidity surveys, for example, can provide data on a disease's natural history, its burden in the population, and the distribution of a disease's risk factors. In the United States, the National Hospital Discharge Survey (45) provides data on short-stay hospitalization for specific conditions; Medicare and Medicare claims data (46) provide morbidity estimates among specific segments of the population (the poor and the elderly); and the National Health and Nutritional Examination Survey (NHANES) (47), an assessment of a nationally representative sample of people conducted through interviews, physical measurements, and biologic samples, provides information on the distribution of common conditions and exposures. Hospital discharge data are available in many countries and have been used, for instance, to assess the contribution of birth defects to pediatric hospitalization (11). These information systems can be particularly powerful when unique identifiers allow investigators to reconstruct the morbidity experience of a well-defined cohort of people with specific birth defects or genetic diseases.

Mortality data are almost universally available from vital statistics records and provide population-based information on survival and cause-specific mortality (7). Limitations of these data include their reliance on coding systems that are not optimized for birth defects and genetic diseases (e.g., International Classification of Diseases [ICD] codes), the often long delay between death and availability of the data, and limited information on risk factors.

Provider surveys are a potential source of data with which to track prevention and screening practices. These surveys are particularly useful if they are conducted on a representative sample and on an ongoing or recurrent basis. One example of such provider surveys is the National Ambulatory Health Care Survey (48), an ongoing nationwide assessment based on a probability sample of ambulatory visits in the United States.

Multiple data sets or linked identifiers have been used in surveillance of birth defects, particularly in Scandinavian countries. For example, data from the National birth defects registry and Cardiology centers in Sweden were linked to study the prevalence of congenital heart defects in Sweden (49), and linked identifiers have allowed researchers in Norway to explore transgenerational risks for congenital anomalies (50). However, the use of multiple linked data sets is still rare in birth-defect surveillance. Although such practice must resolve fundamental issues of confidentiality and privacy, it would represent an efficient use of the limited resources available for birth defect surveillance.

Special Considerations in Birth-Defect Surveillance

Surveillance of birth defects poses specific challenges that stem from the nature of the outcomes under study. These include pregnancy termination, data confidentiality and privacy, targeting of specific populations at increased risk for specific birth defects, and birth defect classification and coding.

Prenatal diagnosis of birth defects and genetic diseases represents a potential opportunity for early treatment, as exemplified by in utero surgery or early postnatal treatment of conditions such as spina bifida or diaphragmatic hernia. However, pregnancy termination of affected pregnancies seriously challenges many functions of birth-defect surveillance, as many such pregnancy terminations occur in settings such as clinics or outpatient surgeries that currently are not incorporated in most surveillance systems. Missing such cases may have profound consequences: birth defect epidemics may be overlooked, the impact of birth defects may be underestimated, and the effectiveness of primary prevention practices may become more difficult to assess. For example, selective pregnancy termination has already changed the birth prevalence of anencephaly and spina bifida in many countries (51), and may complicate the assessment of the effectiveness of National folic acid campaigns (52). With the increasing availability of ultrasonography, it not unreasonable to expect that other birth defects will be similarly influenced by selective pregnancy terminations. For example, in some areas such an impact is already being seen for severe heart defects such as hypoplastic left heart and pulmonary atresia (53–55). However, incorporating data on pregnancy terminations into many current birth-defect surveillance systems may not be easy, particularly in those countries where these procedures take place in many specialty clinics and physicians' offices rather than in a few major hospitals. In addition, issues of confidentiality and privacy are likely to play a major role in determining whether these data are shared with the surveillance system. These considerations are compounded in countries where pregnancy termination is not legal.

The debate on privacy and confidentiality also affects in general the collection, use, and linkage of birth-defect data that include individually identifiable information. The ethical, social, and legal ramifications are complex for both individuals and society. An innovative approach (see Chapter 27 of this volume) has framed the debate in terms of social risk, defined as the danger that an individual will be economically or socially penalized should he or she become identified with a disfavored medical condition (56). Such social risk involves both the threat of risk (attitudes that threaten social harm) and the perception of risk (as it exists among those with the condition), and both play a role in the acceptance of a monitoring system (see Chapter 27). In practice, the complex determination of social risk, whether real or perceived, ensures that adequate protection will have to involve not only legal measures (e.g., laws against discrimination) but also societal changes aimed at reducing or reversing socially harmful behavior and a systematic move to improve health care access and coverage.

It has long been recognized that particular subgroups of the population may be at higher risk for birth defects and single-gene disorders than the general population. Some of these at-risk groups may be defined by socioeconomic level or ethnicity; spina bifida, for example occurs more frequently in some low-income groups and in some Hispanic populations (31,32,57,58). Thus, surveillance and prevention efforts that target these populations might be particularly effective in reducing the burden of birth defects. Such efforts, however, may prove challenging. Poorer people, for example, may be less likely to obtain health care and thus be identified by the surveillance system, particularly in the absence of universal health coverage. In addition, if they are also part of a linguistic minority, they may be overlooked in mainstream surveys that do not accommodate linguistic diversity.

Once affected infants are identified and information is collected, the surveillance system is faced with the complexities of coding and classification. Ideally, codes must be specific and unique, to ensure a one-to-one correspondence between the essential features of a child with birth defects and the codes. The coding scheme should also reflect a developmentally meaningful classification to maximize the etiologic and pathogenetic homogeneity of the case-groups. Such a coding system should also be widely used to facilitate data sharing and collaborative studies. No current system, however, has all three attributes of unique and specific codes, mechanistic classification, and universal use. Although most monitoring programs and registries use the World Health Organization's International Classification of Diseases (ICD), there are many variations. Because ICD codes encompass many human diseases, they are not sufficiently detailed for many rare conditions and specialized purposes, including birth-defect surveillance. For example, omphalocele and gastroschisis are currently assigned the same code, although these two abdominal wall defects have different epidemiologic features, etiologic factors, and probably pathogenesis. Relatively few syndromes have a specific code, and even well-known disorders such as Beckwith-Wiedemann syndrome are assigned a generic code (759.89, "other specified anomalies"). Finally, many anomalies that are often termed "minor" but whose presence is often of diagnostic importance in many teratogen-induced conditions cannot be easily coded with ICD codes, as exemplified by the nail and digital anomalies seen in the fetal hydantoin syndrome (59,60).

To overcome some of these limitations, some organizations, including the British Paediatric Organization (BPA), the U.S. Centers for Disease Control and Prevention (CDC), and EUROCAT, have developed extensions of the ICD codes for birth defects. A few programs and international organizations use "homemade" coding systems in preference to ICD, usually for specific activities such as surveillance of multiple congenital anomalies (19).

Some limitations of current coding could be overcome by minor revisions. Others, however, reflect more fundamental problems of classification rather than coding, and are due to the incomplete and evolving knowledge of normal and abnormal development. The challenge to birth-defect classification and coding is devising and disseminating a system that is sufficiently detailed to capture the basic differences among the outcomes that it monitors yet flexible enough to incorporate new findings.

Using Surveillance Data Effectively
The public health value of surveillance depends in large part on how the information generated from the data is disseminated. The goal is to generate information that is timely, easily accessible, and readily understandable.

Timeliness is central to a surveillance system's ability to promote disease control and prevention. Timeliness is a relative concept, and it may be useful to distinguish among data that are needed immediately, recurrently (e.g., once a year), or only on a long-term basis (22). Data that are needed immediately, or as close to "real time" as possible, might include public health emergencies: the occurrence of birth defects due to known teratogens (e.g., rubella or thalidomide) or to otherwise preventable conditions (e.g., maternal phenylketonuria), or birth defects clusters. In such cases, prompt intervention may improve the outcome of affected infants, identify other people at risk, suggest potential teratogens, and detect failures of prevention (e.g., why a pregnancy occurred during treatment with thalidomide, or what factors contributed to the failure of the phenylalanine-free diet). This level of timeliness requires accepting provisional data and the possibility of false alarms.

Conversely, some information may need to be evaluated and distributed not as quickly. For example, final figures on occurrence rates, on the contribution of birth defects to infant mortality and hospitalization rates, or the results of folic acid consumption surveys might be disseminated annually or semiannually. Typically, such data would be used in planning and evaluating health policies and practices. Finally, accumulated and revised data should be appropriately stored for long-term analysis of trends and for research.

Ease of access to data from birth defects surveillance is also an important consideration. Access is often limited because surveillance data are rarely published in well-known medical journals, with some exceptions (61). Surveillance data are often published, if at all, as annual reports with limited circulation. Access is sometimes facilitated by joint publication (62), though limited distribution often remains a problem. However, the Internet is changing the situation drastically, because of its ability to reduce the time and cost of producing, distributing, and accessing reports, and to link information from multiple sites. Already surveillance reports are available on the Internet (see, for example, www.icbd.org), and this trend is likely to continue.

Surveillance data should also be readily understandable. Unused or misinterpreted data are useless at best, and can be misleading. Identifying and understanding the target population, defining the data and their sources, using common data format to allow comparisons with other sources, and providing informative summary figures are considerations relevant not only to traditional surveillance data but also to nontraditional data generated by the evolving public health genetic programs. For example, like the prevalence of a birth defect can be monitored, so can the risks and benefits of genetic testing. Such data on genetic testing is currently difficult to find and to understand. Both the medical community and the public would benefit from having such data coherently summarized in an ongoing, systematic fashion. These data can be usefully presented by various sources using a common format, for example in terms of the analytic validity, clinical validity, and clinical utility of each genetic test (63). Thus, practical information would be provided, and the lack of data for specific parameters and genetic tests would be highlighted. In the process, the quality of the sources must be evaluated, and the final data provided in manners that are appropriate to the different target populations, such as the community of health care providers or the general public.

Current Challenges Of Birth Defects Surveillance: The Case Of Spina Bifida

Spina bifida exemplifies how surveillance data can contribute to evaluating the impact of a major birth defect and reducing its burden of morbidity and mortality. Spina bifida is a congenital anomaly of the central nervous system that can cause death and severe disability (64,65). Some complications of spina bifida that now occur can be prevented (32,66). The occurrence of spina bifida could be reduced by half or more if women consumed sufficient amounts of folic acid before conception and in early pregnancy (32,67). Additional cases could be prevented by strictly controlling maternal diabetes (68) and by avoiding certain drugs such as valproic acid. Genetic variation could also contribute to the risk for spina bifida (32,69).

Surveillance of spina bifida has traditionally focused on monitoring occurrence rates, most often relying on birth-defect registries with access to birthing hospitals, and sometimes, in the absence of such registries, on alternative data sources such as vital records. As already mentioned, this traditional approach is seriously undermined by the significant proportion of affected pregnancies that are prenatally detected and electively terminated (51). Also, the genetic and environmental determinants of spina bifida are not commonly monitored, and if they are, these data are usually not integrated with the traditional surveillance activities. Finally, surveillance of morbidity and mortality, especially beyond infancy, is rarely done (32).

A comprehensive approach to spina bifida surveillance should encompass multiple components, including a network of population-based birth-defect registries with access to data sources on prenatal diagnosis and pregnancy terminations. These birth-defect registries might also collect storable genetic specimens such as blood spots or cheek swabs from the infant and parents for use in the study and monitoring of the genetic determinants of spina bifida. Surveillance systems should also record information on potentially preventable exposures that could be used to counsel couples, to reduce the risk for a further affected pregnancy in the same family, and to track the effectiveness of policies and campaigns aimed at reducing the number of preventable cases. Vital statistics data linked to the registries would provide information on survival, while linked hospital discharge data would enhance surveillance of co-morbid conditions. Furthermore, provider and population surveys should track the attitudes, knowledge, and use of prevention measures, such as daily use of folic acid, preconceptional control of diabetes, or avoidance of certain drugs around the time of conception and in early pregnancy.

Public Health Genetic Programs: Emerging Need For Population Data

For many years the focus of public health genetics program was newborn screening. In recent years, however, the explosive growth of genetic knowledge has given rise to new questions that require timely and accurate answers. For instance, what data are needed before a new genetic test (e.g., for MCADD—medium-chain acyldehydrogenase deficiency) is considered for newborn screening? How does one evaluate whether a genetic test is safe, effective, and cost-efficient? How does one assess and monitor the genotype and phenotype frequency associated with known and newly discovered mutations in different populations? How can one promote and implement the collection, and use of genetic information that is socially, legally, and ethically acceptable? With the increasing interest in evaluating prevention effectiveness, even traditional activities have come under renewed scrutiny. For example, what impact does current genetic screening for sickle cell disease have on rates of disease, complications, disability, and death in the population? Are known prevention measures such as penicillin prophylaxis applied effectively throughout the population?

As in the case of birth defects, public health genetics can supply crucial information about single-gene disorders that can be used to define and monitor problems, evaluate prevention measures, detect changes in screening practices, and facilitate planning. Many of the issues discussed in connection

with birth-defect surveillance are also relevant to the debate on the integration of genetics into public health—the integration of data sources and disease
registries; the complexities of coding and classification; the ethical, social, and
legal ramifications; and the need for timely and easily accessible data. Certain
aspects of single gene-disorders, however, demand specific considerations. For
example, because the genotype frequency of a single-gene disorder is relatively
stable, ongoing monitoring should focus on the disease phenotype and on the
rate of complications, disability, and mortality. Moreover, the specific ethical,
social and legal ramifications of using genetic information in public health surveillance must be carefully examined (see Chapter 27 in this volume). Genetic
testing also becomes a central issue, as advances in genomic research lead to
the development of new genetic tests. An expert panel from academia, industry, and government has recommended that genetic tests be evaluated according to their analytic validity (the ability of the test to classify the genotype),
clinical validity (the ability of the test to predict the disease phenotype), and
clinical utility (the modification of the clinical phenotype associated with the
use or non use of the test) (63). Such information would help medical professionals, public health officials, and the public evaluate the safety and effectiveness of genetic tests that are finding their way from a research setting to
clinical practice.

Integrating Genetics into Public Health: Two Case Studies

Two single-gene conditions, phenylketonuria (PKU) and MCADD, illustrate
the emerging data needs of public health programs that use genetic information. In many ways, PKU exemplifies many issues associated with single-gene
disorders in the newborn screening programs for which prevention measures
are available (e.g., a low phenylalanine diet). The goals of surveillance in
this setting should include evaluating and monitoring morbidity, disability,
and mortality in people with the disorder, as well as the population-wide
effectiveness of prevention measures. For PKU, such monitoring would
involve tracking infants identified through newborn screening programs;
integrating information on neurologic, psychologic, and social outcomes
from pediatricians, hospitals, developmental disability registries, and special
needs programs; and following affected women to provide reproductive
counseling.

Timeliness is crucial. The birth of a malformed child from a mother with
uncontrolled PKU should quickly lead to appropriate referrals for the mother
and child and to an assessment of the prevention program. By identifying what
steps lead to uncontrolled metabolic PKU in the mother, other cases might be
averted, e.g., by providing better dietary advice and by free distribution of
foods low in phenylalanine.

The example of PKU also suggests that it may be useful to reevaluate the
role of the newborn screening in public health programs. Although tradition-

ally not viewed as monitoring systems, newborn screening programs possess some of the features commonly associated with population-based surveillance, such as complete population coverage. The quantity and quality of medical data, however, is limited. Thus, the public health usefulness of newborn screening programs could be enhanced either by expanding the functions of such programs or by integrating them with other public health information systems. In addition, newborn screening programs would benefit from a formal surveillance evaluation that would assess their sensitivity, flexibility, acceptability, and timeliness (70,71).

Newly identified single-gene disorders provide additional challenges to medical and public health professionals. For example, if a genetic test is available for a newly identified disorder, the question might, and often does arise of whether it should be included in newborn screening programs. Medium-chain acyldehydrogenase deficiency (MCADD), a recently identified disorder of fatty-acid metabolism, exemplifies this situation. MCADD has been associated with an increased risk for infant deaths that in some cases might be decreased by appropriate feeding practices (72). Whether to include MCADD in the newborn screening program has sparked a debate that includes parents, manufacturers of the test, and medical professionals. Although a comprehensive analysis of this debate is beyond the scope of this chapter, it should be noted that for MCADD and other newly identified conditions the lack of data is even greater than for PKU. There is little or not data on frequency of the major mutations in different populations, on the association of specific genotypes with premature mortality and other health outcomes, on the role of gene-environment interactions in modulating disease risk, and the natural history associated with the genotype. Expanding surveillance systems to include this condition could contribute substantially to the knowledge needed to make data-based decisions about screening.

Concluding Remarks

Although public health surveillance has been implemented in different forms for several decades, evolving scientific and social conditions currently challenge its ability to monitor and prevent disease. These changes, however, also offer new opportunities. For example, prenatal diagnosis of birth defects can lead either to earlier treatment or to pregnancy termination. The development of new genetic tests may contribute to earlier detection of potentially harmful mutations and to earlier treatment or prevention of the disease. However, indiscriminate use of genetic tests could be harmful. In both settings, the challenge for modern public health programs is to generate useful, timely, and accessible information, and to make such information available to public health officials, medical professionals, policy makers, and the public. Such information will contribute to a constructive and informative debate that should ensure that advances in birth defects and genetic research translate into a real benefit to individuals and the community, within the boundaries of ethics and the law. The crucial tests will be whether surveillance will manage to expand from monitoring occurrence rates to tracking broader measures of impact (e.g., morbidity, disability, and mortality) as well as disease risk factors, and whether surveillance systems will effectively integrate into public health programs, so that the information can be used to control and prevent disease and promote health.

References

1. Baird PA, Anderson TW, Newcombe HB, Lowry RB. Genetic disorders in children and young adults: a population study. Am J Hum Genet 1988;42:677–693.

2. Czeizel A, Sankaranarayanan K. The load of genetic and partially genetic disorders in man. I. Congenital anomalies: estimates of detriment in terms of years of life lost and years of impaired life. Mutat Res 1984;128:73–103.

3. Chavez GF, Cordero JF, Becerra JE. Leading major congenital malformations among minority groups in the United States, 1981–1986. MMWR CDC Surveill Summ 1988;37:17–24.

4. Kalter H, Warkany J. Medical progress. Congenital malformations: etiologic factors and their role in prevention (first of two parts). N Engl J Med 1983;308:424–431.

5. Boyle CA, Yeargin-Allsopp M, Doernberg NS, et al. Prevalence of selected developmental disabilities in children 3–10 years of age: the Metropolitan Atlanta Developmental Disabilities Surveillance Program, 1991. MMWR CDC Surveill Summ 1996;45:1–14.

6. Infant mortality—United States, 1993. MMWR Morb Mortal Wkly Rep 1996;45:211–215.

7. Yang Q, Khoury MJ, Mannino D. Trends and patterns of mortality associated with birth defects and genetic diseases in the United States, 1979–1992: an analysis of multiple-cause mortality data. Genet Epidemiol 1997;14:493–505.

8. Cunniff C, Carmack JL, Kirby RS, Fiser DH. Contribution of heritable disorders to mortality in the pediatric intensive care unit. Pediatrics 1995;95:678–681.

9. Hudome SM, Kirby RS, Senner JW, Cunniff C. Contribution of genetic disorders to neonatal mortality in a regional intensive care setting. Am J Perinatol 1994;11:100–103.

10. Ling EW, Sosuan LC, Hall JC. Congenital anomalies: an increasingly important cause of mortality and workload in a neonatal intensive care unit. Am J Perinatol 1991;8:164–169.

11. Yoon PW, Olney RS, Khoury MJ, et al. Contribution of birth defects and genetic diseases to pediatric hospitalizations. A population-based study. Arch Pediatr Adolesc Med 1997;151:1096–1103.

12. Economic costs of birth defects and cerebral palsy—United States, 1992. MMWR Morb Mortal Wkly Rep 1995;44:694–699.

13. Waitzman NJ, Romano PS, Scheffler RM. Estimates of the economic costs of birth defects. Inquiry 1994;31:188–205.

14. Lenz W. Malformations caused by drugs in pregnancy. Am J Dis Child 1966;112:99–106.

15. Källén B, Hay S, Klingberg M. Birth defects monitoring systems accomplishments and goals. In: Kalter H (ed). Issues and reviews in teratology. New York and London: Plenum Publishing, 1984, pp. 1–22.

16. Khoury MJ. Relationship between medical genetics and public health: changing the paradigm of disease prevention and the definition of a genetic disease. Am J Med Genet 1997;71:289–291.

17. Källén B. Epidemiology of human reproduction. Boca Raton, FL: CRC Press, 1988.

18. Khoury MJ, Holtzman NA. On the ability of birth defects monitoring to detect new teratogens. Am J Epidemiol 1987;126:136–143.

19. Khoury MJ, Botto L, Mastroiacovo P, Skjaerven R, Castilla E, Erickson JD. Monitoring for multiple congenital anomalies: an international perspective. Epidemiol Rev 1994;16:335–350.

20. Lynberg MC, Edmonds LD. Surveillance of birth defects. In: Haperin W, Baker EL, Monson RR (eds). Public health surveillance. New York: Van Nostrand Reinhold, 1992, pp. 157–172.

21. Thacker SB, Berkelman RL. History of public health surveillance. In: Haperin W, Baker EL, Monson RR (eds). Public health surveillance. New York: Van Nostrand Reinhold, 1992, pp. 1–15.

22. Thacker SB, Stroup DF. Future directions for comprehensive public health surveillance and health information systems in the United States. Am J Epidemiol 1994;140:383–397.

23. Castilla EE, da Graca Dutra M. Limb reduction defects and coastal areas (letter). Lancet 1994;343:1034.

24. Mastroiacovo P, Botto L, Fusco D, Rosano A, Scarano G. Limb reduction defects and coastal areas (letter). Lancet 1994;343:1034–1035.

25. Botting BJ. Limb reduction defects and coastal areas (letter). Lancet 1994;343:1033–1034.

26. Paulozzi LJ, Erickson JD, Jackson RJ. Hypospadias trends in two US surveillance systems. Pediatrics 1997;100:831–834.

27. Paulozzi LJ. International trends in rates of hypospadias and cryptorchidism. Environ Health Perspect 1999;107:297–302.

28. Carlsen E, Giwercman A, Keiding N, Skakkebaek NE. Declining semen quality and increasing incidence of testicular cancer: is there a common cause? Environ Health Perspect 1995;103 (Suppl 7):137–139.

29. Carlsen E, Giwercman A, Skakkebaek NE. Declining sperm counts and increasing incidence of testicular cancer and other gonadal disorders: is there a connection? [editorial]. Ir Med J 1993;86:85–86.

30. Giwercman A, Carlsen E, Keiding N, Skakkebaek NE. Evidence for increasing incidence of abnormalities of the human testis: a review. Environ Health Perspect 1993;101 (Suppl 2):65–71.

31. International Clearinghouse for Birth Defects Monitoring Systems. Time trends 1974–1996: anencephaly, spina bifida, and Down syndrome. In: Botting B, Castilla E, Mastroiacovo P, Siffel C (eds). Annual report 1998. Rome: International Centre for Birth Defects, 1998, pp. 100–101.

32. Botto LD, Moore CA, Khoury MJ, Erickson JD. Neural-tube defects. N Engl J Med 1999;341:1509–1519.

33. Mastroiacovo P, Bertollini R, Corchia C. Survival of children with Down syndrome in Italy. Am J Med Genet 1992;42:208–212.

34. Erickson JD. Risk factors for birth defects: data from the Atlanta Birth Defects Case-Control Study. Teratology 1991;43:41–51.

35. Valproic acid and spina bifida: a preliminary report–France. MMWR Morb Mortal Wkly Rep 1982;31:565–566.

36. Robert E, Guibaud P. Maternal valproic acid and congenital neural tube defects (letter). Lancet 1982;2:937.

37. Bjerkedal T, Czeizel A, Goujard J, et al. Valproic acid and spina bifida (letter]. Lancet 1982;2:1096.

38. Firth HV, Boyd PA, Chamberlain P, MacKenzie IZ, Lindenbaum RH, Huson SM. Severe limb abnormalities after chorion villus sampling at 56–66 days' gestation. Lancet 1991;337:762–763.

39. Mastroiacovo P, Botto LD, Cavalcanti DP, et al. Limb anomalies following chorionic villus sampling: a registry based case-control study. Am J Med Genet 1992; 44:856–864.

40. Olney RS, Khoury MJ, Alo CJ, et al. Increased risk for transverse digital deficiency after chorionic villus sampling: results of the United States Multistate Case-Control Study, 1988–1992. Teratology 1995;51:20–29.

41. Firth H. Chorion villus sampling and limb deficiency—cause or coincidence? Prenat Diagn 1997;17:1313–1330.

42. Yang Q, Khoury MJ, James LM, Olney RS, Paulozzi LJ, Erickson JD. The return of thalidomide: are birth defects surveillance systems ready? Am J Med Genet 1997;73:251–258.

43. Lynberg MC, Khoury MJ, Lammer EJ, Waller KO, Cordero JF, Erickson JD. Sensitivity, specificity, and positive predictive value of multiple malformations in isotretinoin embryopathy surveillance. Teratology 1990;42:513–519.

44. International Clearinghouse for Birth Defects Monitoring Systems. Contributing monitoring systems. In: Botting B, Castilla E, Mastroiacovo P, Siffel C (eds). Annual report 1998. Rome: International Centre for Birth Defects, 1998, pp. 25–39.

45. Graves EJ, Gillum BS. National Hospital Discharge Survey: annual summary, 1994. Hyattsville, MD: National Center for Health Statistics, 1996.

46. Bright RA, Avorn J, Everitt DE. Medicaid data as a resource for epidemiologic studies: strengths and limitations. J Clin Epidemiol 1989;42:937–945.

47. Ezzati TM, Massey JT, Waksberg J, Chu A, Maurer KR. Sample design: third National Health and Nutrition Examination Survey. Vital Health Stat 2 1992:1–35.

48. Woodwell DA. National ambulatory medical care survey: 1995 summary. Hyattsville, MD: National Center for Health Statistics, 1997.

49. Pradat P. Epidemiology of major congenital heart defects in Sweden, 1981–1986. J Epidemiol Community Health 1992;46:211–215.

50. Skjaerven R, Wilcox AJ, Lie RT. A population-based study of survival and child-bearing among female subjects with birth defects and the risk of recurrence in their children. N Engl J Med 1999;340:1057–1062.

51. International Center for Birth Defects, World Health Organization, EUROCAT. World atlas of birth defects. Geneva: WHO, 1998.

52. Rosano A, Smithells D, Cacciani L, et al. Time trends in neural tube defects prevalence in relation to preventive strategies: an international study. J Epidemiol Community Health 1999;53:630–635.

53. Smythe JF, Copel JA, Kleinman CS. Outcome of prenatally detected cardiac malformations. Am J Cardiol 1992;69:1471–1474.

54. Allan LD, Cook A, Sullivan I, Sharland GK. Hypoplastic left heart syndrome: effects of fetal echocardiography on birth prevalence. Lancet 1991;337:959–961.

55. Daubeney PE, Sharland GK, Cook AC, Keeton BR, Anderson RH, Webber SA. Pulmonary atresia with intact ventricular septum: impact of fetal echocardiography on incidence at birth and postnatal outcome. UK and Eire collaborative study of pulmonary atresia with intact ventricular septum. Circulation 1998;98:562–566.

56. Burris S. Law and social risk of health care: lessons from HIV testing. Albany L Rev 1998;61:831–895.

57. Little J, Elwood M. Ethnic origin and migration. In: Elwood JM, Little J, Elwood JH (eds). Epidemiology and control of neural tube defects. New York: Oxford University Press, 1992, pp. 146–167.

58. Prevalence of spina bifida at birth—United States, 1983–1990: a comparison of two surveillance systems. MMWR Morb Mortal Wkly Rep 1996:15–26.

59. Hill RM, Verniaud WM, Horning MG, McCulley LB, Morgan NF. Infants exposed in utero to antiepileptic drugs. A prospective study. Am J Dis Child 1974;127:645–653.

60. Speidel BD, Meadow SR. Maternal epilepsy and abnormalities of the fetus and newborn. Lancet 1972;2:839–843.

61. Birth defects surveillance data from selected states, 1989–1996. Teratology 2000;61:86–158.

62. International Clearinghouse for Birth Defects Monitoring Systems. Annual report 1999. Rome: International Centre for Birth Defects, 1999.

63. Holtzman NA, Watson MS. Promoting safe and effective genetic testing in the United States: final report of the task force on genetic testing. www.nhgri.nih.gov/Elsi/TFGT_final/ 1998.

64. Lynberg MC, Khoury MJ. Contribution of birth defects to infant mortality among racial/ethnic minority groups, United States, 1983. Mor Mortal Wkly Rep CDC Surveill Summ 1990;39:1–12.

65. Shibuya K, Murray CJL. Congenital anomalies. In: Murray CJL, Lopez AD (eds). Health dimensions of sex and reproduction. Boston: Harvard University Press, 1998, pp. 455–512.

66. Kinsman SL, Doehring MC. The cost of preventable conditions in adults with spina bifida. Eur J Pediatr Surg 1996;6(Suppl 1):17–20.

67. Czeizel AE, Dudas I. Prevention of the first occurrence of neural-tube defects by periconceptional vitamin supplementation. N Engl J Med 1992;327:1832–1835.

68. Reece EA, Sivan E, Francis G, Homko CJ. Pregnancy outcomes among women with and without diabetic microvascular disease (White's classes B to FR) versus nondiabetic controls. Am J Perinatol 1998;15:549–555.

69. Shields DC, Kirke PN, Mills JL, et al. The "thermolabile" variant of methylenetetrahydrofolate reductase and neural tube defects: an evaluation of genetic risk and the relative importance of the genotypes of the embryo and the mother. Am J Hum Genet 1999;64:1045–1055.

70. Klaucke DN. Evaluating public health surveillance. In: Teutsch SM, Churchill RE (eds). Principles and practice of public health surveillance. New York: Oxford University Press, 1994, pp. 158–174.

71. Klaucke DN. Evaluating public health surveillance systems. Public health surveillance. New York: Van Nostrand Reinhold, 1992, pp. 26–41.

72. Wang SS, Fernhoff PM, Hannon WH, Khoury MJ. Medium chain acyl-coA dehydrogenase deficiency (MCADD). HuGE Reviews 1999;www.cdc.gov/genetics/hugenet/ MCAD.htm.

8

Surveillance for hemophilia and inherited hematologic disorders

J. Michael Soucie, Frederick R. Rickles, and Bruce L. Evatt

Hemophilia refers to a group of rare hereditary disorders of blood coagulation. The most common are defects of clotting factors VIII (hemophilia A) or IX (hemophilia B) and affect approximately 1 in 10,000 and 1 in 40,000 people in the United States, respectively (1). The combined prevalence for these two single-gene, single-protein, X-chromosome-linked defects is estimated to be 13 cases per 100,000 males or approximately 17,000 cases in the United States. People with hemophilia exhibit varying degrees of factor deficiency, which correlate with their disease severity, and about 40% have the severe (<1% of either factor VIII or factor IX) form of the disorder. Among the congenital bleeding disorders, von Willebrand disease (vWD) is the most common, affecting perhaps as much as 1%–3% of the American population (2–4).

Before the 1980s, hemophilia-associated morbidity, mortality, and disability were due to excessive bleeding, particularly into weight-bearing joints and the central nervous system. The median age of death for individuals with hemophilia was about 11.4 years from 1831 to 1920, but had reached the mid-20s by 1960. During the 1960s and 1970s, a better understanding of the medical basis of the disorders and improved therapy in the form of clotting-factor concentrates lowered mortality and yielded nearly normal life expectancy for such people. Since 1982, however, the AIDS epidemic, the result of HIV-transmission from infected plasma-derived clotting factor, has had a significant impact on mortality (5,6).

Treatment for the severe forms of hemophilia A and B and for their associated complications place large demands on health care resources. The annual cost of highly purified, viral-inactivated or recombinant clotting-factor concentrates for the treatment or prevention of bleeding in those with severe hemophilia can approach $150,000 per patient. Treatment for the preventable complications of the disease increase health care costs substantially beyond this fixed cost of replacement therapy (7), thus impacting significantly on the total U.S. health care budget. Conservative estimates suggest that the current cost of hemophilia care in the United States (including the cost of replacement product) may be as high as $1 billion annually.

Several important considerations influence the design of adequate health care delivery systems for persons with hemophilia. First, hemophilia care is very specialized and appropriate training and experience is needed to avoid poor therapeutic decisions that can lead to severe disability and mortality. Second, because the disease is rare, maintaining the availability of trained and experienced physicians often can be achieved only by concentrating patient care into specialized centers. Third, when complications occur, they are extremely expensive to treat, which places a premium on a preventive approach to care. Finally, the organization of care must be structured to enable optimal delivery of care and allocation of resources.

Based on these considerations, in 1975 the federal government established a network of specialized hemophilia treatment centers (HTCs) designed to provide a public health approach to the care of persons with hemophilia by integrating prevention and clinical practice. The goals of this approach were to (1) reduce the complications of the bleeding disorders in this population; (2) reduce the number of hospitalizations; (3) normalize life expectancy; (4) enable them to maintain a state of health adequate for employment; and (5) reduce the demands on the health care system by providing comprehensive primary and secondary rather than tertiary care. This centralized direction of care not only provided a means of coordinating health care resources but also a way of evaluating outcomes among individuals with rare diseases. This information could then be used to improve services and ensure that effective programs were maintained. In addition, it was hoped that such a system could serve as a model for health care delivery for other chronic diseases.

Need for Data

Data are essential in establishing and maintaining good health care delivery systems. In the early 1970s, data from hemophilia patients were used to show that many of the disabling effects and much of the early mortality caused by hemophilia could be reduced or prevented by providing training for patients in self-therapy and home care. In the United States, these data served as the basis for the comprehensive care approach that was implemented in the HTC system. These data also provided the justification for applying similar principles of care to hemophilia populations in other developed countries, thus doubling the life span of those affected.

After the HTC system was established data were needed to (*1*) plan local health care strategies and set priorities; (*2*) target specific problems; (*3*) motivate government agencies to take action; (*4*) disseminate accurate information to the press; (*5*) gain financial support; (*6*) mobilize the patient community for action; and (*7*) measure the impact of the program to justify the continued support of government and private organizations.

To collect these data, however, a surveillance system was needed. To develop the system, a working group comprising epidemiologists, clinicians, and other individuals with knowledge of the issues important to the hemophilia community was formed. This group established the goals for the surveillance system, selected the type of system that would be used, and determined what data would be collected. Other steps included identification of necessary resources, establishment of functional systems, and the development of a data collection instrument.

Considerations for Data Collection in the Hemophilia Population

Because hemophilia is a chronic disease of low prevalence, developing surveillance and other data collection systems presents special challenges. Most surveillance systems are designed to work with acute diseases or highly prevalent chronic diseases. Registry systems are one logical approach; however, because of privacy issues, including those raised during the HIV epidemic, a registry system for hemophilia has not been established. Other traditional sources of surveillance information, such as death certificates, voluntary reporting, and surveys, provide some types of information but are limited by issues such as timeliness and the degree of participation.

Two sources of data that may be appropriate for hemophilia are medical record reviews and active case reporting as part of a health care system. Each of these methods has its limitations. Medical record review is time-consuming and costly and can only provide retrospective data. The major issue complicating active surveillance is the need for an elaborate, organized reporting network within the health care system. Such a network requires a high level of motivation and a common sense of purpose within system participants.

To achieve a common sense of purpose, a prevention program should seek a consensus on potential uses of data, types of surveillance models that might be used as a pattern for the system, and what data may be available. Generally, two types of approaches are most commonly used: the public health database system and the clinical study database system. The former comprises the minimal amount of data necessary to measure trends and identify specific problems, whereas the latter consists of extensive data sets. For most applications, the public health database system is the most practical.

The process of identifying data needs and uses is done by a group that includes consultants or participants representing the patient community, and representatives from public health and other organizations that will use the data. This group will determine the direction and type of system to be used, and the content of the data collection instrument. Because these representatives often have competing needs, the availability of resources will determine which needs will be addressed. Although the practicality of collecting data for each need should be reviewed, such a review should occur only in the latter stages of the group's discussion so as not to inhibit ideas.

Selection of Data Collection System and Content

To select the most appropriate system for data collection, the program should review existing surveillance systems models with regard to their suitability for collecting data on the hemophilia population, set priorities for surveillance content, and devise potential surveillance questions for each priority content area to be addressed by the system. Once these issues have been addressed, the type of system needed often becomes apparent.

The discussion of possible data collection systems and content should also consider the following aspects: location of data, barriers to data collection, cost of data collection, extent of data, and the sensitivity and validity of the data. The program will have the most difficulty achieving agreement on the data collection instrument. Before being included in the data collection instrument, each data topic should be discussed thoroughly and given priority according to a criteria scale established beforehand. The volume of data desired will likely exceed that which might realistically be collected, and the priority scale will allow only the most valuable data to become part of the collection system. While the group will want to proceed directly to the composition of questions to be included on the instrument, such an approach may be disastrous. We have found the following approach to this process to be the most efficient and effective:

1. State the goals of the data collection. These goals should be the driving force for determining what data are to be collected. Collect data only for specific needs and uses as defined by these goals. Possible goals might include:

   a. Determine the prevalence and incidence of hemophilia (e.g., disease manifestation, demographics).

   b. Study the occurrence of complications and the use of health care resources over time (e.g., nature/type of complications, source of medical care).

   c. Develop population-based data on the social and economic impact of hemophilia and its complications (e.g., medical care, hospitalizations, lost days of work).

d. Detect emerging situations that require intervention.

e. Understand the demographics of HIV/AIDS.

2. Identify the data topics needed to meet the stated goals. These topics will be chosen based upon the priority criteria previously determined by the group. The topics should be specific and data should be obtainable using the resources available. Trying to collect data that require more resources than available will be very discouraging and may cause the entire system to fail. Limit the data elements to the minimum required to answer the questions. The data system is not a medical chart; its success will depend upon its simplicity.

3. Establish definitions for each data topic. These definitions will determine what data will be collected and the minimum amount of data necessary and will ensure that the data are uniform. For instance, if hemophilia is defined differently among participants, then the data are not compatible. This step will also allow data to be abstracted by individuals of varied training backgrounds. The definitions will determine the guidelines for inclusions of data. No questions should be developed until these definitions are determined.

4. Develop the data items. This is a key step in the development of a useful and effective data collection tool. There are many aspects to constructing a data collection instrument that contribute to its effectiveness in obtaining the best possible information in the most efficient and effective way. It is crucial that epidemiologists, statisticians, or others with experience in designing data collection instruments have a role in this process. An additional consideration at this point is to make sure that all data requested by the instrument will be available in the setting in which the instrument will be used. For example, it is unreasonable to expect that individuals working in a clinic will be able to provide information that is only available in a hospital.

5. Field-test the data instrument. This step, which should be done by the participating centers, is crucial in determining the feasibility of collecting the needed data. Field testing will often identify problems with missing data, definitions, and interpretation of results. After the field test, the definitions and data collection instrument should again be modified to correct any problems encountered.

Establishing a Functional System

The first phase in establishing a functional system is to determine the logistics. The *who*, *what*, *where*, and *how* must be evaluated according to available resources. In many respects, the broad scheme will be primarily determined by the criteria previously discussed and the types of resources available for the system.

Planning the details is the most time-consuming task. Many details have to be considered. Will the personnel be volunteers or salaried? Who will abstract the data? How will errors be detected? What are the communication channels? Who will do the analysis? How will conflicts in data be resolved? How will the data be tabulated? How will the data collection forms be printed? Who will pay for postage? How and to whom will the results be communicated? How and by whom will personnel involved in data collection and management be trained? Who will provide technical assistance?

Surveillance Programs for Hemophilia in the United States

The goals of data collection for the hemophilia public health program in the United States are to determine the burden of disease, the source and extent of health resources utilized, and the level of disability and death produced by the disease burden. In addition, the program needs a monitoring system to evaluate the impact of programs directed at reducing these burdens. Especially important issues include blood-transmitted infectious agents and the level of joint and liver disease resulting from chronic bleeding episodes or as a complication of blood-borne infectious agents.

To accomplish these goals, two different systems are utilized, the Hemophilia Surveillance System (HSS) and the Universal Data Collection System (UDC). Each was designed for specific purposes and provides valuable information to federal agencies and health care providers to improve the health care of people with hemophilia by prevention and early intervention.

Hemophilia Surveillance System (HSS)

The HSS is an active public health surveillance system that identifies and collects data on all patients with hemophilia A and hemophilia B in six states. The states include Colorado, Georgia, Louisiana, Massachusetts, New York, and Oklahoma, which comprise approximately 20% of the U.S. hemophilia population (1). Operation of the system is through state health departments collaborating with hemophilia treatment centers and hemophilia associations in these states. Beginning in 1995, surveillance staff in each state, under the authority of the state health department, implemented methods of case finding best suited for a given locality. Standardized data are abstracted from medical and clinical records and include demographic and basic clinic information, detailed information on source of care and reimbursement, number of bleeding episodes and the amount and sources of clotting factor used, the results of testing for exposure to infectious diseases, information from comprehensive assessment of joints, and complete information on all hospitalizations. Data are also collected concerning the immediate and underlying causes of death for individuals who die during the surveillance period. The data are stored in local databases and periodically transmitted without patient identifiers to the CDC for analysis. All transmitted data are screened for omissions, inconsistencies, and possible abstraction or data entry errors.

Because this system is extremely labor-intensive and expensive, it was envisioned to collect data for only 5 years. However, it has already provided invaluable, previously nonexistent data on the hemophilia population and their health care needs as well as information on target areas for prevention. It has also provided information demonstrating the effectiveness of the comprehensive care approach to hemophilia care in reducing mortality.

Universal Data Collection (UDC) System

Universal Data Collection (UDC) is a nationwide surveillance system developed in response to a congressional mandate to the CDC to reduce or prevent the complications of bleeding disorders. Designed to prospectively collect a uniform set of clinical and outcome data, it focuses primarily upon blood-borne diseases and joint disease. Begun in May 1998 and conducted by the CDC's Hematologic Diseases Branch, UDC will eventually supplant other surveillance activities in this community such as the HSS.

Data for UDC are gathered at federally funded HTCs across the United States. The HTC staff obtain information on participant demographics, bleeding disorder diagnosis, treatment regimens and factor replacement products used, history of illness due to and treatment for or vaccination against blood-borne infections, and history of joint disease and its affect upon daily activities. Staff perform joint range-of-motion measurements and draw blood for testing for hepatitis A, B, and C viruses and HIV-1 and HIV-2. Participation is voluntary and open to anyone who meets at least one of the following criteria:

1. Age 2 years or older and diagnosed with a bleeding disorder due to congenital deficiency or acquired inhibitors in which any of the coagulation proteins are missing, reduced, or defective and have a functional level of less than 50%.
2. Age 2 years or older with von Willebrand disease diagnosed by a physician.

Individuals with thrombophilia, coagulation protein deficiencies due to liver failure, or an exclusive diagnosis of a platelet disorder are specifically excluded. They must consent to both data collection and blood testing in order to participate. The goal is to collect a complete set of information and a blood specimen from each participant annually.

Staff complete an Annual Visit form and a Laboratory form for each participant each time he or she participates. A Registration form acknowledging consent is also completed once for each participant. For eligible HTC attendees who decline to participate, staff complete a Patient Refusal form. The Registration, Annual Visit, and Patient Refusal forms are sent to the CDC where information is entered into the UDC database. The Laboratory form is not used for data collection by the CDC but is used by the hepatitis testing laboratory when interpreting test results; the form is routed to this lab by way of the serum bank with aliquots of the blood specimens. Personal identifiers of participants are not reported to the CDC or the hepatitis testing lab. Instead, the HTC generates a random, yet unique and unchanging, identification number for each participant using computer software supplied by the CDC. All communications among the CDC, the hepatitis lab, and the HTC concerning the participant are conducted using this anonymous number. Only the HTCs maintain a list linking the identification number with the patient.

Blood specimens (plasma) are collected and shipped to the CDC serum bank in Lawrenceville, Georgia. The first aliquot of each specimen (as well as any remaining after allocation for routine screening) is banked at this facility to create a specimen pool that may be accessed if special viral investigations become necessary. Additional aliquots are distributed to the HIV testing laboratory at the CDC in Atlanta, Georgia, and to the Eugene B. Casey Hepatitis Laboratory at Baylor College of Medicine in Houston, Texas. Appropriate enzyme-linked immunosorbent assay (EIA) and Western blot tests are performed for HIV-1 and HIV-2. In rare cases, additional tests, such as the P1 and P2 protein dot blot tests, may be employed to distinguish the HIV subtypes. Testing for hepatitis A, B, and C is performed as outlined in the attached testing algorithms. Results of serologic assays are entered into the UDC database and reported to the HTC for use in patient care.

Analyses of these data will be directed toward identifying and describing the occurrence of complications among various subgroups of the hemophilia community so that prevention efforts can be appropriately initiated and implemented. Reports of these analyses will be periodically distributed for dissemination to all participating HTCs. Results of viral testing will be used to determine prevalence and seroconversion rates of viral infection among those with bleeding disorders, as well as to monitor for significant increases that might prompt special investigations. At regular intervals, the data collected from each of the 12 federal hemophilia treatment center regions will be distributed in electronic form to the coordinators of each region for distribution to the HTCs for their use.

Prevention of transfusion-transmissible infectious diseases is a high priority for public health programs in patients with hereditary bleeding disorders. The

UDC system will provide an "early warning system" for the nation's blood supply by establishing a serum bank on all HTC patients participating in the program, thereby allowing the CDC to respond quickly to concerns regarding potential contamination of the blood supply. The UDC and HTC network will provide an important model for testing prevention effectiveness in patients with hereditary bleeding disorders and for following their health outcomes. These mechanisms will allow the CDC, in collaboration with health care providers in the HTCs, state health agencies, the National Hemophilia Foundation, the Federal Drug Administration (FDA), the Maternal and Child Health Bureau of the Health Resources and Services Administration (HRSA), and the National Heart Lung, and Blood Institute (NHLBI), to quickly test and implement aggressive prevention strategies developed for virtually any of the complications of hereditary bleeding disorders.

Summary

Surveillance programs for patients with hereditary bleeding disorders have been deployed widely by the CDC across the United States through a network of interactive programs in state departments of public health and in hemophilia treatment centers. These surveillance programs are providing valuable information for the design and implementation of prevention strategies, which have been developed in collaboration with other involved health care agencies, health care providers, and patient advocacy groups. This powerful prevention coalition can use this unique system to respond rapidly to public health problems among individuals with hereditary bleeding disorders.

References

1. Soucie JM, Evatt B, Jackson D, and the Hemophilia Surveillance System Project Investigators. The occurrence of hemophilia in the United States. Am J Hematol 1998;59:288–294.

2. Montgomery RR, Coller BS. Von Willebrand disease. In: Colman RW, Hirsh J, Marder VJ, Salzman EW (eds). Hemostasis and thrombosis: basic principles and clinical practice (2nd ed). Philadelphia Lippincott, 1994, pp. 134–168.

3. Rick ME. Diagnosis and management of von Willebrand's syndrome. Med Clin North Am 1994;78:609–623.

4. Miller CH, Lenzi R, Breen C. Prevalence of von Willebrand's disease among US adults. Blood (abstract). 1987;70(Suppl):377a.

5. Chorba TL, Holman RC, Strine TW, Clarke MJ, Evatt BL. Changes in longevity and causes of death among persons with hemophilia A. Am J Hematol 1994;45:112–121.

6. Eyster ME, Schaefer JH, Ragni MV, et al. Changing causes of death in Pennsylvania's hemophiliacs 1976–1991: impact of liver disease and acquired immunodeficiency syndrome (letter). Blood 1992;79:2494–2495.

7. Smith PS, Teutsch SM, Shaffer PA, Rolka H, Evatt BL. Episodic versus prophylactic infusions for hemophilia A: a cost-effectiveness analysis. J Pediatr 1996; 129:424–431.

9

Public health assessment of genetic predisposition to cancer

Steven S. Coughlin and Wylie Burke

Cancer prevention and control efforts have traditionally focused on modifiable risk factors for cancer such as cigarette smoking and diet and on screening for disease precursors such as dysplastic nevi and cervical dysplasia (1). However, both the identification and the evaluation of inherited risk are likely to play an increasingly important role in cancer prevention strategies (2–5).

In recent years the focus has shifted from rare cancer syndromes—for example, Li-Fraumeni syndrome and Von Hippel Lindau syndrome—to common adult-onset disorders that are important causes of morbidity and mortality (6). Examples discussed in this chapter include the identification of mutations in the hMSH2 and hMLH1 genes as causes of susceptibility to colorectal cancer and mutations in the BRCA1 and BRCA2 genes identified as causes of susceptibility to breast and ovarian cancer.

The identification and modification of environmental risk factors among people with an inherited susceptibility to cancer is a new paradigm for cancer prevention and control (2,5). For example, genetic testing for colorectal cancer may improve the predictive value of environmental factors such as high-fat diet, inadequate intake of vegetables and fruit, and physical inactivity (4). The identification of gene–environment interactions in the etiology of breast cancer could result in preventive and therapeutic interventions for women at risk for the disease (3). For instance, interactions might be identified between ATM gene mutations and nongenetic factors such as ionizing radiation and cigarette smoking (7). Genetic tests for other conditions may allow for the identification of subgroups of individuals who are more or less likely to benefit from preventive strategies that are of uncertain value in the general population, such as prostate specific antigen (PSA) testing for prostate cancer.

Genetic Polymorphisms and Cancer Susceptibility

Polymorphisms Versus Mutations

Highly penetrant mutations, such as those in the BRCA1 or hMSH2 gene, are the most prominent examples of genetic traits causing a cancer predisposition. However, polymorphisms, or common genetic variants, may also cause an increased risk for disease (8,9). Only a few examples of this phenomenon have been documented, but with progress in mapping the human genome (10), more are likely to be found. Mutations that produce small increases in risk—that is, low-penetrance mutations—are also likely to be found. The distinction between a polymorphism and a low-penetrance mutation is somewhat arbitrary, and is based on prevalence: Genetic alterations are generally considered polymorphisms if their prevalence is greater than 1%.

The number of cancer cases caused by genetic polymorphisms and low-penetrance mutations (in combination with environmental exposures) is likely to be much higher than the number of hereditary cases caused by mutations of high-penetrance mutations, (3,4,11) because the latter are much less common in the population than are genetic polymorphisms that may be linked to cancer.

Three multiple gene "superfamilies" (cytochrome P450s, N-acetyltransferase, and glutathione-S-transferase genes) are briefly described below because of their importance to cancer genetics and public health. These polymorphically expressed genes may be positively (or inversely) associated with susceptibility to cancer and to several other diseases because of their important role in the detoxification (or activation) of xenobiotics and environmental chemicals (9,10). Studies that have examined associations with genetic polymorphisms and specific cancer sites (for example, breast, colorectal, and lung) are discussed later in this chapter.

Cytochrome P450 Enzymes

Cytochrome P450 enzymes are a multiple-gene "superfamily" that plays an important role in the detoxification of xenobiotics such as polycyclic aromatic hydrocarbons, benzo(a)pyrene, arylamines, and heterocyclic amines (12). Although P450 cytrochromes provide a line of defense against exposure to environmental chemicals, carcinogens may be activated by P450 metabolism. Cytochrome P450 enzymes are primarily expressed in the liver and in other tissues (8,12). Of these, the CYP1A1 gene (aryl hydrocarbon hydroxylase genotype), located on chromosome 15q, codes for aryl hydrocarbon hydroxylase (AHH) (8). The AHH catalyzes the mono-oxygenation of polycyclic aromatic hydrocarbons to phenolic products and epoxides that may be carcinogenic. The CYP2D6 gene (debrisoquine hydroxylase genotype) is located on chromosome 22q and codes for debrisoquine hydroxylase (8,12). Debrisoquine hydroxylase metabolizes a variety of drugs and other xenobiotics. Like other polymorphically expressed P450 enzymes, it may activate procarcinogens or, conversely, detoxify carcinogens (8).

N-*Acetyltransferase-1 and -2*

The *N*-acetyltransferase-1 (NAT1) and *N*-acetyltransferase-2 (NAT2) genes are located on chromosome 8q (8). Both are polymorphically expressed in a variety of tissues. The NAT2 detoxifies or, conversely, activates aromatic amines found in tobacco smoke such as 4-aminobiphenyl (13). Both phenotypic assays and genotypic assays for NAT2 can be used to classify individuals as rapid or slow acetylators.

Glutathione-S-*Transferase*

The glutathione-*S*-transferase-M1(GSTM1) gene is located on chromosome 1 and the gene for glutathione-*S*-transferase-T1 (GSTT1) is located on chromosome 11q (8). Glutathione-*S*-transferases detoxify a variety of carcinogens and cytotoxic drugs (for example, benzo(*a*)pyrene, monohalomethanes, and solvents) by catalyzing the conjugation of a glutathione moiety to the substrate (14). The incorporation of glutathione increases the molecule's water solubility and excretability (8). Individuals who are homozygous carriers of deletions in the GSTM1 or GSTT1 genes may have a higher risk of cancer because of their impaired ability to metabolize and eliminate carcinogens (14).

Breast and Ovarian Cancer Susceptibility Genes

Breast cancer is the most common cancer among U.S. women (15). For 1998, about 178,700 new cases will be diagnosed and 43,500 women will die from the disease (15). Although less common than breast cancer, ovarian cancer is also an important cause of premature mortality and morbidity in women. Two of the strongest risks factors for breast cancer are age and family history (16,17). Women who have a first-degree relative with breast cancer have a twofold to threefold increased risk of developing breast cancer. However, the degree of risk is greatest when the affected relative is diagnosed at a young age and at or near average risk when the affected relative is elderly at the time of diagnosis. Approximately 20% of breast cancer patients have a family history of the disease (18). Of these cases, only a small minority have features characteristic of high-risk families, such as early age at onset, bilaterality, and occurrence in multiple generations (19).

Breast cancer is likely to be etiologically heterogenous, as are other chronic diseases (23). However, the overall contribution of genetic factors to these cancers is likely to be considerable. Mutations in the BRCA1 and BRCA2 genes are well-established but rare causes of increased cancer susceptibility (3). Other genetic traits, such as ATM gene mutations and genetic polymorphisms, are likely to account for a genetic predisposition to breast cancer in a larger number of people, though their effect on individual risk may be smaller (3,16).

BRCA1 and BRCA2 Gene Mutations

The BRCA1 gene, on chromosome 17, and the BRCA2 gene, on chromosome 13, were initially identified through linkage studies in families with early-onset familial breast and ovarian cancer (20,21). Multiple different BRCA1 and BRCA2 mutations have been identified in such families. These advances led to the rapid development and commercialization of genetic tests for breast cancer susceptibility.

Laboratory Testing for BRCA1 and BRCA2 Gene Mutations. Because of the heterogeneity of BRCA1 and BRCA2 mutations, laboratory testing for all possible mutations is challenging. False-positive results may occur as a result of benign polymorphisms that are not associated with an increased risk for breast cancer (30). Most of these are missense mutations that do not result in a change in protein structure. Frame-shift or nonsense mutations, which account for about 90% of known BRCA1 mutations, are assumed to predispose to disease because of their effect on protein structure; most produce truncation of the protein product (22). False-negative results of genetic testing may also occur, because testing for hundreds of mutations is not practical with current technology. Some mutations in families with a cancer predisposition linked to a specific BRCA locus remain to be identified, possibly because they occur in noncoding regions of the gene.

Several methods can be used to detect mutations. Direct DNA sequencing can detect sequence variation. Manual sequencing is labor-intensive for a large gene such as BRCA1 or BRCA2 but rarely misses mutations in the coding sequence (23). Single-strand conformation polymorphism (SSCP) assay does not detect all sequence changes but can detect most DNA sequence variation; fragments that have shifted mobility on SSCP gels can then be sequenced to determine the exact nature of the DNA sequence variation (23). Once a mutation is known, allele-specific oligonucleotide hybridization can be used to rapidly screen many samples for that same mutation.

Clinical Significance of BRCA1 and BRCA2 Gene Mutations. Nearly all published studies of mutations in the BRCA1 and BRCA2 genes have involved members of high-risk families. Research entry criteria have typically included multiple family members with early age at onset of cancer or multiple tumors, and pedigrees meeting stringent criteria for autosomal dominant inheritance of cancer predisposition (24). Women from such cancer-prone families who test positive for a BRCA1 or BRCA2 gene mutation may have very high lifetime risks of cancer. Estimates of the penetrance in these high-risk families indicate that the lifetime risk of breast cancer in mutation carriers is similar for both genes (84% cumulative risk by age 70 for BRCA2 compared to 85% for BRCA1) (24,25), but that the risk of early breast cancer is some-what lower for BRCA2 (28% cumulative risk by age 50 compared to 51% for BRCA1). The estimated risk of ovarian cancer is also lower for BRCA2 (27% cumulative risk by age 70 compared to 66% for BRCA1). Men who are carriers of mutant BRCA1 and BRCA2 alleles are at increased risk for prostate cancer and also can transmit the cancer susceptibility gene mutation to their children (25). Breast cancer in men has been seen in association with mutations from both genes, but are more commonly found with BRCA2 mutations. The cancer risk for BRCA2 carriers may also include pancreatic cancer (25).

Carrier Frequency of BRCA1 and BRCA2 Gene Mutations. Using infer-ential procedures, Struewing et al. (26) estimated that the overall carrier fre-quency of BRCA1 gene mutations is 1 in 500 in the general U.S. population (95% confidence interval [CI]: 1 in 300 to 1 in 800). A similar estimate (1 in 833, or between 1 in 500 and 1 in 2000) was obtained by Ford et al. (27).

Population-based studies indicate that BRCA1 and BRCA2 mutations are a rare cause of breast cancer. Studies in North Carolina and Washington found low rates of BRCA1 mutations among women with breast cancer. In the North Carolina study disease-related BRCA1 mutations occurred in 3.3% of white breast cancer patients of all ages (95% CI = 0%–7.2%) and in 0% in black breast cancer patients (28). Young age at diagnosis by itself did not predict BRCA1 carrier status in this population. In white women, the prevalence of BRCA1 mutations was increased among cases with a family history of ovarian cancer or of four or more relatives with breast cancer (with or without a family history of ovarian cancer) (28). The Washington study found BRCA1 muta-tions in 12 of 193 women (6.2%) with breast cancer before age 35, unselected for family history (29).

Similarly, among women with early breast cancer identified through a reg-istry in the United Kingdom, mutations of BRCA1 or BRCA2 were found in only 5.9% of those diagnosed before age 36 and in only 4.1% of women between the ages of 36 and 45 (30). Because some mutations may be missed by current molecular techniques, investigators estimated that the true per-centages of mutation carriers were 9.4% and 6.6%, respectively, for the two age groups; even with this correction, BRCA1 and BRCA2 mutations accounted for only a small proportion of breast cancer cases (30).

Some BRCA1 and BRCA2 mutations occur with increased frequency among certain ethnic groups. The 185delAG mutation in the BRCA1 gene and the 6174delT mutation in the BRCA2 gene are each found in about 1% of persons of Ashkenazi Jewish descent (26,31,32). The 999del5 mutation in the BRCA2 gene occurs in about 0.6% of the general population of Iceland (33). All these mutations have been found in cancer-prone families; they have also been found in cancer patients with less dramatic family histories of cancer. Estimates of penetrance for the mutations found in Ashkenazi Jewish populations, derived from a volunteer survey and from clinical case series, indicate a lifetime risk of breast cancer of 37% to 56% (34–36). The 6174delT mutation has been observed less frequently than 185delAG among Jewish women with early-onset breast cancer, so it may be less penetrant at early ages (26,31,32). A population-based study of the 999del5 mutation in Iceland indicates a lifetime risk of breast cancer of 36% (33).

Interactions of BRCA1 and BRCA2 Gene Mutations with Modifiable Risk Factors for Breast Cancer. The variable age at onset of hereditary breast cancer and the incomplete penetrance of BRCA1 or BRCA2 gene mutations suggest that other host or environmental factors may modify the expression of these traits (37). Data are scant on the role of environmental risk factors for breast cancer among women with BRCA1 or BRCA2 gene mutations. For example, the risks and benefits of estrogen replacement therapy or oral contraceptives in women who carry these cancer susceptibility gene mutations are largely unknown (38), although one study found that women carrying BRCA1 or BRCA2 mutations experienced a reduction on ovarian cancer risk with oral contraceptive use, similar to the risk reduction seen among women in the general population (39). Data are also lacking about the value of lifestyle modifications, such as a low-fat diet, adequate intake of vegetables and fruit, and regular exercise for these women.

Also, uncertainty exists about treatment recommendations for women with BRCA1 or BRCA2 gene mutations. The only available means of primary prevention identified so far are prophylactic mastectomy and oophorectomy. The value of chemopreventive therapy, such as tamoxifen or raloxifene, in women who carry these breast and ovarian cancer gene mutations is unknown. A task force convened by the NIH Cancer Genetics Studies Consortium (CGSC) suggested annual mammography and annual or semiannual clinical breast examination, beginning at age 25 to 35 years, for women who have BRCA1 and BRCA2 mutations, but noted that these recommendations are based upon expert opinion and are not of proven benefit (38). The CGSC task force also recommended ovarian cancer screening with pelvic ultrasound and serum CA-125 measurements (38), again based on expert opinion. Research aimed at improved measures to reduce risk in genetically susceptible individuals was identified as a high priority by the task force (38).

ATM Gene Mutations

Ataxia-telangiectasia (A-T) is an autosomal recessive neurologic syndrome associated with unusual sensitivity to ionizing radiation (40,41). Homozygotes have about a 100-fold greater risk of cancer (mostly leukemia, lymphoma, and other cancers arising in childhood and adolescence) as compared with the general population (41,42). Women who are heterozygous carriers of mutations in the gene for A-T (referred to as the ATM gene) have been reported to have an increased risk of breast cancer (40,43). Easton (43) obtained a pooled relative risk estimate from four studies of 3.9 (95% CI 2.1 to 7.2). More recent studies that have employed molecular techniques have provided inconsistent evidence of a role for ATM gene mutations in patients with breast cancer. Estimates of the heterozygote frequency of ATM gene mutations in the general population, obtained using estimates of the total number of individuals with A-T in the population, have ranged from 0.5% to 2.8% (43,44). The ATM gene was cloned and sequenced in 1995 after the disease was mapped to a region of chromosome 11 in linkage studies (45). More than 100 mutations of the ATM gene have been reported to date.

Public Health Impact of ATM Gene Mutations. Data on the association between ATM mutations and breast cancer are conflicting. Swift et al. (46) examined cancer incidence and mortality among 1599 adult blood relatives of patients with A-T and 821 of their spouses, in a sample of 161 families with A-T. The estimated risk of cancer of all types among heterozygous carriers of ATM gene mutations, as compared with noncarriers, was 3.8 in men and 3.5 in women ($p < 0.005$). The relative risk of breast cancer among women was 5.1 ($p < 0.01$) (46).

In a series of unrelated breast cancer cases with a family history of breast cancer and/or a family history of tumors previously associated with A-T homozygosity or heterozygosity, 3 of 88 (3.4%) of the breast cancer patients had a germ-line mutation in the ATM gene (47). Athma et al. (48) determined the ATM gene carrier status of 775 blood relatives in 99 A-T families using DNA linkage studies. They found 33 women with breast cancer who could be genotyped; of these, 25 were ATM heterozygotes compared with an expected number of 14.9 (odds ratio = 3.8, 95% CI 1.7 to 8.4) (48). For the 21 breast cancers with onset before age 60, the odds ratio (OR) was 2.9 (95% CI 1.1 to 7.6) and for the 12 cases with onset at age 60 or older, the OR was 6.4 (95% CI 1.4 to 28.8).

Conversely, in a study of 401 women with early-onset breast cancer (onset before the age of 40), using a protein-truncation assay, Fitzgerald et al. (49) found no evidence for a role for the ATM gene in the cases studied. Only two mutations (representing 0.5% of the cases) were found in the ATM gene, as compared with only 1% (2 of 202) of the convenience (blood donor) controls (49).

One possible explanation for these conflicting findings across different studies is that ATM gene mutations confer susceptibility to breast cancer only in later life, or only in combination with an exposure such as ionizing radiation (50). False-negative test results or chance variation could also account for this inconsistency.

Polymorphisms Associated with Breast Cancer Risk

The *N*-acetyltransferase-2 genetic polymorphisms have been examined in relation to cigarette smoking and breast cancer susceptibility in women

(13,50–53). No consistent pattern has emerged. In a study by Ambrosone et al. (13), risk for breast cancer was increased among cigarette smokers having the slow acetylator genotype.

Genes that code for cytochrome P450 enzymes involved in the metabolism and transport of estrogen may influence breast cancer risk in women (11). For example, the CYP17 A2/A2 and A2/A1 genotypes have been associated with a young age at first menstruation and an increased risk for breast cancer (54). In a nested case-control study of Asian, African-American, and Latino women in Los Angeles and Hawaii, the OR associated with the A2 allele was 2.5 (95% CI 1.07–5.94) for regional or metastatic breast cancer (54). Because the allele is common in the population (roughly 40%), the risk for breast cancer attributable to this genetic polymorphism may be substantial (perhaps as high as 29% if preliminary findings are confirmed).

No consistent pattern has emerged from molecular epidemiology studies of breast cancer that examined associations with CYP1A1, CYP2D6, or GSTM1 (8), perhaps because of ethnic differences in the frequencies of these alleles or population differences in other risk factors for breast cancer (55).

Colorectal Cancer Susceptibility Genes

Colorectal cancer is one of the most common cancers among U.S. men and women (15). In 1998, an estimated 131,600 new cases will be diagnosed, and 27,900 men and 28,600 women will die from the disease. About 95% of colorectal cancer cases are sporadic and occur outside of the well-described syndromes (56). About 10% of U.S. adults have a first-degree relative with a history of colonic cancer. Such persons have a twofold to threefold increased risk of developing colon cancer (57). Most people with a family history of colorectal cancer lack the pedigree characteristics of autosomal dominant inheritance of cancer predisposition (56). Further, colorectal cancer, similar to other chronic diseases, is likely to have multiple causes, and no single gene is likely to account for a significant attributable fraction of colorectal cancer cases.

The inherited syndromes of colorectal cancer can be roughly divided into those that exhibit colonic polyposis (e.g., familial adenomatous polyposis [FAP] and related syndromes) and those that do not (56–58). The nonpolyposis syndromes include hereditary nonpolyposis colorectal cancer (HNPCC). Those with the nonpolyposis syndromes may have some adenomatous polyps, but these are fewer (56). While the adenomatous polyposis syndromes account for only about 0.5% of colonic cancer cases, the nonpolyposis syndromes may account for 5% or more (56). Familial cases outside of the syndromes may account for 10% to 30% of colonic cancer cases.

Familial Adenomatous Polyposis

Familial adenomatous polyposis (FAP) is an autosomal dominantly inherited disease that occurs in only about 1 in 10,000 people (56). Individuals with this condition develop hundreds to thousands of adenomatous polyps of the colon at a young age, and colonic cancer occurs at an average age of 39 years (57). Total colectomy and mucosal proctectomy is recommended because of the extreme risk for colonic cancer (57). The disease is caused by highly penetrant mutations of the adenomatous polyposis coli (APC) tumor suppressor gene on the long arm of chromosome 5. Individuals in most families with FAP have distinct mutations of the APC gene, and these mutations are almost always associated with truncation of the APC protein (i.e., frameshift or nonsense mutations). Some APC mutations cause additional distinctive clinical features in addition to polyposis (56).

Hereditary Nonpolyposis Colorectal Cancer (HNPCC)

HNPCC, which is much more common than FAP, also occurs in an autosomal dominant fashion (58). HNPCC affects about 1 in every 200 to 400 people in the United States, which makes it one of the most common autosomal dominantly inherited diseases (59). Colon cancer occurs at an average age of 45 years in these individuals (56). The clinical criteria for diagnosis of HNPCC are three family members who have colon cancer (two of whom are first-degree relatives of the third person), colon cancer cases spanning at least two generations, and at least one case diagnosed before age 50 (58). In addition to an increased risk of colorectal cancer, women with HNPCC have an increased risk of endometrial cancer, and other cancers, including ovarian and urinary tract cancers, have been observed in some families (60).

The discovery of DNA abnormalities associated with genomic instability (referred to as *microsatellite instability*) in people with HNPCC led to findings of a defect in the DNA mismatch repair system (61). The hMSH2 mismatch repair gene was identified and cloned in 1993, shortly after a region on chromosome 2p was associated with HNPCC (62,63). A second mismatch repair gene associated with colorectal cancer, hMLH1, was subsequently identified on chromosome 3p (64).

It is now known that HNPCC is caused by germline mutations of any of four (or more) DNA mismatch repair genes (hMSH2, hMLH1, PMS1, and PMS2; others may exist). The first two of these genes account for about 80% to 90% of HNPCC cases, and the others account for only a small fraction of cases (65,66). Linkage and mutational analyses have suggested that hMSH2 is the gene most commonly associated with HNPCC, accounting for 50% to 60% of HNPCC cases; hMLH1 accounts for an additional 30% of HNPCC cases (67). These genes code for proteins that normally repair mutations introduced by the DNA polymerase during cell replication. Mismatch repair dysfunction accelerates the accumulation of mutations in tumor suppressor genes and oncogenes (e.g., *ras*, APC, and p53), thereby speeding the development of malignancy (67,68).

Estimates of the cancer risks associated with hMSH2 and hMLH1 mutations are derived from families characterized by an early age of onset and/or multiple tumors and that meet stringent criteria for HNPCC established for research purposes (60,69). Individuals from families with HNPCC (including those who test positive for a hMSH2 or hMLH1 gene mutation) may have a cumulative risk for colorectal cancer as high as 35% by age 50 and 80% by age 70 (60,67). However, such estimates may be biased upward, because the people selected for study had a family history of cancer. Estimates of the carrier frequency of hMSH2 and hMLH1 gene mutations among those who do not have a family history of colorectal cancer are currently lacking.

Because of the heterogeneity of hMSH2 and hMLH1 mutations, laboratory testing for all possible mutations is difficult for those not from families at high risk for colorectal cancer. False-positive results may occur as a result of missense mutations that are not associated with an increased risk for colorectal cancer. Frameshift or nonsense mutations are likely to predispose carriers to disease (22). False-negative results will also occur in population screening as tests for all possible hMSH2 and hMLH1 mutations are not feasible on a large-scale basis.

Polymorphisms Associated with Colorectal Cancer Risk

Genetic polymorphisms might account for why some people are more sensitive than others to environmental carcinogens or cancer promoters associated with colorectal cancer, such as a diet high in red meat and low in fiber (4). In the Physicians' Health Study, for example, men with the homozygous mutation of the gene associated with reduced activity of 5-methyltetrahydrofolate, the primary circulating form of folate, had half the risk for colorectal cancer of men with the homozygous normal or heterozygous genotypes (70). Among men who drank little or no alcohol, those with the homozygous mutation genotype had an eightfold lower risk than did those with the homozygous normal genotype (OR 0.12, 95% CI 0.03–0.57), and those who were moderate drinkers had a twofold lower risk (OR 0.42, 95% CI 0.15–1.2) (70). These results suggest that the gene mutation reduces colorectal cancer risk and that high alcohol consumption or low folate intake may negate some of the protective effect.

Polymorphisms in *N*-acetyltransferase have also been examined in relation to cancer of the colon and rectum (71,72). This enzyme catalyzes the formation of mutagenic substances from foods such as cooked meat and fish. People in whom acetylation is fast are at increased risk for colorectal cancer in some but not all studies (71–73). Molecular epidemiology studies have also suggested that glutathione-*S*-transferase-M1 genotypes may be associated with susceptibility to colorectal cancer (14).

A polymorphism of the APC gene (I1307K), recently reported to be present in 1 in 17 Ashkenazi Jewish people, may be associated with an increased risk of colorectal cancer in that population (74). This mutation does not directly alter the function of the APC gene but appears to make it unstable and prone to acquire mutations during cell division. In the initial report, a risk relationship was suggested by differences in the frequency of the mutation among Ashkenazi Jewish controls and those with colorectal cancer identified in referral centers (6% vs. 10%) and also between controls and a small subset of case subjects who had a positive family history of colorectal cancer (6% vs. 28%). Additional studies are consistent with a weak association between this polymorphism and colorectal cancer as well as a potential association with breast or other cancers (75–77), but this association cannot yet be considered proven.

Lung Cancer Genetic Susceptibility

Lung cancer is a major public health problem and an important part of the worldwide pandemic of smoking-related death and disability. In 1998, an estimated 93,100 deaths from lung cancer will occur among men in the U.S., and an additional 67,000 deaths from lung cancer will occur among U.S. women (15). The overall contribution of genetic factors to lung cancer is difficult to discern because of the strong associations with cigarette smoking and other environmental exposures (78).

The familial aggregation of lung cancer, which has been well-documented by results obtained from several studies, is not fully explained by the familial aggregation of smoking (79,80). Although most segregation analyses of lung cancer have not provided strong evidence for cancer-predisposing mutations (80), a recent segregation analysis (81) in 337 extended pedigrees provided evidence that a mendelian gene is segregating in these families. The estimated frequency of the high-risk allele was 2%; carriers were estimated to have a RR of lung cancer of 17.3 compared with noncarriers (81). In a population study by Sellers et al. (82,83), the pattern of lung cancer occurrence in families with lung cancer was consistent with mendelian codominant inheritance for early age-at-onset of a rare autosomal gene.

Various studies have examined polymorphically expressed genes in relation to lung cancer risk including those that code for cytochrome P450 enzymes, *N*-acetyltransferases, and glutathione-*S*-transferases (8,78,84). These have included transitional studies of convenience samples of lung cancer cases and controls, and industry-based and population-based studies. Some transitional studies have examined both polymorphically expressed genes and genetic markers of exposure such as DNA adducts in relation to lung cancer risk (14,84).

Cytochrome P450 enzymes activate benzo(a)pyrene and may activate or metabolize other carcinogens found in cigarette smoke (8). Lung cancer cases have been reported to have higher levels of AHH activity as compared with controls, although negative results have been obtained in some studies (84). The results of more recent studies that have looked for associations with CYP1A1 genotypes have also been inconsistent, perhaps reflecting ethnic differences in the frequency of high-risk alleles. Kawajiri et al. (85) reported that Japanese patients with lung cancer were more likely to carry an isoleucine to valine mutation in the CYP1A1 locus. The Msp1 allele has also been associated with lung cancer in Japanese individuals. Studies in Caucasian populations have had negative results, however.

Poor metabolizers of debrisoquine, those unable to metabolize environmental agents via the CYP2D6 pathway, have been reported to have a higher risk of lung cancer, but the strength of the association with this phenotype has varied across studies, and some studies have failed to find an association (78). Some investigators have suggested an interactive effect with cigarette smoking (84). A consistent pattern has not emerged from more recent lung cancer studies that have looked for associations with CYP2D6 genotypes.

McWilliams et al. (86) carried out a meta-analysis of ten case-control studies of GSTM1 deficiency and lung cancer risk and obtained a pooled OR of 1.4 (95% 1.2–1.7). In their meta-analysis, an association was found for each of the three major histologic subtypes of lung cancer (squamous cell carcinoma, adenocarcinoma, and small cell lung cancer) (86). Studies to date have provided little evidence of an interactive effect between GSTM1 genotype and CYP1A1 in relation to lung cancer risk (14). Exposure to cigarette smoke and dietary factors such as low vitamin C intake may influence the importance of GSTM1 genotypes to lung cancer risk. Although the strength of the association between lung cancer and GSTM1 deficiency is likely to be modest at best, this gene could still account for a substantial number of lung cancer cases in the population because of the high frequency of GSTM1 deficiency in the general population.

Although N-acetyltransferase-2 detoxifies or activates aromatic amines found in tobacco smoke, studies of lung cancer have often failed to find an association with acetylator phenotype. Oyama et al. (87) examined NAT2 genotype in 124 Japanese patients with lung cancer and in 376 controls; the slow acetylator genotype was present in 17 (14%) of the lung cancer patients as compared with 40 (11%) of the controls (OR = 2.0; $p = 0.05$).

Somatic mutations such as $p53$ tumor suppressor genes and ras oncogenes are common in lung tumors and activation of myc oncogenes has been reported in small cell carcinomas of the lung (78). Tumorigenesis in the lung is likely to involve a complex series of molecular genetic changes leading to the transformation of normal cells to malignant cells. These genetic changes in the lung that occur during tumorigenesis are somatic events that may be partly a consequence of lung cancer rather than a cause (78).

Prostate Cancer Genetic Susceptibility

The public health burden of prostate cancer is substantial. In 1998, an estimated 184,500 new cases of prostate cancer and 39,200 deaths from prostate cancer occurred, making it the most frequent cancer in males (15). The incidence of prostate cancer is nearly twofold higher in African-American men than in Caucasian men, and mortality is similarly elevated. Environmental factors implicated as possible contributors to prostate cancer risk include high fat diet and vasectomy (88). A genetic contribution to prostate cancer risk has also been documented, but knowledge of the molecular genetics of prostate cancer is still limited.

As with breast and colon cancer, familial clustering of prostate cancer has been observed (89–91). A family history of a brother or father with prostate cancer increases the risk of prostate cancer two- to threefold, with the risk inversely related to the age of the affected relative (91–93). A family history of prostate cancer also increases risk of breast cancer in female relates (94). The association between prostate and breast cancer risks is explained in part by the increased risk of prostate cancer observed among male carriers of BRCA1 and BRCA2 mutations (25,95).

Families demonstrating autosomal dominant transmission of isolated susceptibility to prostate cancer have been observed, and they have been estimated to account for 9% of prostate cancer cases (90). Studies of such families have led to the identification of a possible genetic susceptibility locus on chromosome 1 (96,97), termed HPC1 (hereditary prostate cancer 1). No significant increases in breast cancer or other cancers were found in these families (98), suggesting that the genetic susceptibility conferred by mutations at this locus differs from that conferred by mutations in the BRCA1 and BRCA2 genes.

Linkage studies suggest the existence of other genetic loci potentially related to prostate cancer susceptibility on chromosomes 6 and 13 (99,100). In addition, polymorphisms in the steroid 5-alpha-reductase type II and androgen receptor genes have been postulated to contribute to prostate cancer risk (11). The genetic contribution to prostate cancer susceptibility thus appears to be complex. No role has yet been defined for genetic screening related to prostate cancer susceptibility.

Melanoma Genetic Susceptibility

The incidence of melanoma has increased markedly in the U.S. and in several other countries in recent decades (101). In 1998, an estimated 41,600 new cases were diagnosed in the U.S., and 4600 men and 2700 women died from the disease (15).

Ultraviolet radiation and intense intermittent Sun exposure resulting in sunburns in childhood are major environmental risk factors for melanoma that may interact with genetic influences. Risk factors for melanoma that have a genetic basis include family history, number of atypical nevi, and pigmentary traits such as blue eyes, fair or red hair, and pale complexion (101). Individuals who have one affected relative have about a twofold increased risk of melanoma; those with two affected relatives have about a fivefold increased risk (101). About 10% of cases occur in persons with a familial predisposition (102).

Genetic studies have suggested that the etiology of cutaneous malignant melanoma is heterogenous and complex. Dysplastic nevi syndrome (atypical mole syndrome phenotype) is a highly penetrant autosomal dominant disorder with underlying predisposition to melanoma (103). Some melanoma-prone families have been reported to have an excess of pancreatic cancer (104). In 1989, Bale et al. (105) reported evidence of linkage between the combined trait of dysplastic nevi and melanoma and genetic markers on the short arm of chromosome 1. More recent studies in other pedigrees have failed to confirm these findings, either for melanoma and dysplastic nevi combined or melanoma alone (101).

A linkage analysis in 11 cutaneous malignant melanoma pedigrees by Cannon-Albright et al. (106) provided strong evidence for a dominant, partially penetrant melanoma susceptibility locus on the short arm of chromosome 9. The gene penetrance was estimated to be 53% by age 80 years. Gene carriers had higher nevus counts and nevus densities (computed from mole size and number) than did those who were not carriers. Among gene carriers, those with melanoma had more sunlight exposure than did those without melanoma, suggesting a gene–environment interaction (107).

The CDKN2A tumor suppressor gene was localized on 9p21 in 1994 (108,109); that chromosomal region had previously been associated with malignant melanoma in linkage analyses and in loss of heterozygosity and cytogenetic studies. The CDKN2A gene codes for a low-molecular-weight cell cycle control protein, p16[INK4A], which inhibits excessive cell proliferation by inhibiting the activity of the cyclin D1-cyclin-dependent kinase 4 or 6 complex (102).

Germline mutations of the CDKN2A gene have been found in roughly one-fourth of melanoma-prone kindreds. In a recent population-based study in Stockholm, Sweden, investigators (110) found mutations of the CDKN2A gene in 7.8% of 64 families with two or more first-degree relatives with cutaneous malignant melanoma. No mutations were detected in 36 families with melanoma in more distant relatives. In 1996, a second melanoma susceptibility gene, CDK4, was identified on the long arm of chromosome 12, suggesting that there are diverse mechanisms of melanoma development in high-risk families. The CDK4 mutations are rare and have only been identified in a few families to date (107).

Conclusions

Studies of genetic susceptibility to common cancers highlight the need for additional population-based molecular epidemiologic research so as to better define the contribution of genetic factors to cancer, and to examine interactions with environmental factors amenable to preventive interventions. The etiology of most cancers is likely to be due to an interaction among a variety of genetic factors and nongenetic risk factors such as smoking, diet, and exogenous and endogenous hormones. As Rebbeck (14) observed:

> The etiology of most commonly occurring cancers cannot be explained by allelic variability at a single locus. Instead, the major burden of cancer in the general population probably results from the complex interactions of multiple genetic and environmental factors over time. An understanding of the interplay of xenobiotic exposures, endogenous physiology, and genetic variability at multiple loci will facilitate knowledge about cancer etiology and the identification of individuals who are at increased risk for developing cancer.

The literature summarized in this chapter highlights gaps in our present understanding of the genetics of common malignancies. Relatively few studies have looked for potential gene–environment interactions, explored associations between two or more genetic polymorphisms, or evaluated interactions between genetic polymorphisms and endogenous risk factors. Studies designed to answer such questions are now underway in Los Angeles, in Hawaii, in North Carolina, and in other localities (11,111). They are likely to be particularly informative because they target geographically defined populations that are racially and ethnically diverse, evaluate incident cancers, and have adequate power sizes to explore ethnic and racial differences in cancer susceptibility. Such research strategies represent an important new direction in cancer genetics.

References

1. Greenwald P. Introduction: history of cancer prevention and control. In: Greenwald P, Kramer BS, Weed DL (eds). Cancer prevention and control. New York: Marcel Dekker, 1995, pp. 1–7.

2. Khoury MJ. From genes to public health: the applications of genetic technology in disease prevention. Am J Public Health 1996;86:1717–1722.

3. Coughlin SS, Khoury MJ, Steinberg KK. BRCA1 and BRCA2 gene mutations and risk of breast cancer: public health perspectives. Am J Prev Med 1998;16:91–98.

4. Coughlin SS, Miller DS. Public health perspectives on testing for colorectal cancer susceptibility genes. Am J Prev Med 1998;16:99–104.

5. Coughlin SS. The intersection of genetics, public health, and preventive medicine (editorial). Am J Prev Med 1998;16:89–90.

6. National Society of Genetic Counselors. Predisposition genetic testing for late-onset disorders in adults: a position paper of the National Society of Genetic Counselors. JAMA 1997;278:1217–1220.

7. Swift M. Ionizing radiation, breast cancer, and ataxia-telangiectasia (editorial). J Natl Cancer Inst 1994;86:1571–1572.

8. Smith G, Stanley LA, Sim E, et al. Metabolic polymorphisms and cancer susceptibility. Cancer surveys. Vol. 25: Genetics and cancer: a second look. Imperial Cancer Research Fund. 1995:27–65.

9. Windmill KF, McKinnon RA, Zhu X, et al. The role of xenobiotic metabolizing enzymes in arylamine toxicity and carcinogenesis: functional and localization studies. Mut Res 1997;376:153–160.

10. Green ED, Waterston RH. The Human Genome Project: prospects and implications for clinical medicine. JAMA 1991;266:1966–1975.

11. Feigelsen HS, Ross RK, Yu MC, et al. Genetic susceptibility to cancer from exogenous and endogenous exposures. J Cell Biochem 1996;25(Suppl):15–22.

12. Strong LC, Amos CI. Inherited susceptibility. In: Schottenfeld D, Fraumeni JF Jr (eds). Cancer epidemiology and prevention (2nd ed). New York: Oxford University Press, 1996.

13. Ambrosone CB, Freudenheim JL, Graham S, et al. Cigarette smoking, N-acetytransferase-2 genetic polymorphisms and breast cancer risk. JAMA 1996;276:1494–1501.

14. Rebbeck TR. Molecular epidemiology of the human glutathione-S-transferase genotypes GSTM1 and GSTT1 in cancer susceptibility. Cancer Epidemiol Biomarkers Prev 1997;6:733–743.

15. Cancer facts and figures 1998, American Cancer Society, Atlanta, GA.

16. Newman B, Millikan RC, King M-C. Genetic epidemiology of breast and ovarian cancers. Epidemiol Rev 1997;19:69–79.

17. Mettlin C, Croghan I, Natarajan N, et al. The association of age and familial risk in a case-control study of breast cancer. Am J Epidemiol 1990;131:973–983.

18. Andersen TI. Genetic heterogeneity in breast cancer susceptibility. Acta Oncol 1996;35:407–410.

19. Xu CF, Solomon E. Mutations of the BRCA1 gene in human cancer. Semin Cancer Biol 1996;7:33–40.

20. Miki Y, Swensen J, Shattuck-Eidens D, et al. A strong candidate for the breast and ovarian cancer susceptibility gene BRCA1. Science 1994;266:66–71.

21. Wooster R, Neuhausen SL, Mangion J, et al. Localization of a breast cancer susceptibility gene, BRCA2, to chromosome 13q12–13. Science 1994;265:2088–2090.

22. Collins FS. BRCA1—lots of mutations, lots of dilemmas. N Engl J Med 1996;334:186–188.

23. Shattuck-Eidens D, McClure M, Simard J, et al. A collaborative survey of 80 mutations in the BRCA1 breast and ovarian cancer susceptibility gene. JAMA 1995;273:535–541.

24. Ford D, Easton DF, Stratton M, et al. Genetic heterogeneity and penetrance analysis of the BRCA1 and BRCA2 genes in breast cancer families. Am J Hum Genet 1998;62:676–689.

25. Easton DF, Steele L, Fields P, et al. Cancer risks in two large breast cancer families linked to BRCA2 on chromosome 13q12–13. Am J Hum Genet 1997;61:120–128.

26. Struewing JP, Abeliovich D, Peretz T, et al. The carrier frequency of the BRCA1 185delAG mutation is approximately 1% in Ashkenazi Jewish individuals (letter). Nat Genet 1995;11:198–200.

27. Ford D, Easton DF, Peto J. Estimates of the gene frequency of BRCA1 and its contribution to breast and ovarian cancer incidence. Am J Hum Genet 1995;57: 1457–1462.

28. Newman B, Mu H, Butler LM, et al. Frequency of breast cancer attributable to BRCA1 in a population-based series of American women. JAMA 1998;279:915–921.

29. Malone KE, Daling JR, Thompson JD, et al. BRCA1 mutations and breast cancer in the general population: analyses in women before age 35 years and in women before age 45 years with first-degree family history. JAMA 1998;279:922–929.

30. Peto J, Collins N, Barfoot R, et al. Prevalence of BRCA1 and BRCA2 gene mutations in patients with early-onset breast cancer. J Natl Cancer Inst 1999;91: 943–949.

31. Roa BB, Boyd AA, Volcik K, et al. Ashkenazi Jewish population frequencies for common mutations in BRCA1 and BRCA2. Nat Genet 1996;14:185–187.

32. Oddoux C, Struewing JP, Clayton CM, et al. The carrier frequency of BRCA2 6174delT mutation among Ashkenazi Jewish individuals is approximately 1%. Nat Genet 1996;14:188–190.

33. Thorlacius S, Struewing JP, Hartge P, et al. Population-based study of risk of breast cancer in carriers of BRCA2 mutation. Lancet 1998;352:1337–1339.

34. Struewing JP, Hartge P, Wacholder S, et al. The risk of cancer associated with specific mutations of BRCA1 and BRCA2 among Ashkenazi Jews. N Engl J Med 1997;336:1401–1408.

35. Fodor FH, Weston A, Bleiweiss IJ, et al. Frequency and carrier risk associated with common BRCA1 and BRCA2 mutations in Ashkenazi Jewish breast cancer patients. Am J Hum Genet 1998;63:45–51.

36. Levy-Lahad E, Catane R, Eisenberg S, et al. Founder BRCA1 and BRCA2 mutations in Ashkenazi Jews in Israel: frequency and differential penetrance in ovarian cancer and in breast–ovarian cancer families. Am J Hum Genet 1997;60:1059–1067.

37. Weber BL, Giusti RM, Liu ET. Developing strategies for intervention and prevention in hereditary breast cancer. J Natl Cancer Inst Monogr 1995;17:99–102.

38. Burke W, Daly M, Garber J, et al. Recommendations for follow-up care of individuals with an inherited predisposition to cancer: II. BRCA1 and BRCA2. JAMA 1997;277:997–1003.

39. Narod S, Risch H, Mosleshi R, et al., for the Hereditary Ovarian Cancer Study Group. Oral contraceptives and the risk of hereditary ovarian cancer. N Engl J Med 1998;339:424–428.

40. Swift M, Reitnauer PJ, Morrell D, et al. Breast and other cancers in families with ataxia-telangiectasia. N Engl J Med 1987;316:1289–1294.

41. Lavin MF, Shiloh Y. The genetic defect in ataxia-telangiectasia (review). Annu Rev Immunol 1997;15:177–202.

42. Morrell D, Cromartie E, Swift M. Mortality and cancer incidence in 263 patients with ataxia-telangiectasia. J Natl Cancer Inst 1986;77:89–92.

43. Easton DF. Cancer risks in A-T heterozygotes. Int J Radiat Biol 1994;66(6 Suppl):S177–182.

44. Swift M. The incidence and gene frequency of ataxia-telangiectasia in the United States. Am J Hum Genet 1986;39:573–583.

45. Rasio D, Negrini M, Croce CM. Genomic organization of the ATM locus involved in ataxia-telangiectasia. Cancer Res 1995;55:6053–6057.

46. Swift M, Morrell D, Massey RB, et al. Incidence of cancer in 161 families affected by ataxia-telangiectasia. N Engl J Med 1991;325:1831–1836.

47. Vorechovsky I, Luo L, Lindblom A, et al. ATM mutations in cancer families. Cancer Res 1996;56:4130–4133.

48. Athma P, Rappaport R, Swift M, et al. Molecular genotyping shows that ataxia-telangiectasia heterozygotes are predisposed to breast cancer. Cancer Genet Cytogenet 1996;92:130–134.

49. Fitzgerald MG, Bean JM, Heqde SR, et al. Heterozygous ATM mutations do not contribute to early onset of breast cancer. Nat Genet 1997;15:307–310.

50. Swift M. Ataxia telangiectasia and risk of breast cancer (letter). Lancet 1997; 350:739–740.

51. Ambrosone CB, Freudenheim JL, Marshall JR, et al. The association of poly-morphic N-acetyltransferase (NAT2) with breast cancer risk. Ann N Y Acad Sci 1995; 768:250–252.

52. Ladero JM, Fernandez MJ, Palmeiro R, et al. Hepatic acetylator polymorphism in breast cancer patients. Oncology 1987;44:341–344.

53. Agundez JA, Ladero JM, Olivera M, et al. Genetic analysis of the arylamine N-acetyltransferase polymorphism in breast cancer patients. Oncology 1995;52:7–11.

54. Feigelson HS, Coetzee GA, Kolonel LN, et al. A polymorphism in the CYP17 gene increases the risk of breast cancer. Cancer Res 1997;57:1063–1065.

55. Kelsey KT, Wiencke JK. Growing pains for the environmental genetics of breast cancer: observations on a study of the glutathione-S-transferases. J Natl Cancer Inst 1998;90:484–485.

56. Burt RW, Petersen GM. Familial colorectal cancer: diagnosis and management. In: Young GP, Rozen P, Levin B (eds). Prevention and early detection of colorectal cancer. London: Saunders, 1996, pp. 171–194.

57. Petersen GM. Genetic epidemiology of colorectal cancer. Eur J Cancer 1995;31A:1047–1050.

58. Lynch HT, Smyrk T, Lynch JF. Overview of natural history, pathology, molecular genetics and management of HNPCC (Lynch syndrome). Int J Cancer 1996;69:38–43.

59. Han HJ, Yuan Y, Ku JL, et al. Germline mutations of hMLH1 and hMSH2 genes in Korean hereditary nonpolyposis colorectal cancer (letter). J Natl Cancer Inst 1996; 88:1317–1319.

60. Vasen HF, Wijnen JT, Menko FH, et al. Cancer risk in families with hereditary nonpolyposis colorectal cancer diagnosed by mutation analysis. Gastroenterology 1996;110:1020–1027.

61. Marra G, Boland CR. Hereditary nonpolyposis colorectal cancer: the syndrome, the genes, and historical perspectives. J Natl Cancer Inst 1995;87:1114–1125.

62. Fishel R, Lescoe MK, Rao MR, et al. The human mutator gene homolog MSH2 and its association with hereditary nonpolyposis colon cancer. Cell 1993;75:1027–1038.

63. Leach FS, Nicolaides N, Papadopoulos N, et al. Mutations of a mutS homolog in hereditary nonpolyposis colorectal cancer. Cell 1993;75:1215–1225.

64. Bronner CE, Baker SM, Morrison PT, et al. Mutation in the DNA mismatch

repair gene homologue hMLH1 is associated with hereditary nonpolyposis colon cancer. Nature 1994;368:258–261.

65. Aaltonen LA, Peltomaki P. Genes involved in hereditary nonpolyposis colorectal cancer (review). Anticancer Res 1994;14(4B):1657–1660.

66. Nystrom-Lahti M, Moisio AL, Hofstra RM, et al. DNA mismatch repair gene mutations in 55 kindreds with verified or putative hereditary non-polyposis colorectal cancer. Hum Mol Genet 1996;5:763–769.

67. Kolodner RD, Hall NR, Lipford J, et al. Structure of the human MLH1 locus and analysis of a large hereditary nonpolyposis colorectal carcinoma kindred for MLH1 mutations. Cancer Res 1995;55:242–248.

68. Cho KR, Vogelstein B. Genetic alterations in the adenoma-carcinoma sequence. Cancer 1992;70(6 Suppl):1727–1731.

69. Voskuil DW, Vasen HFA, Kampman E, et al. Colorectal cancer risk in HNPCC families: development during lifetime and in successive generations. Int J Cancer 1997;72:205–209.

70. Ma J, Stampfer MJ, Giovannucci E, et al. Methylenetetrahydrofolate reductase polymorphism, dietary interactions, and risk of colorectal cancer. Cancer Res 1997; 57:1098–1102.

71. Bell DA, Stephens EA, Castranio T, et al. Polyadenylation polymorphism in the acetyltransferase 1 gene (NAT1) increases risk of colorectal cancer. Cancer Res 1995;55:3537–3542.

72. Shibuta K, Nakashima T, Abe M, et al. Molecular genotyping for N-acetylation polymorphism in Japanese patients with colorectal cancer. Cancer 1994;74:3108–3112.

73. Roberts-Thomson IC, Ryan P, Khoo KK, et al. Diet, acetylator phenotype, and risk of colorectal neoplasia. Lancet 1996;347:1372–1374.

74. Laken SJ, Petersen G, Bruber SB, et al. Familial colorectal cancer in Ashkenazim due to a hypermutable tract in APC. Nat Genet 1997;17:79–83.

75. Frayling IM, Beck NE, Ilyas M, et al. The APC variants I1307K and E1317Q are associated with colorectal tumors, but not always with a family history. Proc Natl Acad Sci U S A 1998;95:10722–10727.

76. Woodage T, King SM, Wacholder S, et al. The APC I1307K allele and cancer risk in a community-based study of Ashkenazi Jews. Nat Genet 1998;20:62–65.

77. Abrahamson J, Moslei R, Vesprini D, et al. No association of the I1307K APC allele with ovarian cancer risk in Ashkenazi Jews. Cancer Res 1998;58:2919–2922.

78. Blot WJ, Fraumeni JF Jr. Cancer of the lung and pleura. In: Schottenfeld D, Fraumeni JF Jr (eds). Cancer epidemiology and prevention (2nd ed). New York: Oxford University Press, 1996, pp. 652–653.

79. Osann KE. Lung cancer in women: the importance of smoking, family history of cancer, and medical history of respiratory disease. Cancer Res 1991;51:4893–4897.

80. Yang P, Schwartz AG, McAllister AE, et al. Genetic analysis of families with nonsmoking lung cancer probands. Genetic Epidemiol 1997;14:181–197.

81. Gauderman WJ, Morrison JL, Carpenter CL, et al. Analysis of gene-smoking interaction in lung cancer. Genetic Epidemiol 1997;14:199–214.

82. Sellers TA, Bailey-Wilson JE, Elston RC, et al. Evidence for mendelian inheritance in the pathogenesis of lung cancer. J Natl Cancer Inst 1990;82:1272–1279.

83. Sellers TA, Bailey-Wilson JE, Potter JD, et al. Effect of cohort differences in smoking prevalence on models of lung cancer susceptibility. Genet Epidemiol 1992;9: 261–272.

84. Economou P, Samet JM, Lechner JF. Familial and genetic factors in the

pathogenesis of lung cancer. In: Samet JM (ed). Epidemiology of lung cancer. New York: Marcel Dekker, 1994, pp. 353–396.

85. Kawajiri K, Nakachi K, Imai K, et al. Identification of genetically high risk individuals to lung cancer by DNA polymorphisms of the cytochrome P450IA1 gene. FEBS Lett 1990;263:131–133.

86. McWilliams JE, Sanderson BJS, Harris EL, et al. Glutathione-S-transferase M1 (GSTM1) deficiency and lung cancer risk. Cancer Epidemiol Biomarkers Prev 1995;4: 589–594.

87. Oyama T, Kawamoto T, Mizoue T, et al. N-acetylation polymorphism in patients with lung cancer and its association with p53 gene mutation. Anticancer Res 1997;17:577–582.

88. Pienta K, Esper PS. Risk factors for prostate cancer. Ann Intern Med 1993;118:793–803.

89. Steinberg GD, Carter BS, Beaty TH, et al. Family history and the risk of prostate cancer. Prostate 1990;17:337–347.

90. Carter BS, Beaty TH, Steinberg GD, et al. Mendelian inheritance of familial prostate cancer. Proc Natl Acad Sci USA 1992;89:3367–3371.

91. Ghadrian P, Howe GR, Hislop TG, et al. Family history of prostate cancer: a multi-center case-control study in Canada. Int J Cancer 1997;70:679–681.

92. Gronberg H, Damber L, Damber JE. Familial prostate cancer in Sweden: a nationwide register cohort study. Cancer 1996;77:138–143.

93. Cannon L, Bishop DT, Skolnick M, et al. Genetic epidemiology of prostate cancer in the Utah Mormon genealogy. Cancer Surv 1982;1:47–69.

94. Sellers TA, Potter JD, Rich SS, et al. Familial clustering of breast and prostate cancers and risk of postmenopausal breast cancer. J Natl Cancer Inst 1994;86: 1860–1865.

95. Ford D, Easton DF, Bishop DT, et al. Risk of cancer in BRCA1-mutation carriers. Lancet 1994;343:692–695.

96. Smith JR, Freije D, Carpten JD, et al. Major susceptibility locus for prostate cancer on chromosome 1 suggested by a genome-wide search. Science 1996;274: 1371–1374.

97. Cooney KA, McCarthy JD, Lange E, et al. Prostate cancer susceptibility locus on chromosome 1q: a confirmatory study. J Natl Cancer Inst 1997;89:955–959.

98. Gronberg H, Isaacs SD, Smith JR, et al. Characteristics of prostate cancer in families potentially linked to the hereditary prostate cancer 1 (HPC1) locus. JAMA 1997;278:1251–1255.

99. Cooney KA, Wetzel JC, Merajver SD, et al. Distinct regions of alleleic loss on 13q in prostate cancer. Cancer Res 1996;56:1142–1145.

100. Cooney KA, Wetzel JC, Consolino CM, et al. Identification and characterization of proximal 6q deletions in prostate cancer. Cancer Res 1996;56:4150–4153.

101. Armstrong BK, English DR. Cutaneous malignant melanoma. In: Schottenfeld D, Fraumeni JF Jr (eds). Cancer epidemiology and prevention (2nd ed). New York: Oxford University Press, 1996, pp. 1282–1312.

102. Goldstein AM, Tucker MA. Screening for CDKN2A mutations in hereditary melanoma. J Natl Cancer Inst 1997;89:676–678.

103. Albino AP. Genes involved in melanoma susceptibility and progression. Curr Opin Oncol 1995;7:162–169.

104. Fraser MC, Goldstein AM, Tucker MA. The genetics of melanoma. Semin Oncol Nurs 1997;13:108–114.

105. Bale SJ, Dracopoli NC, Tucker MA, et al. Mapping the gene for hereditary

cutaneous malignant melanoma-dysplastic nevus to chromosome 1p. N Engl J Med 1989;320:1367–1372.

106. Cannon-Albright LA, Godgar DE, Meyer LJ, et al. Assignment of a locus for familial melanoma, MLM, to chromosome 9p13–p22. Science 1992;258:1148–1152.

107. Greene MH. Genetics of cutaneous melanoma and nevi. Mayo Clin Proc 1997;72:467–474.

108. Kamb A, Shattuck-Eidens D, Eeles R, et al. Analysis of CDKN2 (MTS1) as a candidate for the chromosome 9p melanoma susceptibility locus (MLM). Nature Genet 1994;8:22–26.

109. Nobari T, Miura K, Wu DJ, et al. Deletions of the cyclin-dependent kinase-4 inhibitor gene in multiple human cancers. Nature 1994;368:753–756.

110. Platz A, Hansson J, Mansson-Brahme E, et al. Screening of germline mutations in the CDKN2A and CDKN2B genes in Swedish families with hereditary cutaneous melanoma. J Natl Cancer Inst 1997;89:676–678.

111. Newman B, Moorman PG, Millikan R, et al. The Carolina Breast Cancer Study: integrating population-based epidemiology and molecular biology. Breast Cancer Res Treat 1995;35:51–60.

10

Public health assessment of genetic susceptibility to infectious diseases: Malaria, Tuberculosis, and HIV

Janet M. McNicholl, Marie V. Downer, Michael Aidoo, Thomas Hodge, and Venkatachalam Udhayakumar

Our understanding of the host genetic factors that influence susceptibility to and the course of infectious diseases is growing rapidly. Even for the most common pathogens, however, we have an incomplete understanding of all the important genes. As sequencing of the more than 100,000 human genes continues and as technologies advance, new discoveries about host genes and their role in infectious diseases are made almost daily. Translating this knowledge into public health actions, particularly those aimed at combating and controlling infectious diseases, is a major challenge. This chapter focuses on this downstream phase of genetics, particularly on how new knowledge can be integrated into existing public health programs and strategies.

It is likely that no one model for this translation phase will serve all public health agencies because the issues surrounding the prevention and control of infectious diseases vary among and within countries. One approach is to integrate host genetic factors into the classical three steps of primary, secondary, and tertiary prevention (1,2). This prevention model is adequate for many diseases, particularly those of a chronic nature. However, it is not comprehensive enough to capture the multiple requirements of an infectious disease public health program. A second approach is to integrate genetics into the areas outlined in the U.S. preventive strategic plan addressing emerging infectious diseases, which was developed by the Centers for Disease Control and Prevention (CDC) (3). This plan emphasizes four areas: (*1*) surveillance and response to identified infectious disease problems; (*2*) applied research integrating laboratory science and epidemiology to optimize public health practice; (*3*) infrastructure and training to support surveillance and research; and (*4*) prevention and control programs. These four areas overlap strongly with the four areas of emphasis outlined in the CDC's strategic plan for translating genetic advances into public health action (4). Because the CDC's plan for infectious diseases has been implemented in the United States for 4 years and has been widely adopted by many international agencies for the control and prevention of infectious diseases globally, we will use this plan to consider how new genetic knowledge may be integrated into infectious disease public health practice. Also, because infectious diseases are worldwide problems, we will examine aspects of host genes and infectious diseases relevant both in the United States and globally.

Three infectious diseases, malaria, tuberculosis (TB), and HIV/acquired immunodeficiency syndrome (AIDS) will be discussed in the context of this paradigm. These diseases are among the top five leading infectious causes of deaths (5), and they are considered emerging or reemerging threats. In addition, and perhaps because of their global impact, more is known about the host genetic factors that influence susceptibility to and severity of these than of other diseases. For each of these pathogens, at least three different host genes that influence disease are known and, frequently, the same gene impacts more than one disease. Many parts of the world, particularly sub-Saharan Africa, have a high prevalence of the three pathogens. Because of its impact on the immune system, infection with HIV increases the risk for and severity of mycobacterial infections (6–8). Moreover, malaria infection may increase the severity of HIV in co-infected individuals because the parasite modifies HIV transcription rates (9). The coexistence of TB, HIV, and/or malaria in many individuals and populations poses unique challenges for public health officials to understand the complex interactions of host genes with other factors influencing the transmission of these pathogens and their disease course. Consideration of these diseases concurrently may lead to integrated perspectives for their prevention and control, for conservation of resources, and for improvements in public health.

Malaria, Tuberculosis, and HIV: Overview

Differences in the modes of transmission, life-cycles, replication rates, and available prevention and control measures for these pathogens influence strategies to discover host genes that influence susceptibility to and severity of the diseases. These differences also influence strategies to incorporate this knowledge into public health practice. Table 10.1 summarizes some concepts that provide a framework for these strategies.

A complete review of host genes and malaria, tuberculosis (TB), and HIV is beyond the scope of this chapter, and the reader is referred to several recent reviews and publications (10–22). We provide a brief description of the data below, some of which is summarized in Table 10.2. Genes that influence susceptibility and severity of disease are distinguished from resistance genes. It is

Table 10.1 Malaria, TB, and HIV/AIDS: Transmission, Prevention and Risk Groups

Disease	Pathogen (type)	Transmission	Prevention	At-Risk-Population
Malaria	*Plasmodium spp.* (parasite)	Vector (anopheline mosquito), blood	Prevent vector contact, chemoprophylaxis	Children and pregnant women in endemic areas; all age groups in nonendemic areas
Tuberculosis (TB)	*Mycobacterium tuberculosis* (acid-fast bacillus)	Aerosol	Reduce exposure, BCG vaccine, chemoprophylaxis	Children, adults, immunocompromised individuals
HIV/AIDS	Human immunodeficieny virus type 1 (HIV-1) (lentivirus)	Sexual contact, blood or blood products	Reduce exposure, chemoprophylaxis	Fetus/neonate (vertical transmission), adolescents, adults

important to note that the same genes or gene families may impact several diseases. It is also important to remember that, to date, most studies of host genes and their impact on these (and other) infectious diseases have been carried out only in certain populations or races. Thus, the relationship between a particular allele and disease susceptibility or severity may not be generalizable to all populations. Moreover, we only partly know the genetic factors that influence each infectious disease. Finally, as discussed in this chapter, limited data are available on the interaction of these genes with each other or with other risk factors or on their attributable risk for a particular outcome.

Malaria

Malaria is a global problem that ranks second only to TB in the total number of human deaths attributable to an infectious agent. It accounts for 300 million to 500 million annual infections, estimated to cause 1.5 million to 2.7 million deaths annually (5), with about 90% of malaria-associated mortality occurring in sub-Saharan Africa (5,23). Malaria outbreaks are becoming frequent in other regions of the world, especially in the newly independent states (24), and cases of imported malaria are more often being reported in the United States and Europe because of increased travel. Malaria is caused by infection with any of the four known plasmodial species: *Plasmodium falciparum, P. vivax, P. ovale*, and *P. malariae*. Most malaria-associated mortality and severe morbidity, such as anemia and cerebral malaria, are attributable to *P. falciparum* (25). Anopheles mosquito vectors account for most malaria transmission, but human-to-human transmission can also occur through blood transfusion. Traditionally, malaria was contained through vector-control programs. But the

Table 10.2 Host Genes, Impact on Infectious Diseases, and Population Frequency

			Impact of Gene/Genotype on Infectious Diseases			
Disease	Gene/Genotype	Chromosome Location	Resistance	Susceptibility	Disease Outcome	Population Frequency	*Refs
Malaria	Duffy antigen negative	1p22.1 and 1q12-q21	+		Total protection against *P. vivax* infection	Africans near 100% Absent in Caucasians and Mongolians	27, 28
	Sickle-cell trait (Hb AS)	11	+		>90% protection against falciparum cerebral malaria, severe anemia and death	Kinshasa, Zaire 26% Ibadan, Nigeria 24% Accra, Ghana 8% Kampala, Uganda 19% Kisumu, Kenya 25%	31–34
	α-Thalassaemia	16pter-p13.3	+		Reduction of risk of severe malaria up to 0.40 in homozygotes, and up to 0.66 in heterozygotes Reduction in risk of hospital admissions due to other infections is 0.36 in homozygotes, and 0.63 in heterozygotes	Tharu, Nepal 80% Vanuatu 8%–38% Papua New Guinea 4%–38%	36, 37 38, 39
	β-Thalassaemia	11p15	+		Partial protection against severe disease in Liberia (*P. Falciparum*)	Variable frequencies in Mediterranean, Middle east, south-east Asia, and Africa	40
	Melanesian ovalocytosis	17q21-q22	+		Band 3 deletion not found in patients with cerebral malaria in Papua New Guinea. Protection against severe disease	Up to 30% in aboriginal population in south-east Asia and Pacific islands Absent in Africans	41, 42

	Gene	Location				Population	Ref.
	G6PD deficiency	Xq28	+		A 46%–58% reduction in severe malaria for both male hemizygotes and female heterozygotes in Gambia	Female heterozygotes in Gambia 13.7% in Kenya 27.3% Male hemizygotes in Gambia 5.9% in Kenya 18.8%	43
	HLA-B53	6p21.3	+		Partial protection (4–50%) against cerebral malaria and anemia	Nigerians 40% Gambians 25% Zambians 21% Zimbabweans 16% South Africans 2% Caucasians and Orientals 0–1%	35
	DRB1*1302	6p21.3	+	+	Protection against severe malaria anemia	Northern Italian 2.97%	**
	TNF-2 homozygote [a polymorphism in the promoter region of TNF-α gene (-308)]	6p21.3-q21.1		+	7-fold increased risk of death and neurologic sequealae due to cerebral malaria	Gambians, TNF-2 allele frequency 0.16	45
	ICAM-1	19p13.3-p13.2	+	+	2-fold increased susceptibility to cerebral malaria	Kenya >30% Caucasians rare or absent	46
TB	Tay-Sachs (TS) gene	15q23-q24	?		No evidence of protection against TB	TS carriers ~4%	60, 61
	HLA-DR2	6p21.3	+	+	DR2 associated with TB severity	DRB1*1501/DRB1* 1502	***
	DRB1*1501†	6p21.3	+	+	DRB1*1501 and DRB1*1502 both associated with severity and radiographic extent of clinical TB	South African blacks 6.4/0.0 Black Americans 8.6/ 0.8 Japanese (Wajin) 6.8/9.2 Highlanders (Papua New Guinea) 14.7/4.5	

(continued)

Table 10.2 (Cont.)

Disease	Gene/Genotype	Chromosome Location	Impact of Gene/Genotype on Infectious Diseases			Population Frequency	*Refs
			Resistance	Susceptibility	Disease Outcome		
	DRB1*1502†			+	DRB1*1501 and DRB1*1502 both associated with drug failure in TB treatment	French 7.1/0.3 German 7.8/1.1 Italian 5.5/2.2 USA white 9.9/0.7 Canadian 10.9/0.6 Indian 12/11.9	
	HLA-DQB1 *0503	6		+	Associated with clinical TB	Cambodians <1% Caucasian US 1.7%	50 **
	NRAMP-1	2q35		+	4-fold increased risk of TB in persons heterozygous for INTR4 and 3'UTR polymorphisms	Allelic frequency in Gambians 3%	17
	IFN-γ R	6q23-q24		+	Both associated with non-TB mycobacterial disease.	No published data	78, 79
	IL 12R (IL 12B1)	19p13.1		+	Only IFN-γ R is associated with adverse events post-BCG vaccination		
	Vitamin D receptor (VDR)	12q12-q14		+	tt homozygosity associated with increased risk of TB disease	t allele frequency in Caucasian 45%	****
HIV	HLA class I/II	6p21.3	+	+	Faster progression associated with alleles B7, B27, DR7, haplotype A1-B8-DR3, and homozygosity status Reduction of vertical transmission with class I disparity	Caucasians 10% B7, 4% B27, 13% DR7 3% haplotype A1-B8-DR3	90

TAP (often in combination with HLA)	6p21	+	Influence on progression	No data on frequency	90
Δ 32 CCR5	3p21	+	Homozygosity associated with resistance to HIV infection	Homozygosity Caucasians <1% Heterozygosity Caucasians 10–20% African Americans 6% Hispanics 7% Native Americans 13%	20
			Heterozygosity associated with delayed progression to AIDS		
CCR2-V64I	3p21	+	Delayed-progression to AIDS	Caucasians 10% Asians 25%	20, 80
SDF 1-3'A	10q11.1	?	Influence on progression	Caucasians 21% Hispanics 16% African Americans 6% Asians 26%	95
TNF-α	6p21.3	?	Long-term nonprogression	No data on frequency	99

* Reference numbers are for the population frequencies. References for the disease outcome are already in the text.

** HLA 1998 Gjertson DW and Terasaki PL eds, American Society for Histocompatibilty and Immunogenetics (ASHI).

*** Proceedings of the 11th International Histocompatibility Workshop and Conference. Yokohama. Japan 1991.

**** Hill AVS, Ruwende C, Corrah T et al. Association of immunognetic variants with susceptibility to tuberculosis in West Africa. Q J Med. 1996; 89: 868.

† DRB1*1501 and 1502 are HLA-DR genotypes that type serologically as HLA-DR2.

emergence of insecticide-resistant vectors and the lack of economic resources to sustain traditional malaria-control programs have led to the reemergence of malaria, even in regions where once it was controlled. Chloroquine, a cheap and effective drug to cure malaria, is no longer useful in most parts of the world because of drug resistance (24). Side effects in glucose-6-phosphate dehydrogenase (G6PD) deficient individuals also limit use of other antimalarials such as primaquine (see below). The reemergence of malaria underlines the urgent need to develop a vaccine that, along with vector-control measures, will control malaria (26).

Malaria Resistance Genes

Duffy Antigen. The Duffy antigen negative genotype is the only genotype known to provide complete protection against *P. vivax* infection (27,28). It is now known that the Duffy antigen is a chemokine receptor (29) essential for the invasion of merozoites into erythrocytes (30).

Hemoglobin S Gene. Homozygosity for a point mutation in the β-globin gene (Hb-S) causes sickle cell anemia (SS) and sickle cell disease. The carrier state for the sickle cell gene (AS genotype) provides partial protection against falciparum malaria as demonstrated in several studies (31–34). In a definitive large case-control study in The Gambia, it was shown to provide at least 90% protection from cerebral malaria, severe anemia, and death (35). The protective association of the AS genotype probably accounts for the high prevalence of the sickle cell gene in malaria-endemic regions of the world.

α-Thalassemia and β-Thalassemia Genes. The thalassemias are genetically complex disorders associated with hemolytic anemia. The great majority of α-thalassemias are caused by deletions of one or more of the duplicated α-chain genes due to nonhomologous crossing over. Like sickle cell anemia, α-thalassemia is more commonly found in malaria-endemic regions. It also decreases malaria-associated morbidity up to tenfold as observed in the Tharu population of Nepal, where it has reached near fixation (gene frequency of 0.8) (36,37). Paradoxically, in Vanuatu, a southwestern Pacific island, the incidence rates of both *P. vivax* and *P. falciparum* malaria were higher in α-thalassemic children than in normal children (38). When compared to normal children, the risk of severe malaria was reduced to 0.40 in α-thalassemia homozygotes and 0.66 in heterozygotes (39). Interestingly, the same study showed that the risk of overall hospital admission was also reduced to 0.36 and 0.63 in homozygous and heterozygous children, respectively. The mechanism associated with this protection is unclear. It has been suggested that this genotype may provide protection against indirect mortality caused by other infections associated with malaria.

Another anemia caused by decreased synthesis of the β-chain of hemoglobin is β-thalassemia. Over 100 different genetic variations ranging from single-point mutations to gene deletion can cause this condition. A case-control study conducted in Liberia showed that β-thalassemia provides partial protection against clinical and severe malaria caused by *P. falciparum* (40).

Melanesian Ovalocytosis. A 27 base-pair deletion in the gene encoding band 3 protein causes an erythrocyte membrane defect resulting in ovalocytosis. This genotype is prevalent in Southeast Asian populations and those of certain islands of the western Pacific. It has been associated with a lower incidence of both *P. falciparum* and *P. vivax* parasitemia (41). It also provides complete protection against mortality associated with severe malaria in children in Papua New Guinea (42).

Glucose 6-Phosphate Dehydrogenase Gene. Over 200 variants of the G6PD enzyme have been described, some of which have been linked to abnormalities of the G6PD gene. Because the gene is located on the X chromosome the abnormalities are sex-linked. G6PD plays a role in protecting red cells from oxidation-induced hemolysis; consequently, individuals with G6PD deficiency are at high risk of hemolytic anemia following exposure to some antimalarials such as primaquine, and several other nonantimalarial antibiotics. G6PD deficiency provides a 46%–58% reduction in risk of severe malaria for both male hemizygotes and female heterozygotes, as demonstrated in a case-control study conducted in children in Gambia (43).

Human Leukocyte Antigen (HLA) Genes. These genes are part of the major histocompatibility complex (MHC) on chromosome 6 and include the HLA class I (A, B, C) and HLA class II (DR, DP, DQ) genes. They code for the HLA molecules that present antigens to T cells. Different HLA alleles influence susceptibility to malaria. In a large case-control study involving children in The Gambia, HLA-B53 and HLA-DRB1*1302 were less frequent among children with severe malaria (44). It has been proposed that the HLA-B53-mediated protection may involve effective cytotoxic T-cell immunity to liver-stage antigens.

Malaria Susceptibility Genes

TNF-α Gene and ICAM-1 Gene. The TNF-α gene complex is also part of the MHC on chromosome 6, and has several polymorphisms, some of which may alter transcription and/or levels of tumor necrosis factor (TNF), an important cytokine in regulating immune responses. In The Gambia, children homozygous for the TNF-2 allele, a polymorphism in the promoter (−308) region of TNF-α gene, have a seven-fold increased risk for death or severe neurologic sequelae due to cerebral malaria (45). Another immune protein, intracellular adhesion molecule-1 (ICAM-1), which is involved in cell-to-cell communication, influences malaria severity. A new variant of the ICAM-1 gene with a point mutation in the *N*-terminal domain has been identified in some African populations, and children homozygous for this variant in coastal Kenya have a twofold greater risk of having cerebral malaria (46). This association may be explained by the ability of ICAM-1 to enhance sequestration of parasitized erythrocytes in cerebral blood vessels as it is a ligand for adhesion of *P. falciparum*-infected erythrocytes to endothelial cells. Further studies on the role of this ICAM-1 variant in the pathogenesis of cerebral malaria will be important.

Tuberculosis

The World Health Organization (WHO) estimates that 7 million to 8 million new cases of TB occur each year around the world, and TB accounts for more than 3 million deaths annually (47). Almost 2 million TB cases each year occur in sub-Saharan Africa, 3 million in Southeast Asia, and more than a quarter of a million in Eastern Europe. One-third of the increase in incidence that has occurred during the past 5 years is related to HIV co-infection (47,48). Tuberculosis is caused by *Mycobacterium tuberculosis*, an intracellular bacterium. The major route of transmission is person-to-person, through aerosols. Although many people become infected with the pathogen (as can be shown by a positive skin test to the purified protein derivative [PPD]), clinical disease develops in only a minority of cases (47,49). Clinical disease includes pulmonary and extrapulmonary disease, and may result in death (50,51). The only TB vaccine that is widely used is the attenuated strain of *M. bovis*, called *bacille Calmette-Guérin* (BCG) (52). Because of the limited efficacy of BCG vaccination (48,52), the reduced incidence and prevalence of TB, as well as the insensitivity of the PPD skin test in distinguishing vaccine, TB, or other mycobacterium-induced exposure in the developed world, widespread use of the BCG vaccine has decreased (53–56). Several challenges for the prevention and control of TB remain, particularly the long half-life of the pathogen (such that prophylaxis and treatment regimes last for months to years) and the development of drug resistance worldwide (57,58). In March 1993, WHO declared TB a global public health emergency (47).

Tuberculosis Resistance Genes

The Hypothesis of Tay-Sachs Gene. As with malaria and the various hemoglobinopathies described above, genetic differences in host susceptibility to other pathogens, including TB, leprosy, syphilis, cholera, measles, smallpox, plague, and intestinal pathogens, are likely to have profoundly modified human genetic composition over the years (59,60). Individuals who lack resistance genes die more often during epidemics, resulting in selection of survivors who have resistance genes (59,60). Endemic infectious diseases such as TB and plague may have greater selective pressure than epidemic diseases (60). For TB, it has been suggested that certain populations, such as Ashkenazi Jews, may have accumulated TB resistance genes, which may also be linked to other

diseases such as Tay-Sachs disease (TS). Some investigators (60) have speculated that the proportion of Ashkenazi Jews who may be resistant to TB is
higher than the frequency (4%) of the carriers for Tay-Sachs disease gene (60).
Whether this gene per se is associated with TB resistance remains to be confirmed. One case-control study comparing death from TB among Jews who
were carriers and noncarriers of the TS gene did not find evidence supporting
that the TS allele is involved in resistance to TB in Ashkenazim (61).

Tuberculosis Susceptibility Genes

Studies of susceptibility to infection with *M. tuberculosis* are made complex
by the fact that the majority of those who become infected with the bacillus
never develop clinical symptoms of TB. Thus, studies using TB cases and uninfected (e.g., PPD negative) controls are unable to identify true susceptibility
genes; rather, these studies may identify genes that are associated with clinical TB disease.

The HLA Genes. Several case-control studies of TB disease, or the severity of TB, have identified associations with HLA class II genes. A study in the
former Soviet Union (62) found an increased frequency of HLA-DR2 and a
reduced frequency of HLA-DR3 in TB patients. Other studies noted HLA-
DR2 associations with susceptibility to pulmonary tuberculosis as well as the
radiographic extent of the disease (63,64). In an association study with sputum
smear-positive TB conducted in Surabaya, Indonesia, the attributable risk
(AR) for TB associated with HLA-DR2 was 36% and with HLA-DQw1 39%
in patients with active TB, whereas HLA-DQw3 had a preventive fraction
of 57% against TB in the controls (65). Interestingly, while some HLA-DR2
positive patients have high levels of IgG antibodies to PPD, the frequency of
HLA-DR2 is higher in anergic patients, and HLA-DR2 may be associated
with reduced cell-mediated responses (62,66). It has also been suggested that
low plasma levels of lysozyme may be one correlate of susceptibility to TB in
DR2-positive patients (67). These data indicate a complex effect of HLA-DR2
in relation to immunity to TB.

Moreover, HLA-DR2 (DRB1*1501 and DRB1*1502) may also be associated with failure of antitubercular drugs (68). Association of HLA-B5
and HLA-DR5 with TB disease has also been reported, (60) whereas in
Cambodians, DQB1*0503 was associated with TB susceptibility (50). In contrast, to these HLA-related findings, a Brazilian family study identified no
linkage of TB susceptibility to HLA genes (69). Investigators speculated that
host vulnerability is under multigenic control with the major susceptibility
locus outside the HLA complex and modifier genes located within the HLA
system.

The NRAMP1 Gene. The NRAMP1 gene was first identified as a candidate gene for TB susceptibility in murine studies that showed its association

with increased susceptibility to mycobacterial and other intracellular infections (70). The function of this gene is as yet unknown. In humans it is associated with susceptibility to a variety of pathogens, including *M. tuberculosis*, *M. leprae*, and *Leishmania donovani* (19,70,71). At least 11 NRAMP1 polymorphisms (72) have been identified in humans. In a West African case-control study, individuals possessing one of four variants [INTR4, 3'UTR, 5'(CA)$_n$ and D543N] of the NRAMP1 gene had an increased susceptibility to clinical TB, and those heterozygous for the INTR4 and 3'UTR polymorphisms had the greatest risk (17). In contrast, analysis of multicase TB families in Brazil showed that gene markers tightly linked to NRAMP1, such as IL8RB and D2S1471, are associated with susceptibility to TB disease, while NRAMP1 itself was not (73). These studies suggest that several genes may influence TB susceptibility, and that their effects may differ in different populations depending on other genetic or environmental factors (19,21,69,73,74). It has been speculated that NRAMP1 genes could also influence the efficacy of BCG immunotherapy in patients with bladder cancer (75).

Cytokine Genes. Some cytokine genes may play a role in TB susceptibility or in influencing the course of TB disease, although no studies have yet reported such associations. However, individuals with mutations in the IL-12 or interferon (IFN)-γ receptors are particularly susceptible to disseminated non-TB mycobacterial diseases (76–78) and, unfortunately, some individuals with IFN-γ receptor polymorphisms develop severe disseminated BCG disease following BCG vaccination (79).

Vitamin D Receptor Gene. The active form of Vitamin D 1,25 dihydroxyvitamin D3 by interacting with the vitamin D receptor (VDR) acts as an immunoregulator (reviewed in 19). The VDR gene polymorphisms T, t, F and f, identified by the Taq1 and Fok1 restriction enzymes have been found to influence bone- mineral density (reviewed in 19; 80–82). Recent studies have shown that tt homozygosity may be associated with a decreased risk of TB disease whereas the combination of genotype TT/Tt and vitamin D deficiency was associated with TB disease and the presence of genotype ff or undetectable serum level of vitamin D was strongly associated with TB disease. Interestingly, the f allele was associated with extrapulmonary disease (83, 84).

HIV/AIDS

As of late 1997, more than 30 million individuals worldwide were reported to be infected with HIV type 1 (HIV-1) or to have acquired immunodeficiency syndrome (AIDS) (85). While the HIV epidemic was first noted in the early 1980s in the United States and Europe, HIV infection of humans occurred in Africa decades earlier (86). Currently, the highest prevalence of HIV is in sub-Saharan Africa and parts of Asia. In 1997 almost 90% of children <15 years of age newly infected with HIV lived in sub-Saharan Africa (590,000 children infected worldwide, of whom 530,000 are African). In the same region almost 30% of childbearing age women are infected with HIV (87). The global burden of HIV disease is expected to worsen with the 16,000 new HIV infections occurring daily (87). The major routes of HIV transmission are through sexual contact, intravenous (IV) drug abuse, or blood products. There is no vaccine to preventing HIV infection, and while new drugs have become available with remarkable effects on decreasing viral burden, delaying progression to AIDS, and reducing transmission from mother to child, their expense limits use in developing countries. The transmission of and course of HIV disease is known to be influenced by several genes, of which the most consistent and widely observed associations have been with HLA and chemokine receptor genes.

HIV Resistance Genes

The HLA Genes. HLA class I allele discordance, or mismatch, between mother and child has recently been shown to reduce vertical HIV transmission by up to tenfold in a Kenyan population (88). Interestingly, the effect of a three-allele mismatch in reducing HIV transmission was greater than the reduction observed with current antiretroviral therapy, suggesting that, if this observation is confirmed in other studies, new HLA-based strategies might be developed to complement antiretroviral therapy to reduce HIV transmission. Recently, heterozygosity for HLA class I alleles has been shown to delay progression of HIV disease to AIDS (89), whereas previous work from many groups has shown that individual, or combinations of, HLA class I (e.g., HLA-B27) or class II alleles are associated with delayed progression to AIDS (90; reviewed in 18,20,91). These effects may be modified by antigen-processing genes such as the transporter associated with antigen processing (TAP) (90; reviewed in 20).

Chemokine Receptors. Chemokines and their receptors are important in cell movement and trafficking in response to inflammation. The receptors are also HIV-ligands, and normal chemokine receptor expression is usually required for HIV entry into cells. There is a very strong association of homozygosity for the Δ32 CCR5 gene (a 32-bp deleted form of the chemokine receptor gene coding for the chemokine receptor, CCR5) with resistance to HIV infection (reviewed in 18,20). However, individuals with this genotype are susceptible to infection with strains of HIV that use other chemokine receptors (reviewed in 18,20). Protection against vertical transmission of HIV from mothers to Δ32 CCR5-homozygous children has not been conclusively demonstrated. Inconsistent associations have been observed with heterozygosity of Δ32 CCR5 and reduced heterosexual or vertical HIV transmission. The Δ32 CCR5 allele is found in up to 20% of some northern European populations, and it is rare or absent in African or Asian populations. This geographical observation and mathematical estimates dating the origin of the deleted CCR5 gene to about 700 years ago have led to speculation that individuals carrying this allele may have had an evolutionary advantage in the face of other infections widespread in Europe during the pre-HIV era (92,93) (reviewed in 18,20,94).

Heterozygosity for Δ32 CCR5, polymorphisms of the CCR5 promoter, of another chemokine receptor gene (CCR2, 64I) and of the gene coding for SDF-1, a ligand for CXCR4, influence the rate of progression of HIV disease (reviewed in 18,20;95). These effects appear to be independent and additive and result in approximately 2 to 4 additional years of AIDS-free survival in those with one or more protective genotypes (95). The close linkage of the CCR5 promoter and the CCR2 gene on chromosome 3 may indicate important evolutionary relationships between these genes (96). Conflicting data for the role of the SDF-1 gene 3′UTR polymorphism in delaying progression to AIDS have been reported and require additional studies in larger and diverse populations (reviewed in 20).

Lewis Blood Group Antigens and Hemoglobinopathies. Blood group secretor status for the Lewis antigens may influence heterosexual transmission of HIV (97), possibly through effects at mucosal surfaces. Individuals with sickle cell anemia (SS) may have a delayed progression of HIV disease to AIDS (98). This observation needs to be confirmed in larger studies, but it may relate to a reduction in the available target cells for HIV replication because of the frequent autosplenectomy observed in SS patients (98).

TNF-α. Inconsistent associations of polymorphisms at the TNF locus have been observed with the rate of HIV disease progression, although one study reported that some microsatellite alleles at the TNFc locus may be associated with slower progression to AIDS (99).

The HIV Susceptibility Genes

No genes that increase susceptibility to HIV infection have been reported. However, the inverse of the HLA associations with HIV transmission and progression to AIDS noted above is true (i.e., a high degree of concordance between mother and infant HLA class I alleles is associated with higher rate of vertical HIV transmission, and homozygosity for HLA class I alleles is associated with more rapid progression to AIDS) (88,89). In addition, individual HLA class I or class II alleles, or combinations of these (e.g., the extended haplotype HLA-A1, B8, DR3) with or without TAP are associated with rapid progression to AIDS, or with particular manifestations of HIV disease such as Kaposi's sarcoma or lymphadenopathy syndromes (reviewed in 18,20,90;91).

Although small numbers of individuals who are homozygous for Δ32 CCR5 have been reported to become HIV infected (e.g., with HIV strains that use CXCR4 for cell entry), paradoxically, once infected, some of these individuals appear to have a very rapid progression of their disease course (reviewed in 18).

Mannose Binding Lectins. Known as MBL or MBP (mannose binding protein) genes, these genes code for MBL, a glycoprotein important in clearance of some pathogens. Levels of MBL appear to be influenced by MBL genotype, and some low-MBL secreting genotypes are associated with more rapid progression to AIDS (100).

New Genes, New Therapies, and New Fields in Host Genetics and Infectious Diseases

As alluded to earlier, most of the genes that influence infectious diseases remain to be discovered. The process of gene discovery is complex, and many approaches can be taken (e.g., using linkage or association studies, and different laboratory tools). These approaches are well described in some recent reviews (11,21,22). Although not a primary focus of the translation phase of genetics discussed in this chapter, public health agencies play an important role in this discovery process, through epidemiological studies, cohort design, data collection, and laboratory studies, often in collaboration with academia or industry. An integrated collaborative approach to both gene discovery and to translating new knowledge into public health action should be rewarding. The translation phase should also be strongly linked to the biologic studies that follow gene discovery, such as functional studies of genes or alleles, and biotechnological studies and advances that translate the functional data into new therapies or interventions.

Pharmacogenetics

Pharmacogenetics is an emerging field of genetics in which pharmacological therapies are optimized based on the individual genetic characteristics (101). For infectious diseases, this field is already providing some important knowledge that influences public health and clinical practice. For example, knowledge of the host's G6PD status is a critical to determining choice of antimalarial drug. Similarly, in the treatment of TB, the isoniazid-associated peripheral neuropathy is known to have a pharmacogenetic basis. People who are slow isoniazid acetylators (102) are at particularly high risk of neuropathy. The rate of acetylation (of isoniazid and many other drugs) is influenced by polymorphisms in the *N*-acetyltransferase gene, NAT2 (60,103).

Conversely, individuals who rapidly acetylate isoniazid may be at greater risk of developing drug failure or drug-resistant mycobacteria when given typical once-weekly isoniazid dosage regimens (104) and may require higher therapeutic doses of isoniazid. Missense mutations of the NAT2 gene are responsible for instability and inefficiency of NAT, and three variants, M_1, M_2, M_3 of NAT2, account for about 95% of slow acetylator status (60). The slow acetylator phenotype is inherited in an autosomal recessive pattern. Thus, slow acetylators are homozygous and rapid acetylators are either homozygous or heterozygous (103). Eskimo, Japanese, and Chinese populations have high frequencies (80%–90%) of rapid acetylator genotypes, whereas some Arab, Indian, and European populations are predominantly (~70%) of the slow acetylator genotype (102). Future studies of drug efficacy or adverse events, particularly when the drugs are gene-targeted therapies (e.g., chemokine-receptor or cytokine based) are likely to incorporate pharmacogenetics into drug trials. The attractiveness of this approach to industry, insurance companies, and public health is obvious: Targeting of drug therapy to appropriate genotypes in the clinic or in populations may lead to cost savings and reductions in adverse events.

Ecogenetics

Ecogenetics is another relatively new discipline that is somewhat related to pharmacogenetics. The field attempts to explain why some exposed individuals develop adverse events following exposure to environmental agents (e.g., carcinogens, foods, insecticides) and how people adapt to the environment in different ways (60). Nutritional factors, toxins, and other environmental factors may alter the host immune response, or cause organ damage in genetically determined ways. For example, host genes influence susceptibility to hepatitis from a number of environmental toxins, and this susceptibility may influence the risk of or severity of hepatitis following exposure to hepatitis viruses. Concurrent consideration of the influence of host genetics on environmental factors as well as directly on pathogens may discover additive or multiplicative interactive effects of genetic and environmental risks on infectious diseases. An advantage of this approach is that many of the environmental risk factors are modifiable through behavior, diet, and other measures.

Translating Knowledge into Public Health Actions

One of the most difficult decisions facing public health officials or agencies is in choosing which genes to target for their infectious disease program, and in deciding which aspects of the program, (e.g., surveillance, applied research, infrastructure, and prevention) should have the highest priority. Before these decisions can be made, certain information is needed for each gene and disease. Of utmost importance is whether safe, effective interventions or preventions for the infectious disease are available that can be targeted to individuals with the genotype (105). Additional information necessary for such decision making includes knowledge of the magnitude of the relationship between the genotype and the outcome, the prevalence of the genotype, the burden of the disease or outcome, the target populations, and the interaction of the genotype with other genes and with other risk factors.

In the face of a rapidly expanding body of knowledge about genes and infectious diseases and the development of new gene-directed therapies, a second challenge is to ensure communication and collaboration between the partners involved in all phases from gene discovery to public health action. Communication is being made easier through online sources and easily accessible databases such as the National Center for Biotechnology Information website, which provides links to many data sources such as the Online Mendelian Inheritance in Man (OMIM) (106), the Cochrane Collaborations including those on HIV/AIDS (107), and proposed networks such as the HuGE Net (108).

In the following sections we consider specifically how current or future knowledge about host genes and infectious diseases may impact and be integrated into the four areas of infectious disease programs for malaria, TB, and HIV, and how they may impact primary, secondary, and tertiary prevention (Table 10.3).

Table 10.3 From Host Genes to Public Health Actions: Prevention and Control of Infectious Diseases

Prevention Strategy for Infectious Diseases	Incorporation of Host Genetic Information
Surveillance and Response	Existing Surveillance Systems Data collection by HuGE Net Population based surveys of the prevalence of genetic factors Surveillance systems of infectious diseases in local and state departments of health and by federal government agencies
Applied Research	Genetic Studies, Genetic Engineering Association and linkage studies, assessment of the interactions between genetics and environmental factors Clinical trails, assessment of the efficacy of or adverse outcomes to vaccines, antibiotics, gene therapy, or other interventions Assessment of new technology Behavioral sciences and program evaluation
Infrastructure and Training	Partnership and Information Dissemination Funding, laboratory support, training of public health professionals, global surveillance network development Information exchange, education of the lay public, and advocacy groups
Prevention and Control	Reinforcement of Classical Measures Primary, secondary, and tertiary prevention

Surveillance and Response

For malaria, TB, and HIV, classical surveillance determines the incidence and prevalence of these diseases and their associated mortality in certain populations. Constant vigilance enables rapid detection of outbreaks. Current reporting systems are typically based on geographic boundaries, with reporting to a centralized state, regional, or national database. Additional surveillance and reporting are performed based on risk groups. For example, HIV surveillance is targeted to risk groups defined by sexual or drug-using practices, whereas TB surveillance is heightened in immunocompromised persons, such as those with HIV/AIDS. The knowledge that certain populations (defined racially, geographically, or otherwise) may have genotypes that increase or decrease risk for infectious diseases may modify classical surveillance and control measures.

For example, the association of particular NAT2 and G6PD genotypes with adverse drug events may warrant particular vigilance for these problems in genetically at-risk populations as well as more systematic surveillance of populations for these and other risk-associated genotypes. This information could also be useful in determining appropriate prophylactic or treatment regimens for certain populations or regions and may be critical to encouraging the pharmaceutical industry to develop new drugs.

Although genotype-based preventions and/or therapies for TB, malaria, and HIV are not currently available for most of the genotypes listed in Table 10.2, new gene-based drugs and vaccines for these diseases are in clinical and preclinical trials and may soon be more widely used. Surveillance of populations for genotypes on which these therapies are based (e.g., HLA-based vaccines and chemokine or cytokine-based therapies discussed below) may allow targeting and optimization of particular vaccines or therapies to the appropriate populations, as well as targeted monitoring of these populations for gene-related adverse events.

When genotype-based prevention and intervention approaches become more widely available for any of these diseases, appropriately designed and collected surveillance information about these genotypes will be required for informed decision making. Population-based as well as risk-group-targeted surveillance might be useful. Data collection could be performed through the use of databases such as National Health and Nutrition Examination Surveys (NHANES) in the United States or through the development of other national or global repositories. The surveillance for genotypes of interest and the development of DNA banks should be based on partnerships among local, federal, and international agencies, and should build on the CDC, USAID (U.S. Agency for International Development), WHO, and other programs for infectious disease surveillance and response (24,109). These programs include strategies for developing networks, collecting efficient data, building laboratory capacity and tools, and studying patterns of disease trends and outbreaks, into which host genetic knowledge and surveillance can be integrated.

Applied Research

The highest priority areas for applied research in relation to translating current knowledge about host genes and HIV, TB, and malaria into public health action relates to development of vaccines, new drugs, and therapies.

Because no effective vaccines exist for HIV, TB, or malaria, development of these vaccines for primary or even secondary or tertiary prevention is an extremely high priority area for public health research. Using knowledge about HLA class I and II disease associations for these diseases and by dissecting the immune response in exposed or infected individuals, vaccines are being developed for TB, HIV, and malaria using a reverse immunogenetic approach (110–114). For example, identification of HLA-B53 as a gene associated with protection against severe malaria (35,44) led to the use of this approach to determine the molecular basis of such protection. This included HLA-binding studies for the rapid identification of immunologically protective cytotoxic T-cell (CTL) epitopes in malarial parasites (115,116).

Based on this information, new synthetic recombinant vaccines have been developed for malaria, and these vaccines may soon undergo clinical trials (117,118). Similarly, studies of individuals infected with HIV or TB, or apparently resistant to HIV, are generating HLA-based data useful for vaccine design (119–121). Tools such as the EpiMatrix algorithm (122) can predict allele-specific or promiscuous HLA-binding epitopes that may be important for developing subunit HIV, TB, or malaria vaccines. These HLA-based approaches may provide new vaccines for HIV and malaria and alternatives to the BCG vaccine for TB. These new vaccines may be live recombinant vaccines (123,124), DNA vaccines (125–127), or others. Population-based HLA allele frequencies generated through surveillance may be relevant for interpreting the overall efficacy of these vaccines and in monitoring vaccine failures as vaccine-induced pressure could result in the loss of binding of pathogen epitopes to the relevant HLA molecule (44,128,129).

In the domain of drugs for the prophylaxis or treatment of TB, HIV, and malaria, several areas of applied research are of high priority. As mentioned above and in the pharmacogenetics section, continued studies of the relationship of host-genotype (G6PD, NAT2) to nonresponse or drug toxicity in the host or to the emergence of drug-resistant pathogens are very important. For example, if confirmed in other studies the recent observation that HLA-DR2 is more strongly associated with the development of drug-resistant forms of TB (68) might suggest that this genotype would be a useful target for surveillance and or intervention programs. An important applied research objective in relation to antibiotics as tertiary prevention might be the development of simple, reliable diagnostic tests that can be used in primary health centers to identify individuals at potential risk for adverse drug reactions or altered drug efficacy (e.g., genotyping for G6PD before using primaquine for malaria or genotyping for HLA-DR2 and NAT2 for TB).

An exciting area of gene-based drug development is in relation to biologic drugs such as chemokines, cytokines or their analogs, and agonists or antagonists of their receptors. As the functions of genes such as NRAMP1 are elucidated, additional new therapies may be added to the armamentarium. For HIV the new chemokine receptor knowledge has led to a burgeoning of therapeutic strategies, including molecular mimics and receptor-blocking drugs (130). In the classical prevention model, these new therapies might provide either primary prevention (e.g., for those at high risk of acquiring HIV infection) or secondary prevention (e.g., treatment of HIV-infected cases). Other secondary preventions based on chemokine receptors, such as bone marrow replacement or gene therapy (94), are potential long-term genetic strategies. For HIV-infected individuals, applied research to determine the efficacy of and any adverse events associated with new receptor-targeted biotechnological drugs will be of vital importance.

Similarly for malaria and TB, where cytokine gene polymorphisms have or may be associated with different outcomes (TNF with malaria, IFN, and IL-12 receptor with mycobacterial diseases), cytokine-based therapies are now being considered and in some cases moving into clinical trials. Already, cytokine treatment of individuals has been shown to result in rapid clearance of non-TB mycobacterial disease (reviewed in 131,132). Drugs that induce or modify cytokine production are also attractive candidates. In the case of TB and HIV co-infection, trials of cytokine inhibitors gave encouraging results but warrant further assessment (133,134). Much applied research effort should be placed in the area of genetic epidemiology, where new candidates are tested, where preliminary gene-pathogen associations are confirmed in larger studies, and where the interactions with other known genes or risk factors can be carefully examined to determine attributable risk.

For malaria, a priority is to investigate the role of host genetics in severe malaria-associated deaths. For example currently 10% to 50% of cerebral malaria patients die despite medical intervention (135). In association study or other types of epidemiological study design, one gene to examine might be the common African polymorphism in the complement receptor 1 [Sl(a⁻)] (136). This polymorphism influences attachment of *P. falciparum*-infected erythrocytes to normal erythrocytes (137), a phenomenon called rosetting, and therefore may influence the risk of cerebral malaria. The inducible nitric oxide synthase gene (INOS), some alleles of which have recently been shown to be associated with the risk of fatal severe malaria (138), should also be further evaluated.

For HIV and TB, one candidate for evaluation is the gene controlling iron overload (e.g., the genes associated with hereditary hemochromatosis (139) or as yet unidentified iron-overload genes) because iron overload appears to impair macrophage function and pathogen clearance. A recent study in Africa suggested that iron overload may explain death from pulmonary TB (140). Because simple cheap measures to reduce iron overload exist (e.g., diet, phlebotomy), investigations of these genes to identify their role in HIV and TB disease are important. Similarly, confirmation and further study of the role of vitamin D receptor genes in HIV or TB disease would also be rewarding, as dietary supplementation with vitamin D might be a simple public health measure to reduce disease risk or severity.

For all three diseases, continued effort in evaluating the role, in disease susceptibility or pathogenesis, of polymorphism in the many cytokine genes that influence the immune response is likely to be fruitful, as biologic therapies are available or are becoming available for IL-2, IL-10, TNF, other cytokines and their receptors.

Infrastructure and Training

Infrastructure and training underlies and is critical in all areas of public health action including surveillance, research, and the eventual development of programs that are targeted to people with certain genotypes. Providing the tools (laboratory, epidemiology, surveillance) needed to perform applied research and gene-based surveillance in state, regional, or other settings will become more important in the future. The rapid integration of molecular diagnostic surveillance of pathogens in many laboratories throughout the world (109) should facilitate this process as many of the tools and techniques are equally applicable to host and pathogen. This infrastructure development is best achieved through integrated efforts of many international and national organizations.

A second challenge is the maintenance and updating of population-based information on the relationship of genes to infectious diseases. Databases and networks such as OMIM and HuGE Net, as previously mentioned, are a crucial part of this infrastructure. One area that is becoming increasingly important is the education of public health officials about the principles of genetics and about current knowledge of how host genes impact infectious disease risk and outcome in individuals or populations. Examples of existing genetic and infectious disease professional education programs are those developed by the CDC, WHO, USAID, the National Institute of Health (NIH), and academia in the form of workshops, conferences, or fellowships.

Prevention and Control

We have already outlined the few situations in which existing prevention and control programs for malaria, TB, or HIV have been impacted by genetic knowledge. Current laboratory and epidemiological research efforts into the relationship of host genes to all aspects of infectious disease prevention and control are moving gene-based prevention and intervention into several public health settings. As more gene-based therapies and strategies emerge based on this knowledge, prevention and control programs can be modified appropriately (Table 10.3).

One element of translating this genetic knowledge into public health action that should be concurrently addressed is the education of the public. For example, it is important that individuals with particular genetic traits are knowledgeable about their risk of developing infectious diseases or adverse outcomes from antibiotics or other therapies. Educational strategies may range from recommendations for individual action (e.g., avoiding certain anti-malarial drugs by G6PD-deficient people) or also recommendations that individuals adhere to traditional public health practices regardless of genotype.

For example, the new findings about chemokine receptor genes and HIV generated public interest in whether genetic testing for the $\Delta 32$ CCR5 gene should be used to predict disease course or select therapeutic strategies. In the absence of adequate attributable risk and population-based information about this genotype and outcomes, or of CCR5-targeted therapies, public health agencies currently recommend adherence to the usual HIV prevention and intervention strategies regardless of genotype (18,100). In addition to this type of education, it is also important to educate the public about the general principles of genetics and infectious diseases (mutations, selection, disease risk). These efforts could be incorporated into other general strategies to translate genetic research into public health actions. For instance, the Ethical, Legal, and Social Implications Program at the U.S. National Human Genome Research Institute has coordinated public retreats and town meetings to provide education and other forums for scientists and the public to discuss the impact of new discoveries in biotechnology and genetic testing and the role of the media in informing the public about genetics (141).

Conclusions

The great challenge of controlling or eradicating HIV, TB, or malaria has remained with us for many years. Basic principles of prevention, treatment, and education in the control of these diseases still remain the cornerstone of achieving this goal, while development of vaccines for these diseases is an urgent need. The discovery of genes that influence susceptibility and outcomes from these infectious diseases provides new opportunities for intervention and prevention and new strategies for vaccine development that may speed us to this ultimate goal. Many models for integrating the genetic knowledge into a public health program for infectious diseases have been proposed, and in this review we have discussed but one. Whatever approach is taken, it is important to remember that the ethical, legal, and social issues described in the early chapters of this book must be addressed in concert with advances in knowledge and opportunities for disease prevention.

References

1. Mausner JS, Kramer S. Epidemiologic orientation to health and disease. In: Mausner JS, Kramer S (eds). Mausner and Bahn epidemiology: an introductory text. Philadelphia: Saunders 1985, pp. 9–13.

2. Khoury M. Relationship between medical genetics and public health: changing the paradigm of disease prevention and the definition of a genetic disease. Am J Med Genet 1997;17:289–291.

3. Centers for Disease Control and Prevention (CDC). Preventing emerging infectious diseases: a strategy for the 21st century. Atlanta, GA: 1998.

4. Centers for Disease Control and Prevention (CDC). Translating advances in human genetics into public health action: a strategic plan. Atlanta, GA: 1997.

5. World Health Organization (WHO). Fifty facts from the World Health Report 1998: http://www.WHO.ORG/whr/1998/factse.htm. 1998.

6. Porter JD. Mycobacteriosis and HIV infection: the new public health challenge. J Antimicrob Chemother 1996;37(Suppl B):113–120.

7. Blenkush MF, Korzeniewska-Kozela M, Elwood RK, Black W, FitzGerald JM. HIV-related tuberculosis in British Columbia: indications of a rise in prevalence and a change in risk groups. Clin Invest Med 1996;19:271–278.

8. Chum HJ, O'Brien RJ, Chonde TM, Graf P, Rieder HL. An epidemiological study of tuberculosis and HIV infection in Tanzania, 1991–1993. AIDS 1996;10: 299–309.

9. Xiao L, Owen SM, Rudolph DL, Lal RB, Lal AA. *Plasmodium falciparum* antigen-induced human immunodeficiency virus type1 replication is mediated through induction of tumor necrosis factor-α. J Infect Dis 1998;177:437–445.

10. McNicholl JM, Cuenco K. Host genes and infectious diseases: HIV, other pathogens and a public health perspective. Am J Prev Med 1999;16:141–154.

11. Hill AVS. The immunogenetics of human infectious diseases. Annu Rev Immunol 1998;16:593–617.

12. Abel L, Dessein AJ. The impact of host genetics on susceptibility to human infectious diseases. Curr Opin Immunol 1997;9:509–516.

13. Weatherall DJ. Host genetics and infectious disease. Parasitology 1996;112 (Suppl):S23–29.

14. Miller LH. Impact of malaria on genetic polymorphism and genetic diseases in Africans and African Americans. Proc Natl Acad Sci U S A 1997;91:2415–2419.

15. Vidal S, Malo D, Vogan K, Skamene E, Gros P. Natural resistance to infection with intracellular parasites: isolation of a candidate for BCG. Cell 1993;73:469–486.

16. Bloom BR, Small PM. Editorial: the evolving relation between humans and *Mycobacterium tuberculosis*. N Engl J Med 1998;338:677–678.

17. Bellamy R, Ruwende C, Corrah T, McAdam KPWJ, Whittle HC, Hill AVS. Variations in the NRAMP1 gene and susceptibility to tuberculosis in West Africans. N Engl J Med 1998;338:640–644.

18. McNicholl JM, Smith DK, Qari SH, Hodge T. Host genes and HIV: the role of the chemokine receptor gene CCR5 and its allele (δ 32 CCR5). Emerg Infect Dis 1997;3:261–271.

19. Bellamy R, Hill A. Genetic susceptibility to mycobacteria and other infectious pathogens in humans. Curr Opin Immunol 1998;10:483–487.

20. Kaslow RA, McNicholl JM. Genetic determinants of HIV infection and its manifestations. Proc Assoc Am Physicians 1999;111:299–307.

21. Hill AVS. Commentaries. Host genetics of infectious diseases: old and new approaches converge. Emerg Infect Dis 1998;4:695–697.

22. Abel L, Dessein AJ. Genetic epidemiology of infectious diseases in humans: design of population-based studies. Emerg Infect Dis 1998;4:593–603.

23. WHO. World malaria situation in 1991. Part I. Weekly Epidemiol Rec 1993;68:245–252.

24. USAID. Reducing the threat of infectious diseases of major public health importance: USAID's initiative to prevent and control infectious diseases. Washington, DC, 1998.

25. Miller LH, Good MF, Milon G. Malaria pathogenesis. Science 1994;264: 1878–1883.

26. Miller LH, David PH, Hadley TJ. Perspectives for malaria vaccination. Philos Trans R Soc Lond B Biol Sci 1984;307:99–115.

27. Miller LH, Mason SJ, Dvorak JA, McGinnis MH, Rothman IK. Erythrocyte receptors for (*Plasmodium knowlesi*) malaria: Duffy blood group determinants. Science 1975;189:561–563.

28. Miller LH, Mason SJ, Clyde DF, McGinnis MH. The resistance factor to *Plasmodium vivax* in blacks. The Duffy-blood-group genotype, fyfy. N Engl J Med 1976;295:303–304.

29. Horuk R, Chitnis CE, Darbonne WC, et al. A receptor for the malarial parasite *Plasmodium vivax*: the erythrocyte chemokine receptor. Science 1993; 261:1182–1184.

30. Miller LH, Aikawa M, Johnson JG, Shiroishi T. Interaction between cytochalasin B treated malaria parasites and erythrocytes: attachment and junction formation. J Exp Med 1979;149:172–184.

31. Allison AC. Polymorphism and natural selection in human populations. Cold Spring Harb Symp Quant Biol 1964;29:137–149.

32. Luzatto L, Nwachuku-Jsrrett ES, Reddy S. Increased sickling of parasitized erythrocytes as mechanism of resistance against malaria in the sickle cell trait. Lancet 1970;i:319–322.

33. Ringelham B, Hathorn MKS, Jilly P, et al. A new look at the protection of haemoglobin AS and AC genotypes against *Plasmodium falciparum* infection: a census tract approach. Am J Hum Genet 1976;28:270–279.

34. Brabin BJ, Perrin L. Sickle cell trait and *Plasmodium falciparum* parasitaemia in pregnancy in Western Province, Kenya. Trans R Soc Trop Med Hyg 1985;79:733.

35. Hill AVS, Allsopp CEM, Kwiatkowski D, et al. Common West African HLA antigens are associated with protection from severe malaria. Nature 1991;352:595–600.

36. Terrenato L, Shrestha S, Dixit KA, et al. Decreased malaria morbidity in the Tharu people compared to sympatric populations in Nepal. Ann Trop Med Parasitol 1988;82:1–11.

37. Modiano G, Morpurgo G, Terrenato L, et al. Protection against malaria morbidity: near-fixation of the alpha-thalassemia gene in a Nepalese population. Am J Hum Genet 1991;48:390–397.

38. Williams TN, Maitland K, Bennett S, et al. High incidence of malaria in alpha-thalassaemic children. Nature 1996;383:522–525.

39. Allen SJ, O'Donnell A, Alexander ND, et al. Alpha+-thalassemia protects chil-

dren against disease caused by other infections as well as malaria. Proc Natl Acad Sci U S A 1997;94:14736–14741.

40. Willcox M, Bjorkman A, Brohult J, Pehrson PO, Rombo L, Bengtsson E. A case-control study in northern Liberia of *Plasmodium falciparum* malaria in haemoglobin S and beta-thalassemia traits. Ann Trop Med Parasitol 1983;77:239–246.

41. Cattani JA, Gibson FD, Alpers MP, Crane GG. Hereditary ovalocytosis and reduced susceptibility to malaria in Papua New Guinea. Trans R Soc Trop Med Hyg 1987;81:705–709.

42. Genton B, Al-Yaman F, Mgone CS, et al. Ovalocytosis and cerebral malaria. Nature 1995;378:564–565.

43. Ruwende C, Khoo SC, Snow RW, et al. Natural selection of hemi- and heterozygotes for G6PD deficiency in Africa by resistance to severe malaria. Nature 1995;376:246–249.

44. Hill AVS, Elvin J, Willis AC, et al. Molecular analysis of the association of HLA-B53 and resistance to severe malaria. Nature 1992;360:434–439.

45. McGuire W, Hill AVS, Allsopp CEM, Greenwood BM, Kwiatkowski D. Variation in the TNF-α promoter region associated with susceptibility to cerebral malaria. Nature 1994;371:508–511.

46. Fernandez-Reyes D, Craig AG, Kyes SA, et al. A high-frequency African coding polymorphism in the N-terminal domain of ICAM-1 predisposing to cerebral malaria. Hum Mol Genet 1997;6:1357–1360.

47. World Health Organization: Tuberculosis fact sheet: http:// www.who.ch/gtb/publications/factsheet/. 1998.

48. Al-Buhairan B, Pacheco M, Nguy N, Friedman R. Vaccine approaches to tuberculosis: http://www.brown.edu/Courses/Bio_160/tb/tbbody.html. 1998.

49. Porter JDH, McAdam KPWJ. The re-emergence of tuberculosis. Annu Rev Public Health 1994;15:303–323.

50. Goldfeld AE, Delgado JC, Thim S, et al. Association of an HLA-DQ allele with clinical tuberculosis. JAMA 1998;279:226–228.

51. Rom W, Garay S. Tuberculosis. Boston: Little, Brown, 1996.

52. Ellner J. The immune response in human tuberculosis—implications for tuberculosis control. J Infect Dis 1997;176:1351–1359.

53. Pedersen JT, Pallisgaard G. Tuberculosis in low prevalence countries: back to the future? Ugeskr Laeger 1995;157:6859–6863.

54. Ballew KA, Becker, DM. Tuberculosis screening in adults who have received bacille Calmette-Guérin vaccine. South Med J 1995;88:1025–1030.

55. Eskild A. Mass vaccination against tuberculosis—is it necessary in Norway? Tidsskr Nor Laegeforen 1994;114:1840–1844.

56. Trnka L, Dankova D, Svandova E. Six years' experience with the discontinuation of BCG vaccination: cost and benefit of mass BCG vaccination. *Tuber Lung Dis* 1993;74:288–292.

57. Pablos-Mendez A, Laszlo A, Raviglione MC, Binkin N, et al. Global surveillance for antituberculosis-drug resistance 1994–1997. N Engl J Med 1998;338:1641–1649.

58. Snider DE, Castro KG. Editorial. The global threat of drug-resistant tuberculosis. N Engl J Med 1998;338:1689–1690.

59. Diamond J. Guns, germs, and steel: the fates of human societies. New York: Norton, 1997.

60. Vogel F, Motulsky AG. Human genetics: problems and approaches. Berlin: Springer, 1997, p. 543.

61. Spyropoulos B, Moens P, Davidson J, Lowden J. Heterozygote advantage in Tay-Sachs carriers? Am J Hum Genet 1981;33:375–380.

62. Khomenko A, Litvinov VI, Chukanova V, Pospelov L. Tuberculosis in patients with various HLA phenotypes. Tubercle 1990;71:187–192.

63. Singh S, Mehra N, Dingley H, Pande J, Vaidya M. Human leukocyte antigen (HLA)-linked control of susceptibility to pulmonary tuberculosis and association with HLA-DR types. J Infect Dis 1983;148:676–681.

64. Brahmajothi V, Pitchappan R, Kakkanaiah V, et al. Association of pulmonary tuberculosis and HLA in south India. Tubercle 1991;72:123–132.

65. Bothamley G, Beck J, Schreuder G, et al. Association of tuberculosis and M. tuberculosis antibody levels with HLA. J Infect Dis 1989;159:549–555.

66. Selvaraj P, Uma H, Reetha A, Xavier T, Prabhakar R, Narayanan P. Influence of HLA-DR2 phenotype on humoral immunity and lymphocyte response to *Mycobacterium tuberculosis* culture filtrate antigens in pulmonary tuberculosis. Indian J Med Res 1998;107:208–217.

67. Selvaraj P, Kannapiran M, Reetha A, Uma H, Xavier T, Narayanan P. HLA-DR2 phenotype and plasma lysozyme, beta-glucuronidase and acid phosphatase levels in pulmonary tuberculosis. Int J Tuberc Lung Dis 1997;1:265–269.

68. Rajalingam R, Mehra N, Jain R, Myneedu V, Pande J. Polymerase chain reaction based sequence-specific oligonucleotide hybridization of HLA class II antigens in pulmonary tuberculosis: relevance to chemotherapy and disease severity. J Infect Dis 1996;173:669–676.

69. Schurr E, Fujiwara T, Rousseau J, et al. Leprosy and tuberculosis. In: HLA 1991. Tsuji K, Aizawa M, Sasazuki T (eds). Proceedings of the Eleventh International Histocompatibility Workshop and Conference, Yokohama, Japan 1991;1:786–789. New York: Oxford University Press, 1992.

70. Skamene E, Schurr E. Infection genomics: Nramp1 as a major determinant of natural resistance to intracellular infections. Annu Rev Med 1998;49:275–287.

71. Abel L, Sanchez FO, Oberti J, et al. Susceptibility to leprosy is linked to the human NRAMP1 gene. J Infect Dis 1998;177:133–145.

72. Buschman E, Vidal S, Skamene E. Nonspecific resistance to Mycobacteria: the role of the Nramp1 gene. Behring Inst Mitt 1997;99:51–57.

73. Blackwell J. Genetics of host resistance and susceptibility to intramacrophage pathogens: a study of multicase families of tuberculosis, leprosy and leishmaniasis in north-eastern Brazil. Int J Parasitol 1998;28:21–28.

74. Shaw M, Collins A, Peacock C, et al. Evidence that genetic susceptibility to *Mycobacterium tuberculosis* in a Brazilian population is under oligogenic control: linkage study of the candidate genes NRAMP1 and TNFA. Tuber Lung Dis 1997;78:35–47.

75. Liu J, Fujiwara TM, Buu NT, et al. Identification of polymorphisms and sequence variants in the human homologue of the mouse natural resistance-associated macrophage protein gene. Am J Hum Genet 1995;56:845–853.

76. Altare F, Durandy A, Lammas D, Emile JF, Lamhamedi S, Le Deist F. Impairment of mycobacterial immunity in human interleukin-12 receptor deficiency. Science 1998;280:1432–1435.

77. de Jong R, Altare F, Haagen IA, et al. Severe mycobacterial and Salmonella infections in interleukin-12 receptor- deficient patients. Science 1998;280:1435–1438.

78. Newport MJ, Huxley CM, Huston S, et al. A mutation in the interferon-gamma-receptor gene and susceptibility to mycobacterial infection. N Engl J Med 1996;335: 1941–1949.

79. Jouanguy E, Altare F, Lamhamedi S, et al. Interferon-gamma-receptor deficiency in an infant with fatal *bacille Calmette-Guerin* infection. N Engl J Med 1996;335:1956–1961.

80. McNicholl J. Host genes and infectious diseases. Emerg Infect Dis 1998;4:1–4.

81. Sainz J, Van Tornout JM, Loro ML, et al. Vitamin-D receptor gene polymorphisms and bone density in prepubertal American girls of Mexican descent. N Engl J Med 1997;337:77–82.

82. Morrison NA, Qi JC, Tokita A, et al. Prediction of bone density from vitamin D receptor alleles. Nature 1994;367:284–287.

83. Bellamy R, Ruwende C, Corrah T, et al. Tuberculosis and chronic hepatitis B virus infection in Africans and Variation in the vitamin D receptor gene. J Infect Dis 1999;179:721–724.

84. Wilkinson RJ, Llewelyn M, Toossi Z, et al. Influence of vitamin D deficiency and vitamin D receptor polymorphisms on tuberculosis among Gujarati Arians in west London: a case-control study. Lancet 2000;355:618–621.

85. World Health Organization. Global AIDS surveillance. 1997;48:357–364.

86. Zhu T, Korber BT, Nahmias AJ, Hooper E, Sharp PM, Ho DD. An African HIV-1 sequence from 1959 and implications for the origin of the epidemic. Nature 1998;391:594–597.

87. UNAIDS. Report on the global HIV/AIDS epidemic. GENEVA, Switzerland: UNAIDS Joint United Nations Programme on HIV/AIDS, December 1997.

88. MacDonald KS, Embree J, Njenga S, et al. Mother–child class I HLA concordance increases perinatal human immunodeficiency virus type I transmission. J Infect Dis 1998;177:551–556.

89. Carrington M, Nelson GW, Martin MP, et al. HLA and HIV-1: heterozygote advantage and B*35–Cw*04 disadvantage. Science 1999;283:1748–1752.

90. Kaslow RA, Carrington M, Apple R, et al. Influence of combinations of human major histocompatibility complex genes on the course of HIV-1 infection. Nat Med 1996;2:405–411.

91. Malkovsky M. HLA and natural history of HIV infection. Lancet 1996;348:142–143.

92. Stephens JC, Reich DE, Goldstein DB, et al. Dating the origin of the CCR5-delta32 AIDS resistance allele by the coalescence of haplotypes. Am J Hum Genet 1998;62:1507–1515.

93. Martinson JJ, Chapman NH, Rees DC, Liu Y, Clegg JB. Global distribution of the CCR5 gene 32-basepair deletion. Nat Genet 1997;16:100–103.

94. O'Brien SJ, Dean M. In search of AIDS-resistance genes. Scientific American 1997;277:44–51.

95. Winkler C, Modi W, Smith MW, et al. Genetic restriction of AIDS pathogenesis by an SDF-1 chemokine gene variant. ALIVE Study, Hemophilia Growth and Development Study (HGDS), Multicenter AIDS Cohort Study (MACS), Multicenter Hemophilia Cohort Study (MHCS), San Francisco City Cohort (SFCC). Science 1998;279:389–393.

96. Mummidi S, Ahuja SS, McDaniel BL, Ahuja SK. The human CC chemokine receptor 5 (CCR5) gene: multiple transcripts with 5'-end heterogeneity, dual promoter usage, and evidence for polymorphisms within the regulatory regions and noncoding exons. J Biol Chem 1997;272:30662–30671.

97. Blackwell CC, James VS, Davidson S, et al. Secretor status and heterosexual transmission of HIV. BMJ 1991;303:825–826.

98. Bagasra O, Steiner RM, Ballas SK, et al. Viral burden and disease progression in HIV-1 infected patients with sickle cell anemia. Am J Hematol 1998;59:199–207.

99. Khoo SH, Pepper L, Snowden N, et al. Tumor necrosis factor c2 microsatellite allele is associated with the rate of HIV disease progression. AIDS 1997;11:423–428.

100. Garred P, Madsen HO, Balsler U, et al. Susceptibility to HIV infection and progression of AIDS in relation to variant alleles of mannose-binding lectin. Lancet 1997;349:236–240.

101. Kleyn PW, Vesell ES. Genetic variation as a guide to drug development. Science 1998;281:1820–1821.

102. Evans D. Genetics factors in drug therapy: Clinical and molecular pharmacogenetics. Cambridge: Cambridge University Press, 1993 p. 211.

103. Ellard GA. Variations between individuals and populations in the acetylation of isoniazid and its significance for the treatment of pulmonary tuberculosis. Clin Pharmacol Ther 1976;19:610–625.

104. Tuberculosis Chemotherapy Centre Madras. A controlled comparison of a twice-weekly and three once-weekly regimens in the initial treatment of pulmonary tuberculosis. Bull World Health Organ 1970;43:143–206.

105. Kaslow R. Host genes and HIV infection: implications and applications. Emerg Infect Dis 1997;3:401–402.

106. McKusik V. OMIM: http://www3.ncbi.nlm.nih.gov/htbin-post/Omim. 1998.

107. Ioannidis JPA, O'Brien TR, Rosenberg PS, Contopoulos-Ioannidis, DG, Goedert JJ. Genetic effects on HIV disease progression. Nat Med 1998;4:536.

108. Khoury MJ, Dorman JS. Editorial: the human genome epidemiology network. Am J Epidemiology 1998;148:1–3.

109. Centers for Disease Control and Prevention. Addressing emerging infectious disease threats: a prevention strategy for the United States. Atlanta, GA, 1994.

110. Davenport MP, Hill AV. Reverse immunogenetics: from HLA-disease associations to vaccine candidates. Mol Med Today 1996;2:38–45.

111. Ward FE, Tuan S, Haynes BF. Analysis of HLA frequencies in population cohorts for design of HLA-based HIV vaccines, in HIV Molecular Immunology Database 1997. Korber B, et al (eds.). Los Alamos National Laboratory, Theoretical Biology and Biophysics, Los Alamos, NM, p. 10.

112. De Groot AS, Jesdale BM, Meister GE, Muni NI, Roberts CGP. Prediction of T-cell epitopes for HIV vaccine development by computer-driven algorithm, in HIV Molecular Immunology Database 1997. Korber B, et al (eds.). Los Alamos National Laboratory, Theoretical Biology and Biophysics, Los Alamos, NM, p. 17.

113. Roberts CG, Meister GE, Jesdale BM, et al. Prediction of HIV peptide epitopes by a novel algorithm. AIDS Res Hum Retroviruses 1996;12:593–610.

114. Meister GE, Roberts CG, Berzofsky JA, De Groot AS. Two novel T-cell epitope prediction algorithms based on MHC-binding motifs; comparison of predicted and published epitopes from *Mycobacterium tuberculosis* and HIV protein sequences. Vaccine 1995;13:581–591.

115. Aidoo M, Lalvani A, Allsopp CE, et al. Identification of conserved antigenic components for a cytotoxic T-lymphocyte-inducing vaccine against malaria. Lancet 1995;345:1003–1007.

116. Doolan DL, Hoffman SL, Southwood S, et al. Degenerate cytotoxic T-cell epitopes from P. falciparum restricted by multiple HLA-A and HLA-B supertype alleles. Immunity 1997;7:97–112.

117. Gilbert SC, Plebanski M, Harris SJ, et al. A protein particle vaccine containing multiple malaria epitopes. Nat Biotechnol 1997;15:1280–1284.

118. Shi Y, Hasnain S, Holloway B, et al. Immunogenicity and in vitro protective efficacy of a recombinant multistage *Plasmodium falciparum* candidate vaccine. Proc Natl Acad Sci 1999;96:1615–1620.

119. Sriwanthana B, Bond KB, Hodge TW, et al. HIV- specified cytotoxic T lymphocytes (CTLs) in Thai exposed uninfected (EU) female sex workers (FSWs) are directed to multiple regions of *HIV-1* subtype E. 12th World AIDS Conference. Geneva, Switzerland, June 28–July 3, 1998; Abstract 31120.

120. MacDonald KS, Castillo J, Joanne EE, et al. Class I MHC polymorphism and mother to child *HIV-1* transmission in Kenya. 12th World AIDS Conference. Geneva, Switzerland, 1998; June 28–July 3, 1998; Abstract 31131.

121. Laumbacher B, Wank R. Recruiting HLA to fight *HIV*. HLA-restricted peptides from HIV-resistant individuals may act as guides to immunogenic regions of viral proteins. Nat Med 1998;4:505.

122. Schafer JR, Jesdale BM, George JA, Kouttab NM, De Groot AS. Prediction of well-conserved *HIV-1* ligands using a matrix-based algorithm, EpiMatrix. Vaccine 1998;16:1880.

123. Balasubramanian V, Pavelka MS, Bardarov SS, et al. Allelic exchange in *Mycobacterium tuberculosis* with log linear recombination substrates. J Bacteriol 1996;178:273–279.

124. Guleria I, Teitelbaum R, McAdam RA, et al. Auxotrophic vaccines for tuberculosis. Nat Med 1996;2:334–337.

125. Lowrie D, Tascon RE, Coeaton MJ, Silva CL. Towards a DNA vaccine against tuberculosis. Vaccine 1994;12:1537–1540.

126. Huygen K, Content J, Denis O, et al. Immunogenicity and protective efficacy of a tuberculosis DNA vaccine. Nat Med 1996;2:893–898.

127. Robinson HL. DNA vaccines for immunodeficiency viruses. AIDS 1997;11: S109–S119.

128. Udhayakumar V, Ongecha JM, Shi YP, et al. Cytotoxic T-cell reactivity and HLA-B35 binding of the variant *Plasmodium falciparum* circumsporozoite protein CD8+ CTL epitope in naturally exposed Kenyan adults. Eur J Immunol 1997;27: 1952–1957.

129. Gilbert SC, Plebanski M, Gupta S, et al. Association of malaria parasite population structure, HLA, and immunological antagonism. Science 1998;279:1173–1177.

130. Cairns JS, D'Souza MP. Chemokines and HIV-1 second receptors: the therapeutic connection. Nat Med 1998;4:563–568.

131. Otlhenhoff TH, Spierings E, Nibbering PH, de Jong R. Modulation of protective and pathological immunity in mycobacterial infections. Int Arch Allergy Immunol 1997;113:400–408.

132. Johnson B, Ress S, Willcox P, et al. Clinical and immune responses of tuberculosis patients treated with low-dose IL-2 and multidrug therapy. Cytokine Mol Ther 1995;1:185–196.

133. Wallis R, Nsubuga P, Whalen C, et al. Pentoxifylline in HIV-1-seropositive tuberculosis: a randomized controlled trial. J Infect Dis 1996;174:727–733.

134. Klausner J, Makonkawkeyoon S, Akarasewi P, et al. The effect of thalidomide on the pathogenesis of human immunodeficiency virus type 1 and *M. tuberculosis* infection. J Acquir Immune Defic Syndr 1996;11:247–257.

135. Warrel DA, Molyneux ME, Beales PF. Severe and complicated malaria (WHO). Trans Roy Soc Trop Med Hyg 1990; 84 suppl. 2:1–65.

136. Moulds JM, Nickells MW, Moulds JJ, Brown MC, Atkinson JP. The C3b/C4b receptor is recognized by the Knops, McCoy, Swain-langley, and York blood group antisera. J Exp Med 1991;173:1159–1163.

137. Rowe JA, Moulds JM, Newbold CI, Miller LH. P. falciparum rosetting mediated by parasite-variant erythrocyte membrane protein and complement-receptor 1. Nature 1997;388:292–295.

138. Burgner D, Xu W, Rockett K, et al. Inducible nitric oxide synthase polymorphism and fatal cerebral malaria. Lancet 1998;352:1193–1194.

139. Feder JN, Gnirke A, Thomas W, et al. A novel MHC class I-like gene is mutated in patients with hereditary haemochromatosis. Nat Genet 1996;13:399–408.

140. Moyo V, Gangaidzo I, Gordeuk V, Kiire C, Macphail A. Tuberculosis and iron overload in Africa: a review. Cent Afr J Med 1997;43:334–339.

141. Dove A. Genetics research on the town hall agenda, courtesy of ELSI. Nat Med 1998;4:545.

11

Public health assessment of genetic information in the occupational setting

Paul A. Schulte and D. Gayle DeBord

Genetic information is information about genes, gene products, or inherited characteristics that may derive from an individual or family member (1). In the workplace, genetic information is usually the product of genetic screening or genetic monitoring, but may also be derived from a person's medical record. This chapter examines the use of genetic information in the occupational safety and health field in terms of practice, research, and regulation (see Table 11.1). In occupational health practice, *genetic monitoring* of workers exposed to various toxicants is analogous to biological monitoring for the presence or effects of any toxicant. Here the issue is to use genetic material or somatic or germline DNA to assess whether exposures or health effects are likely to have occurred. *Genetic screening*, in contrast, is rarely practiced but is aimed at identifying an asymptomatic person with a particular inherited genetic characteristic who is likely to develop a health effect related to work. For the most part, genetic screening related to occupational diseases involves hereditary characteristics that have an influence in conjunction with a particular exposure but which do not confer a risk on their own. At the present time, little scientific evidence has been found to support a link between unexpressed genetic factors and a person's ability to perform job functions. From a public health perspective, genetic monitoring and screening raise very different issues (2,3).

Genetic monitoring has many of the same strengths and limitations of any type of toxic effect monitoring such as assessing blood lead, carboxyhemoglobin, or liver-function assays. In these situations, the genetic effect must be validated for the exposure or disease—that is, the relationship between the genetic effect and exposure or disease must be known before it is used. Moreover, as with all monitoring, attention needs to be given before the

Table 11.1 Genetic Information in Occupational Safety and Health

	Practice	*Research*	*Regulation*
Genetic monitoring	Analogous to biological monitoring to detect exposure or early health effects	To develop and validate markers of exposure or early effect	Not in regulations, but could be included as early-warning indicator
Genetic screening	Rarely used but use could increase	To identify genetic characteristics that increase risk of occupational disease	Not in OSH regulations, but laws protect workers from inappropriate uses
Information from medical records	Genetic information in a medical record may have utility assessing occupational disease risks	Rarely used	Used in compensation legislation; not in occupational safety and health standards

monitoring to the following issues: Who is going to be monitored? Why? What are individuals told to encourage them to participate? How, to whom, and when will the results be communicated? What follow-up actions will occur for those monitored with regard to the workplace.

Genetic screening in the workplace presents more difficult public health issues than genetic monitoring (4–7). With this effort, the emphasis is not, as in genetic monitoring, on exposure effects; rather, it is on the probability that a person with a particular genetic characteristic is at risk of a disease or an occupational disease (2). For a genetic marker assay to be useful in genetic screening, it must have a high predictive value. Beyond that, a broad range of ethical, legal, and social concerns must be addressed before such a test is considered for use: Not the least of these is that genetic screening is usually described as screening for "susceptibility," which seems to some a pejorative term that somehow places blame on the person with the genetic characteristic (8). Nonetheless, molecular genetics may improve our understanding of the etiology of occupational disease. Ethical and legal issues that protect workers' rights, yet allow use of this information to prevent occupational disease, need to be explored. The question is how to use such information fairly and effectively. The major issue for society is to balance a person's right to work with an employer's responsibility of protecting workers from job-related disease (9).

Genetic research must address many of the same issues as genetic screening and genetic monitoring. In research, there are scientific issues in developing and validating genetic markers in the laboratory and then in the field prior to use in epidemiologic research. Ethical issues should also be addressed before these markers are employed in the field. These markers can be used in toxicologic research to identify mechanisms involved in toxicant exposure–disease relationships. In epidemiologic research the markers can be used as effect modifiers on which to stratify exposure–disease relationships. In the process of testing and using genetic markers in human populations, a range of technical and ethical questions should be considered. These include determining performance characteristics of the assay and optimal handling conditions of biological specimens. In addition, there are ethical requirements placed on the researcher in obtaining participation, interpreting and communicating results, and maintaining privacy and confidentiality.

Genetic markers have been rarely used in the workplace, and only one incident of their use has been tested in the courts. Employers have attempted to use one genetic marker for gender, the absence of a Y chromosome (or male gender), to exclude workers from employment in the lead industry. But that approach was rejected by the courts on the basis that the Occupational Safety and Health Act requires a safe and healthful workplace for all workers [United Automobile, Aerospace and Agricultural Implement Workers of America v. Johnson Controls, Inc. 499 US 187 (1991)] (10). However, knowing that occupational risks can be avoided by acting on genetic information, an employer may still be tempted to develop strategies for using such information to make employment decisions, even though the onus is on employers to provide safe workplaces.

Genetic information may ultimately find the greatest utility in quantitative risk assessments, where it can provide mechanistic information that could be an aid in extrapolation from high to low exposures and from animals to humans in assessing risks (11,12). The limiting factor is how to use genetic information in risk assessments; thus far there are few examples. No formal guidelines exist for incorporating genetic endpoints into quantitative risk assessments.

Occupational Health Practice

To date, genetic monitoring and genetic screening are not used very widely or routinely in industry (2). However, pressure to apply new techniques is likely to increase in the next decade (13). Use of these markers raises several questions: What are the goals of monitoring? What are the costs and benefits? Different biomarkers will be appropriate for different goals, such as exposure assessment, hazard surveillance, group risk assessment, or individual risk assessment. Before use in occupational health practice, the marker must be validated for each of the applications.

Genetic Monitoring
Genetic monitoring involves the periodic evaluation of an exposed population, and it is not unlike most other forms of biological monitoring (14).

Genetic monitoring is ascertaining whether a person's genetic material has been altered over time, thus indicating exposure or providing an early warning of possible health effects. Using changes in genetic materials as exposure indicators has been well studied (15,16). Not only has genetic monitoring been used to assess damage from occupational exposures, but also from other environmental exposures and lifestyle habits such as smoking. The benefits of a monitoring program include (1) identifying a risk for the exposed group as a whole or for individuals; (2) targeting work areas for evaluation of safety and health practices; and (3) detecting previously unknown hazards—thus possibly decreasing health costs for employers, insurance companies, and society in general. In an Office of Technology Assessment survey conducted in 1989 of Fortune 500 companies, only one company reported currently conducting genetic monitoring (2). Five companies reported past use of genetic monitoring and two companies reported future consideration of genetic monitoring.

Ever since the late 1980s, an exponential increase in knowledge about human genetics has occurred because of the rapid progress of the Human Genome Project and technological advances in molecular biology techniques. An increase in the recognition of genetic factors in disease may present many new opportunities for prevention, detection, and treatment of occupational diseases. Adverse health effects have been associated with mutagenic toxic agents (17). These mutations occur at a significant rate above normal background levels. The relationship among genetic damage, mutation, and cancer is becoming clearer. Several types of genetic damage such as mutations and chromosomal aberrations have been associated with various cancers and tumor development in somatic cells. Most research has focused on somatic cell changes. Effects in germ cells are harder to decipher because such effects may not be seen for several generations.

Many different techniques exist for genetic monitoring. Changes can be detected on the molecular or chromosomal level by measuring DNA adducts, mutation levels, sister chromatid exchanges, micronuclei formation, DNA stability, and chromosome aberrations. At the molecular level, DNA adducts have shown much promise. Most initiating carcinogens or their metabolites can bind to DNA bases or other macromolecules forming adducts. Adducts related to the carcinogen can be measured in tissues, exfoliated cells, peripheral blood, and urine (17). A disadvantage of using adducts as a monitoring tool is that adducts are usually measured in a surrogate tissue rather than the target tissue. In addition, DNA adduct levels are dynamic, changing with various Phase I and Phase II enzyme activities, DNA repair, cell turnover, and the chemical stability of the adduct itself.

Somatic mutations in reporter genes may also have potential for genetic monitoring and have been shown to increase after exposure to toxic agents (18). Two of the most widely studied are glycophorin-A (GPA) and hypoxanthine phosphoribosyltransferase (HPRT). Glycophorin-A is a glycoprotein on the membrane of red blood cells. It is a polymorphic gene (M and N alleles) with 50% of the population being heterozygous. The assay measures the frequency that the M form is not expressed on red blood cells in a heterozygous person (19). The HPRT mutants can be selected, since cells with normal HPRT activity are susceptible to cytotoxicity by 6-thioguanine. These assays are highly sensitive but lack specificity for selected exposures. The relevance of these mutations to cancer is not known, but they may serve as a sentinel event for carcinogenesis.

Sister chromatid exchange (SCE) involves the breaking and rejoining of similar matching segments of DNA so that the function and viability of the cell is not compromised. The SCEs have been shown to be most useful in assessing exposure for carcinogens that form DNA adducts that are easily detected in peripheral blood (15). However, a relationship between SCEs and a health effect has not been established, thus limiting their usefulness as predictors of health risk.

Micronuclei are small fragments of DNA or chromosomes apart from the main nucleus. They indicate previous chromosomal aberrations (CAs). Micronuclei can be assayed in peripheral blood lymphocytes and in exfoliated cells from buccal mucosa and the urinary tract (19). The advent of fluorescence in situ hybridization (FISH) technology for detecting micronuclei formation will increase the speed, specificity, and sensitivity of this assay (20).

The CAs include the breaking and rearrangement of parts of chromosomes. Many different types of toxic agents can cause formation of CAs and can be used as a general biological marker to document exposure (15). As with micronuclei, FISH technology has revolutionized this assay, increasing the speed of analysis, efficiency of the assay, and improving its sensitivity (19). Of the three cytogenic markers—SCEs, micronuclei, and chromosomal aberrations—only the aberrations have been shown to be group risk factors for cancer (21,22).

Two other assays evaluate DNA stability. The first is the single-cell gel electrophoresis assay (COMET), which detects low molecular weight DNA as a result of DNA strand breaks. Advantages to this assay are (*1*) it is on the individual cell level; (*2*) any cell population can be used; and (*3*) the assay is sensitive, simple, and cost-effective (23). Another DNA stability assay that may have potential for genetic monitoring is the DNA repair assay (Challenge assay) (15). This assay is based on the premise that cells exposed to hazardous agents may be compromised in their ability to repair further insult to their DNA. Cells previously exposed to environmental agents are challenged a second time by exposure to radiation in the G_0 or G_1 phase of the cell cycle. Cells with higher levels of CAs are not able to cope with the challenge.

For genetic monitoring (as with any biomonitoring) to be useful in the workplace it should be considered within the traditional hierarchy of controls and integrated with the other elements of health and safety programs. The hierarchy of controls establishes primary prevention by substitution and source of exposure controls before secondary or tertiary prevention. Exposure controls can be evaluated by genetic monitoring for biomarkers of exposure or exposure effects or by ambient and breathing zone monitoring. These biomarkers can also be sources of risk estimates that can be used along with morbidity and mortality statistics. If genetic biomarkers are to be useful in the workplace, they need to meet a minimum criteria, as shown in Table 11.2. Various medical surveillance requirements are included in 17 Occupational Safety & Health Administration standards, but only three of these (those for arsenic, lead, and cadmium) require specific medical monitoring; none require genetic monitoring.

Before using genetic biomarkers in monitoring workers, a plan should be in place to determine what will happen to workers with results in the extremes of the distribution of results (2,8,14). Will there be repeat monitoring, diagnostic evaluation, environmental remediations, or medical removal? One concern by critics of genetic monitoring is that the resultant action will focus only on the worker and not on changing the environment (2). Clearly, both types of actions may be warranted. The hierarchy of controls and the principles of the OSHA legislation require emphasizing changing the workplace environment by process modification, engineering controls, and, in some cases, personal protective equipment. However, a person with genetic monitoring results in the extremes of the distribution of group results may need further assessment and follow-up actions. Because many genetic markers can be influenced by nonworkplace exposures, genetic monitoring should be accompanied

Table 11.2 Minimum Criteria for Genetic Tests

Genetic Monitoring
    Acceptable level of sensitivity and specificity
    Acceptance by population being monitored
    Established linkage to exposure or disease
    Protections for privacy and confidentiality
    Notification of participants
    Plan for addressing abnormal results

Genetic Screening
    Acceptable predictive value and reliability
    Protections for privacy and confidentiality
    Goals of screening should be specified
    Equal access and/or random participation
    Linkage of genetic factor to job requirements and duties
    Demonstration that genetic factor is a bona fide qualification for adequate job performance
    Definite plan for use of the data

Adapted from Murray (47) and Lappe (48).

by questionnaire to assess workers' other exposures (which could include residential ambient air, second jobs, behavioral practices, hobby exposures, and so forth). The goal of this assessment should be to explain the workplace results rather than blame the workers for their exposures.

A genetic monitoring result may require that a particular worker be moved from one job location to another. This is known as *medical removal*. This practice has been used with traditional biological monitoring, such as for lead in blood where a health risk is associated with a certain blood level, and where exposure controls are difficult to implement in a timely fashion. With measures like blood lead or zinc protoporphyrin, which are continuous, an employer may have more options than with a discrete measure such as an acquired $p53$ mutation, which is either present or absent.

One issue with medical removal is whether an employee will retain the same pay rate and benefits. This issue is termed *rate retention* and was mandated in the lead standard [(24) CFR 1910.1025 (k) (1)]. A known association, as seen with lead and disease, does not yet exist with most markers that might be used in genetic monitoring. However, a growing body of data has linked cytogenetic markers and somatic mutations in reporter genes with cancer risks in groups of workers (18). Whether this risk would apply to individuals in those groups has not been established. This highlights a confusion in the literature between group risk assessment and individual risk assessment. Epidemiologic research identifies risks for groups and not individuals in the groups. Individual risk functions can be calculated from group risk data when there are individual risk variables (25), but this is not commonly practiced. The potential exists for establishing individual risk profiles based on exposure factors, data from tests on effects of exposure (including genetic monitoring), and hereditary characteristics. Still, this will only be a probalistic determination, much like insurance company ratings of individuals with high risk factors. This kind of risk profiling will put further pressure on insurers and employers to remove or exclude workers rather than correct environmental exposures.

Genetic monitoring of workers requires considering what information workers should be given about the monitoring (so that they participate) and about their test results (26,27). The question of who has access or should have access to the results of genetic monitoring data needs to be considered before implementation of the testing. Participants should be informed about the access that others have to their data.

The question for society and policymakers on the horizon is: Does genetic monitoring indicate a health problem, a potential health problem, or compensable damage? The answers to this question will be affected by the state of science and public policy. At present, genetic monitoring is not validated widely as indicating individual risk of disease or a compensable condition. This situation could change as additional research is conducted.

Genetic Screening

Genetic screening in the workplace could be used in job placement or relocation to ensure that employers place workers most susceptible to a specific risk in the least hazardous environments (2). It could also be used to provide information to prospective or current employees so that they can decide if they wish to work in a particular environment.

Two types of genetic information might be used in occupational genetic screening. One is information about single genes that are strongly associated with rare diseases—for example, the HLA-B27 gene and ankylosing spondylitis, or the gene for hereditary diseases like the retinoblastoma gene (RBI) and eye cancer. In contrast, and more relevant to the occupational environment, are genes that code for enzymes involved in the metabolism (Phase I or Phase II) of occupational toxicants or carcinogens. These genes have multiple alleles and are sometimes called "metabolic polymorphisms." (A *polymorphism* is defined as a gene for which more than 1% of the population has a "variant" nonmajority allele.) They generally do not confer risk on their own but only in combination with a specific exposure (28,29). Examples are CYP2D6 and B(a)P exposure in lung cancer and *N*-acetytranferase-2 (NAT2) and aromatic amines in bladder cancer.

As was noted, genetic screening is rarely used in industrial medical practice because most genetic tests have not been validated—that is, their predictive value for occupational disease has not been determined. The 1989 survey of Fortune 500 companies showed that 12 were using biochemical genetic screening, and none were using direct DNA screening (2). Moreover, the ethical, legal, and social issues surrounding routine genetic screening of workers (mostly before employment or job change) have not been adequately debated. Nonetheless, in most jurisdictions, employers are not prohibited from requiring genetic screening, even if sufficient evidence does not exist for using such information as the basis of employment (1). Even if employers do not use genetic screening, they may still have access to medical records of employees and prospective employees. Employers may be able to learn if these individuals have predispositions to some diseases, although most of these predispositions probably will not pertain to occupational risks. Generally, for the workplace, genes for enzymes that are polymorphic with variants having different metabolic capabilities are likely to be candidates for genetic screening. The rationale is that workers with a particular characteristic can be excluded from exposure or will decide to exclude themselves, and these actions will result in prevention of occupational disease. This assumption may not always be correct, as was determined for one candidate for genetic screening [*n*-acetyltransferase (NAT) phenotype—discussed later].

Genetic screening to prevent workplace disease may have a range of controversial, ethical, and social effects that could include violating the decision-making autonomy of workers and promoting discrimination of racial and ethnic groups with a particular genetic characteristic (26,30). Moreover, the attempt to focus on a single metabolic polymorphism, such as NAT, fails to acknowledge that the body's processing of a xenobiotic toxicant requires numerous genes and enzymes. In the near future, however, new high-throughput technologies may allow for the simultaneous analysis of hundreds or thousands of genes, gene segments, and expression products (31). Statistically and functionally analyzing these multiple markers and interpreting them will be a major methodological problem and may raise new ethical and social issues.

However, as more is learned, it should be possible to identify more realistic combinations of genes and expression products that may provide a profile of individual risks of a given exposure. These technological advances will need to be considered against a backdrop of workers' and employers' rights and responsibilities. Workers have rights to self-determination, privacy, access to their results, and to employment. Employers have the responsibility to provide safe and healthful workplaces. When useful and valuable information can affect occupational risks, it is not likely to be ignored (4). The question is what policy and social controls will be implemented to avoid workers being unfairly and prejudicially treated. Currently, the laws to protect abuse of genetic screening and monitoring data are perceived as few, cumbersome, and difficult to enforce (8). These may include the Civil Rights Act, Title VIII (which prohibits discrimination based on race, religion, gender, and natural origin); the Americans with Disabilities Act (ADA) (which prohibits discrimination on the basis of a disability); and the National Labor Relations Act (which determines what subjects can be bargained).

The question with the ADA is whether a genetic trait is considered a disability. Most genes with polymorphisms for metabolic enzymes are not disease risks by themselves but indicate risk only with exposure. The ADA indicates that to qualify as a disability a condition must "substantially limit an individual in a major life activity." Whether being at risk in a particular job meets this definition is yet to be determined.

Another law, the Health Insurance Portability and Accountability Act, may provide some protection to workers because they will not be as readily subject to health insurance restrictions due to a preexisting genetic condition. This also remains to be widely tested. In addition, numerous laws against genetic discrimination are being considered in various state legislatures (4,9).

Research

Subsequent to development in the laboratory, research involving genetic information is generally along the lines of validating an assay, developing it for use, or determining the role of a genetic marker as a risk factor for disease.

Laboratory Validation

Validity of a marker in the laboratory generally means that the procedure or test responds in the presence of a marker and does not respond in its absence. The first step in laboratory validation is characterization of a genetic marker. Assessing the following characteristics are crucial: dose response, marker persistence, variability within and among individuals, correlation with other markers, and correlation with a critical response (32).

In developing a procedure for use in genetic monitoring, certain characteristics of the procedure must also be known. The test should be sensitive (i.e., it measures the desired effect at low levels of change). The test must have a high degree of accuracy or specificity. Accuracy is the "trueness" of the result. The test must also have precision, which is reproducibility of standards throughout the analyses.

Genetic tests for monitoring are subject to a great deal of variability, because the body actively collects, distributes, and eliminates xenobiotics (32). Repair of damaged DNA also occurs, which adds to the variability. Laboratory procedures can have three basic sources of error: (*1*) technical variability or error in laboratory measurement, (*2*) biological change from time to time in the person, and (*3*) biological changes among individuals (33). Technical variation is largely a result of instrumentation, reagents, and human error in sample labeling, preparation, and test performance (34). Technical variability must be determined to minimize its effect on discerning true differences. The contribution of the variation about biologic changes in an individual or among individuals can be factored in if characteristics and confounders of a genetic marker have been established.

Technical variability can be controlled using appropriate quality-assurance procedures. The first step is to develop a written standard operating procedure that specifies details of the reagents, storage conditions, equipment, sampling and analytical procedures, and calibration and quality-control methods (35). Changes should not be made to the operating procedures unless the impact on sensitivity, accuracy, and precision is known. An operating procedure is critical for monitoring tests so that the same procedure is maintained for subsequent analyses. Using an operating procedure also aids in identifying and minimizing laboratory drift (a change in response with time). Preparing quality-control samples at the beginning of analysis can also determine laboratory drift.

Protocols need to be established for collecting and documenting the samples. Timing the collection of the sample may depend critically on what the test is measuring. Protocols also need to be developed to establish transportation and storage procedures in the preanalytic phase. It is generally accepted that samples should be coded so that the identity or case of exposure of the person's samples is not known to the analyst.

Another important way to decrease technical variation is laboratory enrollment in a proficiency testing program. Proficiency testing increases the confidence in the results generated by that laboratory. In the absence of a formal proficiency testing program, which may be the case if the test used is not in routine use, comparison of results with other laboratories may suffice. Finally, laboratory validation, including an evaluation of technical variability, must be accomplished before a procedure is even considered for genetic monitoring or genetic screening. Establishing a quality-assurance program is essential before any monitoring program is put in place.

Population Validation

Subsequently, an assay must to be validated in terms of its utility in various population groups. This process entails understanding interperson variability according to demographic and behavioral characteristics, determining the underlying prevalence of the marker, and identifying the optimal handling and logistic considerations. Ultimately, validation requires determining the predictive value and attributable proportion (36). Critical in population validation is that exposure assessment should receive as much attention as marker measurement (37). Moreover, in research particularly, whole assay techniques are being developed, and thus some degree of genetic risk factor misclassification will almost inevitably occur in population-based studies. Evaluation of the phenomena in the context of marker prevalence is important in explaining disparate findings in the literature (38).

Many issues of using genetic markers in research are similar to their use in occupational medical practice. The greatest difference is that, in research, less certainty exists about the meaning of the markers, hence the need for the research. Moreover, much of the research is to establish specifications, performance characteristics, and mechanistic information about the marker or the assay, and this has no specificity about individual or group risks. At this level of uncertainty, much debate is triggered concerning what subjects and, in some cases, their close relatives as well should be told about research during recruitment, when reporting test results, or when reporting study results. Debate ranges from proposals to report only clinically relevant findings to proposals to report all results regardless of their relevance for individual risk or health. The issue is further exacerbated by technological and scientific developments that lead to the ability to identify new markers and assays long before their "meaning" is known. This advance, coupled with the increasing practice of storing or banking biological samples containing DNA, presents some unusual logistical and ethical dilemmas (29,39).

Historically, when research subjects agreed to participate in studies, they routinely agreed or were not aware that specimens were going to be stored for subsequent and generally related research. The recent explosion of data about genetic assays has provided researchers with many new opportunities for testing specimens for a wide range of genetic characteristics. The following questions arise: To what extent is further consent required from the initial participants? What feedback on subsequent tests is appropriate? The latter question depends in part on the nature of the initial informed consent. Was the consent to a specific assay, or to broader research questions, a research topic, or area? Were banking and results notification mentioned? Some have argued that in the workplace genetic research setting, informed consent is practically an impossibility in that neither the investigator nor the participant is truly informed of the meaning of the research, or the extent of social or legal jeopardy to which a participant might be subject (40). Also, the consent is often seen as being given within a coercive framework tied to the power relationships in the workplace.

In addition, little research has been conducted to assess whether research participants have subsequently been harmed by stigmatization, job or insurance discrimination, psychological loss of self-esteem or in other ways. Some anecdotes supporting these contentions have been noted. The lack of research on the deleterious effects of participating in investigations with genetic components may not indicate the size of the problem but rather the difficulty in assessing it.

Another problem area is researcher and commercial efforts to market assays before they are validated (41). This stems in part from researchers' conducting poorly designed studies (in terms of sample size, control for bias, and confounding), and then failing to conduct the necessary follow-up work to determine the degree to which the finding is generalizable to other populations. Much of the problem is based on overinterpreting the results of a single small study by the researchers and inappropriate implication by scientific journals, translational newsletters and services, and ultimately by the popular press. Another interpretation problem is the incorrect practice of attributing the cause of complex social and biological phenomena to single-gene explanations.

Regulation

Genetic monitoring or screening and the use of genetic markers are not currently proscribed in workplace regulations, but such efforts are not prohibited. Although some occupational health standards require certain biomonitoring, much debate continues about whether future standards will require genetic testing (screening or monitoring) (9,13). This situation could change as more validated markers become identified and as more is learned about the genetic role in occupational disease. Society is faced with a difficult issue. As one observer (9) has noted: "If society's goal is to protect the welfare of workers, is it a basic contradiction of this goal, as embodied in both statutory law as well as common law, to interpret antidiscrimination laws as protecting the rights of ostensibly healthy individuals to eventually decide to disable themselves in the name of freedom of choice?" Most regulations involving genetic testing or use of genetic markers will most likely be of the protective variety, namely to prevent civil rights abuses involving genetic information. At present, no uniform protection exists against the use or misuse of, or access to, genetic information in the workplace (1). However, federal legislation such as HR 2215, The Genetic Nondiscrimination in the Workplace Act. Was proposed but not passed in 1997. Often, the laws that have been passed have not been related to genetic factors that would interact with workplace exposures, but rather to genetic conditions that of themselves rarely might lead to prematurely reducing an employee's ability to work.

In the conclusion to a visionary book (1988) on variation in human susceptibility, Hornig (42) stated that the central public policy question is: "How should variation in the sensitivity of groups and individuals be taken into account in occupational laws and regulations?" Historically in the occupational arena, susceptibility has not been a major factor in determining permissible exposure levels. The Occupational Safety and Health Act (OSHAct) requires that a standard should be set "which most adequately insures, to the extent feasible, on the basis of the best available evidence, that no employee will suffer material impairment of health or functional capacity." Moreover, a policy strategy that focuses on the worker instead of the workplace, while counter to the spirit of the OSHAct also may not be as effective as it might appear.

For example, the preventive advantage of preselecting and removing individuals who are slow acetylators (with a particular allele for NAT) from a workforce was compared with removing a chemical bladder carcinogen from the work environment. For the worker removal, the attributable proportion was 25% for a twofold association (OR = 2) and 43% for an eightfold association (OR = 8), whereas for removing the carcinogen, the attributable proportions were 50% and 88%, respectively (given that the whole excess risk is not concentrated only among the slow acetylators) (30,43). (*Attributable proportion* is the fraction of the association that can be accounted for by the genetic factor.) Thus, in the above example, removing the carcinogen would account for a larger reduction in the cancer risk than removing the worker.

The use of genetic screening would reinforce the trend in the health promotion field to focus only on those employees identified as "at-risk." This approach can be contrasted with a public health approach that recognizes that most people will have a variety of genetic, environmental, and behavioral risk factors that can contribute to occupational disease. Focusing on just one subgroup can miss many others (44). The extent to which it is possible to identify genetic subgroups that will suffer material impairment may have an impact on the interpretation of the law. Moreover, the implication of such capabilities to identify subgroups leads to arguments for genetic screening, which could result in denying career opportunities to some people and result in their being labeled "unfit." From an employer's perspective, using genetic information to prevent occupational disease or injury may be worthwhile and cost-effective. From the worker's perspective, the potential loss of opportunity and the emphasis on excluding the worker rather than controlling the workplace is unfair and inappropriate.

Additionally, excluding people with a particular genotype does not assure that individuals with another genotype who replace them still will not have some risk. Also taking part in this debate are the insurers who argue that they should be able to use all risk factors—exogenous and endogenous—in considering insurance risks (45). These are the debates that are likely to occur in the next decade.

Workers' compensation is the existing legal framework for protecting workers. Within this framework, the role of a genetic trait as part of the etiology for an occupational disease will depend on a jurisdiction's statutory definition (9). Generally, claimants must prove that the disease is work-related and not one of the "ordinary diseases of life." For example, if a worker had a gene for thalassemic anemia that was activated by lead exposure in the workplace, whether it was compensable would depend on whether this is an ordinary disease of life for this worker just by virtue of his genotype (9). Conversely, it might be argued that such a condition might not have been triggered without the workplace exposure.

Another area where genetic information may impact regulation is in the area of qualitative and quantitative risk assessments. The current requirements for various regulatory agencies is to be able to describe the level of risks and the effect of recommended reduction of exposures [Industrial Union Department v. American Petroleum Inst., 448 USC 607, (1980)] (10). Risk assessment is the practice of determining the extent to which a hazard causes a risk, injury, or disease. It involves establishing the existence of an exposure–response relationship and the area of no or lowest observed effect levels. This can be accomplished qualitatively or by statistical and mathematical modeling.

For example, quantitative risk assessment (QRA) entails extrapolating risks from animal species to humans and from high to low exposures. The use of genetic information can possibly enhance QRAs by providing mechanistic information to judge the appropriateness of extrapolating between species and to describe biological conditions with high and low doses (12,46). There is a great deal of uncertainty in QRA because of the lack of data and the need to make assumptions about relationships between species, and the nature of the exposure–response relationship at low exposures. Understanding the role of genetic factors and impact of xenobiotics may provide more useful information for risk assessors to recommend occupational safety and health standards.

References

1. Rothenberg K, Fuller B, Rothstein M, et al. Genetic information and the workplace: legislative approaches and policy challenges. Science 1997;275:1755–1757.

2. Office of Technology Assessment. Genetic monitoring and screening in the workplace. Washington, DC: U.S. Government Printing Office, 1990; OTA-BA-455.

3. Barrett JC, Vainio H, Peakall D, Goldstein BD. Joint report: 12th meeting of the scientific group on methodologies for the safety evaluation of chemicals: susceptibility to environmental hazards. Env Health Perspect 1997;105(Suppl 4):699–737.

4. Rothstein MA. Genetic secrets: a policy framework. In Rothstein MA (ed). Genetic secrets: protecting privacy and confidentiality in the genetic era. New Haven, Yale University Press, 1997, pp. 451–495.

5. Omenn GS. Predictive identification of hypersusceptible individuals. J Occup Med 1982;24:369–374.

6. Ashford NA. Medical screening in the workplace: legal and ethical considerations. Semi Occup Med 1986;1:67–79.

7. VanDamme K, Castelan L, Heseltine E, et al. Individual susceptibility and prevention of occupational diseases: scientific and ethical issues. J Occup Environ Med 1995;37:91–99.

8. Bingham E. Ethical issues for genetic testing for workers. In: Mendelsohn ML, Mohr LC, Peeters JP (eds). Biomarkers: medical and workplace applications. Washington, DC: John Henry Press, 1998, pp. 415–422.

9. Richter J. Taking the worker as you find him: the quandry of protecting the rights as well as the health of the worker with a genetic susceptibility to occupational disease. Maryland J Contemp Issues 1997;8:189–236.

10. USC. United States code. Washington, DC: U.S. Government Printing Office.

11. Hattis D. Use of biological markers and pharmacokinetics in human health risk assessment. Environ Health Perspect 1991;90:229–238.

12. McClellan RO. Risk assessment and biological mechanisms: lessons learned, future opportunities. Toxicology 1995;102:239–258.

13. Gochfeld M. Susceptibility biomarkers in the workplace: historical perspective. In: Mendelsohn ML, Mohr LC, Peeters JP (eds). Biomarkers: medical and workplace applications. Washington, DC: John Henry Press, 1998, pp. 3–22.

14. Schulte PA, Halperin WE. Genetic screening and monitoring in the workplace. In: McDonald JC (ed). Recent advances in occupational health. Edinburgh, Scotland: Churchill Living Stone, 1987, pp. 135–154.

15. Huessner JC, Ward JB Jr., Legator MS. Genetic monitoring of aluminum workers exposed to coal tar pitch volatiles. Mutat Res 1985;155:143–155.

16. Sorsa M. Genetic monitoring: experiences, possibilities, and applications in occupational health practices. Int J Occup Environ Health 1996;2:554–556.

17. Wild CP, Pisani P. Carcinogen-DNA and carcinogen-protein adducts in molecular epidemiology. In: Toniolo P, Boffetta P, Shuker DEG, Hulka B, Pearce N (eds). Application of biomarkers in cancer epidemiology. Lyon, France: International Agency for Research on Cancer, 1997; IARC Scientific Publications No. 142, pp. 143–158.

18. Albertini RJ, Hayes RB. Somatic cell mutations in cancer epidemiology. In: Toniolo P, Boffetta P, Shuker DEG, Hulka B, Pearce N (eds). Application of biomarkers in cancer epidemiology. Lyon, France: International Agency for Research on Cancer, 1997; IARC Scientific Publications No. 142, pp. 159–184.

19. Moore LE, Titenko-Holland N, Quintana PJE, Smith MT. Novel biomarkers of genetic damage in humans: use of fluorescence in situ hybridization to detect

aneuploidy and micronuclei in exfoliated cells. J Toxicol Environ Health 1993;40: 349–357.

20. MacGregor JT, Farr S, Tucker JD, Heddle JA, Tice RR, Turteltaub KW. New molecular endpoints and methods for routine toxicity testing. Fundam Appl Toxicol 1995;26:156–173.

21. Hagmar L, Brøgger A, Hansteen IL, et al. Cancer risk in humans predicted by increased levels of chromosomal aberrations in lymphocytes: Nordic study group on the health risks of chromosome damage. Cancer Res 1994;54:2912–2922.

22. Hagmar L, Bonassi S, Stromberg U, et al. Chromosomal aberrations in lymphocytes predict human cancer: A report from the European Study Group on cytogentic biomarkers and health (ESCH). Cancer Res 1998;4117–4121.

23. MacGregor JT, Tucker JD, Eastmond DA, Wyrobek AJ. Integration of cytogenetic assays with toxicology studies. Environ Mol Mutagen 1995;25:328–337.

24. CFR. Code of federal regulations. Washington, DC: U.S. Government Printing Office, Office of the Federal Register.

25. Truett J, Cornfield J, Kannel W. A multivariate analysis of the risk of coronary heart disease in Framingham. J Chronic Dis 1967;20:511–524.

26. Soskolne CL. Ethical, social, and legal issues surrounding studies of susceptible populations and individuals. Environ Health Perspect 1997;105(Suppl 4):837–841.

27. Schulte PA, Haring Sweeney M. Ethical considerations, confidentiality issues, rights of human subjects, and uses of monitoring data in research and regulation. Environ Health Perspect 1995;103(Suppl 3):69–74.

28. Grandjean P (ed). Ecogenetics: genetic predisposition to the toxic effects of chemicals. London: Chapman and Hall, 1991.

29. Hunter D, Caporaso N. Informed consent in epidemiologic studies involving genetic markers. Epidemiology 1997;8:596–599.

30. Vineis P, Schulte PA. Scientific and ethical aspects of genetic screening of workers for cancer risk: the case of the n-acetyltransferase phenotype. J Clin Epidemiol 1995;48:189–197.

31. Lockhart DJ, Dong H, Byrne MC, et al. Expression monitoring by hybridization to high-density oligonucleotide arrays. Nat Biotechnol 1994;14:1675–1680.

32. Schulte PA, Talaska G. Validity criteria for the use of biological markers of exposure to chemical agents in environmental epidemiology. Toxicology 1995;101:73–78.

33. Vineis P, Schulte PA, Vogt RF Jr. Technical variability in laboratory data. In: Schulte PA, Perera FP (eds). Molecular epidemiology: principles and practices. San Diego: Academic Press, 1993, pp. 109–135.

34. Stites DP. Laboratory evaluation of immune competence. In: Stites DP, Terr AI (eds). Basic and clinical immunology. Norwalk, CT: Appleton & Lange, 1991, pp. 312–318.

35. Gompertz D. Quality control of biomarker measurements in epidemiology. In: Toniolo P, Boffetta P, Shuker DEG, Rothman N, Hulka B, Pearce N (eds). Application of biomarkers in cancer epidemiology. Lyon, France: International Agency for Research on Cancer, 1998; IARC Publication No. 142, pp. 215–222.

36. Schulte PA, Perera FP. Validation. In: Schulte PA, Perera FP (eds). Molecular epidemiology: principles and practices. San Diego: Academic Press, 1993, pp. 79–107.

37. Rothman N. Genetic susceptibility biomarkers in studies of occupational and environmental cancer: methodologic issues. Toxicol Lett 1995;77:221–225.

38. Rothman N, Stewart WF, Caporaso NE, Hayes RB. Misclassification of genetic susceptibility biomarkers: implications for case-control studies and cross-population comparisons. Cancer Epidemiol Biomarkers Prev 1993;2:299–303.

39. Clayton EW, Steinberg KK, Khoury MJ, et al. Informed consent for genetic research on stored tissue samples. JAMA 1995;274:1786–1792.

40. Samuels SW. The Selikoff Agenda and the Human Genome Project: ethics and social issues. In: Samuels SW, Upton AC (eds). Genes, cancer, and ethics in the work environment. Beverly Farms, MA: OEM Press, 1998, pp. 3–9.

41. Nelkin D, Tancredi L. Dangerous diagnostics. The social power of biological information. New York: Basic Books, 1989.

42. Hornig DF. Conclusion. In: Brain JD, Back BD, Warren AJ, Shaikh RA (eds). Variations in susceptibility to inhaled pollutants. Baltimore: The Johns Hopkins University Press, 1988, pp. 461–471.

43. Vineis P, Schulte P. Attributable risks and genetic predisposition (letter). Clin Epidemiol 1996;49:599.

44. Rose G. Sick individuals and sick populations. Int J Epidemiol 1985;14:32–38.

45. Brockett P, Tankersley S. The genetics revolution: economics, ethics, and insurance. J Business Ethics 1997;16:1666–1676.

46. Bois FY, Krowech G, Zeise L. Modeling human interindividual variability in metabolism and risk: the example of 4-aminobiphenyl. Risk Analy 1995;15:205–213.

47. Murray TH. Genetic screening in the workplace: ethical issues. J Occup Med 1983;25:451–454.

48. Lappe M. Ethical issues in testing for differential sensitivity to occupational hazards. J Occup Med 1983;25:797–808.

III
EVALUATION OF GENETIC TESTING

12

Medical and public health strategies for ensuring the quality of genetic testing

Michael S. Watson

Genetic testing and related genetic services have been available for decades. In their earliest forms, genetic tests were either based on complete, though low-resolution, analyses of the human genome by way of chromosome analysis or on the analysis of gene products in biochemical genetic tests to identify patients with metabolic disease. Services were often provided by clinician-scientists who both defined the specialty of medical genetics (see footnote) and provided most of the services. The disorders for which the tests were of clinical utility tended to be both rare and severe. Initially used as diagnostic tools, biochemical genetic tests were rapidly integrated into many state newborn screening programs, and cytogenetics was integrated into prenatal screening programs. Voluntary quality-assurance programs were developed by professionals in the field.

Over the past 10 to 15 years, significant changes have made medical genetics among the most exciting and rapidly evolving areas of medicine. We have moved from testing for rare diseases to testing for common disease susceptibilities and from low-resolution chromosome overviews of the genome to increasingly focused molecular assessments at the single nucleotide level. In 1995, more than 80,000 molecular diagnostic tests for heritable disease were performed, nearly double the number in 1994 (1). As we continue through what amounts to a technological revolution in a field that affects most other areas of medicine, against the backdrop of a rapidly changing health care delivery and oversight system in the United States, it becomes increasingly important to actively define and pursue measures that will ensure safe and effective

---

The American Board of Medical Genetics was established as the 24th primary specialty board of medicine by the American Board of Medical Specialties in 1991.

genetic testing for the public. This chapter will discuss the issues facing this field, including physician and public education, laboratory quality, and the still ill-defined standards by which decisions are made regarding the transition of research information into clinical investigation and on to standard-of-care service. To understand the issues that must be addressed to assure quality testing, some knowledge of the practice and information on its place in health care delivery are valuable.

The Test and the Testing Service

As was clearly stated by the National Institutes of Health and Department of Energy (NIH/DOE) Task Force on Genetic Testing (TFGT) (2), a genetic test is more than just the laboratory test itself. It is part of a broader testing service that encompasses patient identification, education and referral, and the ultimate delivery of the test results and their interpretation to those tested. Systems exist within which greater focus can be brought to the laboratory technical issues; however, preanalytic issues, such as recognition of risks and appropriate referral and delivery of accurate and balanced information to patients, are areas for which significant concerns have been expressed.

The Delivery System for Genetic Services

Medical genetics services are commonly provided as part of a multidisciplinary patient assessment. Genetic evaluation is complicated by the fact that it commonly involves families, but health care delivery systems are directed at individuals. Within a single family, there may be individuals lacking health care coverage, and those with coverage may be under managed care or in fee-for-service systems. Family members may be required by payers to receive their services from providers contracted to their programs, complicating the delivery of a family-based medical service.

It is generally accepted that insufficient "genetics" manpower and the large population that may access these services in the future will necessitate that many types of providers have knowledge of and experience in the practice of genetics, with primary-care physicians forming the front lines for patient identification. However, a recent study of the knowledge gap resulting from the recent and explosive expansion of the field indicates that geneticist physicians are able to answer nearly 95% of questions presented in genetic knowledge questionnaires as compared to 74% for nongeneticist physicians (3). Among these nongeneticist physicians, there is a clear decrease in knowledge among those graduating medical school prior to 1970. Few primary-care physicians were exposed to genetic services because these were directed at rare diseases.

It is this knowledge gap that underlies many of the difficulties in delivering genetic services. Lack of familiarity compounded by increasing demands on time may render primary-care physicians less effective in providing front-line identification of those at risk; hence, while the educational process continues, genetics laboratories will have a greater responsibility for ensuring appropriate and informed use of genetic tests than for other types of tests.

Types of Tests and Intended Uses

It is becoming increasingly apparent that genetic variation, both normal and abnormal, underlies much of human disease; however, the magnitude of this genetic contribution varies from negligible to deterministic. As such, the very definition of a genetic test can have broad implications. The definition of "genetic testing" offered by the TFGT had several goals: (*1*) to be semantically correct such that any test (molecular, cytogenetic, or biochemical) providing information derived from the human genome and its expression is included; and (*2*) to not be so broad that virtually every test available be encompassed under the definition (2). To meet the second goal, the TFGT recommended that consideration be given to the magnitude of the genetic contribution to avoid encompassing common tests, such as cholesterol screening, with a relatively small contribution to the genetic factors of disease development in the great majority of people.

The types of genetic tests are broad both technically and in their use. When performed in high-quality laboratories, they are highly sensitive in detecting the types of abnormalities they are designed to detect. Unfortunately, mutations come in many varieties, can be distributed in or around coding sequences, and are found in genes ranging in size from small to large (4). Depending on the types of mutations characteristic of a particular gene, the analytically very sensitive test may have high to low clinical sensitivity. This is often because a significant proportion of patients have mutations in genes yet to be identified or have disease that is not associated with highly penetrant single gene(s). Multiple techniques are often needed to thoroughly analyze a particular gene. Even so, there are individuals who have mutations that haven't been identified, even in some of the most thoroughly studied genes.

Furthermore, a single gene may be associated with seemingly unrelated diseases or phenotypes (pleiotropism), or a disease or phenotype may be caused by mutations in more than one gene (heterogeneity). For instance, the ApoE gene has been implicated as a risk factor for development of dementias, including Alzheimer disease (5,6), is associated with hyperlipidemia, and is a risk for coronary artery disease (7). In many instances, the expression of a particular mutation is impacted by other genes (polygenic), which may alter penetrance and disease severity.

The aforementioned discussion of the potentially wide range of uses of the same genetic test focuses on abnormalities arising in the germline; however, the uses of some genetic tests extend to nonheritable somatic changes, as seen with testing for mutations in the p53 gene (8). Abnormalities in *p53* detected by identical methods can inform about the staging of a tumor in somatic tissues, an application not necessarily constrained by concerns about the interpretation of results in a human genetics context, or about heritable changes associated with a diagnosis of Li Fraumeni syndrome (9). Testing for inherited mutations may be further extended to the prenatal setting, both uses that require results to be interpreted in the context of inherited human disease. Inherent in the discussion of *p53* is the concept that a disorder may be either noninherited or inherited. Understanding test results and their implications in such scenarios will require a sense of these two etiologies and the proportion of cases with particular clinical indications that are heritable.

The range of phenotypes in individuals carrying identical mutations can be broad (*variable expressivity*). Multiple genes may be acting in concert to cause a phenotype (*polygenic*) or may require an environmental (*multifactorial*) interaction to be expressed in an individual. Heterogeneity of genes with mutations that can result in a particular phenotype requires that laboratories and clinicians work closely together. For some patients, clinical presentation may direct the sequence through which genes should be asessed. Among individuals with breast cancer, the presence of an individual in the family who is a male with breast cancer or a female with ovarian cancer may indicate that the testing should begin with BRCA1 or BRCA2 (10–12). Additional information as to the family history may also impact the interpretation of results, particularly when the test gives negative results and residual risk is uncertain. As laboratories move through the genes that may be related to the disorder at decreasing frequency, communication between laboratory and clinical providers will be important.

The fact that these tests have multiple intended uses has been among the most difficult of issues to address. Few would argue with the diagnostic use of a test for an individual affected with a particular disorder; however, some concern has been raised about the use of the same test in unaffected presymptomatic individuals from families segregating the disease-related gene(s), and still others raise concerns when the test is for susceptibility, particularly in the absence of treatment interventions.

Other concerns arise when the test is a population screening tool. As technology becomes less costly, the focus will shift from analytic aspects of a test to defining the appropriate situations in which a test is to be used. Finally, it is important to remember that we remain quite ignorant about the primary and secondary roles that any particular gene product may play, including those of genes with disease-associated mutations.

Genetic tests may be used as diagnostic tools or screening tools in the presymptomatic (people who are now unaffected, but will be affected later in life) or those predisposed (people at risk but not assured of being affected) to developing a certain disease. Such tests may be used prenatally, postnatally, or postmortem. They may be used to identify carriers with reproductive risks or people who are themselves at risk of developing disease. Furthermore, they can target individuals, families, well-defined populations, or entire populations.

New Test Development

Genetic tests are developed in stages, which encompass both the analytical and clinical aspects of the tests. The initial stage is a research stage during which an association between mutations in a gene and a particular phenotype are established. Even if the research indicates an association, it may not necessarily have resolved the magnitude of this relationship nor its impact on outcome, particularly when disease prediction in otherwise normal individuals is intended.

In fact, it is an inherent bias in medical genetics that disease-causing genes are identified in people with the disease and that those most severely affected are most likely to access health care. At present, no standards exist to guide the decision of whether or not the relationship is of a magnitude sufficient to justify moving to a clinical investigative stage. This transition seems to be the most contentious. It must be recognized that the information needed to determine the relationship's significance may be interpreted only in the context of knowledge of a patient's disease state as well as pedigree structure. The issue is less whether the test–disease relationship should be more carefully evaluated, but how one evaluates it both fairly and with maximum education of those involved. This includes (*1*) what a test will or will not do, (*2*) how the results may positively and negatively affect them, and, equally important, (*3*) what the results do and do not mean. Rather than constraining this stage of development, we must determine the most fair and effective ways of ensuring safe and informed participation in this stage. Institutional review boards (IRBs) must adapt to the scientific and clinical needs of studies involving genetic testing.

During the final stage of development, namely accepted clinical practice, many additional factors, which translate into clinical utility, come into play. These include cost-benefit analyses of the information gleaned from those tested and its contribution relative to other clinical or laboratory information used to assess the relevant condition. In genetics, the cost-benefit analysis is a quickly shifting target attributable to rapid changes in technology that reduce costs and the similarly rapid move toward treatments resulting from knowl-edge of the genetic etiology of the disorder.

To gain a better understanding of the potential steps in test development where oversight or standards development may be appropriate, a brief overview of the development and transition of various uses of genetic tests for cystic fibrosis can be illustrative. Some steps may be amenable to an external assessment of validity, whereas others may require defined standard(s) around which laboratory practice can proceed.

Genetic testing for cystic fibrosis (CF) became possible in 1985 (13) with the identification of markers linked to the disease-causing gene. At that time, Southern blotting methods were used, and the test was limited to affected indi-viduals and their families. Only about 80% of cases were informative and therefore amenable to linkage analysis in the family. Between 1986 and 1988 more and closer linkage markers became available, such that 85% of families were informative for testing (14). By 1989, the cystic fibrosis transmembrane regulatory (CFTR) gene had been identified, and six relatively common disease-associated mutations were known (15). At that point, direct testing or linkage could be used to assess affected individuals and their families, and the possibility existed that populations (newborns, couples, ethnic groups, and others) could be studied. Interested parties generally agreed that a larger pro-portion of patients should be identifiable before moving into either carrier screening or other screening strategies (16).

Concurrently, methods for mutation detection were becoming more directed and less labor-intensive, and improved mutation scanning methods were available. By 1990, tests were available for 10 to 20 of the 115 known mutations; by 1993, 30 of 330 mutations were commonly included in tests, and by 1997, 60 of 600+ mutations were commonly part of tests. Current tests include 72 of the 700+ known mutations. Nevertheless, most of the remaining mutations are rare or "private mutations" present in single families (17). As nucleic acid chips (18) and other microarray technologies develop, all or most mutations may become easily testable. Until that time, providers must appreciate the pace at which these tests are evolving. Today's mutation test for CF may include 80 mutations, whereas next year's test may include hundreds. Analytical sensitivity for those mutations included in the panel will be very high, regardless of the number of mutations tested; however, clinical sensitivity will increase as additional mutations are added to the panel.

It is unlikely that regulatory bodies will have sufficient expertise or the interest in assessing every disease-causing mutation. Rather, standards will develop for the scientific and clinical criteria that must be met for the mutation to be considered disease-causing. Major changes in technology will be validated independently of specific diseases, and their use in individ-ual diseases will be determined by their ability to detect the range of mutations characteristic of that disorder. In any case, it is important to understand that for those whose mutations are identified, the test may have great value, while to those lacking one of the established mutations, the test is of limited or no value. However, once a mutation is identified within a family, both carriers and noncarriers in that family may benefit from testing. Balancing the interests of the two becomes an important consideration.

Test Validation

Two aspects of genetic tests require validation. Under the Clinical Laboratory Improvement Amendments of 1988 (CLIA '88) (19), analytical validity must be established for any new test put into service after September 1993. In this context "new" refers to any test new to that laboratory, regardless of whether it is a test that has been possible in the past. Demonstration of scientific and clinical validity, however, is not required under CLIA '88. The Food and Drug Administration (FDA) provides oversight of manufactured kit-based tests including assessment of analytical validity and clinical validity and utility, whereas CLIA is the lone oversight body for tests using reagents developed in laboratories. When a new test not previously available in laboratories is developed, scientific validity and analytical validity must be established. Because new genetic tests are infrequently developed as kits that might be within the purview of the FDA and are commonly in-house-developed assays, they are unlikely to be subjected to significant external review of scientific validity and clinical utility, aside from that presented in the peer-reviewed literature. In such an environment, test availability may be confined to those tests with external funding to support testing and controlled through the availablity of reimbursement for the testing.

As illustrated in the CF testing example, analytical and clinical validity are independent of one another. At the outset, linkage tests were analytically valid and brought useful clinical information to many of those tested diagnostically and their families. In the hands of well-trained laboratory personnel, the tests were highly accurate; however, questions about clinical utility were numerous, though often a function of cost. Over time, the linkage test was supplanted by other highly analytically accurate tests; however, although a CFTR mutation analysis test may be very accurate in detecting a particular mutation, its overall clinical utility is a function of the number of mutations assayed. Translated into practical terms, a test is highly analytically accurate and of high clinical utility when the mutation is found. When the mutation is not found, the test is still analytically accurate, but the clinical utility is limited to those with informative test results. The accompanying list shows a number of recommendations that TFGT recently (2) offered for test validation.

- The genotypes to be detected by a genetic test must be shown by scientifically valid methods to be associated with the occurrence of a disease. The observation must be independently replicated and subject to peer review.
- Analytical sensitivity and specificity of a genetic test must be determined before it is made available in clinical practice.
- Data to establish the clinical validity of genetic tests must be collected under investigative protocols.
- In the clinical validation phase, the study sample must be drawn from a group of subjects representative of the population for whom the test is intended.
- Formal validation for each intended use of a genetic test is needed.
- Before a genetic test can be generally accepted in clinical practice, data must be collected to demonstrate the benefits and risks that accrue from both positive and negative results.
- No clinical laboratory should offer a genetic test whose clinical validity has not been established, unless it is collecting data on clinical validity under either an IRB-approved protocol or a conditional premarket approval agreement with the FDA.

Several features of genetic tests must be considered when determining the type and methods of validation needed for any particular test. For the most part, genetic technologies ask laboratory questions for which no predicate test exists; hence, there is no preexisting test, other than a clinical diagnosis, that would be considered a "gold standard" against which the new test can be compared.

The approach to analytical validation will vary with the question to be answered by the test. When used for population carrier screening in individuals either pregnant or planning pregnancy, the tests will likely focus on mutations of known clinical consequence. The use of genome scanning methods may be precluded as the interpretation of ions not known to be disease causing would be beyond a screening program. However, in a diagnostic setting in which the likelihood of a mutation in a particular gene that might harbor any of a large number of mutations is high, scanning methods are likely to be used and the results interpreted.

Diagnostic assays should be tested for their ability to detect specific mutations known to occur in significant proportions of affected individuals. Similarly, the analytical technique that identifies the mutations must be validated; however, because some mutations will be rare or even confined to a single kindred, not all disease-causing mutations can be anticipated. There is a need to define a set of standards based on the science of genetics (e.g., what distinguishes pathological mutations from normal variations) that can be used to characterize a test and should be met for applicable test results to be considered valid. Included would be criteria for defining a disease-related mutation based on specific criteria (e.g., the type of variation, the functional domain in which the variation occurs, whether the change leads to protein truncation, and so forth). Difficulties interpreting sequence variations commonly arise during the early phases of investigative testing and will continue even after a test is considered "accepted." Expert-based practice-of-medicine judgments will be made about the clinical relevance of any previously unknown, rare, or private mutation. Practitioners' knowledge of human genetics will be factored into decisions of whether the mutation meets certain yet-to-be defined standards of a "pathological" mutation (e.g., gain or loss of function; mode of inheritance).

In addition, it is likely that professional organizations will be actively involved in cataloguing both gene-disease relationships and mutation-disease relationships. As has been apparent during the evolution of a CF test, throughout the evolution of the test there will be points when major technical breakthroughs necessitate that new methods be validated. Fortunately, as these points arise, there will be "gold standards" against which the new method can be compared. The highest standards and qualifications should be met by laboratories offering assays capable of identifying variations whose significance must be determined by the laboratory.

Additional clinical utility questions arise when genetic tests become screening tools. Many of these issues are population-based and are being faced at present owing to the recommendation of attendees of a recent NIH Cystic Fibrosis Consensus Conference that all couples pregnant or considering pregnancy should be offered CF carrier screening (20). Despite disease incidences in ethnic groups ranging from 1/3330 (Caucasian) to 1/32,100 (Asian American), the attendees recommended that testing be offered to all couples. Further complicating the screening process are the differing frequencies of the various mutations in these populations (17,20). Most of the mutations identified in CF patients have been among Caucasians because of their high disease frequency. Common mutations in the Caucasian population account for about 83% of the known mutations for that group; however, in African-American populations, these same mutations account for only about 52% of disease-causing mutations. In Native Americans, only about 25% of mutations are those common in Caucasians. Although issues of increasing population admixture and programmatic simplicity underlined the decision to offer screening to all couples, much work needs to be done to develop appropriate materials to help both physicians and patients (*1*) appreciate the likelihood of the patient carrying a mutation, (*2*) understand the range of mutations that the test to be requested will include, and (*3*) understand test results.

When tests for mutations are to be part of screening programs, it is important that they are validated both clinically and analytically. The lack of a standardized mutation battery of known clinically relevant mutations was an obvious problem when preconception CF couple carrier screening was recommended. Some laboratories offered only a single mutation for the test, which may be of some value in narrow ethnic groups or in families known to carry the specific mutation, but very inadequate for screening (21). Rarely do laboratories indicate the intended use of their test to allow referring providers to determine whether the test is intended for diagnosis or screening.

Individual risk assessment can be complicated by factors such as diseases or phenotypes in the proband, family history, and ethnicity. Though some factors impart high risk, others with more moderate associations should not necessarily trump other risks or evidence against risks. A Bayesian approach to risk calculation (22) may be the better approach to risk assignment, allowing for a more uniform absolute risk cutoff as an indication for testing. A case against CF screening in Asian Americans because of the very low incidence of CF in that population can be made; however, it is likely that this aspect of risk will have to be part of educating the patient prior to deciding whether testing is appropriate for that individual.

Population concerns are also reflected in the interpretation of genetic test results. In conditions such as Gaucher's disease for which four mutations are routinely tested in laboratories, clinical sensitivity is about 97% in those of Ashkenazi Jewish ancestry but only 75% in other ethnic groups (23,24). Tested individuals clearly have different residual risks of carrying a mutation after testing negatively for the core set of four mutations, depending on ethnicity. Until mutations that are restricted to or more or less common in various ethnic groups are identified, quantified, and incorporated into testing panels for disorders in which there is a wide population variation, there will be an inequality in the informativeness of tests among ethnic groups. The information made available to patients and physicians must include such distinctions.

Given that a wide array of caveats may be applied to the interpretation of test results as tests develop through the investigative stage, it is important that institutional review boards (IRBs) be involved in study development. Although it is clear that there is wide variation in the expertise and knowledge of IRBs, their role in protecting study participants from research-related risks is important; however, because IRBs focus on the research plan rather than the results, an improved approach to acquiring and evaluating data during the investigative stage would be beneficial. Because the results of common disease testing, particularly for disease susceptibility, are often probabilistic, it may take years to acquire the outcome data needed to fine-tune the clinical performance characteristics (e.g., clinical utility) of a particular test. In rare disease testing, it may never be possible to identify sufficient numbers of patients to allow performance characteristics to be defined at a level needed for common or moderately frequent disease tests. In both settings, it is unlikely that any manufacturer will be sufficiently motivated by the market potential or be able to develop clinical trials of a size sufficient to address these long-term outcome issues independently. Hence, some thought must be given to bringing the Humanitarian Device (25) considerations of the FDA into line with the Orphan Drug Program considerations (26). Again, paradigms other than disease versus nondisease will be required to factor in considerations such as unaffected carrier states, susceptibilities, and so forth. As we pursue the information needed to maximize test result interpretation, we must avoid overly restricting access to genetic testing and must find ways to facilitate technology assessment and new technology reimbursement.

Clearly, there is a need for any association of mutations in a gene with a disease to be scientifically and clinically validated. This will most likely occur through evidence in the peer-reviewed literature and should include, at a minimum, confirmation of the association from at least two independent groups, or, if the disease or risk factor is sufficiently common, at least two other peer-reviewed publications. It is important that tests for disease susceptibility or prediction be developed in clinical trial programs or that alternative means to collect outcome information over the long term be developed.

Furthermore, the analytical techniques by which the mutations are identified should meet similar criteria. After their scientific and clinical validity is established, it is likely that tests will progress to the investigative stage of testing. Important at this stage is determining whether heterogeneity is likely, an important consideration in defining the caveats of the investigative testing for those who decide to participate. When testing involves genes with allelic heterogeneity, it is likely that the first versions of the test will include the mutations most common to the ethnic groups included in the original studies. For many genes, there is likely to be a substantial proportion of rare or private mutations; therefore, validation requirements will begin to change according to the reason for testing (i.e., diagnostic vs. screening).

A remaining aspect of test development is the parallel process of assessing the specific nongenetic risks and interventions that may be relevant to those testing positive for susceptibilities. In the absence of proven interventions, reproductive decision making is likely to be the recourse. Many endpoints at which interventions will be assessed will require significantly large populations and may require long time periods to reach. Similarly, large populations will be needed to assess the contribution to disease development of various implicated nongenetic risk factors. It is unlikely that any single manufacturer will be able to run trials of populations of sufficient size to answer such questions independently. Coordinated data collection through consortia similar to the National Human Genetics Research Institute's Cancer Genetic Studies Consortium or the Cancer Genetics Network will facilitate the acquisition of compatible data to address such questions.

The Current Regulatory Environment

As previously discussed, the FDA has had a limited role in overseeing genetic testing. Few tests have been kit-based, particularly for heritable disease testing, with most being developed in laboratories using either general laboratory reagents or reagents made by the laboratories themselves. To gain regulatory control over the unregulated products that laboratories use to build a test, the FDA has established the Analyte Specific Reagent (ASR) category of devices (27), a system requiring manufacturers to inform the FDA that the product is being sold for incorporation into in-house-developed tests and ensures Good Manufacturing Practice (GMP). To date, the FDA has chosen not to exercise its perceived mandate to regulate laboratories themselves; such an expansion of its role would be costly and would lack precedent.

Undoubtedly, tests will increasingly move toward kit-based systems and the FDA's role will expand. The development of regulatory standards to be used to increase oversight will be most effective when the standards developed by those trained to provide these services are considered. Such standards are needed to guide development of appropriate oversight; however, it must be realized that how the tests are used is just as, or more important than, the laboratory issues. Regulating intended use has a long and unsuccessful history; estimates are that nearly 40% of FDA-approved drugs are prescribed for uses other than those for which they had been approved (23).

For the most part, uses not stated in the labeling materials accompanying the product are distinct from those for which the product was approved. The "off-label" uses in genetic testing are more likely to be related to magnitude of risk. Individuals with the most severe features of their disease (e.g., early age of onset, strongly positive family history, severe phenotype) are most likely to have mutations in genes associated with that disease, whereas those with only a subset of the most common disease features will be less likely to yield abnormal test results. Those identified through various types of population screening (e.g., ethnic groups, entire populations) have the least chance of harboring mutations in a disease-associated gene. This is quite apparent when BRCA1 and BRCA2 testing is being considered. The chance that a mutation in these genes is present in the 50-year-old woman with breast cancer is considerably lower than that of the 50-year-old woman with ovarian cancer and an accompanying strong family history of early-onset breast and ovarian cancer (10). Families selected because they reflect the most severe features of the disease are more likely to have higher penetrance of the mutations carried.

The designated system for overseeing laboratory practices is described in CLIA '88 (19). Both FDA regulations and CLIA requirements establish quite different levels of oversight. The FDA has traditionally overseen the manufacture of products used in testing, holding them to a high standard of both technical and clinical validity. The CLIA regulations have been considerably less stringent, with a focus on personnel, quality control and assurance, and analytical validity. To ensure safe and effective use of genetic testing, a balance must be struck between these two approaches; however, in its most complex forms, genetic testing has a significant "practice of medicine" component that has been difficult to encompass in regulatory programs. The regulatory balance will be further enhanced by significant private-sector efforts to address education and training in genetics and to develop standards for providing services.

In addition to quality control (QC) and quality assurance (QA), the CLIA also defines the areas of testing for which proficiency testing is required. Currently, there is no requirement under CLIA for proficiency testing in any area of genetic testing; however, the Genetic Testing Subcommittee of the Clinical Laboratory Improvement Advisory Committee is reviewing the state of laboratory practices in genetics so as to focus better the preanalytic and postanalytic components of testing, as well as the programs available for QA and interlaboratory comparison. Well-established QA programs for genetic testing have been offered by the College of American Pathologists (CAP) and the American College of Medical Genetics (ACMG), and proficiency testing should be required of all such laboratories.

The rapid development of genetic testing, the difficulty in developing regulatory oversight, and the need for interpreting highly complex information dictate significant involvement of professional organizations at many levels. These characteristics of genetic testing explain the success of CAP/ACMG programs, which maintain a significant educational component in the Laboratory Accreditation Programs and involve highly trained individuals directly involved in delivering genetic services. Flexible programs with access to skilled professionals are critical to the oversight of evolving high-complexity testing areas such as genetics. Standards of practice will be established by professionals and their related professional organizations. Standards of practice for genetic testing laboratories have been promulgated by the ACMG (28) and are generally reflected in the inspection criteria of the CAP.

The multidisciplinary nature of genetic testing services and the many points within the delivery process where one can directly impact QA may require new paradigms for oversight and offer further support for the recent formation of the Secretary's Advisory Committee on Genetic Testing (SACGT) of the U.S. Department of Health and Human Services to (*1*) assess the progress toward addressing the recommendations of the TFGT, (*2*) to identify new areas of concern, and (*3*) to redirect efforts for recommendations that are not being adequately addressed.

Laboratory Quality

Personnel
The highest personnel standards should be met by a laboratory or those conducting genetic tests when genetic tests are used in heritable disease testing.

A number of such recommendations offered by the TFGT (2) are shown in the accompanying listing. Results of tests for infectious diseases or acquired changes are often applicable to only the individual tested and lack familial consequences, which allows the laboratory to be more technically focused. Results are commonly integrated with other types of testing results to arrive at patient-management decisions; however, when testing involves the constitutional genome, preanalytical and postanalytical components, including result interpretation, are critical to ensure appropriate testing and result communication. Often, the interpretive component is dependent on the laboratory director's training.

A laboratory's range of techniques may be tiered by complexity and have some relationship to personnel standards. The highest standards should be met for tests that may identify rare or private gene sequence variations, and which will have to be assessed for the likelihood that they are disease related. Patients may have previously described mutations of known clinical significance or the result may be of a previously unknown change. Interpretation of these results will depend on the laboratory director's knowledge of human genetics and the ability to communicate effectively with clinicians.

An equally demanding task is testing for disease susceptibility in otherwise normal individuals. Genetics knowledge should be required of all genetics laboratory directors and should be a required component of their training programs. The techniques used by the laboratory as well as the intended uses of those techniques can be indicators of those types of services requiring the highest standards. Tests for heritable diseases in the diagnostic setting may require greater expertise, and tests directed at screening will require a well-integrated delivery system with skilled laboratorians and well-defined follow-up systems.

Although the FDA can restrict the performance of genetic tests to individuals able to document particular types of training, the development and oversight of personnel standards falls under the CLIA '88 regulations. Because the regulations are driven by techniques and methods—and molecular biological methods can be applied to both human and nonhuman (e.g., infectious agents) genomes for acquired or heritable disease traits—it has been difficult to define the necessary educational and training requirements for applying these methods to heritable human disease. The need for high standards in particular areas of genetic testing should go beyond the lowest common denominator, that being the technical component of the tests. Neither should the technically similar but quite different interpretive aspects of infectious disease or acquired disease testing be held to the requirements for heritable disease testing. A system of assessing technical issues and clinical impact of a test could be extended to clinical laboratories offering genetic testing services. It would be similar to the triage approach of the FDA in stratifying tests by complexity and impact on those tested.

Limited problems specific to laboratories were identified by the TFGT (2). Most involved issues related to demonstrating competency of both the staff and the laboratory. Although there remains only one recognized certification board specific to genetic testing—the American Board of Medical Genetics—it is unusual for federal regulation to be driven by laboratory directors' specific board certifications or areas of training. Genetic testing laboratory technologists lack training program opportunities. Most technologists are trained on the job. Incorporation of genetic testing technologies into laboratory technologist training programs would enhance the overall skills of genetic testing facilities. If current recommendations fail to resolve the problems identified in laboratories, the only recourse will be to tighten personnel standards.

FEATURES OF GENETIC TESTING DRIVING PERSONNEL
REQUIREMENTS

- Directors and technical supervisors in laboratories performing high-complexity (genetic) tests must have formal training in human and medical genetics documented by certification from an organization that assesses knowledge of human and medical genetics as part of its certification process.
- Tests that can be used for purposes of predicting future disease should be given a CLIA rating of "high complexity."
- Training programs for laboratory technologists need more human and medical genetics content.
- Until a CLIA-recognized genetics specialty is established, laboratories performing DNA- or RNA-based tests should choose to participate voluntarily in the College of American Pathologists (CAP) molecular pathology program, including the CAP/American College of Medical Genetics (ACMG) molecular genetics surveys. The public should have access to results of a laboratory's participation in these programs.
- Heritable disease genetic test results must be interpreted and results written in a form that is understandable to the nongeneticist health care provider.

Provider Competency

It is clear that relatively weak links in the chain of a genetic testing service exist in the preanalytic and postanalytic parts of the service. To improve provider competency in this area, the recommendations given in the accompanying list have been made for curriculum development and training (2).

GENETICS EDUCATION NEEDS AND COMPETENCY
DETERMINATION

- Basic genetics curricula need to be developed for medical school and residency training to ensure broad-based knowledge of human and medical genetics.

- Intermediate-level genetics curricula need to be developed for individuals from specialties (oncology, cardiology, pediatrics) having significant proportions of patients and should be offered through medical school and residency training programs or continuing education programs.
- Hospitals and managed-care organizations should require evidence that providers are competent to serve as intermediates between patients and genetic testing services when tests to assess future risks are employed.
- The genetics components of the U.S. Medical Licensing Examination (USMLE Steps 1, 2, and 3) should be improved and should be independently evaluated and scored to ensure provider competency.
- Schools of nursing, public health, and social work need to strengthen the genetics components of their training programs.
- Internet information sources specific to rare diseases should be developed and promulgated to facilitate differential diagnosis, referral, or consultation.

That providers are in a more labor-intensive position, with less time available for continuing education, may be the greatest barrier to improving competency. Maximum advantage of "educable moments" when providers seek information for managing patients care should be taken to increase provider competency in genetic testing and may be facilitated by including references or informational materials with results. Providing clinicians with brief pretest educational materials would be of significant value when reviewing testing indications and posttest educational materials that enhance test result interpretation by providing broad overviews of the test and implications of various results. The pace of development and improvement in knowledge of genetic diseases, susceptibilities, and associated risks dictate that this information be frequently updated and readily accessible. These resources would greatly facilitate developing and implementing of clearinghouses and hotlines for providing genetic testing information.

Private Sector, Government Partnerships

In many ways, the decision to avoid undue regulation of genetic testing in recent years stemmed from several concerns: the potential to stifle development in an area as rapidly evolving as genetic testing; difficulty regulating clinical practice; and a relative paucity of documented errors in laboratories operating under the highest standards currently available. The formation of SACGT, which will include representatives from various interest groups (consumers, payers, professionals, industry, others), further points to the recognition that regulation alone may not be the preferred recourse to the spectrum of concerns about genetic testing. Accepted standards of practice should drive regulation development rather than the other way around. Clearly, professionals involved in service provision, board examination development, educational materials development, and research are important contributors to a shared goal of providing safe and effective genetic testing services to the public. The broad social and ethical considerations surrounding genetic testing point to the need for direct public involvement.

Conclusions

Scientific and clinical communities, industry, government, and consumers will all have to work together to ensure safe and appropriate use of genetic testing. With the rapid and recent evolution of genetic testing and its implications for common diseases and susceptibilities, the education of medical students and the continuing education of providers are both critically important to the transition of safe and effective tests into practice. The broad range of potential intended uses or target populations for genetic tests may require new paradigms for oversight.

Any use to which genetic tests are applied should be validated before conducting clinical trials, with fine-tuning of performance characteristics and assessment of clinical utility occurring during trials. Both technologies and tests require validation. As tests evolve, yet-to-be developed standards should be part of the clinical decision-making process required for interpreting the significance of sequence variations not commonly encountered in a particular gene. Additionally, some standardization of data collection during investigative stages of testing will facilitate technology transfer in genetic testing.

Aside from improving education and training requirements for laboratory personnel and developing more kit-based testing systems, there is limited room for improving the laboratory components. The critical importance of test interpretation may ultimately necessitate education and training requirements in that area. Clearly, greater focus on test result interpretation can be added to the CLIA '88 regulations, and proficiency testing can be mandated for laboratories offering these services. As kit-based tests begin to reach the marketplace, the FDA can greatly enhance its role in regulating both uses and users of these tests; however, given the range of genetic disease incidence and susceptibility, it will be important to remain cognizant of the thousands of rare genetic diseases for which tests cannot necessarily be constrained by the requirements for common disease testing.

The "practice-of-medicine" component of genetic tests makes them quite different from many other tests that have a straightforward positive or negative result. This component also has limited the development of regulatory oversight and identification of the areas of laboratory practice that can be regulated; hence, a focus on training and educating laboratory personnel is important and can be addressed in the CLIA regulations. Some preanalytic and postanalytic components of the test might also be impacted through CLIA and heightened state and local oversight. Ultimately, testing can be significantly enhanced by developing standards around which critical laboratory decisions can be made about introducing new tests, the quality of information in test marketing, and the reporting of results. Practitioners will have to take responsibility for ensuring that accurate information about the positive and negative implications of testing and results are readily available for patients and physicians.

Those involved in the multidisciplinary delivery of genetic services will most likely have the greatest impact on quality of genetic services. Some states have established significantly higher and more specific standards for genetic testing laboratory services. To maximize those benefits, there may be a need to develop similar requirements for the providers referring tests to the laboratory. Development of comprehensive centers for genetic testing may be an effective way of ensuring the full complement of services needed. Accreditation of the centers could be either voluntary or mandated if needed.

Finally, the TFGT offered the first assessment of the state of affairs in genetic testing in the United States. Concerns requiring attention are found in test development and transition into service, laboratory testing, and the delivery system in which services are provided. Attention to whether or not expressed goals and recommendations are being met would offer significant guidance to those charged with similar tasks in the future and ensure that the goals of safe and effective genetic testing continue to be pursued.

References

1. ACMG. American College of Medical Genetics Survey of American Board of Medical Genetics Certified Molecular Geneticists, 1996.

2. Task Force on Genetic Testing. Holtzman NA, Watson MS (eds). Promoting safe and effective genetic testing in the United States. Final Report. Bethesda, MD: National Institutes of Health, 1997.

3. Hofman K, Tambor E, Chase G, Geller G, Faden R, Holtzman N. Physician knowledge of genetics and genetic tests. Acad Med 1993;68:625–632.

4. Antonarakis SE. Mutations in human diseases: nature and consequences. In: Rimoin DL, Connor JM, Pyeritz RE (eds). Emery and Rimoin's principles and practice of medical genetics (3rd ed). New York: Churchill Livingston, 1996, pp. 53–65.

5. Saunders AM, Strittmatter WJ, Schmechel D. Association of apolipoprotein E allele E(epsilon)4 with late-onset familial and sporadic Alzheimer's disease. Neurology 1993;43:1467–1472.

6. Roses AD. Apolipoprotein E affects the rate of Alzheimer disease expression: beta-amyloid burden is a secondary consequence dependent on ApoE genotype and duration of disease. J Neuropathol Exp Neurol 1994;53:429–437.

7. Utermann G. (1986). The ApoE-system: genetic control of plasma lipoprotein concentration. Ad Exp Med Biol 1996;201:262–272.

8. Masuda H, Miller C, Koeffler HP, Battifora H, Cline MJ. Rearrangement of the p53 gene in human osteogenic sarcomas. Proc Natl Acad Sci USA 1987;84:7716–7719.

9. Malkin D, Jolly KW, Barbier N, et al. Germline mutations of p53 tumor-suppressor gene in children and young adults with second malignant neoplasms. N Engl J Med 1992;326:1309–1315.

10. Easton DF, Ford D, Bishop DT, and the Breast Cancer Linkage Consortium. Breast and avarian cancer incidence in BRCA1-mutation carriers. Am J Hum Genet 1995;56:265–271.

11. Ford D, Easton DF. The genetics of breast and avarian cancer. Br J Cancer 1995;72:805–812.

12. Easton DF, Bishop DT, Ford D, Crockford GP, and the Breast Cancer Linkage Consortium. Genetic linkage analysis in familial breast and ovarian cancer. Am J Hum Genet 1993;52:678–701.

13. Tsui L-C, Buchwald M, et al. Cystic fibrosis locus defined by a genetically linked polymorphic DNA marker. Science 1995;230:1054–1057.

14. Zielinski J, Tsui L-C. Cystic fibrosis: genotypic and phenotypic variations. Annu Rev Genet 1995;29:777–807.

15. Riordan JR, Rommens JM, Kerem B, et al. Identification of the cystic fibrosis gene: cloning and characterization of complementary DNA. Science 1989;245: 1066–1073.

16. American Society of Human Genetics. The American Society of Human Genetics Statement on cystic fibrosis screening. Am J Hum Genet 1993;46:393.

17. Cutting G. Cystic fibrosis. In: Rimoin DL, Connor JM, Pyeritz RE (eds). Emery and Rimoin's principles and practice of medical genetics (3rd ed). New York: Churchill Livingston, 1996, pp. 2685–2717.

18. Lipshutz RJ, Fodor SPA, Gingeras TR, Lockhart DJ. High-density synthetic oligonucleotide arrays. Nat Genet Suppl 1999;21:20–24.

19. Public Law 100-578: Clinical Laboratory Improvement Amendments [CLIA] of 1988. 1988;42 U.S.C. 263a.

20. Genetic testing for cysticfibrosis. NIH Consensus Statement Online. 1997 April 14–16;15:1–37.

21. Grody WW, Desnick RJ, Carpenter NJ, Noll WW. Diversity of cystic fibrosis mutation-screening practices. Am J Hum Genet 1998;62:1252–1254.

22. Young ID. Risk estimation in genetic counseling. In Rimoin DL, Connor JM, Pyeritz RE (eds). Emery and Rimoin's principles and practice of medical genetics (3rd ed). New York: Churchill Livingston, 1996, pp. 521–533.

23. Beutler E. Modern diagnosis and treatment of Gaucher's disease. Am J Dis Child 1993;147:1175–1183.

24. Horowitz M, Tzuri G, Eyal N, et al. Prevalence of nine mutations among Jewish and non-Jewish Gaucher disease patients. Am J Hum Genet 1993;53:921–930.

25. Public Law 100-290: Orphan Drug Amendments of 1988. 1995; U.S.C. Sec 360cc(a) (abstract).

26. Public Law 97-414: 1995; U.S.C. Sec. 360aa et (abstract).

27. Federal register 1996;61(51):10484–10489.

28. Watson MS (ed). American College of Medical Genetics. Standards and Guidelines: Clinical laboratory genetics (2nd ed). Bethesda, MD: ACMG, 1999.

13

Newborn screening quality assurance

W. Harry Hannon, L. Omar Henderson,
and Carol J. Bell

In 1961, blood collected as a dried spot on filter paper was first introduced by Dr. Robert Guthrie in New York for testing newborns for phenylketonuria (PKU) (1). He coupled the specially collected specimen with a unique bacterial inhibition test that he developed for phenylalanine (2). This combination of easily transportable specimens and inexpensive tests made large-scale testing for PKU possible. The first case of PKU detected by this procedure occurred in a pilot study in New York after the testing of 800 newborns (1). The first application of the population-based newborn screening for PKU using this unique specimen collection and test system was initiated in Massachusetts in the fall of 1962 with the testing of most newborns in the state (3). The successful introduction of dried-blood spots (DBSs) for PKU screening led to the development of population screening of newborns nationwide with the use of blood drops collected by a heel stick and absorbed into filter paper. The ease of transporting the DBSs made them ideal specimens for large-volume testing by regionalized laboratories for population-based screening.

Today, newborn screening is the largest genetic testing effort in the nation and is primarily performed by state public health laboratories. The detection of treatable, inherited metabolic diseases is a major public health responsibility. Screening tests are designed to sort newborns who probably have a disease from those who do not. These tests are not intended to yield a diagnostic testing outcome. However, effective screening of newborns, with the use of DBS specimens collected at birth, combined with follow-up diagnostic studies and treatment, helps prevent mental retardation and premature death. These blood specimens are routinely collected from more than 95% of all newborns in the United States. State public health laboratories or their associated laboratories routinely screen DBS specimens for inborn errors of metabolism and other disorders that require intervention.

In 1975, the Committee for the Study of Inborn Errors of Metabolism, National Academy of Sciences, stated that greater quality control of PKU screening is essential and recommended that a single laboratory within the Centers for Disease Control and Prevention (CDC) be responsible for maintaining the proficiency of the regional laboratories testing newborns for PKU (4). For more than 20 years, the CDC, along with its cosponsors, the Health Resources and Services Administration and the Association of Public Health Laboratories, has conducted research on materials development and has assisted laboratories with the quality assurance (QA) for these DBS screening tests. The heart of these efforts, the Newborn Screening Quality Assurance Program (NSQAP), is a voluntary, nonregulatory program designed to help participating laboratories evaluate and improve the quality of their testing and to foster the standardization of newborn screening services nationwide. The success of any external proficiency-testing (PT) program depends on the full participation of all laboratories that have similar responsibilities. Most laboratories that test DBS specimens participate voluntarily in the NSQAP. Quality assurance services of the NSQAP primarily support newborn screening tests performed by state laboratories; however, the program also accepts other laboratories, manufacturers of test kits, and international participants.

Newborn screening for PKU and congenital hypothyroidism is carried out in all 50 states, the District of Columbia, and Puerto Rico (5,6). Galactosemia and hemoglobinopathies (e.g., sickle cell disorders) are the disorders that are next most frequently screened for. The number and type of other disorders that are screened vary from state to state. One private laboratory offers supplemental testing for over 20 disorders.

Quality Assurance

Quality assurance (QA) is an active system of setting criteria for the quality of performance required for each step in the overall newborn screening process to ensure adequate confidence in each procedure. Quality control (QC) is the mechanistic procedure for monitoring adherence to the set QA criteria, for establishing corrective action when the criteria are not met, and for documenting the assay's performance and corrective actions taken (7). The QA and QC operations are complex because of the number of steps, facilities, and personnel involved. Centralization of screening facilities and operations reduces the complexity somewhat and produces a more controllable operation and a system with reduced risk for failures. Although laboratories serve as the focal point for the identification of presumptive positive cases, both the laboratories and the analytical methods they use constitute only one of the QA elements in the screening process (7).

Laboratory QA criteria are set primarily for three steps associated with analytical performance: ensuring adequate specimen volume, eliminating false-negative identifications, and minimizing the number of false-positive detections to a cost-effective range. By applying QC principles to analyses, the laboratory staff can monitor analytical variables, and if the analytical system fails, can effectively target corrective steps to ensure quality and improve performance. Laboratories primarily use two types of QC applications to monitor their QA criteria: internal and external actions. *Internal* QC is referred to as *bench-level QC* and is an important process for routinely monitoring the stability of the analytical performance. *External* QC is most often referred to as *PT*. Regularly participating in an external PT program and keeping records of this performance are the best means by which laboratories can show their quality of performance. Internal and external QC efforts are complementary activities and key elements of any laboratory QA system (7).

An effective QA system must be based on realistic criteria for high-quality analytical and overall laboratory performance. This permits a laboratory to set and monitor, through its QC parameters, the daily achievement rate of these standards of performance. A fully operational QA system also allows for interlaboratory comparisons of analytical precision and relative bias. Performance criteria for the newborn screening laboratory must be predetermined and recorded as part of the written QA protocol. The QA system enables the laboratory to qualitatively rate the validity and credibility of its performance.

All newborn screening testing must be done by facilities licensed by their respective states and must meet the requirements of the Clinical Laboratory Improvement Amendments of 1988 (CLIA'88). As part of these requirements, a screening laboratory must meet certain criteria for QC and must participate in PT programs. Proficiency testing is used to evaluate the quality of the measurement process on a periodic basis, usually quarterly. Thus, PT specimens are to be handled and analyzed the same as patient specimens. Laboratories must satisfactorily participate in a Health Care Financing Administration (HCFA)-approved PT program (if available) for each method they use to analyze human specimens. In the absence of an HCFA-approved PT program for newborn screening, the NSQAP enables laboratories to meet the CLIA quality-assurance requirement for verifying test accuracy. If a PT program is not available for a specific newborn screening test, laboratories must have a system for verifying the accuracy and reliability of their test results at least twice a year. Laboratories can develop a self-administered PT program using available reference methods and materials. This PT program will be administered by a QA officer who is not in the participating laboratory. The laboratories must then document their performance in this self-administered type PT in a QC manual, which is available for review.

In addition, HCFA-approved PT providers must meet set criteria. One requirement is the availability of a performance-grading scheme. The analytical values of DBS assays for newborn screening cannot be reasonably applied to the grading of tests because of the intrinsic variance (e.g., spot size, hematocrit, elution) of the specimen type, the inherent purpose of screening, and the sorting of the population tested. Therefore, error judgments for a grading scheme for screening laboratories should be based on either the presumptive clinical assessment or the sorting of positive and negative outcomes.

Newborn Screening Quality Assurance

The Newborn Screening Quality Assurance Program (NSQAP) at the CDC in Atlanta, Georgia, provides services for laboratories that use DBS specimens to perform newborn screening tests. The mission of this program is to improve interlaboratory comparability and to work toward interlaboratory standardization. Current participants include newborn screening laboratories, confirmatory testing laboratories that use DBS tests, diet-monitoring laboratories, and manufacturers of testing products. The NSQAP interacts with state-affiliated newborn screening programs and the manufacturing community to (1) maintain laboratory methods, (2) evaluate and distribute reference and QC materials, (3) evaluate QC systems available to user laboratories, (4) conduct training and/or provide consultative services, and (5) develop mechanisms for the voluntary evaluation of laboratory performance, the transfer of new and improved technology, and the evaluation of programs that screen for hypothyroidism, PKU, other inborn metabolic disorders, and hemoglobinopathies. Figure 13.1 shows the number of program participants in the QC and PT program components for each disorder. The NSQAP provides QC materials, PT services, and technical support to 64 domestic screening laboratories, 20 manufacturers of diagnostic products, and 122 laboratories in 33 foreign countries.

Quality assurance programs enable screening laboratories to achieve high levels of technical proficiency and maintain continuity despite changes in commercial assay reagents while maintaining the high-volume specimen throughput that is required. Laboratories that misclassified a PT specimen are provided immediate notification and consultation to resolve the analytical problem. Through interactive efforts, NSQAP and screening laboratories continually strive to improve program services to better meet the growing and changing needs of newborn screening activities in the public health community and to help ensure equivalent high-quality testing by these programs nationwide. Besides the two DBS distribution components, the program con-

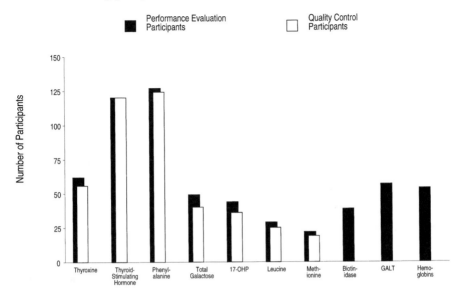

Figure 13.1 The number of participants for components of the quality assurance program in 1998.

tains a filter-paper evaluation component for the QA of this product. Methods developed by the NSQAP are used to evaluate and compare different production lots of filter paper from commercial sources.

Filter-Paper Matrix

Although the DBSs were used successfully in semiquantitative assays (i.e., bacterial inhibition assays) for newborn screening, the DBS matrix encountered mixed reports of adequate performance when quantitative assays for congenital hypothyroidism were introduced. A significant problem was that the variance contributions of the filter-paper matrix were not realized fully; consequently, they were not minimized and contained for use in quantitative assays. Standardizing the filter-paper matrix for performance parameters has contributed substantially to our confidence in its reliability and to the acceptance of DBSs as a specimen matrix for a variety of new applications and technologies.

The collection of DBS specimens for newborn screening and other related applications requires special grades of commercially manufactured paper as a unique whole-blood collection matrix. In the United States, only papers approved by the Food and Drug Administration (FDA) are acceptable for blood collection for clinical tests. Critical to proper and effective use of this matrix is an ongoing assessment and evaluation of new production lots as they are manufactured, as well as the monitoring of problems identified with individual lots in use by state-affiliated newborn screening programs. Because the paper-punch size selected from a blood spot is used as a volumetric sample for quantitative analysis, a high degree of uniformity is essential.

The NSQAP and the two FDA-approved manufacturers have reached an agreement whereby the NSQAP is provided with statistically valid sample sets from each new production lot of filter paper for evaluation by standardized procedures (8) before the new lot is released to the user community. Each year the NSQAP evaluates, with the extensive cooperation of manufacturers (Schleicher & Schuell, Keene, NH; Whatman, Fairfield, NJ), new lots of paper approved by the FDA for blood collection. Each manufacturer is responsible for establishing its own evaluation laboratory using the same procedures as those used by the NSQAP.

After all parties conducting independent evaluations of the filter-paper lot agree that the lot is acceptable, the lot is released for distribution. The independent evaluations by the NSQAP are an impartial and voluntary service offered as a function of the QA program and do not constitute preferential endorsement of any product over other specimen-collection papers approved by FDA.

The specific role of the NSQAP in this evaluation process includes (1) evaluating manufactured lots of filter-paper products for physical parameters, serum absorption volume, homogeneity, and absorption time; (2) monitoring the performance of new production lots relative to previous lots; (3) maintaining criteria for certification of paper lots used by screening laboratories; (4) maintaining a controlled historical storage center of papers previously approved for newborn screening; and (5) reporting the outcomes of these evaluations to the user community. Standardization is required both for within-lot and lot-to-lot performance of filter paper to help ensure reliable analytical transitions and comparability of calibrators, patient specimens, and QC materials. The volumetric aliquots of serum contained in a punch size from a DBS are affected by several variables, including the paper thickness, the volume of blood applied, the humidity, the printing process used to produce blood-collection forms, the handling during specimen collection, the blood absorption time, and the storage environment for the paper (9,10).

In the future, other commercial sources of FDA-approved filter paper for specimen collection may become available in the United States. Theoretically, if the performance criteria (8) are met, the transition between commercial sources of paper should not be different from the transition between lots from the same source. Because screening programs have limited experience with the impact of multiple sources of filter paper on performance, they should sort the specimens by filter-paper source for analysis and closely monitor performance parameters until they are confident in the new product. Soon the screening community could be coping with calibrators, patient specimens, and control materials on filter paper from different commercial sources. The screening programs must be cautious and include monitoring for each parameter in their QC operations.

Specimen Collection

Most of the specimen-collection facilities have selected DBS specimens collected by a heel stick as the method of choice for newborn screening. However, procedures are also available for applying blood collected in capillary tubes and by dorsal vein puncture onto the preprinted circles of filter paper. Although these methods are not the preferred choice, they are now considered to be rational alternatives to direct application from the newborn's heel-stick site (7). The DBS has the advantage of being simple and easy to handle as well as posing fewer biological hazards than liquid specimens.

A national standard has been developed for the uniform collection of quality DBS specimens from newborns (8). This standard specifically defines how to collect blood onto filter paper, specifications for the specimen matrix, specimen shipping requirements, and other parameters. Screening laboratories routinely monitor the quality of collected specimens against their established criteria of acceptance and rejection. The primary justification for refusing to analyze a specimen and declaring it unacceptable is that its analysis may yield unreliable, misleading, or clinically inaccurate values for a particular analyte. Because, by this definition, unacceptable specimens give no usable information, such specimens should not be analyzed; and those responsible for collecting the specimens should be informed so that an acceptable specimen can be obtained as soon as possible (8). The collection of unacceptable specimens delays the analysis and potentially the treatment of affected newborns.

Quality Control and Performance Evaluation

The NSQAP prepares and distributes to laboratories worldwide more than 250,000 DBSs each year. The manufactured DBS materials must simulate, as closely as possible, the actual specimens for the assay systems. Dried-blood materials that are prepared for QC and PT are certified for homogeneity, analyte accuracy, stability, and suitability for all assays from different commercial sources. The NSQAP distributes DBS materials used in screening tests for congenital hypothyroidism, PKU, galactosemia, congenital adrenal hyperplasia, homocystinuria, maple syrup urine disease (MSUD), biotinidase deficiency, and hemoglobinopathies. These materials must be stable under the routine conditions of shipment, laboratory logistics, analysis, and storage, and must be homogeneous enough that their variance will not contribute significantly to the analytical variance of the methods and their detection outcomes. The concentration of analyte in the control materials must cover the range of normal and abnormal specimens tested by the screening process and include a low-level analyte specimen with which to monitor the analytical sensitivity of the methods (7).

The NSQAP prepares "zero-base" whole-blood pools for DBS materials by gently mixing washed, outdated Red Cross-packed red blood cells with clean-filtered serum to yield a whole-blood pool with a hematocrit of 55%. Portions of the pool are enriched with the desired analyte at predetermined concentration levels. Each portion is then uniformly applied to approved filter-paper cards in 100 μL aliquots, air-dried horizontally overnight, packed in sealed bags with desiccant, and stored at −20 °C. Blood collected from any source, including cord blood, that is prepared for use in the production of QC and PT materials must be negative for HIV, hepatitis, and other infectious agents. Documentation of the source, composition, homogeneity, and stability of all DBS materials and the procedure(s) used to assign their expected or target values are available upon request from the NSQAP. Specimens from newly prepared production lots of DBS materials are checked for stability and tested to ensure their homogeneity and the accuracy of their assigned concentration values.

To ensure that laboratories receive representative sheets of the production batch, the NSQAP uses a random number table to select the set of DBS sheets for each laboratory. The QC shipments are distributed semiannually and include the blood-spot sheets, instructions for storage and analysis, and data report forms. Data from five analytical runs of each lot and shipment are compiled in both the midyear and annual summary reports that are distributed to each participant. The reported QC data are summarized and show the analyte by series of QC lots, the number of observations, mean values, and the standard deviations (SDs) by kit or analytical method.

In addition, NSQAP uses a weighted linear regression analysis to examine the comparability by method of reported versus enriched concentrations. Results of the linear regression analyses (Y-intercept and slope) for all lots within an analyte set are summarized in the reports. The mean value and the within-laboratory and total SDs are calculated for each concentration within a QC lot for a specific analyte. The summarized QC data provide information about method-related differences in analytical recoveries and method-related biases. Because each QC lot series is prepared from a single batch of hematocrit-adjusted, nonenriched blood, the endogenous concentration of a given analyte is the same for all specimens in a lot series. The Y-intercept of the regression analysis for reported values provides a measure of the endogenous analyte concentration.

For amino acid–enriched DBS materials, participants measure the endogenous concentration levels by analyzing the nonenriched QC lots (the base pool). The values for the Y-intercept and the base pool are similar for most methods. Ideally, the slope should be 1.0, and most slopes calculated for reported data are close to this value. Because the endogenous concentration is the same for all QC lots within a series, it should not affect the slope of the regression line among methods. Generally, slope values substantially different from 1.0 indicate that a method has an analytical bias. Figure 13.2 shows an example of mean values of reported results for phenylalanine measurements by different methods used for linear regression analysis. These data, routinely compiled by NSQAP, help participants understand the performance of different methods and to select appropriate test methods and kits in the future.

For the PT component, designing evaluation materials that fairly assess a screening laboratory's performance is difficult because of the variable cutoff values both within and among laboratories. The NSQAP analyzed this problem and concluded that the only equitable method by which all laboratories could be evaluated is one that is based on the first decision level (cutoff) for separating test results that require follow-up testing from negative test results that do not. This initial decision (cutoff) value should be an important part of the routine reporting scheme for all participants even though it will differ among laboratories. All PT panels contain five blind-coded specimens,

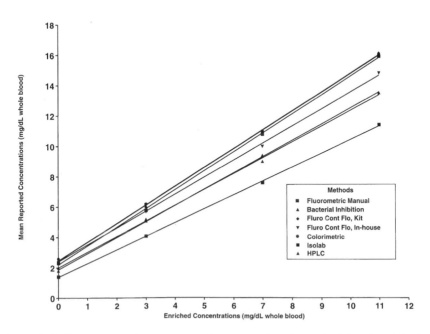

Figure 13.2 Comparison of mean reported concentrations by method for phenylalanine quality-control materials.

each consisting of 100 µL blood spots. Specimens in the PT panels either contain endogenous levels or are enriched with predetermined levels of thyroxine, thyroid-stimulating hormone, phenylalanine, total galactose, 17α-hydroxyprogesterone, leucine, or methionine. Special separate panels for biotinidase deficiency and galactose 1-phosphate uridyltransferase deficiency are prepared with purchased blood from donors with enzyme deficiencies. The DBS specimens for sickle cell disorders and other hemoglobinopathies are prepared from residual cord blood provided to the QA program by the Alabama and Georgia newborn screening programs.

In quarterly reports the NSQAP summarizes the quantitative data and clinical assessments for all data received from PT program participants by the due date. Because some of the pools in a routine PT survey represent a unique donor specimen, differences in endogenous materials in the donor specimens are important parameters for assessing performance and method-related differences. Presumptive clinical classifications (based on quantitative data) of some specimens may differ by participant because of specific clinical-assessment practices. Only the qualitative assessments are reported for the sickle cell disorders and other hemoglobinopathies. Table 13.1 shows the results for phenotype and clinical assessment misclassifications reported for hemoglobinopathies in 1998.

For those participants who provide their cutoff values, the NSQAP applies these cutoffs in the final appraisal of the error judgment. The errors for qualitative assessments in the PT component are split into *misclassifications* and *transcription errors*. Transcription errors, which continue to be a major error component in the PT surveys, are monitored to provide an indication of attention to detail by laboratory personnel. Using 1998 data, the number of false-positive misclassifications exceeded the number of transcription errors and false-negative misclassifications for most disorders. The NSQAP calculates the rates for false-positive classifications on the basis of the number of negative specimens analyzed; the false-negative classifications are based on the number of positive specimens analyzed. Screening programs are designed to avoid

Table 13.1 Errors Reported by Participants of the Sickle Cell Disease and Other Hemoglobinopathies Program in 1998*

Transcription errors	0.1%
Phenotype misclassifications	1.0%
Clinical assessment misclassifications	0.9%
Labs making transcription errors	1
Labs misclassifying specimens	5
Labs correctly classifying specimens	47

* Total of 52 laboratories, 1040 assayed specimens.

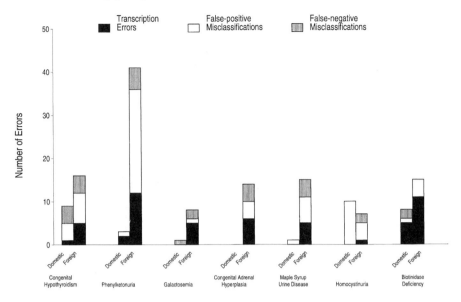

Figure 13.3 The summary of performance evaluation errors by domestic and foreign laboratories in 1998.

false-negative reports; this precautionary design, however, may be the cause of many of the false-positive classifications (11). False-positive classifications are a cost-benefit issue and a credibility factor with follow-up programs (11). False-positive rates should be monitored and kept as low as possible. Figure 13.3 shows the total number of classification and transcription errors made by domestic and foreign laboratories that screened for selected disorders in 1998. For most disorders, the number of errors was greatest for foreign laboratory participants.

Mass Spectrometry and DNA Methods

The introduction of tandem mass spectrometry to newborn screening has greatly expanded the potential number of disorders detectable by routine newborn screening with the DBS specimen. Over 15 disorders could be added to the present screening profiles, some of which raise many issues about follow-up and treatment of affected newborns. The most important of these disorders appears to be medium-chain acyl-CoA dehydrogenase deficiency (MCAD), a defect in the oxidation of fatty acids. The reported prevalence of MCAD is 1 in 10,000 (12). However, no external QA program is now available for the measurement of acylcarnitines by tandem mass spectrometry for detection of these disorders. Laboratories using tandem mass spectrometry will need to operate and document QA efforts within their respective facilities according to the CLIA regulations for situations where no PT programs are available (13). A laboratory must have a system for verifying the accuracy and reliability of its test results at least twice a year. If a laboratory performs the same test on different instruments or methodologies, a mechanism must be established to evaluate and define the relationship between test results. The laboratory must have documentation of all QA activities, including problems and corrective actions taken, and must maintain accurate record-keeping (13).

Only a few state newborn screening programs do DNA testing for cystic fibrosis (CF), but there is a growing interest by other programs. Specimens used to monitor the quality of testing should closely simulate the actual routine clinical specimen. Historically, these materials have been prepared by analyte enrichment (or spiking of normal base biological matrices) or from materials obtained from donors afflicted with the disorder or genetic defect being tested for. Presently, two PT surveys (non-HCFA approved) operate with worldwide participation for QA of CF testing: the CAEN QA Survey (France) and the Human Genetics Society of Australasia's Newborn Screening Quality Assurance Program (New Zealand) (14). The Australasian QA Program offers PT services for DNA testing for CF (ΔF508). However, the preparation method for DNA QA materials used in these programs does not appeal to some participants because detection depends on the compatibility of the primers used in the ΔF508 assay with the amplicons. Determining the number of DNA mutations screened for as part of CF detection and whether QA materials can effectively simulate these mutations are unanswered questions. Efforts are ongoing to improve these QA test materials so that they provide better method harmonization and better simulation of the CF mutations.

The development of simulated materials through specific DNA-probe spiking of specimens is problematic for assessing the equivalency of performance for all test systems. Materials that harmonize for all test systems are essential to performance assessments of DNA tests. This is a difficult challenge because of the underlying analytical variables; but until such PT materials with the required mutations are developed, meaningful performance data are difficult to gather both for the CF test and for other emerging DNA tests for newborn screening. One possible solution to this dilemma is the development of unique evaluation processes for DNA tests. Perhaps such a process could assume that a laboratory's performance on any one mutation test adequately measures its performance on all similar DNA testing performed during the PT assessment window. This and other possible options need study and development by experimental trials within the DNA-testing community.

Banking of Leftover DBS Specimens

With the expanding interest in the use of DBSs for DNA testing, newborn screening programs are faced with many decisions regarding leftover patient specimens. Advances in mechanisms to obtain sufficient quantities of DNA from DBSs and to apply the polymerase chain reaction (PCR) technology allow numerous genetic tests to be performed on a single DBS (15). Presently, a few states have retained more than a million leftover specimens. The length of storage time varies among national screening programs. Figure 13.4 shows, by state, the length of time that leftover specimens are stored.

The value of retained DBSs is directly related to the documentation and care with which they are stored (16,17). When newborn screening programs decide to store leftover DBSs for lengthy intervals, scientifically sound and justifiable approaches must be used in all aspects of storage. To ensure the validity of stored specimens, operators of the program should develop a storage policy and design a QA system. If the analytes (mutations) for which the DBSs are being saved are known, then appropriate assayed QC materials should be included (16). All QC materials must be handled and stored with the specimens under identical processing conditions. The QC materials should be randomized in the storage system to prevent location bias. Compromised or potentially tainted specimens have no scientific value. Flow-charting the

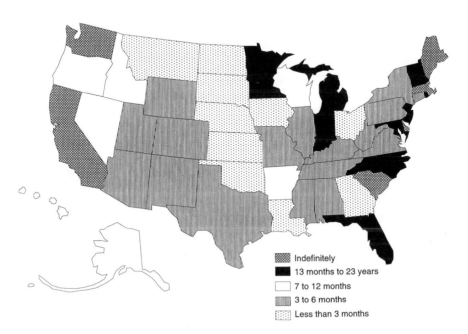

Figure 13.4 The length of time that leftover newborn screening dried-blood-spot specimens are kept by state screening programs.

process and using bar code identifications are useful in tracking the specimen. Systems for easy access and retrieval should be design components of the storage system. A program should also document storage conditions for QA records. Uncontrolled storage and release could produce compromised specimens and other problems.

In addition, screening programs should formalize operations for handling leftover specimens; however, only a few programs have written guidelines for the release and use of stored specimens (16). Consent requirements for extended use of screening specimens are unclear. Some programs use informed refusal or lack of dissent. Clarifications of the legal and ethical questions are important to the use and release of leftover DBS specimens (16).

Summary

External QA programs provide participants with information on the specificity of methods used, on accuracy of calibration systems in use, and on their and other participants' overall compliance with specific performance quality goals (7). Reliance on the technical consultative and statistical support services of sponsoring PT surveillance programs and on shared data and expertise among screening laboratories is vital for improved analytical performance of individual laboratories as well as for interlaboratory standardization. Laboratory testing goals for newborn screening are met through the analysis of only a single DBS specimen from each newborn. The time frame for this critical testing and assessment is limited, and the outcome of a false-negative result has serious medical and legal consequences (18). External QC testing must meet special criteria that define the quality of results needed to make a clinical decision and must vary with the disorder screened for, the analyte measured, and the method used.

Moreover, these statistical interpretations of short windows of observations for analytical test results are not altogether satisfactory and must be balanced by rigorous review and evaluation procedures for all internal and external QC measures (7). Each step must be thoroughly documented to facilitate review and evaluation, more readily identify sources of analytical error, and effectively resolve detected problems. Good QA practices and quality improvement ensure that all data, conclusions, and reports derived from those data are technically sound and legally defensible (18).

Finally, QA programs are designed to help screening laboratories achieve excellent technical proficiency and maintain confidence in their performance while processing large volumes of specimens daily. The NSQAP continually strives to produce certified DBS materials for reference and QC analysis, to improve the quality and scope of services, and to provide immediate consultative assistance. Through the interactive efforts with participants, the NSQAP and other QA programs aspire to meet the growing and shifting needs arising from the rapidly changing profile of national newborn screening efforts and from the introduction of advanced technologies applied to DBS testing.

Acknowledgments

We thank the staff members of the NSQAP for their dedication and service to our program participants worldwide: Barbara Adam, Ricky Alexander, Kami Borsellino, Sarah Brown, Hugh Gardner, Roberta Jensen, Dr. Joanne Mei, Nancy Meredith, and Dr. F.W. Spierto.

Use of trade names is for identification only and does not imply endorsement by the Public Health Service or the U.S. Department of Health and Human Services.

References

1. Guthrie R. The origin of newborn screening. Screening 1992;1:5–15.

2. Guthrie R, Susi A. A simple phenylalanine method for detecting phenylke-tonuria in large populations of newborn infants. Pediatrics 1963;32:338–343.

3. MacCready RA. Phenylketonuria in screening programs. N Engl J Med 1963; 269:52–56.

4. National Academy of Sciences. Genetic screening: programs, principles, and research. Washington, DC: National Academy Press, 1975, p. 91.

5. Hiller EH, Landenburger G, Natowicz MR. Public participation in medical policy-making and the status of consumer autonomy: the example of newborn-screening programs in the United States. Am J Public Health 1997;87:1280–1288.

6. Newborn Screening Committee, Council of Regional Networks for Genetic Services (CORN). National Newborn Screening Report—1995. Atlanta (in press).

7. Slazyk WE, Hannon WH. Quality assurance in the newborn screening labora-tory. In: Therrell BL Jr (ed). Laboratory methods for neonatal screening. Washington, DC: American Public Health Association, 1993, pp. 23–46.

8. Hannon WH, Boyle J, Davin B, et al. Blood collection on filter paper for neona-tal screening programs (3rd ed): approved standard. Wayne, PA: National Committee for Clinical Laboratory Standards, 1997. NCCLS Document LA4-A3.

9. Slazyk WE, Phillips DL, Therrell BL Jr, Hannon WH. The effect of lot-to-lot vari-ability in filter paper on the quantification of thyroxin, thyrotropin and phenylalanine in dried-blood specimens. Clin Chem 1988;34:53–58.

10. Arends J. Neonatal screening using dried blood spotted on filter paper: method-ological factors which contribute to imprecision. In: Therrell BL Jr (ed). Advances in neonatal screening. Proceedings of the 6th International Neonatal Screening Symposium; 1986 Nov 16–19; Austin, TX. Amsterdam: Elsevier Science Publishers, 1987, pp. 549–550.

11. Therrell BL Jr, Panny SR, Davidson A, et al. U.S. newborn screening system guidelines: statement of the Council of Regional Networks for Genetic Services. Screening 1992;1:135–147.

12. Ziadeh R, Hoffman EP, Finegold DN, et al. Medium chain acyl-CoA

dehydrogenase deficiency in Pennsylvania: neonatal screening shows high incidence and unexpected mutation frequencies. Pediatr Res 1995;37:675–678.

13. *Federal register*. 1992, Feb 28;57(40):7150–7185.

14. Centers for Disease Control and Prevention. Newborn screening for cystic fibrosis: a paradigm for public health genetics policy development—proceedings of a 1997 workshop. MMWR 1997;46 (No. RR-16):13–14.

15. McCabe ERB. Utility of PCR for DNA analysis from dried blood spots on filter paper blotters. PCR Methods Appl 1991;1:99–106.

16. Therrell BL Jr, Hannon WH, Pass KA, et al. Guidelines for the retention, storage, and use of residual dried blood spot samples after newborn screening analysis: statement of the Council of Regional Networks for Genetic Services. Biochem Mol Med 1996;57:116–124.

17. McEwen JE, Reilly PR. Stored Guthrie cards as DNA banks. Am J Hum Genet 1994;55:196–200.

18. Andrews LB (ed). Legal liability and quality assurance in newborn screening. Chicago: American Bar Foundation, 1985, pp. 29–73.

IV

DEVELOPING, IMPLEMENTING, AND EVALUATING POPULATION INTERVENTIONS

14

Public health needs assessment for state-based genetic services delivery

Robert M. Fineman and Debra Lochner Doyle

In 1976, Public Law 94-278 established a national genetic disease program, "The National Sickle Cell Anemia, Cooley's Anemia, Tay-Sachs, and Genetic Diseases Act." Using funds from PL 94-278, state health departments, medical genetics providers, and others worked together to develop statewide systems for genetic health care services. The purpose of these systems was to prevent premature death or disability related to genetic risk factors by establishing statewide genetic health care systems that would be accessible to all residents. These systems included early identification, referral, evaluation, screening, diagnostic testing, and genetic counseling, as well as education for health and social services providers and the general public. In Washington State, as in many other states, public health dollars were allocated to support a statewide, regional genetic clinic system whose staff provided genetic services and education.

In 1988, an Institute of Medicine report entitled "The Future of Public Health" challenged state and local health departments to return to their roots by refraining from paying for direct clinical services and giving more attention to the public health core functions of assessment, policy development, and quality assurance (1). At the same time, health care reform began its sweep across the United States in the form of managed care, creating additional concerns for genetic service providers, patients, payers, and others. Many people feared that managed-care practices would raise barriers to access to specialty services, while insurers and health care purchasers worried about escalating health care costs. Simultaneously, the field of genetic medicine began evolving at an unparalleled pace, increasing the need for clinical services and education.

To address all of these issues, state governments, like corporations and businesses, began adjusting in an effort to be competitive and meet the needs of various target groups. In doing so, they placed significant emphasis on knowledge-based decision making, strategic planning, and policy setting. In fact, consultants advising business leaders identified the capacity to perform quality needs assessments as an important core competency of a knowledge-based organization (2). In regard to public health genetics, needs assessment can be defined as a process whereby local, state, and national agencies identify genetic health care problems (including health status and risk factors) and resources, evaluate the resources and how effectively they are being used, and present the results of these analyses to decision-makers and others (3).

Recognizing that a needs assessment is "the process of evaluating the problems and solutions identified for a target population," one can easily see its inherent value for both the private and public sectors (4,5). Needs assessments have rapidly become an important component of all public and private organization strategies, and they must precede policy development and assurance activities.

This chapter will review three basic types of needs assessment: the discrepancy, marketing, and decision-making models. In addition, we will review examples of genetic needs assessments from different states and discuss their importance. Frequently, needs assessments include individual case reports to highlight specific problems or issues in individuals, families, and communities; however, such case reports will not be presented here.

Getting Started

First and foremost, clarifying the question to be answered is essential to any needs assessment. This clarification may help to establish the parameters, or scope, of the project irrespective of which model of needs assessment is used. Additional factors that will play a role in determining scope as well as methods are resources and timelines. How much money has been allocated for the project? The cost of performing a needs assessment varies according to its nature and scope. For example, who will do the assessment? Will it be the responsibility of one individual, a team of individuals, done "in-house" or contracted out? Is there a set time for when the results of the assessment must be determined for use in other organizational efforts?

Addressing these questions should help to determine the model most appropriate for the needs assessment as well as possible methodologies. For example, if little money is available for the project, then the needs assessment staff may by necessity be forced to work with existing data as opposed to collecting new data. Some of these factors will be more readily apparent in the various examples provided within this chapter. In addition, pointers on

Table 14.1 Do's and Don'ts for Performing a Successful Statewide Needs Assessment

Do's	*Don'ts*
1. Have/know your budget. 2. Have realistic limits on your purpose/ questions. 3. Take advantage of advisors. 4. Review the literature. 5. Seek data from existing sources. 6. Recognize your target audience when communicating results. 7. Present the findings in a "'reader-friendly" fashion.	1. Don't cut corners unnecessarily. 2. Avoid "scope creep."* 3. Don't do it alone. 4. Don't rely solely on existing databases. 5. Don't delay reporting results. 6. Don't use technical jargon and acronyms.

*Expansion of the needs assessment beyond allocated resources.

completing a successful statewide needs assessment are summarized in Table 14.1.

The Discrepancy Model

The *discrepancy model*, sometimes called the *gap model*, is the most common approach used for needs assessment. In fact, it was used in all of the statewide genetic needs assessments published to date. These include assessments conducted in Washington, Nevada, Connecticut, Arizona, Texas, South Dakota, Hawaii and Ohio (6–13). The discrepancy model typically involves three steps:

1. Setting goals for an "ideal" system. (What should the system look like?);
2. Evaluating performance measures of the current system (What does the system look like now?); and
3. Identifying gaps between the ideal and the current systems.

Oftentimes, identified experts are surveyed to accomplish the first step: goal setting. A "Delphi" process of this type can be used to reach consensus and might include key or expert informant interviews and/or telephone or written surveys. Regardless of the methodology used, the end result should be a description of what the "experts" perceive to be the desired system. Note that "expert" as used here is a fairly broad term that refers to anyone likely to be involved in providing information, perceptions, or opinions. For example, "experts" in genetic services could include patients, families, community representatives, genetic service providers, primary-care providers, researchers, hospital administrators, or third-party payers including Medicaid.

The second step is to describe the existing system. Perhaps the most important factors to remember are the purpose of the assessment and the questions that need to be addressed. A well-framed question or project purpose will help identify potential databases (e.g., birth, death and fetal death certificate registries, hospital records, and so forth), and may help delineate other options or methods for collecting data needed to answer specific questions.

It is always prudent to seek data from existing databases first. For a statewide genetic needs assessment, existing sources could include data collected and maintained by the state health, social services, education, or law enforcement agencies. Because these databases are frequently developed for purposes other than addressing genetic health care issues, they usually will not be sufficient to meet all of the needs of a genetic needs assessment, and additional data collection will likely be required.

The third and final step in the discrepancy model is to compare the ideal or desired system for delivering genetic services with the system that currently exists. A "need" is identified when a performance measure of the current system fails to meet the projected performance of the ideal system. It is worth noting that the discrepancy model does not typically identify solutions to problems. The accompanying example describes how the discrepancy model was used for South Dakota's statewide genetic needs assessment.

USE OF THE DISCREPANCY MODEL

In 1995, the South Dakota Department of Health undertook a statewide genetic needs assessment. The three goals of the assessment were to:

- Evaluate past activities.
- Examine present roles and activities.
- Create a strategic plan to better address the genetic health care needs of women, infants, and children.

The health department contracted with the Great Plains Genetics Services Network (GPGSN) for technical assistance. Approximately $4400 was budgeted for two consultants to work with designated state health department staff members. A list of questions drafted to guide the process included the following:

1. Are there certain basic standard services that "must" be provided?
2. What types of genetic services in South Dakota are needed by mothers and children to promote maternal and child health?
3. Where should these services be provided?
4. What resources exist for providing and funding these services?
5. How can these services be provided in an efficient, cost-effective, and "user-friendly" manner?

To address these questions, the consultants interviewed staff members from the South Dakota Department of Health, the Birth Defects and Genetics Center at the University of South Dakota School of Medicine,

Indian Health Services, lay organizations, and a number of physicians and consumers. When pertinent and feasible, they asked for reports or further documentation from the interviewees. In addition, the consultants reviewed existing data in the annual report of the state's Title V agency, looked at copies of the state health department's contracts with genetic clinics, and examined quarterly reports (service utilization data) of genetic clinics, and the current Maternal and Child Health Block Grant application, which included statewide demographic information. On the basis of this information, the consultants were able to provide the state health department with a formal report that summarized the needs assessment process, described the existing genetic health care delivery system (including specific gaps), and recommended ways of expanding services and exploring alternative funding sources.

In summary, the procedures used by the consultants clearly exemplify the three-step process in the discrepancy model. The consultants utilized information collected from many "experts" to articulate what genetic service delivery in South Dakota should look like. They next reviewed existing data sources and, when possible, obtained additional data that described the existing system. Finally, they compared the "real" with the "ideal" systems and identified genetic service areas that were thought to be insufficient.

The Marketing Model

This type of needs assessment, which is termed the *marketing model*, helps an agency learn about and adapt to the needs of client populations or target groups. It focuses on the fit between the needs of target groups and the agency's ability to promote and fulfill those needs. A major component of the marketing model approach is the notion of *exchange*. The target groups obtain one or more things they need or want in exchange for one or more things they are willing to give up. Thus, a marketing model needs assessment can help create and implement a future bartering situation for resources such as time, money, expertise, or some sort of product. The exchange helps fulfill the needs and wants of the individuals and agencies involved, and usually includes four important components: product, price, place, and promotion.

In October 1994, the Genetic Services Section of the Washington State Department of Health (DOH) received a grant from the Maternal and Child Health Bureau to create and implement a user-friendly, statewide genetic education program for primary-care providers (PCPs). Included in the grant application for this genetics education project was the proposed use of a marketing model needs assessment. The accompanying example describes how a marketing model needs assessment was used to improve the outcome of this project.

USE OF THE MARKETING MODEL

Initially, a survey was mailed by state DOH staff members to several thousand PCPs throughout Washington State to inquire about their interest in participating in a genetic education program. They were asked what type of genetic information they would be interested in receiving and the best way for them to receive it. In addition, more than 50 professionals and consumers (key informants) representing a variety of target groups were interviewed regarding what they perceived to be the genetic education needs of PCPs. On the basis of the results obtained, a curriculum entitled "Genetics & Your Practice" was developed and marketed, and included free continuing medical education (CME) credits for physicians. Medical geneticists and genetic counselors from around the state conduct the training sessions, which are scheduled for grand rounds, large state meetings that PCPs are likely to attend, and at other venues. Also, the state DOH and the University of Washington established a statewide toll-free genetic resource line for PCPs. These actions were undertaken as a direct result of the information gleaned from the marketing model needs assessment. A few of the comments generated from that assessment are included below.

Patients/consumers said they wanted:

- Access to parent and/or peer support-group information and other resource information.
- Help in giving information to their families (and others such as schools, social services, and judicial and legal systems), and access to genetic health care services for other family members.

PCPs said they wanted:

- Easy access to genetic health care information.
- To know how genetic health care information is relevant and applicable to their practice.
- A coordinated education program provided locally by good teachers, at no charge, with free continuing medical education (CME) and continuing education (CE) credits, and at times and locations that are convenient for them to attend.

Genetic health care specialists said they wanted:

- The state DOH and others to set up and maintain all of the logistical aspects of the genetics education project and to pay them (the specialists) appropriately for their time and travel to educate (train) PCPs.
- A readily available supply of all educational/resource materials (including a trainer's manual and all information that will be given to the PCPs).

Other interested stakeholders (staff members from 15 to 18 local and statewide agencies, organizations, and institutions) said they wanted:

- An appropriate curriculum for PCP education that can either be integrated into existing courses and/or be taught as a stand-alone course.

Genetic Services Section staff members and Washington State Genetic Advisory Committee members said they wanted:

- To increase PCP knowledge and use of genetic health care services statewide, as well as their utilization of additional medical, social, educational, and other services that patients with birth defects or genetic diseases usually need.

Because a marketing model needs assessment was performed as part of this education project, appropriate training materials were developed that focused on what the target groups wanted, training sessions were coordinated to meet the needs of the trainers and PCPs, and an "information-on-demand" 1-800 resource line was implemented. Since the beginning of 1996, more than 3500 PCPs and others in Washington State have participated in one or more "Genetics & Your Practice" training sessions, with a trainee satisfaction rate of 90%+. There is little doubt that the marketing model needs assessment played a significant role in the success of this project. It not only provided background information for developing products, but also maximized information exchange among target groups, improved organizational planning, and increased overall efficiency, thereby saving time and valuable resources. Finally, the assessment helped everyone involved in this genetic education project feel like a full partner in it.

The Decision-Making Model

The *decision-making model* is the most complex of all needs assessment models. This model assumes that decision-makers are naturally biased when they encounter multidimensional needs assessment data. Therefore, in the decision-making model, values and their role in the needs analysis are made explicit. The values assigned reflect how important the person assigning the value (i.e., the decision-maker) views the available information when making a decision about a particular issue. While it is generally the decision-maker who assigns the values, the values of others may also be used in this model.

Unlike the discrepancy model, which focuses on needs identification, or the marketing-model, which uses bartering as a means to achieve its ends, the decision-making model emphasizes the final aspect of the needs assessment process—deciding on a course of action. Some may question how this process can be considered a needs assessment since it focuses on deciding upon a course of action based on needs that have been predetermined or assigned. However, given the definition provided earlier in this chapter, that a needs assessment is the process of evaluating the problems *and solutions* identified for a target population, it is clear that the decision-making model fits within this definition.

The three steps in the decision-making model are: (*1*) problem-modeling, (*2*) quantification, and (*3*) synthesis. In this model, needs identification occurs during the *problem-modeling* phase. The problem is defined and framed by options and attributes. The options are the choices the decision-maker(s) has, while the attributes are the actual measurements gathered for needs identification. The decision-maker's values are reflected during the *quantification* stage. To do this, first the raw measurements are transferred by the decision-maker into utilities or the seriousness of need for that attribute. Next the attributes are assigned a weight. It is in the assigning of weights that the decision-maker's value of an attribute is identified.

Finally, during the *synthesis* step an overall need index is calculated by multiplying the weights and utilities and summing the products across attributes. The largest need will carry the highest index for an option. It is important to recognize that no single indicator or criterion will measure a construct precisely. However, multiple indicators of need are more likely to reflect accurately the problem or construct (14).

Although the decision-making model has not been used in any of the statewide genetic needs assessments published to date, staff members of the Genetic Services Section of the Washington State DOH have used a version of this type of needs assessment to help in allocating resources to Washington's regional genetic clinics. The process used is described in the accompanying example.

USE OF THE DECISION-MAKING MODEL

In March 1998, members of the Genetic Services Section staff asked the Washington State Genetic Advisory Committee to help establish an equitable plan for allocating available financial resources to the regional genetic clinics. The "problem" or need was determined to be a lack of criterion, or a documented method, for allocating available funds to the regional genetic clinics (the problem-modeling phase). To address this issue, the Advisory Committee requested that data be compiled that reflected the following:

- The number of patients seen and the reasons for referral to the various clinics around the state.
- A map depicting which counties were served by the clinics.
- County population demographics.
- Information on how other states allocate resources.
- A line-item budget for the Genetic Services Section indicating the available fiscal resources.

Using these data, the Advisory Committee reached a consensus that a funding formula with multiple variables would be the most equitable method of allocating resources. Specific variables in the funding formula that the Advisory Committee wanted to have addressed included the following:

- Staffing needs of genetics clinics (based on the number of families served).
- The length of time a family is required to wait to get an appointment.
- The number of people in a county who speak no English or who have English as a second language.
- The level of education (less than 12 years, 12 years, more than 12 years) of residents within a county.
- The number of complex cases seen in the clinic each year.

The last three variables were included because patients in these categories usually require significantly more patient-contact hours. Data were compiled for each of these variables. However, when reviewing these data, state DOH staff members expressed concerns about two issues: (*1*) the waiting-list factor would tend to penalize rural clinics that intentionally host only four or five genetic clinics per year with a medical geneticist in attendance; and (*2*) because there is overlap among clinics serving multiple counties, the county-specific data would not be very accurate. Because of these concerns, the Advisory Committee assigned very low utility scores to these two variables.

As it was clear that the Advisory Committee valued highly the attribute of "patient-contact hours," an alternative measurement was sought. Specifically, certain reasons for referrals were categorized as complex cases. For example, in the prenatal clinical setting, referrals for an abnormal prenatal ultrasound, family history of a metabolic disorder, or a known history of a chromosomal abnormality were all considered complex cases. In addition, all new, nonprenatal patients referred for genetic evaluations were designated as complex cases. Based on the service-utilization data provided by the clinics, the percent of complex cases was determined. In addition, each clinic's staffing needs were documented. The percent of complex cases (adjusted to 1) was weighted three times greater than the staffing needs, again using state DOH staff as the decision-makers (the quantification phase).

Based on the data compiled and the discussions that ensued throughout the process, a funding formula was created (the synthesis phase) and available financial resources were divided among the genetics clinics.

Again, all the steps required for the decision-making model were employed in the example illustrated—problem-modeling, quantification, and synthesis. In this instance, the problem was defined as a need to identify an equitable means of distributing financial resources, and options for addressing the problem were modeled using available data. Next, measurements that included values of decision-makers were quantified, and the results were synthesized to give priority to the available options.

Communicating the Results of the Needs Assessment

Communicating the results of a needs assessment is critical if the information is to be used effectively in policy development. Assessors should consider several issues when reporting their findings. First, who is the intended audience? Frequently, this is the decision-maker or policymaker. Because these people are typically busy and may or may not be sophisticated about data or research findings, the report writer needs to communicate the findings succinctly and in nontechnical terms. Furthermore, creative formatting can be effective in highlighting the facts or the information that the report writer wants the reader to understand (9). In addition, by including highlights in a brief executive summary (usually no more than one to four pages), the writer has a better chance of succinctly conveying the desired information. It is also important to recognize that needs assessments capture data during a specified time frame. Lengthy delays in reporting the findings can result in the data being called into question. Therefore, it is advisable to report needs assessment findings in a timely fashion.

Tips for Completing a Successful Statewide Needs Assessment

Tips for successfully completing a statewide genetic needs assessment can be gleaned from each of the examples cited above. (Refer to Table 14.1 for a summary of some important issues about performing a successful, statewide genetic needs assessment.)

The Value of a Statewide Genetic Needs Assessment

There are numerous advantages to performing a statewide genetic needs assessment. The most obvious ones are that the data collected can be used for strategic planning, allocation of resources, and making decisions affecting policy. However, there are additional advantages that may not be so obvious. For example, in Washington State the completion of the statewide genetic needs assessment also resulted in an increased level of awareness and appreciation of genetic health care issues in the state DOH where the Genetic Services Section resides. This increased understanding proved to be instrumental in preserving funds for the statewide regional genetic clinics during times of significant cutbacks in state general funds used to pay for clinical services.

In addition, numerous partnerships have been formed both inside and outside the agency because the partners recognized shared goals, priorities, and areas of concern derived from our needs assessment activities. Data collected as part of the Washington State genetics needs assessment have also been used successfully to foster equity in consumers' access to services, and in the allocation of resources to our genetic health care providers. Finally, the needs assessment has been useful in strategic planning efforts and the development of grant applications.

Summary

In this chapter we described three basic types of needs assessments and presented examples of how they can be used to evaluate state-based genetic health care services. We also provided tips for successfully planning and conducting genetic needs assessments, and for effectively communicating the results of needs assessment activities.

The Human Genome Project should be completed in the first decade of the 21st century. The knowledge it will bring to basic sciences and clinical medicine is destined to have a major impact on medicine, industry, agriculture, law, society in general, and the environment. While some people view the revolution in genetics with great concern, others regard it as exciting and filled with opportunities.

Various public and private agencies, organizations, and institutions are charged with protecting residents from health hazards, and preventing premature death, disability, and needless suffering. How emerging genetic technologies will impact society politically, financially, ethically, legally, socially, and medically can and should be measured by public and private agencies. Collectively, the stage is set to answer a host of questions that will require data collection and evaluation in order to make knowledge-based decisions that will promote healthy outcomes. One important way to do this is by using needs assessment techniques as outlined in this chapter because, if performed properly, they can help ensure that future policy development and assurance activities will promote improved individual, family, and community outcomes.

References

1. Institute of Medicine. The future of public health. Washington, DC: National Academy Press, 1988.

2. Tecker G, Eide K, Frankel J. In pursuit of a knowledge-based association. American Society of Association Executives, 1996.

3. Keppel KG, Freedman MA. *What is assessment?* Public Health Manage Prac 1995;1:1–7.

4. McKillip J. Need analysis: tools for the human services and education. Applied Social Research Methods Series (Vol. 10). Newbury Park, CA: Sage Publications, 1987.

5. Witkin BR, Altschuld JW. Planning and conducting needs assessments: a practical guide. Thousand Oaks, CA: Sage Publications, 1995.

6. Genetic health care in Washington: assessment of services and perceptions and establishment of a statewide plan. Olympia, WA: Washington State Department of Health, December 1997.

7. Coulombe E. A genetics needs assessment for the state of Nevada. NV: Nevada State Health Division, Family Health Services Bureau, December 1992.

8. Borenstein P, Greenstein RM. Needs assessment: clinical genetics services for the underserved of greater Hartford. September 1989–May 1990. Division of Human Genetics, Department of Pediatrics, University of Connecticut Health Center, Farmington, CT.

9. Genetic health care in Arizona: a plan for the 21st century. Phoenix: Arizona Department of Health Services, 1998.

10. McCabe ERB, Patterson PJ, Botsonis H, et al. Needs assessment for genetic services in Texas. In: Paul N, Kavanaugh L (eds). Washington, DC: National Center for Education in Maternal and Child Health, 1990, pp. 54–58.

11. Christianson C. A review and evaluation of South Dakota's genetics program, 1995. Unpublished manuscript.

12. Assessing the needs for a system of genetic services. Honolulu: State of Hawaii, Pacific Southwest Regional Genetics Network, November 1993.

13. Regional comprehensive genetic program in Ohio: genetic state plan and report to the community. Columbus: Ohio Department of Health, 1998.

14. Cool TD, Campbell DT. Quasi-experimentation: design and analysis of issues for field setting. Chicago: Rand McNally, 1979.

15

Access to genetic services in the United States: A challenge to genetics in public health

Jane S. Lin-Fu and Michele Lloyd-Puryear

Dramatic advances in genetics in recent decades have opened many opportunities for understanding and promoting health, lowering mortality and morbidity, and preventing diseases. These advances, however, have also posed a grave challenge to the U.S. health care system, which is still neither accessible nor affordable to all. At a time when cost constraint is given top consideration in health care planning, the need to develop the infrastructure for a relatively new type of service—genetic services—has attracted little attention, despite the high visibility of the Human Genome Project. If the United States takes no action to systematically build the needed service infrastructure and incorporate this new knowledge and technology into the American health care system, genetic services will trickle into our health care much the same way as prenatal screening has been incorporated thus far. Integrating genetic services into health programs is a formidable task not only because of the lack of an appropriate infrastructure, but also because certain basic conceptual conflicts and dilemmas first must be resolved.

Access: What It Does and Does Not Offer

The word *access* is defined as "the ability, right or permission to approach, enter, speak with, or use admittance; a way or means of approach" (1). But in the discourse on health care, access to care is often thought of as a virtual magic bullet that can resolve most inequities in a seriously flawed health care system and eliminate the health disparities in health status and health outcomes for minority populations. Implied in this somewhat naive concept is the assumption that adequate services exist and that all people would

273

receive essentially equal treatment if only they had equal access to those services.

However, before one can benefit from any health services, including genetic services, such services must first be *available* and also *culturally appropriate* and *acceptable, particularly to racial and ethnic minorities, in addition to being accessible and affordable*. These elements do overlap, but the focus of each is different. Before examining access to genetic services, this chapter will first explore whether the systems of a service infrastructure needed to meet the rise in demand for genetic service resulting from the Human Genome Project are *available*. Access also cannot be discussed without considering the *genetics literacy* of the American public, which is a prerequisite if patients are to make truly informed decisions and preserve their autonomy. Unless these equally important components are in place, any attempt to broaden access to genetic services will have a limited impact and may even be hazardous to the less-informed population.

Assuring Availability of Genetic Services

Building a Genetic Services Infrastructure

A rational approach to ensuring proper and timely harvest of the fruits of the Human Genome Project is to legislatively mandate and fund, *concurrent with this research effort*, a national genetic services development program and a national public genetics literacy program. The purpose of the genetic services development program would be to systematically prepare the U.S. health care infrastructure (both public and private) to translate new genetic knowledge and technology into human services under well-defined ethical, scientific, and legal guidelines. The purpose of the literacy program would be to conduct an intense nationwide public education program to improve the genetics literacy of the public. Such a genetics literacy program would require congressional commitment and strong national leadership, as well as close coordination of a broad coalition of federal, state, and local public health agencies; professional and private organizations concerned with genetics, public health, primary-care as well as specialty-care providers; institutions of higher learning concerned with the education and training of health professionals; education organizations; consumer advocacy and support groups; minority and other community organizations; and news and other communication media.

The systems of an infrastructure for genetic services will require not only sufficient numbers of genetics professionals, particularly those trained in genetic counseling and public health, but also a well-prepared community of primary-care providers (physicians, nurses, midwives, physician assistants). The involvement of primary-care practitioners in genetics is pivotal, for the vast majority of patients are unaware of the genetic nature or component of their illnesses and do not seek help directly from genetics specialists. Instead, they usually consult primary-care providers first. Even when patients are aware of the genetic nature of their conditions, under the rapidly expanding managed-care plans, they must first see and undergo triage by their primary-care providers. Thus, such providers should serve as a link between patients and genetic specialists.

Despite this important potential role, however, studies have found that few primary-care providers are ready to take on this new task (2,3). And given that there is a genetic basis for virtually all diseases, including cardiovascular diseases, diabetes, learning disabilities, mental illness, and cancer, formal linkages should also be established between the genetics community and subspecialty-care providers such as oncologists, cardiologists, and psychiatrists, as well as other service providers, including social workers, psychologists, and consumer support groups. Clearly, health care providers need education and guidance in understanding not only the scientific advances in genetics, but also the ethical, legal, and psychosocial implications of these advances. They also need to know that the way medicine is practiced has to change as genetics moves to the forefront of health care (2–4).

A firm partnership needs to be promoted between the genetics community and public health programs at federal, state, and local levels. Because most public health officials have thus far shown little interest in genetics, it is important to educate workers in the field on the public health implications of recent advances in genetics. However, careful deliberation on how genetic services will be delivered in the context of public health must precede any effort to initiate new programs (see section on public health later in chapter). Other important activities include a nationwide genetics laboratory quality-assurance and proficiency-testing program, expanded state birth-defect registry activities, well-designed epidemiological surveys, and research projects. In addition, the United States should establish a centralized genetics resource center easily accessible via both electronic and other modes of communication. The center should provide up-to-date genetics research findings and other information relevant to clinical application and in separate formats appropriate for health professionals and for the general public. It could also coordinate educational activities between federal and state public health agencies.

Also needed is major federal leadership along with funding to improve the genetics content of all school curricula, from elementary grades through graduate schools involved in educating and training health professions. Consultation and cooperation of the news media, science reporters, television producers, publishers, and other communication specialists are also critical in improving the general genetics literacy. It is important that public education in genetics be conducted in collaboration with and under the leadership and the supervision of health authorities who can ensure that the information is accurate and unbiased (3,4).

Limited Federal Activities Without Legislative Mandate and Fiscal Support

In the United States, genetic services are currently being provided in multiple settings (such as community clinics, academic health centers, public health departments, commercial laboratories, and private practice) without any systematic approach, oversight, or assessment of what will be needed in the future. And despite the apparent need to build an infrastructure for genetic services and prepare the American public for the advances made by research, Congress has neither issued a legislative mandate nor appropriated money for these activities. This tragic failure of the United States to develop a broad cohesive national plan for building a genetic services infrastructure and providing public education *concurrent* with research under the Human Genome Project reflects one of the biggest blind spots in recent U.S. health care policy and planning.

To date, federal agencies interested in developing genetic services have relied on a small amount of discretionary funds appropriated under a broad mandate. For example, for almost two decades, with a budget of $7 million to 9 million annually, the Maternal and Child Health Bureau (MCHB) of the Health Resources and Services Administration (HRSA), U.S. Department of Health and Human Services (DHHS), has supported multiple projects directed at the development of genetic services. The MCHB program stimulated and provided support to initiate statewide newborn sickle cell screening programs. In collaboration with the Centers for Disease Control and Prevention (CDC) and the Association of Public Health Laboratory Directors, the MCHB established a quality assurance and performance evaluation program to improve the state newborn screening systems.

In addition, funding has been provided to improve comprehensive follow-up care of infants with sickle cell disease identified by newborn screening programs and to integrate the various types of health services within a community or geographic area for infants and children with sickle cell disease. The MCHB has supported demonstration projects to provide counseling for individuals and families affected by thalassemia; to increase the use of genetic services by Southeast Asian refugees; to develop peer-support groups for young adults with genetic disorders; to overcome ethnocultural barriers and increase access to and utilization of genetic services for populations confronted by language and cultural barriers; to produce culturally sensitive genetics education materials in different languages; and to initiate model programs that provide transition from pediatric care to adult family and specialty-care for young adults with genetic disorders.

Additionally, the MCHB encouraged the formation and provided funding for ten regional genetics networks, the Council of Regional Networks for Genetic Services, and a consumer organization, the Alliance of Genetic Support Groups, to assist states in developing genetic services and to forge close partnerships among public health officials, primary- and subspecialty-care providers, and consumers. Most recently, the MCHB funded the establishment of a National Newborn Screening and Genetics Resource Center and for states, planning grants for the development of state genetics plans. Using MCHB Block Grant funds, the states have devoted varying amounts to develop state-level genetic services. In the early 1990s, the MCHB initiated grants to set up genetics education for primary-care providers. Some of these educational materials are now freely available via the electronic media.

Although the MCHB has accomplished much, its annual budget of about $9 million is woefully inadequate compared with the $300 million for the Human Genome Project. Other federal public health agencies such as CDC and the ELSI (Ethical, Legal and Social Implications) program of the National Human Genome Research Institute (NHGRI) also have devoted a limited budget toward public education, public policy development, and other services. But the lack of specific appropriations to systematically plan and build the needed service infrastructure nationwide has resulted in an inadequate number of genetic specialists, as well as a primary-care and a public health workforce ill prepared to incorporate genetics into their practices.

Current U.S. Genetics Human Resources

In August 1998, the American Board of Medical Genetics (ABMG) reported that it had issued 1990 certificates to qualified physicians or those with doctoral degrees: 917 in clinical genetics, 147 in medical genetics, 159 in clinical biochemical genetics, 491 in clinical cytogenetics, 227 in clinical molecular genetics, and 49 in clinical biochemical/molecular genetics. Because a person may be certified in more than one area, one can assume that the number of board-certified geneticists is fewer than 1990 (American Board of Medical Genetics, personal communication, 1998). Of these 1990 certificates, 630 have been issued since 1990 (3; American Board of Medical Genetics, personal communication, 1998). In addition to these doctoral-level geneticists, 1070 board-certified genetic counselors have been approved by the ABMG, or by the American Board of Genetic Counseling (ABGC), ever since it took over the responsibility of certifying this specialty in 1993 (American Board of Medical Genetics, personal communication, 1998). For a nation of more than 270 million people, fewer than 3000 board-certified genetics specialists (not all of whom are in clinical work) can hardly be expected to meet the need for services resulting from the Human Genome Project. Without even exploring other parts of the genetic services infrastructure, one must seriously question whether the United States has enough qualified geneticists and genetic counselors to meet the needs of the entire population.

The lack of genetics human resources to translate progress into human services is particularly troubling in view of the remarkable advances in molecular biology, automated sequencing, and information processing that have markedly reduced the time and the cost of genetic testing. And as direct marketing of genetic tests has already begun, genetic counseling by qualified personnel with no commercial interests in the tests is critical if the public is to make informed decisions about being tested (3,4).

Among primary-care providers, inadequate preparation in genetics is compounded by the severe time constraints imposed on virtually all service providers and by a lack of reimbursement for cognitive services such as genetic counseling. Thus, it is doubtful that the U.S. health care system has sufficient human resources to meet the needs for genetic services created by progress made under the Human Genome Project (3–5).

Barriers to Access

Even if sufficient genetic services were available, providing universal access to such services remains a grave challenge. Advances in genetic medicine and technology may further widen the gap in health care access between people of different socioeconomic strata. Although deterrents to such access include insurance, socioeconomic, geographic, ethnocultural, psychosocial, genetics literacy, and logistical barriers (e.g., need for transportation, baby-sitting services), this chapter limits it discussion to those barriers associated with genetics literacy, insurance, and ethnocultural differences.

Low Genetics Literacy of the American Public
A 1990 National Science Foundation survey found only 7% of Americans to be scientifically literate (6). In its 1992 survey, the March of Dimes found that a majority of respondents knew little or nothing about genetic testing or gene therapy (7). Promoting access to genetic services for a population with very little or no knowledge of genetics is comparable with inviting computer-illiterate people into a state-of-the-art computer room expecting them to use and benefit from this modern technology. Without some degree of genetics literacy and a clear understanding of the limitations and the potential risks involved in genetic testing (such as insurance and employment discrimination, psychological trauma, intrafamilial conflict, and social stigmatization), people cannot make truly informed decisions about using genetic services.

Health Insurance Barriers
Health insurance presents a special problem in genetics. Many patients either have no health insurance or are underinsured. Others find that their condition is not covered by their insurance plans. Still others are afraid to use their insur-

ance for genetic testing, fearful that the test results might compromise their future ability to get insurance coverage not only for themselves but possibly for their family members. The dramatic expansion of the use of "gatekeepers" within the health insurance industry adds yet another dimension to this already complicated issue of insurance coverage. Timely referrals to appropriate subspecialists, such as geneticists, may or may not be made, depending on both the genetic competency of the primary-care providers and the sound judgment of these "gatekeepers" (3–5).

In 1997, an estimated 43.4 million people, or 16.1% of the U.S. population, had no health insurance coverage. Among those with insurance, most (70.1%) were covered by private insurance, and 61.4% had employment-based insurance. Government programs accounted for 24.8% and military insurance for 3.2% of the coverage (8).

Not surprisingly, lack of health insurance was more common among the lower socioeconomic strata. Despite the existence of government programs such as Medicaid and Medicare, 31.6% of such individuals, or 11.24 million people, had no health insurance. Among those with annual incomes of under $25,000, 25.4% had no health insurance compared with 8.1% among those with incomes of $75,000 or more. Minorities had a relatively high rate of noncoverage: 34% among Hispanics, 21.5% among blacks, and 20.7% among Asian Americans and Pacific Islanders, as compared with 12% among non-Hispanic whites and 15% of whites. The foreign-born had a much higher rate of noncoverage (24.3%) than did native-born (14.2%), and among noncitizens, 43.6% were uninsured. The less educated are also less likely to have health insurance: 26% of those without a high school diploma but only 8.2% of those with a bachelor's degree had no coverage (8).

In addition, people of prime reproductive age (18 to 44 years old) consistently had lower rates of health insurance than did those younger or older. For example, 30.1% of those aged 18 to 24 had no coverage compared with 15% of those younger than 18 and 14.1% of those aged 45 to 64 (8).

Thus, the most vulnerable populations—minorities, the poor and near-poor, the less educated, and the foreign-born—are those most likely to have no health insurance. But lack of such coverage is only one dimension of a complex problem that must be resolved before genetic services truly can be accessible. In addition to those without health insurance, many more are underinsured, with coverage limited to basic health services that may not pay for genetic services, as is the case with the state Children's Health Insurance Program (CHIP). In 1996, 15% of all American children and 23.8% of poor children had no health insurance coverage (9). The new CHIP affords states an unprecedented opportunity to extend coverage to low-income uninsured children. For the most part, however, states have not structured the CHIP with particular attention to youngsters with special health needs, nor have they included in the coverage items such as screening tests beyond vision screening (9). Genetic services may therefore not be *affordable* even to those with health insurance.

People with genetic disorders also face a problem not usually shared by those with other disorders: the potential impact of genetic information on their future insurability and/or insurance premium. Such information also has potential insurance implications for one's offspring and other family members. In other words, people who obtain genetic services through their insurance coverage may face genetic discrimination and the loss or limitation of future insurance coverage or coverage at an exorbitant premium (3–5).

The issue of insurance discrimination against individuals with or at risk for genetic disorders stems from the fact that many insurance companies use medical information about a person's risk for disease and death in determining insurance eligibility, limitations of coverage, and the insurance premium. Ironically, genetic tests now allow people to determine their genetic susceptibility to certain diseases such as breast and colon cancer and cardiovascular diseases, a development that has important implications for prevention and treatment strategies. But it is precisely the genetic information made possible by these remarkable tests that might compromise someone's ability to obtain health insurance in the future, as well as create the possibility of discrimination in other areas such as life and disability insurance, employment and educational opportunities, and mortgage or other long-term loans (3–5).

Both the Task Force on Genetic Information and Insurance (5) and the Task Force on Genetic Testing of the NIH-DOE Working Group on Ethical, Legal, and Social Implications of Human Genome Research (4) have recommended that genetic information should not be used to deny health care coverage or to otherwise discriminate. But such recommendations are hardly protective without proper legislative backing. Although several bills have been introduced in Congress, federal legislative protection against genetic discrimination does not exist. State laws aimed at genetic discrimination vary widely in their coverage, and not all states have such legislation.

Ethnocultural Barriers

Culture plays a central role in determining one's health beliefs, attitudes, and behavior, but few health care providers take note of this fact or realize that "health" is a cultural concept that may be defined differently in different cultures. Nor are many aware that the health care system itself is a cultural system designed and administered largely according to the mainstream culture. In genetics, cultural consideration is particularly important for several reasons. Although the knowledge that certain diseases run in families spans all societies, beliefs about causation of familial diseases and birth defects vary considerably. Cultural attitudes toward reproduction, pregnancy, childbirth, diseases, and disabilities also differ among different ethnic populations. Moreover, culture comes into play in provider–client interaction and communication, which are both key parts of genetic counseling. People from cultures that expect authority figures (such as health care providers) to give clear directions often find nondirective genetic counseling utterly confusing and even bewildering (10–12).

In 1998, the four population groups recognized by U.S. federal programs as minorities (black or African American, Hispanic or Latino, Asian American and Pacific Islander, and American Indian and Alaskan Native) together numbered 73.96 million, or 27.5% of the total population. Between 1970 and 1990, the minority population grew at a rate about three times that of the total population. This faster rate of growth is expected to continue. The U.S. Census Bureau projects that minorities will account for about one-third of the U.S. population by the year 2010 and almost one-half of the population by 2050. In 1990, about 8% of the U.S. population were foreign-born, but by 1998, the population had increased to 10% (10,13). Given these demographic trends in the United States, attention to ethnocultural barriers is paramount to achieving universal public access to services.

Among the various ethnocultural barriers to health care access, a linguistic barrier is the most important and visible. In the 1990 census, 13.8% of the U.S. population, or 31.8 million people, aged 5 years and older, spoke a non-English language at home. Among these, 4.8 million (15.2%) did not speak English very well, and 1.8 million did not speak English at all. About 8 million households are reported to be linguistically isolated (households where no one, 14 years or older, spoke English only and no one who spoke a non-English language spoke English very well). Linguistic barriers are more common in some states than others. In six states (AZ, CA, HI, NM, NY, TX), 20% or more of the population spoke a non-English language at home. New Mexico and California led with rates of 35.5% and 31.5%, respectively (14).

Despite the importance of ethnocultural barriers in deterring access to and proper use of health services, the U.S. health care system is poorly prepared to break down these barriers. Cultural competency is not a licensing requirement for health professionals, and properly trained medical interpreters are virtually nonexistent in most clinical sites that need them. Interpretation is often left to young children, relatives, or friends who are not qualified for the task. In genetics, the need for a proper professional interpreter is even more important because of the sensitive nature of the issues to be discussed and the need for privacy and confidentiality of information exchanged (10,11).

Also deeply troubling is the fact that the genetics community in the United States includes few minorities, even though in 1998, about one-quarter of the population consisted of racial and ethnic minorities. With the exception of Asian Americans and Pacific Islanders, minorities are severely underrepresented. A 1998 survey conducted by the American Society of Human Genetics (Jane Salomon, American Society for Human Genetics, personal communication, September 1998) found that of 4810 U.S./Canadian members who responded, 83.8% were white and 12.5% were Asian American or Pacific Islanders, but only 1.1% were black, 0.7% Hispanic, and 0.6% American Indian, Eskimo or Aleut (1.1% reported as "other"). Even more striking is the 1998 survey conducted by the National Society of Genetic Counselors, which found that 93% of its members were white and 4% were Asian Americans or Pacific Islanders. Blacks and Hispanics each accounted for only 1%, and no one reported as American Indian or Alaskan Native (15). This lack of minority representation further limits the access of minorities to culturally sensitive and relevant genetic services. More important, it also means a lack of input from minority communities in shaping public policies and planning genetic research and services.

Genetics and Public Health: Meeting the Challenge

Thoughtful deliberation is required to translate new knowledge and technology from genetic research into clinical service, especially as delivered in public health programs. Genetic epidemiologic information from carefully designed studies is needed to understand how genetic factors interact with each other and with environmental factors, how disease becomes manifested, and how morbidity and mortality can be prevented. But such studies may be fraught with many ethical, legal, and psychosocial issues that must be resolved first if pitfalls are to be avoided (16,17). With the uncovering of a genetic basis for most common diseases, one can envision expanded genetic services integrated broadly into public health programs. However, before that expansion can be properly instituted, many challenges lie ahead.

Persistence of an Obsolete View on Genetic Disorders
Genetic diseases gained recognition in public health with the introduction of the newborn screening program for phenylketonuria (PKU) in the early 1960s. This public health program resulted from intense pressure put on state legislatures by advocates like Dr. Robert Guthrie, by parents, and by organizations excited at the prospect of preventing mental retardation. State laws mandating such screening became the foundation of this public health program. In 1972, the Sickle Cell Anemia Control Act thrust another genetic disease into public health programs. But poor public understanding of the disease compounded by misguided legislation mandating premarital and preschool testing in some areas and poorly planned programs led to public confusion and insurance and employment discrimination against those with the sickle cell trait. The disastrous results of this well-intended but poorly planned public health genetics program raised questions about genocide and caused many minorities, particularly African Americans, to be highly skeptical of public health genetics programs (18–20).

State newborn screening programs quickly expanded to include other metabolic errors and later, nongenetic diseases such as toxoplasmosis and HIV infection. Today the number of diseases screened for varies from state to state; however, all states, the District of Columbia, and Puerto Rico screen for PKU and hypothyroidism (3,21). Still viewed largely as a genetics program, newborn screening is unique in that it operates under state mandates and statutes, most of which do not require informed consent. Parental dissent is generally permitted, and parents can refuse testing for their children. Maryland and Wyoming are the only two states that require informed consent. States have made efforts to educate parents about the program but neither provide nor require pretesting genetic counseling (3,21).

Ever since PKU and sickle cell screening were introduced, many advances have been made in clinical genetics, including prenatal screening for hemoglobinopathies, for metabolic and other disorders, and for prenatal triple marker screening for neural tube defects and chromosomal anomalies. However, for many people in public health, PKU is still seen as the prototypical genetic disorder, in which a mutation in a single gene causes a rare disease. Generally viewed as rare diseases, genetic disorders are still seen by many as not highly relevant to the public health community.

Complicating this obsolete view is the fact that two key questions remain to be answered: *How should genetic disorders be defined? Should all genetic mutations be considered genetic disorders?* Not all genes follow simple patterns of inheritance. Some mutated genes, although inherited, show no effect unless other genes are also mutated or the person with those mutated genes is exposed to certain environmental factors. Therefore, predicting a person's risk for disease on the basis of his or her genetic makeup becomes difficult. Many of the disorders displaying complex patterns of inheritance or gene-gene or gene-environment interaction, such as breast and prostate cancer, hypertension and coronary heart disease, and diabetes, are already of public health interest (3,4,16). Will genetic medicine change our approach to the treatment and prevention of such common diseases? Should a public health approach based on genetic medicine be introduced in public health programs for these diseases? Are public health programs prepared to take on this challenge?

Nondirectiveness in a Highly Directive Program

Public health programs have traditionally been highly directive. That is, public health authorities give clear instructions on what the public should do, such as eating a balanced diet, receiving vaccines at certain times, obtaining a Pap smear and mammography, and quitting smoking. Are public health programs ready to depart from this long-held tradition of being highly directive and begin administering a program whose central tenets include personal autonomy, informed decision making, and nondirective counseling? Will public health authorities agree that preserving patients' personal autonomy is more important than the possible public health benefit of population-based screening? And should there be any exceptions to this rule? If so, what criteria should be applied?

Some careful and thorough rethinking is also due in the genetics community. The principle of nondirectiveness in genetic counseling is not embraced worldwide, and whether genetic counseling can be totally nondirective has been seriously challenged, given the counselor's personal perspective (3,4). Moreover, is not counseling about alcohol intake and diabetes control during pregnancy and mammography screening for breast cancer already directive in the United States? Now that genetics has moved into common multifactorial diseases in which early intervention may modify disease outcome, and many tests for genetic susceptibility are now feasible, does not directiveness have a place in genetic counseling? If so, under what circumstances should it be acceptable and how does one continue to safeguard the personal autonomy of patients who must make reproductive and other choices as part of genetic testing?

Primary Prevention: A Potentially Dangerous Approach in Public Health Genetics

It is an axiom in public health that primary prevention is always better than secondary or tertiary prevention. But if public health is to expand its role in delivering genetic services, it must be willing to part with this principle under certain circumstances. Primary prevention still has a place in genetics. For example, promoting a folic acid intake among women of reproductive age to lower their risk of having offspring with a neural tube defect is a perfectly acceptable public health primary prevention strategy. But the primary prevention of genetic diseases—more specifically, genotypic prevention—may seem dangerously close to eugenics and genocide (20,22). It is critical to bear in mind that during the first two decades of this century, thousands of people deemed by the eugenics movement to be "unfit" were "eugenically sterilized" in the United States (20). Today, the goal of premarital or prenatal screening for recessive traits for sickle cell anemia and thalassemia in the United States is not to prevent the birth of individuals with these diseases or to reduce the incidence of these diseases. Genetic screening is not intended as a tool for the primary prevention of genetic disease. Rather, genetic screening and counseling are intended to give the population at risk the information needed to make informed choices and prepare for the outcome of their decision.

The approach taken in the United States differs from some instituted elsewhere. In Cyprus, where thalassemia is highly prevalent in the general population and does not affect minority populations disproportionately, thalassemia screening is not identified with a minority population as is hemoglobinopathy screening in the United States. In the United Kingdom and in the United States, where both sickle cell anemia and thalassemia disproportionately affect minority groups, the need for sensitivity to the fear of eugenics and for the preservation of personal autonomy has been extensively discussed (18,20,22,23).

Because genetics is about all human beings, the appropriateness of primary prevention of genetic diseases through reproductive choices should not be viewed as an issue that concerns only minorities. The importance of safeguarding personal autonomy and self-determination and ensuring equity in a free society should concern all who uphold human rights. Moreover, the public health genetics community must be sensitive to people with disabilities and be careful not to offend or violate the rights of those disabled by genetic disorders. Pronouncing a public health policy to reduce the incidence of certain genetic diseases by preventing the birth of individuals with these disorders is to publicly declare that people with these disorders are less desirable than others and that their births should be avoided (18–20,22,23).

Cost-Benefit Analysis of Genetic Programs

Cost-effectiveness is a key consideration in all public health programs. Undoubtedly programs such as newborn screening for PKU and hypothyroidism have been highly cost-beneficial. Likewise the early identification of newborns with sickle cell disease followed by penicillin prophylaxis and comprehensive care has significantly reduced mortality and morbidities from this disease. Presumably, the early detection of individuals with increased genetic susceptibility to certain disorders such as coronary heart disease or breast cancer, followed by close monitoring and early intervention, can improve their outlook as well (3,4). However, cost-benefit ratios may present a problem in some genetics programs.

If we accept the premises that genetic counseling must be nondirective, particularly counseling about reproductive choices and decisions to be tested, and that genetic programs must respect the patient's right not only to know but also not to know about specific genetic information, then the conventional method of measuring cost-benefit ratios of programs becomes problematic. For example, genetics programs should not measure the cost of providing prenatal genetic testing and counseling against the number of women who eventually agree to have amniocentesis or chorionic villus sampling or decide to terminate their pregnancy when an affected fetus is detected. Programs also should not measure the cost of screening for a recessive trait against the number of homozygote births that are prevented (4,8). Will public health programs, which have traditionally boasted of high cost-benefit ratios in programs such as vaccination and injury prevention, be able and willing to accept this change in attitude and practice? Will public health authorities deviate from conventional cost-benefit analysis and consider providing the public a basis for informed decision making as a sufficient justification for funding a program?

Ensuring Personal Autonomy: Informed Decisions and Confidentiality

No broad-based genetic testing program should be implemented before sufficient resources are available for public education and genetic counseling prior to testing and follow-up services after testing. Nor should any population-based genetics programs be initiated without safeguarding the ethical principles of patient autonomy, equity, and privacy (3,4). With the current shortage of genetic counseling resources, time constraints on provider–client interaction, and the low genetics literacy of the public, one must seriously question whether most patients in a large-scale public health genetic testing program can be expected to make truly informed decisions; this question is especially applicable to socioeconomically vulnerable populations. Safeguarding the autonomy of this population is particularly important as this population may be easily swept into a publicly promoted health program with little or no understanding of the options and the risks involved. Even if informed consent is introduced, will this be merely a sham formality to cover up a poorly informed decision? Another critical issue is the confidentiality of genetic information. Without clear legislative and regulatory protection against discrimination based on genetic information, public health authorities must proceed with extreme caution in initiating any broad-based genetic testing program. The fiasco from the sickle cell testing of the early 1970s must not be repeated (3,4,18–20,22,23).

Race and Ethnicity in Public Health Genetic Programs

In the United States, although racial designation in census data is based on self-identification, racial classification in the social context has no biological basis. Despite this illogical and offensive approach, the U.S. census and other governmental data sources continue to tabulate data according to race and ethnicity as defined by the 1977 U.S. Office of Management and Budget Directive No. 15.

The incidence of diseases often varies among different racial and ethnic populations, and it is common for public health programs to target high-risk groups who often are minorities. Although the method of reaching out to each community should be culturally appropriate, the actual test and treatment or prevention measures used are generally the same for all racial and ethnic groups. This "one-size-fits-all" approach, however, may present a problem in public health genetic programs.

In planning for public health genetics programs, not only must one bear in mind that the frequency of genetic disorders is often very different in different populations and the genotype–phenotype correlation may vary from group to group, but common mutations for the same genetic disease often differ among racial and ethnic populations. A single public health policy on a genetic disease for all racial and ethnic groups may be neither prudent nor ethical. The 1997 National Institutes of Health Consensus Development Statement on Genetic Testing for Cystic Fibrosis (CF) (24) is a clear example.

The statement recommended that genetic testing for CF should be offered to adults with a positive family history of CF, to partners of people with CF, to those seeking prenatal care, and to couples planning a pregnancy. It did not recommend offering the CF test to the general population. The statement acknowledged the wide range of test sensitivity in different population groups using current technology; nonetheless, it made no special recommendation for groups for whom the current CF test is of extremely low sensitivity. In the United States, the incidence of CF is much higher among European Americans (1/3300) than among African Americans (1/15,300) or Asian Americans (1/32,100). Because of differences in mutation, the sensitivities of current CF tests vary widely, ranging from 90% to 95% among Americans of European ancestry to 30% among Asian Americans. Thus, offering CF testing to couples planning for a pregnancy or women seeking prenatal care, regardless of race or ethnicity, utilizing tests for the predominant mutations in Americans of European ancestry would have an extremely low cost-benefit ratio in certain minority populations such as Asian American and Hispanic (25).

More important, offering a genetic test of extremely low sensitivity to certain racial and ethnic populations raises the ethical issue of equity and questions the wisdom of such across-the-board genetics public policy for all U.S. populations. In CF testing, assuring true informed decision through effective counseling is a particular challenge for the Hispanic and Asian American populations. These two minority groups have the lowest test sensitivity (57% in Hispanics and 30% in Asian Americans) yet both have a very high proportion of immigrants who face severe linguistic and cultural barriers in accessing any service. Because offering a genetic test of 30% to 50% or even 75% sensitivity in a broad-based program should have been unacceptable to most public policymakers, one must question what is an acceptable sensitivity level when genetic testing is recommended without regards to race and ethnicity? If one truly considers all human beings as equal, regardless of race and ethnicity, then shouldn't public health policies and programs on genetic testing seek a test sensitivity of 90% to 95% for all racial and ethnic groups and not just for the majority population? If this is deemed impractical, and public health programs decide to offer a test with less than 90% sensitivity to certain minority populations, is this ethical and how should people in these communities be counseled? Is equity in fact achievable in "one-size-fits-all" genetics public policies?

Conclusions

Recent research in genetics has greatly enhanced our understanding of the role of genetics in health and diseases, expanded the scope of medical genetics, and offered remarkable potential for promoting health and improving quality of life. But these highly successful research activities have not been accompanied by concurrent and systematic efforts to build the needed infrastructure for genetic services and resources and improve the genetics literacy of the American public. Because a genetic basis has been demonstrated in many if not most common diseases, public health agencies and organizations should explore how genetic services can be integrated into their programs. However, in addition to the need to develop an appropriate infrastructure, many conceptual as well as practical issues must first be resolved. Weighing the history of eugenics earlier in the 20th century and the disastrous sickle cell screening experience of the 1970s, any effort to initiate public health genetic testing must be carefully planned with input from the communities targeted and proceed with extreme caution to avoid past mistakes and new pitfalls.

Acknowledgment

The authors thank Ms. Kaye Vander Ven and Dr. Marie Mann for their careful editing and thoughtful comments and to Ms. Carrie Diener for her help with library research.

References

1. Fexner SB, Hauck LC (ed). Random House unabridged dictionary (2nd ed). New York: Random House, 1993.

2. Hoffman KJ, Tambor ES, Chase GA, Geller G, Faden RR, Holtzman NA. Physician knowledge of genetics and genetic tests. Acad Med 1993;68:625–632.

3. Andrews LB, Fullarton JE, Holtzman NA, Motulsky AG (eds). Assessing genetic risks: implications for health and social policy. Washington, DC: National Academy Press, 1994.

4. Holtzman NA, Watson MS (eds). Promoting safe and effective genetic testing in the United States. Bethesda, MD: National Institutes of Health, 1997.

5. NIH-DOE Working Group on Ethical, Legal, and Social Implications of Human Genome Research. Genetic information and health insurance: report of the task force on genetic information and insurance. Bethesda, MD: National Institutes of Health, 1993.

6. Miller J. The public understanding of science and technology in the United States, 1990. Report to the National Science Foundation. Washington, DC: National Academy of Science, 1992.

7. March of Dimes Birth Defects Foundation news release. White Plains, NY: September 29, 1992.

8. U.S. Bureau of the Census. Health insurance coverage. Washington, DC: Author, 1998.

9. Fox HB. States' CHIP policies and children with special health care needs. Washington, DC: Maternal and Child Health Research Center, October 1998.

10. Lin-Fu JS. Making genetic services and education culturally relevant: Proceedings of the Conference on Genetic Services: Developing Guidelines for the Public's Health, Washington, DC, February 16–17, 1996. Atlanta, GA: Council of Regional Networks for Genetic Services, 1997.

11. Lin-Fu JS. Ethnocultural factors in genetic counseling: The Asian-Americans as a model. Presentation at the Conference on the Thalassemias: Diagnosis, management, Future Perspective for Therapy, New York Hospital–Cornell Medical Center, New York, May 15, 1989.

12. Fisher NL. Cultural and ethnic diversity: a guide for genetics professionals. Baltimore, MD: The Johns Hopkins University Press, 1996.

13. U.S. Bureau of the Census. Annual population estimates of the United States by age, race and Hispanic origin. Washington, DC: Author, 1998.

14. U.S. Bureau of the Census. Statistical abstract of the United States (116th ed). Washington, DC: U.S. Government Printing Office, 1996.

15. Schneider, KA. The 1998 professional status survey. Perspect Genetic Counsel 1998;20:S1–S8.

16. Khoury M, Yang Q. The future of genetic studies of complex human diseases: an epidemiological perspective. Epidemiology 1998;9:350–354.

17. Bondy M, Mastromarino C. Ethical issues of genetic testing and their implications in epidemiologic studies. Ann Epidemiol 1997;7:363–366.

18. Bowman JE. The road to eugenics. Univ Chicago Law School Round Table 1996;3:491–517.

19. Scott RB. Historical review of legislative and national initiatives for sickle cell disease. Am J Pediatr Hematology/Oncology 1983;5:346–351.

20. Kevles DJ. In the name of eugenics: genetics and the use of human heredity. New York: Knopf, 1985.

21. Hiller EH, Landenburger G, Natowicz MR. Public participation in medical policy making and the status of consumer autonomy: the example of newborn screening programs in the United States. Am J Public Health 1997;87:1280–1288.

22. Juengst ET. Prevention and the goal of genetic medicine. Hum Gene Ther 1995;6:1595–1605.

23. Atkin K, Ahmad WIU. Genetic screening and haemoglobinopathies: ethics, politics and practice. Soc Sci Med 1998;46:445–458.

24. National Institutes of Health. Consensus development statement: genetic testing for cystic fibrosis. Bethesda, MD: Author, 1997.

25. Haddow JE, Palomaki GE, Bradley LA, Doherty RA. Screening for cystic fibrosis. JAMA 1998;279:1068–1069.

16

Community genetics in The Netherlands

Leo P. Ten Kate

Community genetics is concerned with the application of medical genetics to the benefit of as many people as is possible and meaningful in the community (1). The term was first used by Bernadette Modell in 1990 (2).

Community genetics differs from *clinical genetics* in many respects. Whereas clinical geneticists are concerned with people and families who come to their clinics with their worries, community geneticists go out to the community in search of individuals who may be at risk but have not yet been identified or helped. Still, when clinical genetic services are unavailable for the members of a community, putting these services into place may be the first concern of the community geneticist. Other community genetic activities include conducting genetic screening, providing genetic education, applying genetics in primary care, providing genetic services for disadvantaged populations, and registering genetic and congenital anomalies.

In this chapter we will review the current situation in the Netherlands, starting with some background information on health insurance schemes, followed by a description of clinical genetics services, and a survey of community genetics services. Then we will consider the prevailing climate of fear and uneasiness regarding genetics in Dutch society at large and among politicians in particular. And finally we will describe the activities of a small band of people who are trying to get community genetics "on the agenda."

Health Insurance Programs

Medical expenses in the Netherlands are divided into normal medical expenses and exceptional costs. Exceptional costs (e.g., for long-term care or advanced treatment) are covered by a compulsory national insurance program under the Exceptional Medical Expenses Act. Normal medical expenses are paid by various insurance arrangements. Slightly more than 60% of the Dutch population is covered by the Health Insurance Act. Individuals whose annual income is below approximately US$32,000 and all recipients of social security benefits are compulsorily insured under this act. About 5% of the population are covered by health insurance programs for public servants, and a little over 30% of the population have private medical insurance. Private health insurance companies have an obligation to accept individuals whose medical expenses are no longer covered by the Health Insurance Act because of a rise of yearly income above US$32,000, irrespective of their medical risk.

Clinical Genetic Services

Recently, the *European Journal of Human Genetics* published a supplement with data on genetic services in 31 European countries, including the Netherlands (3,4). Each review gives information on a country's background, its health service setting, history of medical genetics, and seven dimensions of the quality of genetic services: their availability; patients access to them; their value in sustaining life; state of the art; their safety; their effectiveness; and consumer satisfaction with the services. The project, named CAGSE (Concerted Action on Genetic Services in Europe), resulted not only in this overview but also in three recommendations: (*1*) ensure in each country the presence of a national medical genetics organization; (*2*) ensure the presence of regional medical genetics centers; and (*3*) ensure provision of training and education (5).

In the Netherlands these recommendations have long since been fullfilled at least in part: The Dutch Society of Human Genetics was founded more than 50 years ago. For a population of about 15.5 million, the country has had eight clinical genetic centers since 1980. Clinical genetics was recognized as a medical specialty in 1987. Undergraduate training for medical and nursing students and genetics training for primary-care teams and other health care workers, however, leave much to be desired.

The eight clinical genetic centers are part of or closely affiliated with the eight academic hospitals in the country. They offer genetic counseling; cytogenetic, molecular, and biochemical diagnosis; fetal sampling; and prenatal ultrasound (see Table 16.1). These services are paid for by the normal medical insurance schemes. There are numerous indications for genetics services on which the clinical genetic centers and the health insurance companies agree.

By the end of 1998, the Netherlands had 60 clinical geneticists; in addition, 12 genetic physicians and 10 genetic associates were in training. Both training

Table 16.1 Approximate Numbers of Clinical Genetic
Activities in the Netherlands, 1997

Activity	No.
Genetic counseling	8,600
Cytogenetic diagnosis	
Postnatal	14,000
Prenatal	13,500
Molecular genetic diagnosis	
Postnatal	18,000
Prenatal	300
Biochemical diagnosis	
Postnatal	19,000
Prenatal	300
Fetal sampling	
Amniocentesis	9,400
Chorionic villus biopsy	3,800
Cordocentesis	100
Fetal ultrasound	9,000
Molecular genetics	18,000

programs are supervised by the Dutch Society of Clinical Genetics, which is part of the Dutch Society of Human Genetics. Both societies have implemented quality-control systems for clinical genetics, clinical cytogenetics, and clinical molecular genetics.

Community Genetic Services

Table 16.2 lists *genetic screening* programs in the Netherlands. Neonatal screening for phenylketonuria (PKU) and congenital hypothyroidism are well established and have a very high coverage rate. Recently, a 2-year pilot program of neonatal screening for congenital adrenal hyperplasia was started in a part of the country. Prenatal cytogenetic diagnosis has been offered to older pregnant women since the early 1970s. At present, the target group consists of women who are over 35 in the 18th week of gestation. One may question, however, whether the latter is really an established practice as the Ministry of Health recently has requested a review to evaluate whether this type of screening is admissible under the Population Screening Act (see below). Offering maternal serum screening or ultrasound screening to detect congenital anomalies is not currently permitted, although there were pilot programs in the past and individual requests can be granted. There is one pilot study on preconceptional screening of cystic fibrosis carriers and one on cascade screening for familial hypercholesterolemia.

Table 16.2 Genetic Screening Programs in the Netherlands

Period in Life	Established	Not Established
Neonatal	PKU, CHT	CAH
Prenatal	Rh	Triple test
	Age-related PCD	US
Preconceptional		CF carriers
Adults		FH

Abbreviations: CAH = congenital adrenal hyperplasia; CF = cystic fibrosis; CHT = congenital hypothyroidism; FH = familial hypercholesterolemia; PCD = prenatal cytogenetic diagnosis; PKU = phenylketonuria; Rh = rhesus bloodgroup; US = ultrasound.

Table 16.3 Some Registries of Congenital Anomalies and Genetic Disorders in the Netherlands

EUROCAT, Northern Netherlands
EUROCAT, Southwestern Netherlands
National Neonatal Registry
National Obstetrical Registries
Registries for several types of hereditary cancer
Registries for specific disorders such as CF, Rb, CH

Abbreviations: CF = cystic fibrosis; CH = chorea Huntington; EUROCAT = European Registration of Congenital Anomalies; Rb = retinoblastoma.

Table 16.3 lists *registries* of congenital anomalies and genetic disorders within the country or within large parts of it. The EUROCAT registries are part of the European network of registries of congenital anomalies and encompass well over 25% of births in the Netherlands. Some information on these disorders, although less detailed, can also be obtained from the national obstetric and neonatal registries. National registries of families with hereditary cancers have been established to monitor periodic follow-up of people at risk within these families.

The national federation of patients and parents' organizations in the field of congenital and genetic disorders, or VSOP, plays an important part in *educating* the public about genetics. The VSOP has developed teaching materials (written and video) for high school students. Recently, a series of lessons on genetics and disease was televised nationally. Nevertheless, the uptake of this information is fragmentary, and genetic illiteracy is widespread, not only in the public at large but also in the medical profession.

In the Netherlands, everyone has his or her own general practitioner. These general practitioners are the gatekeepers to secondary facilities, including clinical genetics services. Unfortunately, many of them have limited knowledge about genetics, and when confronted with a patient who wants to have information, they tend to counsel in a directive manner and to value prevention more highly than informed decision making (6). Recommendations on developing standards and protocols, made by the Dutch Society of Clinical Genetics to the National Society of General Practitioners, have not been acted upon so far.

There are about 1.5 million immigrants in the Netherlands, many from countries bordering the Mediterranean Sea, but also from Indonesia, Surinam, and the Netherlands Antilles. The number of carriers of hemoglobinopathies is estimated at about 100,000 (7). Because marriages tend to be within ethnic groups, some of which also have a preference for intermarriage among relatives, the risk for autosomal recessive disorders in the offspring is increased. Despite this increased risk, people from ethnic minorities seem to make less use of clinical genetics services than does the rest of the population. Screening programs for sickle cell disease or for carriers of hemoglobinopathies have not been tried for fear of discrimination (7).

Genetics and Society

Although people in the medical profession and families with genetic disorders generally recognize the potential benefits of discoveries made by genetic research, the public at large often reacts to these discoveries with fear and disapproval. The media, many politicians, and some ethicists and sociologists are especially apt to overemphazise possibilities for misuse in the future.

One way of dealing with controversial issues is to organize a social debate. In the Netherlands, there is a special organization, the Rathenau Institute, founded by the Ministry of Education and Sciences, but scientifically independent, whose mission is to contribute to the social debate and the formation of political opinion on issues that are the result of, or are connected with, scientific or technological developments, including the ethical aspects of such developments (8). The first social debate organized by this institute was on predictive genetic research and took place in 1994 and 1995. At present, a debate on predictive medicine, to which genetic testing contributes substantially, is in preparation. The impact of these activities appears modest if judged only by the number of people actively involved and the amount of media coverage. However, the debates' influence on political opinion and therefore on political decisions could be substantial.

An example of a government action where debate might be useful is the Population Screening Act, which came into force in 1996. In this act, screening is defined as a direct or indirect offer of testing. The act describes three situations in which such an offer is forbidden unless one is licensed by the Ministry of Health: (*1*) screening for cancer, (*2*) screening by means of ionizing radiation, and (*3*) screening for severe diseases or abnormalities for which no treatment or prevention is possible (abortion, although legally permitted, is not regarded as prevention). A license for the third category can only be granted if this is warranted by exceptional circumstances. This extra condition of exceptional circumstances was introduced during parliamentary discussion by the Confessional party, which was strong and in power at that time, but has since lost many supporters.

Although the aim of the act (to protect people from potential psychological or physical risk) is praiseworthy and although a licensing system is an appropriate means of achieving such an aim, the act itself is a disaster. The main reason for this is that it uses terms like "offer," "severe," "treatment," and "exceptional," which are inexact and cause frequent problems in interpretation. An example of such an interpretation problem is the following: Offering genetic testing to family members of patients with genetic diseases (e.g., Duchenne muscular dystrophy) is regarded as the standard of care as these family members or their children run high risks, and may want to take appropriate measures to prevent harm. However, a strict interpretation of the Population Screening Act would regard this as an offer to screen for an untreatable disease, which is forbidden. The problem has been solved temporarily by differentiating between informing and offering testing to family members in the course of assisting an individual request for help at one side, and cascade screening at the other side.

Another problem arising from the Population Screening Act has already been indicated above. Maternal age has been regarded as a valid indication for prenatal cytogenetic diagnosis ever since the early 1970s, and over 13,000 pregnant women receive prenatal testing yearly. Still, clinical genetic centers had to apply for a licence for offering this testing recently. So far no definite licence has been granted, and the matter is being studied in a Health Council Committee.

Notwithstanding all the problems with the Population Screening Act, two good things surfaced. First, the discussion in Parliament made it painfully clear that decisions at this level are made by people who lack sufficient knowledge of the issues at stake. When asked whether screening for carriers of severe, incurable, autosomal recessive disorders was also subject to the prohibition of this law, the then-Minister of State answered that this clearly was the case as there is no treatment for carrier status. Second, to find out in which cases licensing would be justifiable, the Ministry of Health asked the Health Council of the Netherlands for a report on genetic screening (9). In response to this request, the Health Council instituted an ad hoc Genetic Screening Committee. The committee considered that "genetic screening should enable people to escape their fate by giving them the freedom to make an informed choice and adopt a chosen course of action which they regard as acceptable." By taking this position, the committee freed itself from the restrictive viewpoint of the legislature and formulated a set of criteria to be met by genetic screening programs (Table 16.4).

Table 16.4 Criteria to Be Met by Genetic Screening Programs*

1. A genetic screening program must relate to a health problem or to a condition that can lead to such a problem in those being tested or in their descendants.
2. The target group of the screening program must be clearly defined.
3. The purpose of the program must be to enable participants to determine the presence or the risk of a disorder or carrier status and to make a decision on the basis of that information.
4. Practical courses of action must be open to participants.
5. Participation in a genetic screening program should be completely voluntary and should be conditional on consent based on good information.
6. The target group should be supplied with good-quality, comprehensible information.
7. A test method suited to the objective of the screening should be available.
8. There should be sufficient facilities for follow-up testing, to carry out the selected courses of action, and to inform and support the participants.
9. The procedures used for the storage of medical information and cellular material must incorporate adequate measures to protect both the personal privacy of participants and their rights regarding their personal data and cellular material.
10. If scientific research is carried out within the framework of screening, participants should be properly informed about this in advance.
11. Provision should be made for continual quality assurance of the effectiveness, efficiency, and safety of the test procedure, any follow-up work, and any information and support given to participants.
12. When weighing the benefits and drawbacks for participants in the program, the final balance should be clearly biased toward benefits. To assist with this evaluation, those proposing a screening program must provide information about:

    a. the prevalence of the disease or disorder in the target group;
    b. the natural course of the disorder, and the variation in the disorder's severity;
    c. those target groups that are eligible for testing and the considerations that led to selection of the proposed target group and the proposed time of life for testing;
    d. the specificity, sensitivity, and predictive value of the test method to be used and the burden that such testing imposes on participants;
    e. the available courses of action if a health problem or carrier status is revealed;
    f. the time allowed by the procedure for consideration and possible implementation of the option chosen;
    g. the potential psychological, social, and other repercussions (both positive and negative) of an offer and of participation or nonparticipation in the screening, both for those to be tested and members of their family and for groups within the community;
    h. the likelihood of erroneous results, the possible consequences of this for participants, and the measures taken to limit any harm that such errors might cause;
    i. guarantees to prevent participants from experiencing unjustified impediments (as a result of their participation or nonparticipation in the screening program or follow-up testing) in obtaining employment or private insurance coverage; and
    j. the costs associated with the screening and with establishing the requisite infrastructure.

*As reported in reference 9.

As shown in Table 16.4, one of the criteria to be met by genetic screening programs (12i) deals with insurance coverage. According to the Medical Examination Act (1997) life-insurance companies are not allowed to ask questions about genetic disorders that are not already manifest in the applicant, nor about testing performed for such disorders or about a family history of genetic disorders unless the amount insured exceeds about US$150,000. Below this amount, insurance companies are not allowed to order tests for these diseases either. The same rules apply to disability insurance if the amount insured stays below 70% of the applicant's income. Similarly, medical examination in connection with a job application is subject to strict rules.

Hope and Encouragement

The work of the Genetic Screening Committee of the Health Council of the Netherlands made it clear that genetics and public health are not incompatible provided that ethical standards such as respecting patient autonomy, providing benefit and no harm, and ensuring justice are followed. At the same time, societal fears about and disapproval of genetics have not disappeared and, in the end, may jeopardize, through political pressure, the delivery of clinical genetic services. Claiming the existence of a seperate field, termed *community genetics*, serves three important purposes.

First, it draws attention to an area where much research is needed, both to find out which proposed new activities are worthwhile and to evaluate those that have already been started.

Second, by fostering strict adherence to ethical principles, it helps to reconcile genetics with societal values. Third, it frees those in clinical genetics services from the conflicts arising from the different aims of clinical and community genetics.

In 1995 a small group of people in the Netherlands decided to form the Community Genetics Initiative Group, with the aim of putting "community genetics on the agenda." The group consisted of three clinical geneticists, one epidemiologist, and two biologists with expertise in genetic education of high school students and college undergraduates. The group currently also includes two general practitioners and a health scientist. The organization's first activity was to form an invitational workshop on community genetics in 1996 (10). Participants were from departments of general practice, clinical genetics, and social medicine; research organizations; patient organizations; and government. The workshop was opened on behalf of the Minister of Health, and the presentations included contributions by an ethicist and a representative of the patient organization, as well as lectures by individuals involved in community genetic activities.

Because of the success of the invitational workshop, scientific meetings, lasting 4 to 6 hours, were organized in 1997, 1998 and 1999. Calls for papers resulted in numerous submissions dealing with screening, psychosocial aspects of genetic testing, genetic education, genetics and primary care, and registration and epidemiologic subjects. Lobbying by one of the members of the original group contributed to the appearance of a new international scientific journal, *Community Genetics*. Invitations to give talks on community genetics are received by members of the group from interested parties, both nationally and internationally. Workshops on Community Genetics were included in the 1999 and 2000 annual meeting of the European Society of Human Genetics and in other international and national meetings.

Why dwell upon our own successes so extensively? Because the Dutch experience might be a model for other countries. And if we can be of any help, we will be glad to do so. The future will show whether our efforts resulted in a permanent place for community genetics or whether they were only a way of whistling to keep our spirits up. But isn't that important as well?

References

1. Ten Kate LP. Editorial. Community Genet 1998;1:1–2.

2. Modell B, Kuliev A. The history of community genetics: the contribution of the haemoglobin disorders. Community Genet 1998;1:3–11.

3. Harris R, Reid M. Medical genetic services in 31 countries: an overview. Eur J Hum Genet 1997;5(Suppl 2):3–21.

4. Ten Kate LP. Genetic services in the Netherlands. Eur J Hum Genet 1997; 5(Suppl 2):125–129.

5. Harris R. Preface: three principles. Eur J Hum Genet 1997;5(Suppl 2):1–2.

6. De Smit D. Information about congenital disorders: an attempt to improve its quality in primary care. Thesis Amsterdam, Vrije Universiteit, 1997.

7. Giordano PC. Hemoglobinopathies in the Netherlands: diagnosis, epidemiology and prevention [partly in Dutch]. Thesis Leiden 1998.

8. The Rathenau Institute and the debate. Annual report 1994.

9. Health Council of the Netherlands: Committee on Genetic Screening. Genetic screening. The Hague: Health Council, 1994; publication no. 1994/22E.

10. Ten Kate LP, Beemer FA, Broertjes JJS (eds). Community genetics: utility and necessity [in Dutch]. Vakgroep Didactiek van de Biologie, Universiteit Utrecht, 1997.

17

Delivery of genetic services in developing countries

Victor B. Penchaszadeh

Close to 80% of the world's population live in countries that have not yet reached the levels of industrialization of developed nations, and they are variously referred to as "third world," "underdeveloped," "less developed," and "developing." Although the latter term was adopted in this chapter, it should be noted that nothing in the economic indices of these countries suggest that they are actually "developing." Developing nations are characterized by low per capita gross national product (GNP), economic dependency, low urbanization, poor technological development, lack of qualified human resources, and a number of other social, demographic, cultural, and health correlates of underdevelopment. However, the division between "developed" and "developing" countries is not always clear-cut, and there are wide differences in economic and social development among developing countries, as well as between population groups within each developing country. Furthermore, significant pockets of underdevelopment and poverty also exist in developed nations. Thus, generalizations about the "developing world" based on statistical averages fail to capture the wide range of realities that are part of underdevelopment.

The control of infectious and nutritional diseases in the developed world and the advances in genetic technology in the last quarter of the 20th century have brought to the foreground the health problems associated with genetic factors. Developing countries, in contrast, still face many environmentally caused diseases correlated with poverty, infections, and malnutrition, and attention to genetic disorders has lagged. An epidemiological transition, however, is occurring in some of these countries, with chronic and congenital conditions steadily increasing their impact on health, and both the prevention and the care of genetic disorders are becoming a public health concern. In this chapter the priorities and organization of genetic services in the developing world are discussed against the background of the realities of underdevelopment.

Economic and Demographic Realities of Underdevelopment

Ninety percent of the 140 million babies born in 1995 were in developing countries (1). Table 17.1 shows some key economic and demographic characteristics of developing nations, grouped in several geographic regions and compared with developed nations. The per capita GNPs of developing nations are 10 to 40 times lower than those of developed countries, and the gap between rich and poor nations is widening. Over the past 30 years the developed countries' share of the world's global GNP increased from 70.2% to 82.7%, whereas that of the countries with the poorest 20% of the world's population declined from 2.3% to 1.4% (1). In addition, developing countries are characterized by an increased concentration of wealth in a smaller proportion of the population than what prevails in developed countries (2).

Only 37% of the population in developing countries is urbanized, as compared with 77% in developed nations, although urbanization is occurring very fast and some of the largest cities of the world are in developing countries (Mexico City, Sao Paulo, Beijing). Access to safe water and adequate sanitation in developing countries is clearly deficient. Although the average number of children per woman (total fertility rate) in developing countries declined from 6.0 in 1960 to 3.2 in 1996, it is still almost twice that in developed nations, where it is 1.7. The combination of high fertility and low life expectancy in developing countries leads to a high proportion of young people (40% of the population is under 18 years of age, as compared with 23% in developed nations) (3). Educational levels in developing countries tend to be low, particularly in women.

Health Conditions and Delivery of Health Care

The populations of developing countries are subjected to heavier burdens of disease than those of developed countries. The larger impact of environmental factors on disease patterns in the developing world is reflected in the distribution of causes of death (Table 17.2).

Although mortality under 5 years of age in developing countries has declined significantly in the last 25 years, its average is still several times higher than in developed nations (Table 17.3). Infant mortality rates vary widely among developing countries, ranging from a low of 9 per thousand in Cuba to

Table 17.1 Selected Demographic Indicators by World Regions

	Total population (thousands) 1995	Percentage of population urbanized 1996	GNP per capita (US$) 1995	Life expectancy (years) 1970	1996	Total fertility rate 1960	1996	Percentage of population with access to safe water 1990–1996	Percentage of population with access to adequate sanitation 1990–1996	Total adult literacy rate (per 1000) 1995	Percentage of primary school children reaching grade 5 1990–1995
Developed countries	838,679	78	25,926	72	77	2.8	1.7	—	—	98	99
All developing countries	4,577,675	38	1,101	53	62	6.0	3.2	70	42	71	75
Sub-Saharan Africa	576,069	32	501	44	51	6.6	5.9	49	44	57	67
Middle East and North Africa	318,201	56	1,710	52	65	7.1	4.5	81	72	59	91
South Asia	1,267,705	27	345	48	61	6.1	3.5	80	33	49	59
East Asia and Pacific	1,797,840	33	1,043	58	68	5.8	2.1	67	35	84	90
Latin America and Caribbean	479,139	74	3,271	60	69	6.0	2.8	77	71	87	74

Source: UNICEF, *The State of the World's Children, 1998.*

Table 17.2 Causes of Death in the Developed and Developing World, 1996

| | Developed World | | Developing world | |
	Percentage	Number of deaths in thousands	Percentage	Number of deaths in thousands
Infectious and parasitic diseases	1.2	151	43	17,161
Cardiovascular diseases	45.6	5,522	24.5	9,778
Cancers	21.0	2,544	9.5	3,802
Respiratory diseases	8.1	979	4.8	1,909
Perinatal and neonatal causes	1.0	119	9.1	3,626
Maternal causes	0	3	1.5	582
Other and unknown causes	23.1	2,798	7.7	3,063

Source: World Health Organization, *World Health Report 1997*.

a high of 171 per thousand in Niger, compared to under 10 per thousand in developed nations (3). Approximately 70% of the 11.6 million deaths of children under 5 years of age that occur annually in developing countries are attributable to five illness groups: acute respiratory infections (19%), diarrhea (19%), perinatal causes (18%), measles (7%), and malaria (5%); malnutrition is an associated cause in 54% of those deaths (4). Forty-two percent of deaths at all ages in developing countries are largely avoidable, whereas only 6% of deaths in industrialized countries are avoidable (4). Adding to this toll, the AIDS pandemic is currently ravaging many developing countries, diverting scarce health resources (5).

In the area of reproductive health, maternal mortality is alarmingly high, reaching apocalyptic figures in Africa, with an average of 477 per 100,000, compared with 13 per 100,000 in the industrialized world (6). Obstructed labor, hemorrhage, and postpartum infection account for almost one-half of maternal mortality. Lack of access to adequate prenatal care, to fertility regulation, and to safe abortion are main contributors to maternal morbidity and mortality. Contraceptive prevalence between 1990 and 1997 was only 54% in developing countries, compared with 72% in the industrialized world (3). The legal restrictions to induced abortion that exist in some developing countries do not deter women from having abortions, but make the procedure unsafe and responsible for a large proportion of maternal morbidity and mortality. Half of the 45 million induced abortions that occur worldwide annually are unsafe; 90% of these unsafe abortions take place in developing countries and account for 13% of maternal deaths (6). In Latin America, the annual rate of unsafe abortions is 41 per 1000 women (compared with only 2 per 1000 in Europe), and 20% of them lead to complications and subsequent hospitalization. (7)

Health expenditures in the developing world are inappropriately low,

Table 17.3 Selected Health Indicators by World Regions

	Under-age 5 mortality rate (per 1000)		Percentage of infants with low birthweight 1990–1994	Percentage of children under age 5 moderately or severely underweight 1990–1997	Contraceptive prevalence (%) 1990–1997	Percentage of births attended by trained health personnel 1990–1996	Maternal mortality rate (per 100,000) 1990	Percentage of central government expenditures allocated to health and defense (1990–1996)	
	1960	1996						Health	Defense
Developed countries	37	7	6	—	72	99	13	12	9
All developing countries	216	97	18	30	54	53	470	4	12
Sub-Saharan Africa	257	170	16	30	15	37	980	5	10
Middle East and North Africa	241	65	11	17	46	62	320	6	21
South Asia	239	119	33	51	38	29	610	2	16
East Asia and Pacific	201	54	11	20	74	75	210	2	14
Latin America and Caribbean	157	43	10	10	64	78	190	5	5

Source: UNICEF, The State of the World's Children, 1998.

Table 17.4 Global Health Expenditures, 1990

Countries and groups of countries	Percentage of world population	Total health expenditure (billions of dollars)	Percentage of GNP spent on health	Per capita health expenditure (dollars)
Industrialized countries	15	483	9.2	1860
Former socialist countries of Europe	7	49	3.6	142
Developing countries	78	170	4.7	41
Latin American and Caribbean countries	8	47	4.0	105
Eastern Mediterranean countries	10	39	4.1	77
India	16	18	6.0	21
China	22	13	3.5	11
Other Asian countries and islands	13	42	4.5	61
Sub-Saharan African countries	10	12	4.5	24
World	100	1702	8.0	329

Source: Word Bank, World Development Report, 1993.

averaging only 4% of the GNP in 1990, compared with 9.2% of the GNP in developed countries (1) (Table 17.4). Comparison of absolute figures is even more impressive, as the GNPs of developing countries are several times lower than GNPs of developed countries (Table 17.1): The total average annual per capita health expenditure in 1990 was US$41 in developing countries, compared with US$1861 in the developed world (1). The actual money available for health for most people in developing countries is even lower, as only half of the total amount spent comes from the public sector. Thus, the averages mask spending inequalities between the well-to-do, who pay high fees in the private sector, and the majority, who rely on the underfunded public sector (1).

Health services in the developing world have substantial structural and functional deficiencies with complex historical, political, cultural, and economic roots (1). Deficient comprehensive health planning and implementation, overlapping functions, and poor coordination compound underfunding. Furthermore, health resources are unequally distributed, with a disproportionate amount going for excessive specialization and high technology in tertiary centers in large cities, at the expense of more cost-effective primary-care services. Those expensive specialized services typically cater to a small, wealthy segment of the population, who enjoy services equivalent to those of people in developed countries. Training of health professionals tends to emphasize individual curative medicine rather than community-based preventive approaches (1).

Frequency of Birth Defects and Genetic Diseases in the Developing World

The prevalence of birth defects and genetic disorders in the developing world is underestimated by a lack of diagnostic capacity and the unreliability of health records and statistics. In addition, recorded diagnoses tend to reflect obviously apparent acute illnesses, rather than basic constitutional conditions that increase vulnerability to infections and malnutrition, leading to an even greater underestimation of congenital conditions (8). In fact, as described below, the global prevalence of birth defects and genetic diseases in the developing world is similar to that in developed countries, albeit with regional variations in frequencies of some conditions.

Congenital Malformations
Congenital malformation registries in Mexico (9), Costa Rica (10), Cuba (11), South America (12), South Africa (13,14) and China (15) show that the prevalence of recognizable malformations among newborns is 2% to 3%. This frequency is similar to that found in the industrialized world (16,17). In the eastern Mediterranean region, limited surveys have shown wide variation in the rates of congenital malformations (18). In any case, detected rates in developing countries must be considered minimum estimates because of these countries' low diagnostic capacities and underreporting. This in turn makes it difficult to compare rates between regions or to determine possible causal factors. Some geographical variations in rates of specific malformations, however, seem to represent true differences. Neural tube defects, for example, are particularly prevalent in China (19), Mexico (9), and Central America (10), probably because of a combination of external factors, such as nutritional deficiencies and exposure to environmental pollutants. Both cleft lip and cleft palate are relatively common among American Indian and Asian populations (15,16), while microtia is frequent in the highlands of Ecuador, South America (20).

Chromosome Abnormalities
Because of sociocultural traditions and limited access to family planning, many women in developing countries continue to reproduce until advanced age. The percentage of births to women over 35 years old averages 11% to 15% in different regions of the developing world, compared with 9% in industrial countries (6). Maternal age-specific rates of Down syndrome in developing countries are similar to those reported in developed countries (8,12–14,21,22). Because of inadequate cytogenetic diagnostic services, there is limited observational data on the frequency of other chromosomal disorders. Nevertheless, some data suggest that the birth prevalence of chromosome disorders is higher in developing than in developed nations, and may reach 3 per 1000 for Down

syndrome and about 6 per 1000 for all chromosome abnormalities (23). These figures are consistent with the higher proportion of births to women of advanced age and the limited access to prenatal diagnosis and selective pregnancy termination.

Consanguinity, Founder Effects, and Genetic Diseases

Marriage between relatives has been practiced customarily for centuries in many populations around the world, where it is deeply rooted in a web of social, economic, and cultural factors. Although the practice has declined in industrial nations, it continues to be very prevalent in numerous areas of the developing world, particularly in parts of Africa, the eastern Mediterranean region, and in southern India, where consanguineous marriages range from 25% to 60% (24–28). To a lesser extent, consanguineous marriages are also common in Brazil (29) (0.6%–9%) and Japan (30) (1.6%–3.9%). Marriage between relatives increases the likelihood of homozygosity among the offspring and is associated with higher risks for stillbirth, neonatal or childhood death, serious congenital abnormality, or some degree of mental retardation (23), and a higher frequency of autosomal recessive conditions and congenital malformations (25,26). Thus, high incidence of consanguineous marriages may contribute to the burden of genetic diseases in some communities in the developing world, particularly in those that are experiencing a significant reduction in infant mortality rates. However, in some communities consanguineous marriages are a traditional custom and an important factor in the social and cultural fabric, contributing to economic and family stability. Hence, efforts to discourage them on genetic grounds seem inappropriate and could even be counterproductive (31).

In a number of regions, particularly in the New World, many populations were originated by a small number of original people (founders), who experienced restricted mobility for many generations. This combination of founder effects and geographic isolation has led to clusters of single-gene conditions, both recessive and dominant (32–39) (Table 17.5). Some of these clusters may represent significant public health burdens, as the needs of hundreds of patients with severe disabling conditions in a small area may impinge upon an already strained health sector, as is the case with spino-cerebellar atrophy in Cuba (37), Huntington's disease in Venezuela (39), and albinism in South Africa (40).

Hemoglobinopathies as a Public Health Problem

The hemoglobinopathies (sickle-cell diseases and thalassemias) constitute the major public health problem posed by genetic conditions worldwide, particularly in the developing world. The beta-S mutation occurred independently on at least four different occasions: three in Africa and one in the Indian subcontinent and Arabia (41). Numerous alpha- and beta-thalassemia mutations

Table 17.5 Some Single-Gene Clusters in Latin America

Locality	Country	Disease	Reference
Aicuna	Argentina	Oculocutaneous albinism	32
San Luis del Palmar	Argentina	Chondro-ectodermal dysplasia	32
Cordoba	Argentina	Gm-1 gangliosidosis	33
Bahia	Brazil	Achondrogenesis II	34
South	Brazil	Acheiropodia	35
Cartago	Costa Rica	Low-tone progressive deafness	36
Holguin	Cuba	Spino-cerebellar atrophy type II	37
Irapa	Venezuela	Spondylo-epiphyseal dysplasia	38
Maracaibo Lake	Venezuela	Huntington's disease	39

originated independently in Africa, Asia, and the Mediterranean basin (42). The abnormal hemoglobin genes were maintained at high frequencies in those populations because they gave carriers a selective advantage in resistance to malaria. The slave trade and later migrations disseminated those mutated genes worldwide. Slightly over 200 million people (about 4% of the world population) carry a potentially pathological hemoglobinopathy mutation, and 250,000 children are born every year with a major hemoglobinopathy, 75% of which are sickling disorders. Ninety-five percent of carriers and affected individuals live in the developing world (21).

In Africa, the average carrier frequency of abnormal hemoglobins (mostly sickling) is 13.3%, with wide regional variations that reach 23.3% in sub-Saharan Africa (8). The estimated birth prevalence of homozygotes for major hemoglobinopathies is 9.2 per 1000, which extrapolates to 162,000 affected children born annually (21,43). In Latin America, abnormal hemoglobins are more frequent in countries with a high proportion of African descent (the Caribbean, Panama, northern Brazil and Guyana, and to a lesser extent Venezuela, Colombia, and Ecuador). In these countries, sickling hemoglobins are more common than thalassemias (44–47). In the Middle East, the most common abnormal hemoglobin is also hemoglobin S, with carrier frequencies ranging from <1% to almost 20% in some areas (18,48). Alpha- and beta-thalassemia genes are also frequent, with carrier frequencies ranging from 1% to 10% (18,48). In Iran, Pakistan, and India, the major type of hemoglobinopathy is beta-thalassemia, with carrier frequencies of 3% to 5% (43). In Southeast Asia and southwestern China, thalassemias are very common, with an average carrier frequency of 11.6% (21,49,50).

Other Single-Gene Disorders
Major single-gene defects in the developing world have a global incidence similar to that in industrialized countries: approximately 3.5 per 1000 births (8). The frequency of individual conditions varies in different regions

according to ethnicity, founder effects, carrier selection, inbreeding, and genetic drift. Thus, some mendelian conditions are particularly frequent in some populations, such as spondylocostal dysplasia among Puerto Ricans (51) and spinal muscular atrophy among Arabs (52). In contrast, other recessive conditions of relatively high prevalence among northern Europeans, like phenylketonuria (PKU) and cystic fibrosis, are less frequent in developing countries.

Multifactorial Conditions

Multifactorial conditions, caused by interactions between genetic predispositions and environmental factors, include most congenital malformations and chronic conditions of children and adults (e.g., diabetes, cancer, obesity, mental illness, and coronary disease). As described previously, the frequency of congenital malformations in developing countries is similar to or higher than that in industrialized nations, most likely because of a combination of exogenous factors such as poor nutrition, prenatal infections, exposure to teratogens, and deficient prenatal care. The prevalence of common multifactorial conditions among adults and children increases as childhood mortality by infections and malnutrition declines and life expectancy rises. Significant proportions of the population in many developing countries are affected by these conditions. Mortality statistics comparing the developed and developing worlds show that although the burden of infections and parasitic diseases is still enormous, cardiovascular conditions and malignancies are also significant (Table 17.2). Morbidity data on other chronic conditions also indicate the growing importance of multifactorial conditions in the developing world.

Epidemiological Transition and the Impact of Genetic Diseases on the Public's Health

The increased prevalence of infections and malnutrition, and the deficiency of resources to address health problems and disabilities, render populations of the developing world more vulnerable to the consequences of birth defects and genetic conditions. Hence, the burden of genetic disorders is actually greater than in developed nations. For example, hemoglobinopathies have tremendous economic, social, and human impact in the developing world (53). Less detailed documentation exists on the toll of human suffering caused by other genetic conditions and birth defects in developing countries, owing to lack of awareness, absence of registries, unreliable statistics, and deficient diagnoses. However, increasing indications show a growing number of people in the developing world experiencing improved living and health conditions, and that the relative impact of congenital disorders and chronic noncommunicable diseases is increasing. Thus, between 1960 and 1996, the average infant mortality rate in developing countries fell from 137 per 1000 to 66 per 1000 livebirths, a more than 50% reduction (3). The reduction has been even greater in Latin America (from 105 to 35 per 1000 livebirths) and in the Middle East (from 154 to 50). Twelve of 22 Latin American countries have infant mortality rates under 30 per 1000 and 3 have rates below 15 per 1000 livebirths (3). In the Middle East and Asia, most countries have infant mortality rates under 50 and several have reduced it to under 30 per 1000 livebirths. In the same period, life expectancy increased by approximately 10 years in most countries (average: from 53 to 62 years; Table 17.1).

The reduction in infant mortality rates denotes a general improvement in most health indicators, as infections and malnutrition are brought under control. This phenomenon is determining an *epidemiological transition*, with birth defects and genetic diseases accounting for an increasing share of morbidity and mortality. Common chronic conditions associated with genetic predispositions, such as diabetes, cancer, coronary disease, and mental illness, are increasing their impact on health. Additional factors contributing to this epidemiological transition are changes in lifestyles, with old traditions giving way to modernization, new dietary habits, increased stress, and urbanization. In Latin America, for example, mortality from cardiovascular diseases and cancer is approaching the rates of developed countries: In 1990 the percentage of deaths from cardiovascular diseases in Latin American countries ranged from 20% up to 46% (compared with 54% in the United States) and the percentage from malignancies ranged from 8% to 25% (compared with 23% in the United States) (54). Similarly, in most Latin American nations, congenital anomalies have risen to the 3rd or 4th place as a cause of infant mortality (54), while birth defects and genetic conditions account for 10% to 25% of pediatric admissions in large cities (55–57). The fact that these disorders require longer hospital stays (56,57) and expensive resources for their care adds to the challenges faced by developing countries in this area.

Delivery of Genetic Services in Developing Countries

Goals and Strategies of Genetic Services

The goals of genetic services everywhere are the prevention, management, and treatment of birth defects and conditions in which genetic factors play a causal role. Various strategies have been developed over the past two decades to achieve those goals, most of which focus on prevention and reproductive options, as therapy for genetic diseases is expensive and not yet very effective (23).

Among the strategies in place are some preventive public health measures directed at subsets of the general population. Preconceptional measures for the primary prevention of birth defects and genetic diseases include rubella immunization, avoidance of exposure to teratogens, folic acid dietary supplementation, and detection of genetic risks by family history and/or carrier detection, followed by genetic counseling. Most commonly, however, detection of genetic risks occurs postconceptionally, and prevention is based in genetic counseling for reproductive options, including voluntary prenatal diagnosis and interruption of affected pregnancies.

Worldwide experience, both in developed and developing countries, indicates that most people, albeit not all, use genetic services to avoid the birth of an affected infant (23). The target population for genetic services may be the entire community (e.g., heterozygote detection of carrier status for a prevalent recessive condition like thalassemia), the prenatal population (e.g., maternal serum screening or fetal ultrasound for Down syndrome risk), or special groups identified by the presence of a particular risk factor (maternal age, family history, exposure to a teratogen, and others). Newborn screening for serious diseases amenable to early and cost-efficient treatment is a prime example of secondary prevention. Services for the care, management, and psychosocial support of patients with genetic diseases and their families are typical secondary and tertiary prevention components of genetic services. More recently, as predisposing genetic factors to common multifactorial disorders are being recognized, programs are implemented to identify those factors in the population. Preventive measures and treatment for conditions such as diabetes, obesity, coronary disease, and some cancers follow the detection of risk factors (23).

Making genetic counseling part of preventive services helps to educate patients about their risks and to make informed decisions, regardless of the type of genetic intervention (diagnostic, predictive, or therapeutic) being considered. Education of the public, of health professionals, and of health authorities about genetic risks and their prevention is another critical component of genetic services.

General Situation of Genetic Services in Developing Countries

In most countries of the world, genetic services are at an early stage of development or may be nonexistent. In developed countries, where both the organization and funding of health services in general are generally adequate, there are still numerous technical, social, ethical, and legal hurdles for the prevention and control of genetic disorders (23). In developing countries, genetic services encounter even more serious challenges, because (a) there remain many unmet needs in other areas of health (such as infections, malnutrition, prenatal care, labor and delivery care, and newborn care); (b) genetic conditions are generally not considered priorities by members of the medical profession or public health officials; (c) genetic services are misperceived as expensive and dealing only with rare diseases; (d) because genetic services are more diagnostic than therapeutic, their preventive value may be perceived as associated with the interruption of affected pregnancies, which is opposed by some traditional sectors of society; and (e) the public is largely unaware of the genetic risks and the possibilities of prevention.

Despite these difficulties, genetic services have been implemented in developing countries starting in the 1970s and 1980s, following similar patterns. These services, initiated by medical geneticists trained in developed countries, have been centered in teaching hospitals in major urban areas, initially as part of research projects and without coordination with related health services. The emphasis has typically been on clinical genetics, dysmorphology, cytogenetics, and prenatal diagnosis of chromosome anomalies (58). In some countries with a high prevalence of hemoglobinopathies, genetic services actually grew out of the programs for the control and management of hereditary anemias (53), as in Cyprus (59,60), Saudi Arabia (61), and Nigeria (62,63). Biochemical genetics laboratories for the diagnosis of inborn errors of metabolism, conversely, are scarce (64,65). A DNA-based diagnosis is only available in a few centers and for a small number of conditions. Referral systems for the study of patients are largely informal (64,65).

As in developed countries (66), prenatal diagnosis in the developing world, is also considered the most practical current application of genetic services, particularly where induced abortion is legal. This is the case in China, Southeast Asian countries, India, South Africa, Cuba, and Cyprus, where government-funded prenatal diagnosis is provided. In addition, in an increasing number of countries, although induced abortion is technically illegal, prenatal diagnosis of fetal abnormalities is an accepted service, and voluntary interruption of affected pregnancies takes place without much government interference. The public's acceptance of this service is directly correlated with educational and economic level, irrespective of religious affiliations. In countries where the public sector does not fund these services, the growing demand for prenatal diagnosis is channeled to the private sector, creating economic barriers to access. These private services, unfortunately, tend to be fragmented, without rational medical indications, with only perfunctory genetic counseling, and no quality control.

With few exceptions, departments of health at city, provincial, and national levels do not have explicit policies for the prevention and management of genetic diseases. Thus, population-based prevention programs are rare. Newborn screening programs for phenylketonuria and congenital hypothyroidism are somewhat developed in Latin America, covering 20% to 30% of births in a few major cities of the region (65). These programs, however, tend to lack the financial resources and organization necessary for the proper follow-up of abnormal initial screening results and the long-term treatment of affected infants. Furthermore, newborn screening laboratory services are usually contracted to private for-profit laboratories without proper quality control or oversight from the state.

A significant deficiency in most of the developing world is the lack of education of health professionals in genetics. Most medical schools in developing countries do not have formal courses in clinical genetics, and physicians at large have a poor grasp of the modern applications of genetics in medical practice.

Despite the obstacles and difficulties noted above, there has recently been a significant increase in the awareness of health officials, medical professionals, and the public at large of the relevance of genetic factors in health. This awareness is translated into an improvement in delivery of some genetic services in the developing world, albeit with wide variations among countries and regions. In Latin America, for example, clinicians and scientists who received medical genetics training abroad eventually developed successful local postgraduate training programs in medical genetics in their countries, and there are currently approximately 500 trained clinical geneticists in the region, largely in major cities (65). These specialists provide an array of genetic services, including genetic counseling, as there are no genetic counselors specifically trained as such. The specialty of medical genetics has been recognized in Mexico, Cuba, Brazil, and Argentina. There are centers of excellence in clinical genetics, cytogenetics, prenatal diagnosis, and in the management of hemoglobinopathies. Molecular diagnosis is slowly developing for a limited number of conditions (64,65).

Over the past 15 years, several meetings of experts in medical genetics from developing countries were convened by the World Health Organization (WHO). A number of recommendations have resulted (18,65,67–71). It is apparent that the differences in goals and strategies for genetic services between the developed and the developing world have more to do with epidemiology, economics, and education than with differences in culture, traditions, and/or religion. Epidemiologic realities determine the priorities of health services (i.e., balance between communicable versus noncommunicable diseases; or between primary vs. tertiary care). In turn, the economy dictates the availability of funds and their allocation, while the education of health professionals and the general public influences promotion and acceptance of different prevention programs.

Selected Examples

Some of the points raised above, and the similarities and differences in approaches to genetic services, are illustrated in the following discussion on selected developing countries.

Genetic Services in Cuba

Health services in Cuba are centrally planned and financed by the state according to national goals, with wide coverage and access free of charge (11).

Health indices are similar to developed nations, with an infant mortality rate of 9 per 1000 and congenital anomalies the second cause of death in that age group (54). Sickle cell disease is a prevalent problem, as 3.7% of the population carries the S mutation (44). In the early 1980s, the National Center of Medical Genetics was created and staffed with medical geneticists trained abroad (11). This core staff, in turn, trained several teams of one pediatrician and one obstetrician for the major hospitals in every Cuban province, where genetic services were established. Prenatal prevention programs addressed mainly sickle cell disease, congenital malformations, and chromosome abnormalities. In the ensuing years, those functions were progressively assumed by trained clinical geneticists (now numbering approximately 100). Genetic services have expanded to include newborn screening for PKU and congenital hypothyroidism, clinical genetics and cytogenetic services in pediatric hospitals, and linkages with other specialties (11).

Sickle cell prevention is based on hemoglobin electrophoresis of pregnant women at 16 weeks of gestation, identification of carrier couples, genetic counseling, and the offer of amniocentesis with the option of voluntary termination of affected pregnancies. A single laboratory in Havana performs all the fetal DNA tests for the S mutation. This program covers close to 90% of the pregnancies in Cuba, and it enjoys high public acceptance (44,72,73).

Prevention of chromosome anomalies is based on the offer of prenatal diagnosis to women over 38 years of age, while prevention of congenital anomalies is based on maternal serum–alpha-fetoprotein analysis (MS-AFP) at 16 weeks of gestation and a routine ultrasound examination at 20 weeks. The MS-AFP assay technology used in Cuba was developed locally at very low cost, and the program covers 95% of all pregnancies (11,64). When fetal chromosome abnormalities or severe malformations are detected, couples are counseled and given the option of pregnancy termination. Between 1982 and 1993, a total of 328,983 pregnancies (approximately 95% coverage) were screened by MS-AFP in the city of Havana (74). A total of 1371 malformed fetuses were detected by amniotic fluid AFP and/or ultrasound, two-thirds of which had neural tube defects (NTDs). In that 12-year period, the birth prevalence of NTDs in Havana fell 90% (74).

All components of the Cuban genetic program are regionalized, with family physicians as the first line of care at the primary level, and a referral network of regional genetic clinics is in place. Biochemical diagnosis of inborn errors of metabolism and molecular diagnosis of HbS, fragile X, and cystic fibrosis are centralized in Havana (11). Currently, all provinces in Cuba have genetic clinics staffed by clinical geneticists and, recently, nurses are being trained in genetic counseling (75).

The goals and methods of the Cuban genetic program have been well accepted by the Cuban population (73), and there has been a significant reduction in the birth prevalence of sickle cell anemia, neural tube defects, severe congenital heart defects, and other serious malformations (11,64). The Cuban approach to prevention and care of genetic disorders and birth defects is based on the identification of main epidemiologic priorities, taking advantage of preexistent health programs, proper regionalization, and development of appropriate technology. Reduction of infant mortality due to infections and malnutrition was a significant previous step, whereas the key factors in the program's success were a clear statement of goals and policies, high-level political support, and an adequate organization of existing resources.

Genetic Services in China

Although there are no detailed national data on genetic diseases or congenital malformations, a high birth prevalence of neural tube defects (NTDs) has been reported in some areas of China (19), while abnormal hemoglobins, mainly alpha- and beta-thalassemias and hemoglobin E, are known to be prevalent in the southern and southwestern provinces (42). A national survey in 1987 estimated that China had 52 million people with disabilities (4.9% of the population), two-thirds of which were due to postnatal diseases and injuries, while the remaining one-third were due to genetic conditions and birth defects (76).

Cytogenetic centers began organizing in the mid-1970s, and chorionic villi sampling was first developed in China in 1975. China has a few genetic professionals concentrated in a small number of facilities in the main cities. The emphasis of these services is on the diagnosis and management of hemoglobinopathies (68–70) and on prenatal diagnosis. Comprehensive clinical genetic services have small coverage, and an extremely wide gap exists between the need and the availability of such services, particularly in rural areas where 69% of the population resides (76–78). Newborn screening for PKU and congenital hypothyroidism has been piloted in only a few centers, with an annual coverage of fewer than 50,000 births; the frequency of PKU is 1 in 17,000 births, and that of congenital hypothyroidism is 1 in 7000 (79).

Fertility regulation is part of the national policy for the control of population growth, and family planning is a constitutional "duty" of couples. The policy of one child per family, however, is enforced with laxity, particularly in rural areas. Induced abortion is legally available and widely used for a variety of reasons, including fetal anomalies (80). As part of the national policy, a "Law on Maternal and Infant Health Care" was recently enacted (81), which includes plans for the prevention of birth defects and genetic diseases by preconceptional and prenatal counseling and diagnosis.

Responding to Western criticism that some provisions of this law were "eugenic" (82), Chinese geneticists argued that although the legislation was originally dubbed the "Eugenics Law," this term in the Chinese language does not have the connotations of racism and enforced interference with reproduction that some in the West attach to it. Rather, it is based in the concepts of "well bearing and well raising" ingrained in Confucian philosophy and is devoid of any racist connotations (76). Implementation of this law will require a huge educational program in genetics for primary physicians and the development of nationwide services for genetic counseling and diagnosis. This policy cannot be judged fairly outside the context of the distinct historical, cultural, health, and economic realities of modern China.

Genetic Services in India

The global prevalence of birth defects and genetic conditions in India is similar to that found in the developed world (83). Hereditary anemias in particular are a common problem, including beta-thalassemia, hemoglobin E, hemoglobin D, and sickle-cell anemia, with wide regional differences (84,85). The average prevalence of beta-thalassemia carriers is 3.3%, which means that 7000 homozygotes and 30 million carriers are born annually (21). In India, where most health care services are the responsibility of the government, clinical genetic services have not had a high priority. Nevertheless, in the late 1970s, clinical departments of university hospitals began providing some level of genetic services. In the early 1980s, the Indian Council of Medical Research moved to create medical centers of excellence and, as part of this policy, by 1985 several dozen genetic centers were established in different parts of India (86). These centers are engaged primarily in clinical genetics, cytogenetics, and prenatal diagnosis. Diagnostic biochemical genetics and molecular genetics laboratories are limited to a few centers. Only a small portion of the Indian population has access to genetic services. Prenatal diagnosis is well accepted by the public and the option of terminating an affected pregnancy is legal. However, its coverage is limited because of economic and educational barriers, with not more than 5% of the need being met (83). Despite these limitations, some well-equipped centers provide prenatal diagnosis of beta-thalassemia with appropriate cost-efficient technology (87). A misuse of prenatal diagnosis for fetal sexing unrelated to medical conditions has been reported, although this practice has been condemned by most geneticists and outlawed by the government (86). Newborn screening is not part of a systematic health policy.

Genetic Services in South Africa

South Africa's population of 34 million has a heterogenous ethnic distribution, with a majority of blacks (74%) of various ethnicities. Its rates of congenital malformations, chromosome abnormalities, and single-gene disorders are similar to those found in developed countries (13,14,88–91). A high frequency of oculo-cutaneous albinism has been reported in some regions (40); PKU is rare in the black population and less frequent among whites than it is in Europe, possibly as a result of the founder effect (88). In contrast, the birth incidence of galactosemia is 1 in 16,000 among blacks, five times higher than in European populations (92). Contrary to the rest of sub-Saharan Africa, the prevalence of hemoglobinopathies is very low (88).

Genetic services in South Africa began developing in the early 1970s following the pattern of individual clinical and laboratory-based services for diagnosis and counseling in academic tertiary centers (88). In 1975, a genetic subdirectorate was established in the Department of Health, which funded the training of a small number of "genetic nurses," although genetic services continued being part of research projects of academic centers and not accessible to the majority black population. There are no newborn screening programs in South Africa.

With the democratic reorganization of the country after the fall of apartheid, the Department of Health has set new priorities for the transformation of the health system, with an emphasis on primary-care and the extension of services to previously underserved black communities, particularly in rural areas (93). Genetic services have been recognized as appropriate components of maternal and child health care, and they are currently being reorganized and extended to primary-care levels, with the goal of increasing their accessibility. Detection of genetic risks at the primary-care level is implemented in some provinces by trained indigenous nurses, supervised by academic centers (94–96). A policy document on genetic services prepared by the Department of Health has listed as national priorities the prevention and management of Down syndrome, neural tube defects, albinism, and fetal alcohol syndrome (97).

Prenatal diagnosis is available in major academic centers, but black women are not fully using these services, possibly for economic reasons as well as lack of information (98). As is the case worldwide, these services typically attract the better-educated members of the middle and upper classes. In 1996, South Africa enacted a liberal abortion law, which may facilitate more extensive use of prenatal diagnosis in the prevention of genetic conditions and birth defects.

Genetic Services in Cyprus

Genetic services in Cyprus have grown out of the need for prevention and control of beta-thalassemia, as 16% of the population are carriers. A plan for prevention was laid out in 1972, with health education, community involvement, carrier detection in the general population, and genetic counseling (59). The program did not influence spouse selection nor reproduction patterns. The availability of prenatal diagnosis in the early 1980s did, however, affect reproduction decisions. Through the involvement of the Greek Cypriot Church, a premarital certificate attesting that the marrying couple had been tested for thalassemia and counseled appropriately became a requirement for marrying in church (there were no attempts to disuade carrier couples to marry, and no results were disclosed to third parties). A comprehensive prenatal diagnosis program followed (59). Over the ensuing years the annual birth incidence of thalassemia homozygotes dropped 97% as a result of campaigns of public education, community participation, genetic counseling, and voluntary prenatal diagnosis followed by the option of pregnancy termination (59,60). Factors contributing to this success include the facts that (a) thalassemia is a very severe condition with a costly and not very effective treatment; (b) Cyprus is a small country and Greek Cypriots enjoy good standards of living, education, and health; and (c) the program was based on public education and was developed with consideration for local cultural practices.

Discussion and Future Perspectives

Public health policies throughout the world for the past quarter century have emphasized the need of clearly defining program goals and extending primary health care to all segments of the population, while linking the primary care level with secondary and tertiary levels in a regionalized manner that makes the best possible use of existing resources (99). The application of that same strategy is key to the implementation of population-based preventive programs for birth defects and genetic diseases, and of patient/family-based genetic services.

To define goals for genetic services in developing nations, efforts must be made to improve knowledge of the impact of genetic disorders in the community. Epidemiological research should be stimulated to provide better data on the prevalence and types of birth defects, genetic diseases, and genetic predispositions to common diseases at the country level. Issues of population structure (i.e., consanguinity, founder effects, cultural and geographic isolation) must be studied to assess their influence on geographical clusters of genetic diseases. The health beliefs, traditions, and social expectations of communities should also be assessed properly before setting program goals.

In addition to being based on sound epidemiologic data, genetic services should always be comprehensive—that is, combining the best possible patient care available in the country with population-based prevention strategies such as public education, screening and control of genetic risks, and genetic counseling (23). Setting the goals of genetic services in the framework of the health and well-being of individuals and families, and not only in public health terms, will increase their acceptability by the public. The risk of a narrow public health approach is the confusion with eugenic goals, which should never be part of the objectives of genetic services.

A key ingredient for success of genetic programs in developing countries is that services extend their coverage into primary-care settings, which is where genetic risks should be identified. To avoid duplication of services and to be as cost-efficient as possible, genetic services must be regionalized, with tertiary centers responsible for specific geographic and/or administrative areas.

Programs at secondary and primary-care levels should be supervised by tertiary centers (58). The insertion of genetic services in the community is a key to the success of any genetic program, particularly in developing countries. This approach of *community genetics* was outlined by the World Health Organization (23) and has led to the formulation of strategies appropriate for the developing world (71).

Another condition for success is the integration of genetic services with general health services, such as family planning, prenatal care, child growth and development monitoring, nutrition, cancer prevention, and others. The health personnel in charge of these programs should also address the genetic components of prevention and care.

Serious efforts should be undertaken in genetic education. Many misconceptions about genetics abound in the developing world that affect the prevention and care of genetic conditions. Undergraduate curricula for the health professions should be updated, and the practical aspects of medical genetics should form part of the clinical teachings. The relationships between genetics and public health, largely neglected in most professional circles, should be addressed in the growing number of schools of public health of developing countries. For the already practicing health professionals, continuing education programs should be developed to familiarize them with the modern concepts of clinical genetics and their application to the prevention of genetic conditions and the care of individuals, families, and populations beset with genetic disorders. Officials in charge of public health programs should be targeted specifically for continuing education in genetics. Conversely, medical geneticists should be educated in public and community health, so that it is recognized that the impact of their services will be much greater when developed at the community-wide level.

It is evident that in developing countries there are insufficient numbers of health professionals and laboratory personnel with the proper training to provide genetic services. Rather than training additional specialized personnel, efforts should be directed toward training in genetics of health professionals such as physicians, nurses, psychologists, and social workers. Genetic counseling should become a tool that all health professionals can apply in practice with the proper supervision.

An important prerequisite for the expansion of programs for the prevention and care of birth defects and genetic diseases is the improvement in prenatal-delivery care and family planning. In addition, preventive actions should focus on specific conditions that are significantly impacting health because of their prevalence and severity, and the feasibility of their prevention. In this regard, the prevention of congenital rubella by immunization of susceptible children should be a priority. Educational and social programs to prevent alcohol consumption during pregnancy will help prevent fetal alcohol syndrome, which has a high prevalence in some populations. Neural tube defects can be partially prevented by the combination of preconceptional folic acid supplementation, maternal serum screening programs, and fetal ultrasound.

Another condition amenable to prevention is Down syndrome, through public education on the importance of maternal age, and family planning to encourage women to complete childbearing by age 35, and implementation of maternal serum antenatal screening. Women of advanced maternal age who become pregnant could be offered chromosome prenatal diagnosis (amniocentesis or chorionic villi sampling), according to availability of resources. These services require comprehensive educational programs, genetic counseling at the primary-care level, and regionalized fetal medicine and laboratory facilities. All programs should have standardized protocols for evaluating their effectiveness.

Newborn services must improve by increasing the proportion of babies born in institutions, and by ensuring that they have a complete physical examination to detect congenital malformations whose outcome can be improved with early intervention, such as congenital hip dysplasia, cleft palate, congenital heart defects, and others.

Some common severe inherited conditions, such as hemoglobin disorders, cystic fibrosis, fragile-X syndrome, hemophilia, and muscular dystrophies, contribute considerably to chronic morbidity in childhood in many developing countries. Prevention and care of affected children and their families in specialized centers may significantly reduce the overall burden due to chronic disease at the community level (53,69).

As was stated above, misconceptions in the population about goals and possibilities of genetic services are common in developing countries. The interest and acceptance of genetic services by the public is directly related to educational level and knowledge about the existence and purposes of services. Thus, it is essential that the public at large be educated about genetic factors in disease and the value of services in their prevention and care. Public education in genetics should be culturally sensitive and take into account the traditions and customs prevailing in society (100). Parent/patient organizations are key to convey the point of view of the patients in programs of prevention and care of genetic diseases. Although the strength and accomplishments of such voluntary groups are not as well known as in developed countries, their growing number and assertiveness will play a major role in shaping genetic services in developing countries.

Accepted international ethical guidelines of public health programs in genetics are as valid in developing as well as in developed countries (101). Major ethical issues in current medical genetic practice are inadequate services and inequitable access to existing services. Furthermore, public health genetic goals cannot override the cultural norms of society nor personal values, beliefs, and reproductive rights of individuals. Thus, preventive genetic services should always be voluntary, respecting autonomous decisions of patients and preceded by proper information in the form of nondirective genetic counseling. Extraordinary care must be taken to avoid stigmatization and discrimination of affected persons (101).

A recent WHO expert group of medical geneticists from developing countries recommended that governments give more priority to prevention and care of birth defects and genetic disorders (71). Emphasis was on primary prevention of selected conditions (congenital rubella, fetal alcohol, NTDs, Down syndrome, and mendelian disorders of high prevalence), and in the development of genetic services based in simple educational and screening actions at the community level, supported by regional networks of secondary and tertiary care level centers. The fate of genetics services in the developing world ultimately rests upon the wisdom and political will of statesmen, public health officials, and medical educators.

Finally, for the right to health care to be meaningful, it should include the prevention and care of genetically determined conditions. Genetic-health professionals in developing countries must act in conjunction with public health officials, other health professionals, parent/patient groups, and other community organizations to achieve an adequate allocation of resources for health care in general and genetic services in particular, making equity the highest priority.

References

1. World Bank. World development report, 1993. New York: Oxford University Press, 1993.

2. United Nations Development Programme. Human development report 1997. New York and Oxford: Oxford University Press, 1997.

3. UNICEF. The state of the world's children, 1998. Oxford and New York: Oxford University Press, 1998.

4. Murray C, Lopez A (eds). The global burden of disease. Cambridge, MA: Harvard School of Public Health, 1996, p. 176.

5. World Bank. Confronting AIDS. Public priorities in a global epidemic. New York: Oxford University Press, 1997.

6. United Nations Population Fund. The state of world population. New York: UNFPA, 1998.

7. The Allan Guttmacher Institute. Clandestine abortion: a Latin American reality. New York and Washington, DC: The Alan Guttmacher Institute, 1994.

8. WHO. Community approaches to the control of hereditary diseases. Report of a WHO Advisory Group on Hereditary Diseases. Geneva, 3–5 October 1985. Unpublished WHO document HMG/AG/85.10. Hereditary Diseases Programme. Geneva: WHO 1985.

9. Mutchinick O, Lisker R, Rabinsky V. The Mexican program of registration and epidemiologic surveillance of external congenital malformations (SPA). Salud Publica Mex 1988;30:88–100.

10. Saborio M. Experience in providing genetic services in Costa Rica. In: Kuliev A, Greendale K, Penchaszadeh VB, Paul, NW (eds). Genetic services provision: an international perspective. Birth Defects Orig Art Ser 1992;28:96–102. March of Dimes Birth Defects Foundation, White Plains, New York.

11. Heredero L. Comprehensive national genetic program in a developing country—Cuba. In: Kuliev A, Greendale K, Penchaszadeh VB, Paul NW (eds). Genetic services provision: an international perspective. Birth Defects Orig Art Ser 1992;28:52–57. March of Dimes Birth Defects Foundation, White Plains, New York.

12. Castilla EE, Lopez-Camelo JS. The surveillance of birth defects in South America: I. The Search for time clusters: Epidemics. Adv in Mutag 1990;2:191–210.

13. Delport SD, Christianson AL. Congenital anomalies in black South African liveborn neonates at an urban academic hospital. S Afr Med 1995;85:11–15.

14. Venter PA, Christianson AL, Hutamo CM, Makhura MP, Gericke GS. Congenital anomalies in rural black South African neonates—a silent epidemic? S Afr Med J 1995;85:15–20.

15. Xiao KZ, Lang ZC, Chen JH, Liu SL, et al. Consecutive three-year birth defects monitoring in Sichuan province. Heredity Dis 1988;5:65–68.

16. ICBDMS. Congenital malformations worldwide: a report from the international clearinghouse for birth defects monitoring systems. Amsterdam: Elsevier, 1991.

17. World atlas of birth defects. Geneva: International Centre for Birth Defects and World Health Organization, 1998.

18. Alwan AA, Modell B. Community control of genetic and congenital disorders. Technical Publications Series, No. 24. Alexandria WHO Regional Office for the Eastern Mediterranean, 1997.

19. Xiao KZ, Zhang ZY, Su YM, Liu FQ, et al. Central nervous system congenital malformations, especially neural tube defects in 29 provinces, metropolitan cities and autonomous regions of China: Chinese Birth Defects Monitoring Program. Int J Epidemiol 1990;19:978–982.

20. Castilla EE, Orioli IM. Prevalence rates of microtia in South America. Int J Epidemiol 1986;15:364–368.

21. Modell B, Bulyzhenkov V. Distribution and control of some genetic disorders. World Health Stat Q 1988;41(3/4):209–218.

22. Zhang SZ, Xie T, Tang YC, Zhang SL, Xu Y. The prevalence of chromosome diseases in the general population of Sichuan, China. Clin Genet 1991;39:81–88.

23. Report of a WHO Scientific Group. Control of hereditary diseases. Geneva: WHO Technical Report Series 865, 1996.

24. Khlat M. Endogamy in the Arab world. In: Teebi AS, Farag TI (eds). Genetic disorders among Arab populations. New York and Oxford: Oxford University Press, 1997, pp. 63–77.

25. Bittles AH, Mason WM, Greene, Rao NA. Reproductive behavior and health in consanguineous marriages. Science 1991;252:789–794.

26. Jaber L, Halpern GJ, Shohat M. The impact of consanguinity worldwide. Community Genet 1998;1:12–17.

27. Devi ARR, Rao NA, Bittles AH. Inbreeding and the incidence of childhood genetic disorders in Karnataka, South India. J Med Genet 1987;24:362–365.

28. Khlat M, Khoury M. Inbreeding and diseases: demographic, genetic and epidemiologic perspectives. Epidemiol Rev 1991;13:28–41.

29. Freire-Maia N. Genetic effects in Brazilian populations due to consanguineous marriages. Am J Med Genet 1989;35:115–117.

30. Imaizumi Y. A recent survey of consanguineous marriages in Japan. Clin Genet 1986;30:230–233.

31. Modell B, Kuliev AM. Social and genetic implications of customary consanguineous marriage among British Pakistanis. Report on a meeting held at the Ciba Foundation, January 15, 1991. London: The Galton Institute, 1992.

32. Castilla EE, Sod R. The surveillance of birth defects in South America: II. The search for geographic clusters: endemics. Adv Mutag Res 1990;2:211–230.

33. Kremer RD, Levstain IM. Enfermedad de Sandhoff o gangliosidosis GM2 tipo-2. Medicina 1980;40:55–73. [Spanish]

34. Quelce-Salgado A. A new type of dwarfism with various bone aplasias and hypoplasias of the extremities. Acta Genet 1964;14:63–66.

35. Freie-Maia A. Historical note. The extraordinary handless and footless families of Brazil: 50 years of acheiropodia. Am J Med Genet 1981;9:31–41.

36. Leon PE, Bonilla JA, Sanchez JR, et al. Low frequency hereditary deafness in man with childhood onset. Am J Hum Genet 1981;33:209–214.

37. Auburger G, Orozco Diaz G, Ferreira Capote R, et al. Autosomal dominant ataxia: genetic evidence for locus heterogeneity from a Cuban founder-effect population. Am J Hum Genet 1990;46:1163–1177.

38. Arias S. Osteochondrodysplasia Irapa type: an ethnic marker gene in two subcontinents. Am J Med Genet 1981;8:251–253.

39. Avila-Giron R. Medical and social aspects of Huntington Chorea in the State of Zulia, Venezuela. In: Barbeau A, Chase TN, Paulson GW (eds). Advances in Neurology, Vol. 1. New York: Raven Press, 1973, pp. 261–266.

40. Kromberg JGR, Jenkins T. Albinism in the South African Negro: II. Prevalence. S Afr Med J 1982;61:383–386.

41. Serjeant GR. Geography and the clinical picture of sickle-cell disease. Ann N Y Acad Sci 1989;565:109–119.

42. Weatherall DJ, Clegg JB, Higgs DR, Wood WG. The hemoglobinopathies. In: Scriver CR, Beaudet AL, Sly WS, Valle D (eds). The metabolic and molecular basis of inherited disease. New York: McGraw-Hill, 1995, pp. 3417–3484.

43. Report of the 7th Meeting of the WHO Working Group on the Control of Hereditary Anemias. Nicosia, Cyprus, 3–4 April 1993 (WHO/HDP/TIF/HA/93.1).

44. Granda H, Gispert S, Dorticos A, et al. Cuban programme for prevention of sickle cell disease. Lancet 1991;337:152–154.

45. Naoum PC, de Mattos LC, Curi PR. Prevalence and geographic distribution of abnormal hemoglobins in the state of Sao Paulo, Brazil. Bull Pan Am Health Organ 1984;18:127–138.

46. Salzano FM. Incidence, effects, and management of sickle cell disease in Brazil. J Pediatr Hematol/Oncol 1985;7:240–244.

47. Martins CSB, Ramalho AS, Sonati MF, Goncalves MS, Costa FF. Molecular characterization of beta-thalassemia heterozygotes in Brazil. J Med Genet 1993;30:797–798.

48. El-Hazmi MAF, Warsy AS. Hemoglobinopathies in Arab countries. In: Teebi AS, Farag TI (eds). Genetic disorders among Arab populations. New York and Oxford: Oxford University Press, 1997, pp. 83–110.

49. Winichagoon P, Fucharoen S, Thonglairoam V, Tanapotiwirai V, Wasi P. Thalassemia in Thailand. Ann N Y Acad Sci 1990;612:31–42.

50. Zeng YT, Huang SZ. Disorders of hemoglobin in China. J Med Genet 1987;24:578–583.

51. Perez-Comas A, Garcia-Castro JM. Occipito-facial-cervico-thoracic-abdomino-digital dysplasia; Jarcho-Levin syndrome of vertebral anomalies: report of six cases and review of the literature. J Pediatr 1974;85:388–391.

52. Al-Rajeh S, Bademosi O, Ismail H, et al. A community survey of neurological disorders in Saudi Arabia. The Thugbah study. Neuroepidemiology 1993;12:164–178.

53. Community Control of Hereditary Anemias. Memorandum from a WHO meeting. Bull World Health Organ 1983;61:63–80.

54. Pan American Health Organization. Health conditions in the Americas. Washington, DC: PAHO 1994.

55. Barreiro CZ, Negrotti T, Penchaszadeh VB. Prevalence of genetic disease in a pediatric referral hospital. Excerpta Med Intl Congr Series 1976;397:60–61.

56. Penchaszadeh VB. Frequency and characteristics of birth defects admissions to a pediatric hospital in Venezuela. Am J Med Genet 1979;3:359–369.

57. Carnevale A, Hernandez M, Reyes R, Paz F, Sosa C. The frequency and economic burden of genetic disease in a pediatric hospital in Mexico City. Am J Med Genet 1985;20:665–675.

58. Penchaszadeh VB. Implementing comprehensive genetic services in developing countries: the case of Latin America. In: Kuliev A, Greendale K, Penchaszadeh VB, Paul NW (eds). Genetic services provision: an international perspective. Birth Defects Orig Art Ser 1992;28(3):17–26. March of Dimes Birth Defects Foundation, White Plains, New York.

59. Angastiniotis MA, Hadjiminas MG. Prevention of thalassemia in Cyprus. Lancet 1981;1:369–370.

60. Angastiniotis MA, Kyriakidou S, Hadjiminas M. How thalassaemia was controlled in Cyprus. World Health Forum 1986;7:291–297.

61. El-Hazmi MAF. Care for people with hemoglobin disorders. World Health Forum 1994;15:165–168.

62. Anionwu EN, Patel N, Kanji G, Rengers H, Brosovic M. Counselling for prenatal diagnosis of sickle cell disease and B thalassaemia major: a four-year experience. J Med Genet 1988;25:769–772.

63. Akinyanju OO, Anionwu EN. Training of counsellors on sickle cell disorders in Africa. Lancet 1989;I:653–654.

64. Penchaszadeh VB, Beiguelman B (eds). Medical genetic services in Latin America. Geneva: WHO publication WHO/HGN/CONS/MGS/98.4, 1998.

65. Penchaszadeh VB, Beiguelman B. Medical genetic services in Latin America: report of a meeting of experts. Pan Am J Public Health 1998;3:409–420.

66. Harris R. Preface and Overview. Genetic services in Europe. Eur J Hum Genet 1997;5(Suppl 2):1–21.

67. Pan American Health Organization. Prevention and control of genetic diseases and congenital defects: report of an advisory group. Scientific Publication 460. Washington, DC: PAHO, 1984.

68. Organización Panamericana de la Salud. Ejecución de Actividades de Salud de Genética en América Latina y el Caribe. Informe de un Grupo de Expertos. Havana, Cuba, 9–11 October, 1987. Internal Publication. Washington, DC: PAHO 1988.

69. World Health Organization. Implementation of cystic fibrosis services in developing countries: report of a joint WHO/International Cystic Fibrosis (Mucoviscidosis) Association Meeting. Manama, Bahrain, 18–19 November 1995. Geneva: WHO publication WHO/HGN/ICF(M)A/WG/95.6, 1995.

70. Pan American Health Organization. PAHO/WHO Consultation on the development of PAHO strategy on congenital disorders. Washington, DC, 7–8 October 1998. Washington, DC: PAHO internal publication, 1998.

71. World Health Organization. Prevention and care of genetic diseases and birth defects in developing countries: report of a joint WHO/World Alliance of

Organizations for the Prevention of Birth Defects Meeting. The Hague, 5–7 January 1999. WHO publication. (in press).

72. Granda H, Gispert S, Martinez G, et al. Results from a reference laboratory for prenatal diagnosis of sickle cell disorders in Cuba. Prenat Diagn 1994;14:659–662.

73. Dorticos-Balea A, Martin-Ruiz M, Hechevarria-Fernandez P, et al. Reproductive behaviour of couples at risk for sickle cell disease in Cuba: a follow-up study. Prenat Diagn 1997;17:737–742.

74. Rodriguez L, Sanchez R, Hernandez J, et al. Results of 12 years' combined maternal serum alpha-fetoprotein screening and ultrasound fetal monitoring for prenatal detection of fetal malformations in Havana City, Cuba. Prenat Diagn 1997;4:301–304.

75. Penchaszadeh VB, Heredero L, Punales-Morejon D, Rojas I, Perez ET. Genetic counseling training in Cuba (Abstract) Am J Hum Genet 1997;61(4) (Suppl: A):1099.

76. Xin M. Ethics and genetics in China. In: Wertz DC, Fletcher JC (eds). Ethics and human genetics: an international perspective (2nd ed). New York: Springer-Verlag. (in press).

77. Lo WHY. Medical genetics in China. J Med Genet 1988;25:253–257.

78. Zeng YT, Huang SZ, Zhang ML. Prenatal diagnosis of thalassemia: experiences at the Shanghai Children's Hospital. Hemoglobin 1988;12(5 & 6):796–800.

79. Zhou ZL. Recent advances of perinatal medicine in China. Chin Med J (Engl) 1995;108(5):387–389.

80. Wang Y, Becker S, Chow LP, Wang SX. Induced abortion in eight provinces of China. Asia Pac J Public Health 1991;5:32–40.

81. Law of the People's Republic of China on Maternal and Infant Health Care. Order of the President of the People's Republic of China No. 33, October 27, 1994.

82. Editorial. Western eyes on China's eugenics law. Lancet 1995;346:131.

83. Verma IC. Control of genetic disorders in India. Paper presented at the joint WHO/World Alliance of Organizations for the Prevention of Birth Defects Meeting. The Hague, 5–7 January 1999.

84. Chaterjee JB. Hemoglobinopathies, glucose-6-phosphate dehydrogenase and allied problems in the Indian subcontinent. Bull World Health Organ 1966;35:837–856.

85. Sangani B, Sukumaran PK, Mahadik C, et al. Thalassaemia in Bombay: the role of medical genetics in developing countries. Bull World Health Organ 1990;68:75–81.

86. Verma IC, Singh B. Ethics and medical genetics in India. In: Wertz DC, Fletcher JC (eds). Ethics and human genetics. New York: Springer-Verlag, 1989, pp. 250–270.

87. Saxena R, Jain PK, Thomas E, Verma IC. Prenatal diagnosis of beta-thalassemia: experience in a developing country. Prenat Diagn 1998;18:1–7.

88. Jenkins T. Medical genetics in South Africa. J Med Genet 1990;27:760–779.

89. Kromberg JGR, Jenkins T. Common birth defects in South African Blacks. S Afr Med J 1982;62:599–602.

90. Kromberg JGR, Christianson AL, Duthie-Nurse G, Zwane E, Jenkins T. Down syndrome in the black population (Letter). S Afr Med J 1992;81:337.

91. Christianson AL. Down syndrome in sub-Saharan Africa. J Med Genet 1996;33:89–92.

92. Manga N, Jenkins T, Lane AB. The molecular basis of transferase galactosemia in the South African black population. SA Society of Human Genetics Congress, Pilanesberg, 18–21 May 1997. Abstract Book: 43.

93. Department of Health of South Africa. White paper for the transformation of the health system in South Africa. Government Gazette, 16 April 1997, Vol. 382, No. 17910. Pretoria, South Africa.

94. Viljoen D, Beighton P, Hitzeroth H. Medical genetics in primary health care. S Afr Med J 1995;85:1–3.

95. Christianson AL, Venter PA, Gericke GS, du Toit JL, Buckle C, Nelson M. Genetics for Africa: experience in the northern province of South Africa 1990–1995 (abstract). Eur J Hum Genet 1998;6(Suppl 1):183.

96. Christianson AL, Modiba J, Venter PA. Clinical case load of a genetic trained nursing sister in a rural South African hospital (abstract) Eur J Hum Genet 1998;6(Suppl 1):183.

97. Subdirectorate of Human Genetics, Department of Health of South Africa. Policy for the prevention and care of genetic diseases at the primary care level. Pretoria, South Africa, 1998.

98. Viljoen D, Oosthuizen C, Van der Westhuizen S. Patient attitudes to prenatal screening and termination of pregnancy at Groote Schuur Hospital: a two-year prospective study. East Afr Med J 1996;73:327–329.

99. World Health Organization. World Health Report 1997. Geneva: WHO 1997.

100. El-Hazmi MAF. Genetic diseases in Arabia: a model for national awareness and care programme. Saudi Med J 1992;13:514–520.

101. World Health Organization. Proposed international guidelines on ethical issues in medical genetic and genetic services. Report of a WHO meeting on ethical issues in medical genetics. Geneva, 15–16 December 1997. Publ. WHO/HGN/GL/ETH/98.1.

18

Genetics and prevention effectiveness

Scott D. Grosse and Steven M. Teutsch

Advances in human genetics require systematic assessment for their rational translation into public health policy and practice. Prevention-effectiveness research is that part of the policy assessment process that addresses trade-offs among harms, benefits, and costs of disease-prevention strategies (1). If one strategy is more effective and costs less than other strategies, and in addition poses no risk of harms, a decision is usually simple. More commonly, though, a strategy that is superior on one or more criteria (i.e., is more effective or less costly) ranks poorly on another. In such cases, the trade-offs need to be calculated with quantitative prevention-effectiveness models. The results can then be used in developing guidelines and making resource allocation decisions.

Prevention effectiveness includes quantitative and qualitative methods of policy analysis. Qualitative issues include the ethical, legal, and social consequences of public choices, such as the differential effects of an intervention on population subgroups. Salient issues related to genetics include informed consent to genetic testing, stigmatization of individuals and groups, discrimination in employment, and access to insurance. These have implications for both public policy and individuals (2). For example, a program of genetic screening acceptable in a society with universal health insurance might pose unacceptable risk to individuals without guaranteed access to health care. These issues are addressed in Part V of this book. Quantitative prevention-effectiveness research integrates methods from economics, health services research, and technology assessment to analyze the cost of illness and the effectiveness, benefits, and costs of public health policies and programs. The most common analytic methods are *decision analysis* and *economic analysis*.

This chapter is intended to help the reader critically evaluate quantitative prevention-effectiveness studies in genetics and to understand their uses and limitations. No prior knowledge of prevention-effectiveness methods is assumed. Therefore, the first part of the chapter consists of an overview of the major types of analysis, definitions, underlying concepts, and rules for carrying out prevention-effectiveness analyses. The second half of the chapter applies these rules to case studies of recent economic evaluations of genetic screening, genetic testing, and genetic-test–specific therapeutic interventions.

Decision Analysis and Expected Values

Decision analysis is used to calculate the expected values of health outcomes resulting from different strategies. An expected value is the average value of an outcome if a choice were repeated numerous times. It is defined as the sum of the products of the values of each event that could occur and the probabilities of each event occurring. For example, the expected value of a gamble that has a one tenth probability of yielding $100 and a nine-tenths probability of yielding nothing is $10 [(0.1 × 100) + (0.9 × 0)]. It is different from the typical yield, which is $0. Whether the value of a gamble is the same as the mathematical expectation depends on one's risk preferences. A risk-averse individual, one who prefers a sure thing to an uncertain outcome with the same mathematical expectation, by definition would place a lower value on an uncertain outcome (3).

Life expectancy is an example of expected value. The future number of years lived by a cohort is calculated by multiplying age-specific survival rates by the number of individuals projected to be alive at the beginning of each age interval to calculate the number alive at the beginning of the next age interval. Life expectancy is calculated as the ratio of the projected number of years lived by all members of the cohort divided by the number of members of the cohort. Life expectancy is not necessarily the same as the life span of a typical individual. For example, a cohort of 100 people aged 60 years would have an additional life expectancy of 5 years if 20 are expected to survive 20 years and 80 are expected to each live for 1 year and 3 months. Use of life expectancies in decision analysis presumes risk neutrality (1). If analysts report the distribution of expected outcomes as well as the expected value, individuals who are risk averse can make their own assessments of the trade-offs.

Building a Decision Model

In setting up a decision analysis, the analyst first creates a decision tree in which each strategy (intervention or no intervention) is assigned a branch (1).

The expected value of each branch is calculated by multiplying the value of each outcome (e.g., years of life expectancy) by the probabilities of those outcomes. The probabilities vary depending upon factors such as choices made, biological factors, test characteristics, and behaviors. Under each strategy, separate branches are specified for each possible event—for example, becoming diseased or remaining healthy. In a disease branch, the average value of all possible outcomes (e.g., death, disability, recovery) is calculated and multiplied by the probabilities of each. The expected value of an intervention branch is the weighted average of the expected values of the disease and nondisease branches. Ultimately, the strategy with the highest expected value is considered the preferred choice.

A standard decision tree model involves discrete time periods and is non-recursive. In contrast, a Markov model allows probabilities to vary by small increments (e.g., annual incidence rates over a period of several decades), and individuals can cycle, that is, repeat states (4). While Markov models may more accurately reflect real-world situations, because of their complexity, they are difficult to document in journal articles. Spreadsheets can be used to approximate the results of a Markov model, as discussed below.

Utility Assessment and QALYs

Life expectancy is only one potential outcome measure in decision or cost-effectiveness analyses. Analyses that consider only life-years as an outcome measure may tend to favor interventions that extend the probability of life at the risk of serious side effects over interventions that are more beneficial in terms of perceived quality of life. For this reason, it is preferable to use an outcome measure that incorporates the potential harms and benefits in terms of health or quality of life among surviving individuals as a result of an intervention. To do this, one needs a common metric integrating morbidity and mortality outcomes. The most commonly used metric of this kind is an index known as *quality-adjusted life years*, or QALYs (5).

The calculation of quality-adjusted life years is based on the use of *expected utilities* to value health outcomes. *Utility* refers to people's values or preferences for different states. If people have stable preferences, it is possible to compute indices that combine the expected utility of living in a state of impaired health with the utility of being alive in good health (3). To calculate quality-adjusted life years, one first multiplies the utility for each health state (U_i) by expected durations of time spent in each state (t_i). The sum of these products is a QALY index. In mathematical terms,

$$QALYs = \Sigma \, U_i \, t_i.$$

One way to derive utility weights for QALYs is to use standard population-based multiattribute scales such as the Quality of Well-being Scale (QWB) or the Health Utilities Index (HUI) (6). If this approach is taken, the next step is to determine the symptoms or characteristics of a condition that correspond most closely to the items on the scale. This approach can work well for analyses of well-defined conditions. It is especially suitable for analyses performed from a societal viewpoint as the scales are often based on community preferences.

The other common way of deriving utility weights is from primary survey data. This approach is particularly well suited for clinical decision analyses. It allows the impact of variation in individual responses on conclusions to be assessed. Several methods can be used to directly elicit preferences about multiple health states (3,6). In the *standard gamble*, individuals are asked to choose between remaining in a state of ill health and undergoing a procedure that will either return them to perfect health or kill them with a defined probability. The probability is varied until the individuals indicate they have no preference between the two choices. In the *time–trade-off* method, individuals are asked how much time in a state of full health they would be willing to trade in return for a longer time alive in less than perfect health.

Economic Analyses

Economic analyses of public health programs are generally identified with calculations of monetary costs. This is a rather narrow perspective, for economic theory is framed in terms of utility maximization, not simply in terms of dollars. One major limitation of many economic analyses is that they do not include the costs of pain and suffering. These are real costs that influence decision making but are left out of economic analyses that focus on accounting costs. These costs are at least partially included in the expected utilities used to calculate QALYs, which constitute another argument in favor of using QALYs as outcome measures for economic evaluations of health interventions.

Economic evaluations of health programs can be classified as partial, intermediate, or full evaluations (7). A *full* economic evaluation incorporates all aspects of the costs and benefits of an intervention. A *partial* economic evaluation consists of one component of a full evaluation. These include decision analyses, which model the effectiveness but not the cost of an intervention. Partial evaluations also include two types of cost-accounting analyses: cost-of-illness and cost-identification studies. Cost-of-illness studies are used to calculate the cost burden of a condition or illness, which sets an upper limit on the economic benefit of a preventive intervention that prevents all new cases of the condition. Cost-identification studies are used to assess the costs of delivering interventions.

There are two primary methods for conducting a full economic evaluation of a health intervention, the most common of which is *cost-effectiveness* analysis (CEA). This type of evaluation gives results in terms of the ratio of cost per unit of improvement in health outcomes achieved. If the net cost of an intervention is negative, the intervention is said to be *cost saving*. In that case, a cost-effectiveness ratio is not meaningful. The other major type of economic evaluation, *cost-benefit* analysis (CBA), converts health outcomes into monetary values. This method is less commonly used in public health because of disagreement over the suitability and validity of methods of putting monetary valuations on health states and life (5).

The health outcome used in the denominator of a cost-effectiveness ratio can be either in the form of physical units, such as years of life saved, or utility indices such as QALYs. Many people refer to an analysis that uses QALYs as the denominator in the outcome ratio as a *cost-utility* analysis (CUA). However, a recent expert panel convened by the U.S. Public Health Service recommends that *all* cost-effectiveness analyses use QALYs whenever possible (6). Use of a standard outcome measure such as QALYs allows analysts to use a common denominator to compare the cost-effectiveness of interventions.

The calculation of a cost-effectiveness ratio can be represented in simplified form as follows. First, assume that an intervention, A, is being compared with a baseline of no intervention, O. The cost-effectiveness of the intervention is the total cost of the intervention plus the cost of illness if the intervention is implemented (Cost of illness$_A$) minus the cost of illness if one does nothing (Cost of illness$_0$) divided by the difference between net outcomes under the intervention (Health outcomes$_A$) compared with the baseline (Health outcomes$_0$).

$$\text{CE ratio} = \frac{\text{Intervention cost} + (\text{Cost of illness}_A - \text{Cost of illness}_0)}{(\text{Health outcomes}_A - \text{Health outcomes}_0)}$$

If more than two alternatives are modeled, each intervention when compared to the baseline yields an *average* cost-effectiveness ratio. In addition, it is important to calculate *incremental* cost-effectiveness ratios that compare the costs and health outcomes of pairs of interventions (1). Interventions that are both more expensive and less effective than other interventions are said to be *dominated* and are excluded from the calculation of incremental cost-effectiveness ratios. Average and incremental cost-effectiveness ratios may yield different conclusions. For example, universal screening of newborns for sickle-cell disease in a population with a low prevalence of the mutation has been reported to have a low (favorable) cost-effectiveness ratio when compared with no screening but a high (less favorable) cost-effectiveness ratio when compared with racially targeted screening (8).

Cost-effectiveness analysis is often confused with *intermediate* economic analyses that examine only short-term outcomes. Ratios such as the cost of screening per person screened or per case identified are often referred to as *estimates of cost-effectiveness*, but this is not correct. A cost-effectiveness estimate requires calculation of all costs, benefits, and harms flowing from the identification of affected individuals. Although one strategy may have a lower cost per person tested or cost per case identified than the other, this is not sufficient to favor one strategy over the other if the two strategies result in different numbers of individuals identified. The higher-cost strategy may be preferred if it results in more cases identified and if the incremental benefit of case identification exceeds the incremental cost. This limitation is not true of *cost-minimization* analyses, which compare interventions such as screening protocols that have approximately the same outcomes to determine which one costs the least to operate (6).

Single numerical estimates of net benefits or cost-effectiveness ratios may provide a misleading sense of precision. Often, not much is known about key parameters such as the magnitude of a protective effect or the costs of an intervention. To clarify the degree of uncertainty and the degree to which policy decisions might have varying effects depending upon the projected benefit and cost of an intervention, prevention-effectiveness studies typically report *sensitivity analyses*. Sensitivity analyses indicate how cost-effectiveness estimates vary under ranges of assumptions about key parameters. Recently, methods used to calculate confidence intervals around cost-effectiveness estimates have also become available. If a specific intervention is favored under a wide range of assumptions, the result is said to be *robust*.

Evaluating a Cost-Effectiveness Study

Readers need to be critical in evaluating prevention-effectiveness analyses, especially economic evaluations (7,9–10). A number of excellent texts on preparing economic evaluations of health interventions have been published (1,5–7). However, the peer-review process does not guarantee that recommended guidelines have been followed. The BMJ Economic Evaluation Working Party has published a checklist for reviewers and editors to use in assessing economic analyses (9). A paraphrased version of the BMJ checklist below condenses and rearranges the original 35 items into a set of 12 questions (Table 18.1). The questions refer to a full economic analysis; some of the questions are not relevant in evaluating a partial economic

Table 18.1 Checklist for Assessing Economic Analyses of Health Interventions

- Is the research question stated and its importance justified?
- Are the alternatives compared clearly described and the rationale for their choice presented? Is an incremental analysis reported for alternative interventions?
- Is the viewpoint (perspective) of the analysis clearly stated and justified?
- Are costs clearly and appropriately defined and sources reported?
- Is the time horizon of costs and benefits stated?
- Is the discount rate stated and justified?
- Are costs reported for specific years, along with details of adjustments for inflation?
- Is the source of effectiveness estimates stated and details of how the estimates were derived presented?
- Are the outcome measures of the analysis and their methods of calculation stated?
- Is a sensitivity analysis reported and the choice of variables and ranges justified?
- Do conclusions address the study question and follow from the data reported?
- Are the conclusions accompanied by appropriate caveats?

evaluation. Definitions of concepts such as *discounting* are explained in the text.

Framing the Study

When framing a prevention-effectiveness study, investigators must address a series of issues. First, they should choose an appropriate study question, a hypothesis that is both testable and likely to contribute to a policy decision if answered. Second, investigators should ensure that all viable, policy-relevant alternatives are included. An evaluation that does not consider *all* viable intervention strategies may yield misleading results, because an excluded option may be more attractive than any of the strategies modeled.

The viewpoint or perspective from which the analysis is conducted must correspond to the study question and the intended audience (8). Public health impact is best addressed by analyses that use the *societal* perspective, which integrates costs experienced by all relevant groups, including the health care system and individuals or families. In the *health care system* perspective, only medical costs are included. The consensus of experts is that this should never be the only perspective used, although it is useful as a complement to the societal perspective (6).

If the audience of a study consists of health care plan managers, a *payer* perspective is appropriate. However, switching of individuals among health plans, which reduces the benefits of prevention to the payer, should be taken into account. Finally, many decision analyses address harms and benefits faced by *individuals*, without considering costs to the health care system or society. This type of clinical decision analysis is valuable for case management but is less useful for drawing inferences for decisions by insurers or public policy makers.

Definitions of Costs

The costs of disease include direct costs, productivity losses (often referred to as *indirect costs*), and intangible costs. Direct costs include medical care, services such as physical therapy or special education, and the time and travel costs of families. Direct costs are calculated after subtracting the usual medical care or education costs incurred by individuals so as not to overstate the benefits of preventing disease. Productivity losses consist of the useful work lost because of disease. These are excluded from analyses that use QALYs as outcome measures to avoid double counting (1). Psychosocial or intangible costs are excluded from cost-effectiveness analyses but may be included in cost-benefit analyses. Intervention costs can also be broken down into direct costs and overhead or indirect costs.

The choice of costs to include should be determined by the analytic perspective. Analyses from the health system perspective include the direct medical costs of disease and the costs of medical interventions but not patient or nonmedical costs. This type of analysis is less demanding of data, but the perspective should derive from the study question, not convenience. The societal perspective should encompass *all* costs associated with an intervention. For example, the costs of screening include all costs that follow upon a positive result, including diagnosis, follow-up, and treatment, as well as the costs of organizing and promoting screening. Published cost analyses often exclude many relevant costs and hence may offer misleadingly low estimates of screening costs.

Charges or list prices are often used to approximate the costs of purchased inputs. This presumes the existence of competitive markets. In noncompetitive markets where there are barriers to entry and relatively few buyers or sellers, costs and prices may diverge. For example, list prices for commercial genetic tests might be multiples of actual resource costs (11). Actual amounts paid by purchasers of health services as recorded in medical claims databases may also be used in place of charges. However, these may understate the costs of providing services because service providers can shift costs to other consumers.

In economic analyses conducted from the societal perspective, costs are estimated on the basis of resources consumed, which are not necessarily the same as payments. Resources are valued at their *opportunity cost*, which is the greatest value that resources could yield if employed elsewhere. For example, the value of time is measured by how much individuals could earn in another activity. Programs that use volunteers or donated or depreciated equipment may have low accounting costs but still incur substantial resource costs. The opportunity cost of time spent being screened or treated or providing care to family members is a major component of patient and family costs.

The most direct source of data on resource costs is *micro-costing* of quantities and unit costs of personnel, supplies, equipment, and so forth (5). Micro-costing is laborious and may lead to underestimates of some types of costs for which detailed data are not available. A less-demanding approach is *gross-costing*, in which accounting data are used. One approach is to multiply stated charges for hospital and physician services by available cost-to-charge ratios to approximate resource costs (6). As already mentioned, payments from medical claims databases can also be used. In general, gross-costing approaches are most commonly used for cost-of-illness estimates, whereas micro-costing is the preferred option for valuing the costs of delivering interventions.

In costing interventions, investigators should clearly state the method they use to allocate shared or overhead costs. They may follow accounting principles in assigning overhead charges to each activity (5). However, in economic analyses, only costs that vary with an intervention are included. *Marginal* costs are costs that vary with the *scale* of the intervention and may include some administrative costs. If the question is whether an intervention is adopted at all, *incremental* costs are relevant (8). Incremental cost is the difference in cost associated with one program or set of interventions and the costs of running another program. The incremental cost of an intervention that expands an existing program, for example, is the additional cost of running the expanded program after subtracting the cost of running the existing program.

Time

The *time horizon* of a study has two elements, the time frame and the analytic horizon (1). The *time frame* is the period over which intervention costs are measured, typically a year. The *analytic horizon* is the period over which costs and benefits associated with health outcomes resulting from early diagnosis and treatment are calculated. The analytic horizon might be a defined period (e.g., 10 or 20 years) or the lifetimes of the individuals receiving the intervention. The latter approach is in general preferred.

If the analytic horizon is longer than a year, costs are *discounted* to account for differential timing. The rationale for discounting includes time preference (people prefer to have benefits sooner) and the opportunity cost of resources (i.e., expected return on investments). As an example of discounting, suppose that an intervention yields $2 million in benefits 20 years in the future. At a discount rate of 5% per annum, the benefits are worth $753,779 today, calculated according to the financial formula for the *present value* of a future sum. If the intervention cost $1 million, the net present value of the intervention would be negative if one used a 5% discount rate but would be positive if one did not employ discounting. In cost-effectiveness analysis, future health outcomes are discounted at the same rate as future costs or monetary benefits in part to avoid favoring interventions that yield health benefits far in the future (1).

Cost-effectiveness studies commonly use discount rates of 3% or 5%. The Panel on Cost-effectiveness in Health and Medicine recommends that estimates of societal time preference and returns to capital are consistent with both numbers, especially a 3% discount rate (6). Because a higher discount rate makes benefits occurring far in the future less attractive, it is important to compare studies using the same discount rate when evaluating interventions with long analytic horizons over which benefits are assessed. Studies conducted from the perspective of specific sectors should use discount rates reflecting the cost of capital and time preference of the group whose perspective is being modeled. For example, an analysis conducted from a payer perspective might use a discount rate that reflects the payer's opportunity cost of capital, which may be much higher than 3% to 5%.

Inflation adjustment is needed to make cost data from different years equivalent. Suppose that one has data on intervention costs from 1994, earnings data from 1990, and budget data from 1998. To make the dollar figures equivalent, one would need to translate each set of data into the same year's dollars. Earnings data are adjusted on the basis of changes in hourly compensation, whereas medical costs are adjusted on the basis of changes in the medical component of the consumer price index. This method of inflation adjustment can overstate the costs of items for which costs either decrease or rise relatively slowly owing to increased technical efficiency in production.

Effectiveness and Outcomes

The source of data on the effectiveness of an intervention is critical in assessing the validity of an analysis (9). Estimates taken from a randomized controlled trial are more reliable than estimates from observational data. The quality of data from observational studies is highly variable. The number of cases, completeness of follow-up, and representativeness of the data should be considered. "Expert opinion" is a less reliable source of estimates of effectiveness. For screening, the accuracy or validity of the screening tests and the effectiveness of the interventions that follow a positive diagnosis need to be considered. The two important test characteristics are *sensitivity*, the fraction of true cases that are detected, and *specificity*, the fraction of unaffected individuals that test negative. Optimistic assumptions about sensitivity and specificity can make a screening intervention appear unrealistically beneficial.

$$Sensitivity = \frac{TP}{TP + FN} \qquad Specificity = \frac{TN}{TN + FP}$$

where

TP = True positives (affected individuals who test positive)

FP = False positives (unaffected individuals who test positive)

TN = True negatives (unaffected individuals who test negative)

FN = False negatives (affected individuals who test negative)

Efficacy, the benefit of an intervention conducted under ideal conditions, differs from *effectiveness*, the expected benefit in routine practice (12). The major cause of divergence between efficacy and effectiveness is *incomplete adherence*, including uptake of screening and adherence to prescribed interventions. Models that assume that everyone offered screening will accept it or come back for follow-up visits and comply with prescribed treatments can greatly overstate the benefits of the intervention.

Investigators should clearly define and justify the outcome measure they use to assess interventions. Expected years of life gained is a commonly used outcome; however, this measure may be problematic for two reasons. First, if there are significant nonfatal outcomes, results may be misleading. For example, focusing on mortality as an outcome overvalues interventions that prevent premature mortality but cause adverse health effects. This problem can be overcome by using quality-adjusted life-years, which allow for the incorporation of harms and benefits into a single outcome measure. Because methods for calculating QALYs have not been standardized, presentation of information on how they are computed is critical to an intelligent interpretation of the study. The second problem with use of expected life years as an outcome measure, which applies to QALYs as well, is that expected values do not reflect individual risk preferences. For individual decision-analysis models, it is desirable to report the distribution of expected outcomes, not just mean values.

Sensitivity Analyses

Accounting for uncertainty is a critical facet of a prevention-effectiveness analysis (1). Estimates of costs and effectiveness are usually imprecise and uncertain. *Sensitivity analyses* are used to quantify the impact of this uncertainty and model assumptions on a finding that a particular intervention is or is not cost saving or cost-effective. This can be done in one of two ways. One way is to vary parameters within ranges of plausible values to see whether results change qualitatively. If not, the results are considered *robust*. The second way is a *threshold analysis* that calculates the value of a parameter that results in a qualitatively different outcome from the base-case analysis. Instead of conducting a sensitivity analysis, it is also possible to calculate confidence intervals for cost-effectiveness ratios based on the distributions of values for each estimate of cost and effectiveness (13).

Most sensitivity analyses report the results of changing just one or two variables at a time, but a broader approach might be better (5). In a one-way sensitivity analysis, researchers vary one parameter at a time within a range of plausible values to see how the outcome of the model changes as the parameter changes. For example, if the estimate of efficacy is a 50% reduction in risk, a range from 30% to 70% could be tested in a sensitivity analysis. In two-way sensitivity analyses, two parameters are simultaneously varied. Although sensitivity analyses indicate which parameters have the greatest influence on results, they may lead to overconfidence in the robustness of results. Often a result is qualitatively unaffected by changes in one or two parameters, but a set of plausible parameter values may reverse the conclusion. To avoid this hazard, researchers may also conduct "worst-case" analyses (5).

Drawing Conclusions

Conclusions should squarely address the study question posed at the beginning of an article and not overgeneralize. For example, an analysis from an individual perspective may not be generalizable to policy or reimbursement questions. External validity of results is dependent upon the representativeness of the data used. For instance, the cost-effectiveness of screening depends upon the prevalence of the condition being screened for, and the results may be valid only for populations with similar prevalences.

Conclusions should also be accompanied by caveats, including recognition of potential harms (10). The conclusion should highlight results, including worst-case analyses, that may have policy implications. The conclusion should indicate the degree to which assumptions about parameters are *conservative* in the sense of making a proposed intervention look less favorable than would other values that could have been chosen. If an intervention is cost-effective even under relatively unfavorable assumptions, greater confidence can be placed in the findings. Finally, in analyses that use QALYs as outcome measures, researchers should discuss how different methods of measuring or weighting preferences could affect the results.

CASE STUDIES OF PREVENTION EFFECTIVENESS AND GENETICS

The remainder of the chapter consists of a critical review of the economic and decision-analysis literature on certain genetic disorders and interventions. The case studies selected for review are prevention-effectiveness analyses of population-based screening for genetic disorders, genetic testing of family members, and prophylactic surgeries contingent on genetic tests, published through the end of 1998. The Task Force on Genetic Testing has defined genetic tests to include not only molecular tests that analyze human DNA, RNA, and chromosomes, but also biochemical tests of proteins and metabolites that can identify diseases caused by variants in single genes (14). The relative advantage of these two types of genetic tests (biochemical vs. molecular or DNA) is an important issue in population screening for genetic conditions. Single-gene conditions, such as PKU or sickle cell disease (SCD), which are already routinely identified through population-based biochemical tests of newborn infants, are not explicitly addressed here.

The first case studies address population screening for two autosomal recessive single-gene conditions: *cystic fibrosis*, a disease that manifests in early childhood, and *hereditary hemochromatosis*, a disease of adults. In autosomal recessive disorders, individuals with two mutated alleles, whether homozygotes (two copies of the same variant allele) or compound heterozygotes (copies of two different variant alleles), are likely to become diseased while heterozygotes may be phenotypically normal. The remaining case studies address susceptibility genotypes for colorectal, breast, and ovarian cancers. In the case of autosomal dominant cancer syndromes, the carrier of a single mutated allele is at elevated risk of disease.

The *penetrance*, or risk of disease associated with a particular genotype, may be an important predictor of the clinical utility and prevention effectiveness of a test or intervention for a genetic disorder. If penetrance is very high, almost all individuals with the affected genotype will eventually become diseased. If penetrance is modest, for each case of disease there may be multiple individuals who do not experience disease. Any harms resulting from identification and/or intervention are borne by all individuals with an affected genotype; however, as benefits occur only for the fraction of cases resulting in phenotypic disease, the ratio of benefit to harm is lower if penetrance is lower.

Cystic Fibrosis

Cystic fibrosis (CF), a disorder of chloride transport across membranes, causes accumulation of mucus in the lungs and pancreas. Repeated infections, poor nutritional status, and lung dysfunction and destruction result from this condition. Cystic fibrosis occurs in 1 in 3000 Caucasian Americans, 1 in 15,000 African Americans, and 1 in 30,000 Asian Americans. Over 500 known mutations on the CF transmembrane conductance regulator (CFTR) gene have been identified. The most common of these is the ΔF508 allele, which comprises two-thirds of CFTR mutant alleles among Americans of European ancestry with CF, although less than half of those among individuals of non-European backgrounds (15).

Identifying infants with CF allows for early initiation of therapy that may ameliorate the progression of disease but does not prevent the development of symptoms. Studies comparing cohorts that were or were not screened at birth indicate that early identification yields benefit in nutritional status and lung function (16). A randomized controlled trial, conducted in Wisconsin with enrollment between 1988 and 1994, reports significantly greater heights for children screened at birth than for affected children who were not identified at birth (17). However, the published results are inconclusive owing to potential selection bias (18). Until the cohort was unblinded at age 4 years, measurements were taken on all affected children identified at birth, including those without symptoms, whereas children from the other arm of the study were measured only after identification on the basis of symptoms.

Newborn screening for CF for a number of years has been conducted in several countries as well as by state newborn screening programs in Colorado and Wisconsin; programs are also being introduced in additional states. Introducing CF screening in state newborn screening programs remains controversial. An expert group convened by the Centers for Disease Control and Prevention (CDC) in January 1997 recommended additional pilot CF newborn screening programs (19), whereas a National Institutes of Health (NIH) Consensus Development Conference in April 1997 recommended *against* newborn CF screening (20).

A full economic evaluation of newborn CF screening has not yet been published. Such a study would require data that are not yet available on costs, benefits, and harms of screening compared to diagnosis on the basis of clinical symptoms. Costs of not screening include the medical tests and procedures employed to rule out other causes before a CF diagnosis is established, as well as the parental anxiety and time involved in this process. Costs of screening include additional medical services provided following an earlier CF diagnosis. A systematic assessment of these costs has yet to be published.

Partial economic evaluations of newborn CF screening have compared two types of screening strategies. The first approach uses elevated immunoreactive trypsinogen (IRT) measures on newborn dried blood spots to identify children needing repeat IRT tests, followed by diagnosis on the basis of a sweat test for those with a second positive IRT test. Ever since the identification in 1989 of mutations on the CFTR gene, many programs have instituted a two-tier screening strategy in which samples with an initial elevated IRT are immediately subjected to a mutation analysis (21,22). This second approach eliminates the need for additional blood samples and requires fewer children to be referred for sweat tests. One disadvantage of this approach is that individuals without the CFTR mutations being tested for will be missed. Another is that carrier status detected by mutation analysis may be unwanted information, and carriers may be subject to stigmatization or discrimination.

Several analyses compare the costs of biochemical (IRT) and biochemical-molecular (IRT/DNA) methods of screening newborns for CF. For example, the incremental cost of adding a CF screening test to a newborn screening panel has been calculated to be $1.09 in Australia (21) and $1.60 in Wisconsin (22), both in U.S. dollars. There is inconsistency across studies in the costs that are included; administrative costs, sweat tests, and genetic counseling are often excluded. One analysis uses cost data from Wisconsin in conjunction with program data from two IRT/DNA programs in Wisconsin and South Australia, and two IRT programs in Colorado and northeastern Italy (23). The analysis follows a health system perspective and uses average costs, including part of the cost of specimen collection. Investigators report that the IRT/DNA screening strategy employed in South Australia costs the least per case identified. This is due to a higher prevalence of CF in Australia; the IRT/DNA strategy is calculated to cost more per child screened. Specifically, the standardized cost per newborn tested for CF was $5.54 in Colorado, $5.68 in Italy, $5.80 in Australia, and $5.96 in Wisconsin, in 1994 U.S. dollars.

An analysis of CF screening costs in New Zealand calculates incremental costs, which is appropriate for a newborn screening program that already collects dried blood spots (24). During a 6-month period in 1995 an IRT/IRT protocol and an IRT/DNA protocol were simultaneously followed. All infants referred for diagnostic testing received genetic counseling and testing, as well as a sweat test, so as to provide conclusive confirmation of CF status. Because identical cases were reported, this is a cost-minimization analysis that compares the costs of two strategies with identical outcomes. When costs are analyzed from the laboratory perspective, IRT/DNA screening is found to be more expensive, $0.88 versus $0.71 per newborn for IRT/IRT, in 1995 U.S. dollars.

The New Zealand study also employs a societal perspective by including parental time costs and provider costs. When all costs associated with CF screening are included, the IRT/DNA method used in New Zealand is found to be less costly, $1.85 versus $3.07 per newborn for IRT/IRT. The lower costs result from fewer infants being recalled for blood draws and sweat tests. This conclusion cannot be validly generalized to other screening and diagnostic protocols, however (24). For example, the provider and parent time costs of the IRT/IRT protocol could be reduced if the second dried blood spot specimen were collected as part of a routine well-baby visit. The costs would also be reduced if only infants with positive sweat test results received genetic counseling and testing. Conversely, screening costs are lower in New Zealand because of the use of in-house IRT assays. Because screening and diagnostic protocols are rarely standardized, it may be misleading to generalize on the basis of cost data from a single program.

Hereditary Hemochromatosis

The most prevalent genetic disorder in the United States is hereditary hemochromatosis (HH), an inborn error of iron metabolism that causes excess absorption of dietary iron and can lead to iron overload. Hemochromatosis has many clinical manifestations, including liver cirrhosis, hepatocellular carcinoma, diabetes mellitus, and cardiomyopathy. The number of individuals affected by clinical hemochromatosis is unknown, because of widespread underdiagnosis. Most individuals who have hereditary hemochromatosis do not display symptoms, and there is disagreement over how best to determine which individuals have the condition. Estimates of prevalence of HH vary depending upon definitions and tests used, as well as the ethnic composition of the population. The most commonly cited estimates of prevalence in the United States are in the range of 2 to 5 per 1000 population (25).

Hemochromatosis is an attractive candidate for population-based screening because of the relatively high prevalence of the condition and the ability to prevent clinical disease with early identification. Treatment consists of phlebotomy to normalize iron stores, followed by regular phlebotomies three or four times a year for life. Treatment appears to prevent morbidity and normalize life expectancy in individuals detected prior to the development of cirrhosis or diabetes (26). Conversely, an expert panel recently concluded that not enough is yet known about the natural history of hemochromatosis to recommend population-based screening (27). In particular, it is not known how many individuals identified through screening would develop clinical disease in the absence of screening.

Unlike in the case of CF, a number of full economic evaluations of screening for hereditary hemochromatosis have already been published. Between 1994 and 1995, six economic analyses of screening for HH using biochemical measures were published; all concluded that HH screening is either cost saving or highly cost-effective (28–33). One of these studies considers testing family members of affected individuals (28). The other five studies address population-based screening of adults for HH, including testing of family members of individuals identified through screening. Two of these studies (29,30) have previously been assessed with regard to criteria for an economic evaluation (8). Three of the five studies are cost-effectiveness analyses that relate total direct costs (intervention costs and averted medical care costs) to changes in life expectancy (29,31,32). In the other two, cost per case identified is the main outcome measure (30,33). These are cost-identification studies, not cost-benefit or cost-effectiveness analyses according to conventional criteria (5).

Relatively few published full economic evaluations meet all of the criteria summarized in Table 18.1. In the case of the HH studies reviewed here, the study question is not framed adequately in terms of modeling a realistic screening intervention. Each of the studies is based on an idealized testing and intervention protocol that assumes that individuals comply fully with recommendations. None of the models allow for the fact that individuals may drop out at various stages of the screening, diagnostic, and treatment process. With attrition or incomplete adherence, the numbers of cases of disease prevented would be smaller than assumed, with adverse implications for calculated cost-effectiveness.

With regard to the second criterion, none of the studies considered a broad range of alternatives. Each compares a single screening strategy with the alternative of no screening. Hence, there is no incremental analysis of the costs and benefits of various screening strategies, and it is not possible to compare their relative cost-effectiveness. Incremental cost-effectiveness, together with other policy considerations, is particularly important in evaluating targeted versus universal screening. Two studies evaluate screening targeted to males (31) or Caucasian males (32) yet do not consider the costs, benefits, and harms accruing to individuals excluded from screening. A potential rationale for racial targeting is that hemochromatosis is much less common among non-Caucasians; for example, one U.S. study reports that the prevalence of hemochromatosis is 3.5 per 1000 among Caucasians and 0.5 per 1000 among non-Caucasians (33). One study (29) reports separate cost-effectiveness ratios for males and females, allowing policymakers to assess the harms and benefits of targeting screening to males.

The analytic perspective is either not stated or is not employed consistently. A public health policy analysis should employ the societal perspective, including costs to individuals, payers, providers, and governments. None of the studies include costs to individuals, even though one of the studies states that a societal perspective was employed (32). Each study restricts itself to direct medical costs, which would be consistent with a health care system or payer perspective. However, coverage of direct medical costs was incomplete; for example, one study omitted costs of hospitalization for complications following liver biopsy (29).

The published hemochromatosis cost-effectiveness analyses all assume that the fraction of those who test positive for HH is the same as the population prevalence. This assumption is valid for a test administered to individuals who have not previously been tested. As the yield on repeat tests of individuals who have already tested negative is presumably quite low, repeat testing must somehow be ruled out. Two studies propose screening either individuals attending physician offices (31) or blood donors (29). The results for these two studies may apply to a one-time intervention but cannot be extrapolated to routine screening as a public health intervention. The other study proposes screening cohorts of men when they turn 30 years of age (32). This strategy could be implemented on a routine basis without reduction in yield in subsequent waves.

Two of the CEA studies use elevated transferrin saturation (TS) as the first screening test, but with different cutoff points (31,32). One study assumes a test, namely unsaturated iron-binding capacity (UIBC), whose test validity has not been established and for which a price was not available (29). Two of the studies address complications from liver biopsy and allow for people to refuse a biopsy (29,32). Two of the studies discount future costs at a 3% rate (29,32), while the other study eschews discounting (31). (See Table 18.2.)

The biggest unknown is the direct medical costs associated with hemochromatosis. This is a function of two factors: the fraction of individuals with untreated HH who develop clinical symptoms, and the cost of treating symptomatic individuals. The studies are in close agreement on the former (0.43–0.50 for males) but differ widely on the latter. One study uses a single cost of $4000 per annum for treating individuals with clinical disease (31), whereas (the other two) report treatment costs for specific symptoms (29,32). There is extremely wide variation in the treatment-cost data. One reports the costs of treating liver cirrhosis as C$1000 per year in outpatient costs and C$50,000 in the last year of life for hospitalization (29). The other assumes that the cost of treating cirrhosis is $250,000 for a liver transplant in 1% of cases (32). The cost of treating hepatocellular carcinoma is given as C$50,000 in the first study and $1000 in the second study. Hospitalization cost for congestive heart failure is represented as C$10,416 in the first study and $45,000 in the second study.

Uncertainty regarding parameter estimates can be addressed through sensitivity analysis. Each of the hemochromatosis studies reports the results of

Table 18.2 Assumptions and Findings of Hemochromatosis Screening Cost-Effectiveness Analyses

	Buffone and Beck (31)	Phatak et al. (32)	Adams et al. (29)
Prevalence of homozygotes	0.0033	0.0030	0.0030
Penetrance (probability of developing clinical disease)	0.50	0.50	0.43 (males) 0.28 (females)
Initial screening test (threshold for TS test)	TS (62%)	TS (55%)	UIBC
Cost of initial screening test	$10.50	$12	C$5
Currency	NR	1990 U.S. dollars	1994 Canadian dollars
Second test frequency	0.30	NR	0.07
Cost of serum ferritin	$13.50	$20	C$27
liver biopsy among those who screen positive	1.0	0.50	0.90
Cost of liver biopsy	$350	$600	C$248
Discount rate	None	3%	3%
Cost per life-year saved	$605	Cost-saving	Cost-saving (males) C$4802 (females)

NR, not reported.

one-way or two-way sensitivity analyses. One of the most critical parameters is penetrance, the proportion of individuals identified through screening who would eventually develop clinical symptoms if undiagnosed. This proportion is usually lower in individuals identified through population-based screening than in clinical studies. One analysis reports that screening men for HH is cost-saving if at least 40% develop symptomatic disease, whereas if the fraction is 20% the cost per life-year saved is just below $10,000 (32). Another reports a threshold of 52.7% for the same variable (31). The study by Adams et al. reports that HH screening is cost-saving in males if the probability of disease symptoms exceeds 0.30 (29). Only one of the studies reports a multivariate sensitivity analysis, restricted to a set of four test validity parameters (31). This study reports that the cost per life-year saved could be as high as $39,410 in the worst-case scenario. If other variables had been included in the worst-case scenario, the cost per life-year saved could have been higher.

The results of the published sensitivity analyses are consistent with HH screening appearing to be cost-effective under a range of assumptions. A number of limitations need to be considered. First, none of the studies calculate the threshold for disease penetrance below which HH screening would be considered *not* cost-effective. For this reason, the question of whether HH screening is cost-effective at low levels of penetrance cannot be answered, even if all other assumptions are accurate. Second, sensitivity analyses only apply to parameters included in the models. The effects of excluding parameters such as patient time costs and adherence to referrals for testing or phlebotomy regimens are not addressed. It is not known whether taking these and other relevant variables into account might reverse conclusions about cost-effectiveness from a societal perspective.

The identification of the HFE candidate gene in 1996 has allowed for molecular tests to be used in screening for or diagnosing hereditary hemochromatosis. Between 60% and 85% of HH cases in the United States are homozygous for the C282Y missense mutation on the HFE gene (25). Smaller numbers of individuals with HH are homozygotes for the H63D missense mutation or complex heterozygotes for the C282Y and H63D mutations. The frequency of the C282Y mutation varies according to ancestral origins and is highest in populations of northwestern European ancestry. A compilation of findings from smaller studies reports that the frequency of C282Y homozygosity among unselected individuals is approximately 5 per 1000 in northern Europeans, less than 1 per 1000 among southern and eastern Europeans (e.g., Italians, Greeks), and extremely rare among non-Europeans (34).

The relative cost-effectiveness of molecular genetic and phenotypic tests for first-stage screening for HH in blood donors has been assessed in a very preliminary way in one study, published in 1997 in abstract form (35). Adams and Valberg conclude that genetic testing, based on detection of C282Y homozygotes, could potentially cost less per case identified than phenotypic testing using transferrin saturation and serum ferritin test. This is the case if the cost of the molecular test is $10, which is less than one-tenth of a typical charge, however (36). The model further assumes that only C282Y mutations would be revealed, even though standard HFE mutation analyses also test for the H63 mutation. Reporting only C282Y homozygotes means that individuals with H63D homozygosity and compound heterozygosity would fail to be diagnosed, and this approach might be regarded as unacceptable on ethical grounds (37). Conversely, reporting all susceptibility genotypes would lead to many more individuals testing positive and being recommended to undergo medical treatment but would result in the identification of relatively few additional cases. Under either strategy, genetic testing of the population of HFE mutations could result in stigmatization and unnecessary treatment of individuals who would never develop symptomatic disease (27).

Mutation analysis on the HFE gene as a diagnostic substitute for liver biopsy has also been addressed in a partial economic analysis from Australia that compares the costs of HH screening strategies in which a C282Y mutation test is or is not included in the diagnostic phase (36). At a cost of $120 for an HFE mutation analysis, compared to $900 for liver biopsy, it is reported that diagnostic costs are less expensive if mutation analysis is substituted for liver biopsy. This assumes that disease penetrance among homozygotes with repeated elevated TS measures is the same as among individuals with elevated iron stores determined by liver biopsy. The analysis does not take into account the availability of other diagnostic methods, including quantitative phlebotomy, for at least some cases. It unrealistically assumes 100% sensitivity of all tests, both biochemical and molecular, and 100% adherence with screening and treatment. Finally, only medical costs are included in the analysis. The likely effect of the exclusion of patient time costs is to understate the advantage of a molecular test, as inclusion of patient time costs can be expected to increase any cost advantage of a protocol that reduces the number of visits.

Inherited Colorectal Cancer Syndromes

At least 10% of cases of colorectal cancer (CRC) are due to Mendelian-inherited genetic disorders (38). The two major forms of inherited CRC syndromes are familial adenomatous polyposis (FAP), associated with hundreds of mutations on the APC gene, and hereditary nonpolyposis colorectal carcinoma (HNPCC), most commonly associated with mismatch repair gene mutations on the hMSH2 and hMLH1 genes. Both are autosomal dominant disorders, so individuals who carry a single variant allele (heterozygotes) are at risk of developing disease, unlike recessive disorders where mutation carriers are generally phenotypically normal. Both FAP and HNPCC are associated with early onset of colon cancer, especially FAP. The APC mutations associated with FAP are thought to have a penetrance of close to 100% by age 50. Prophylactic removal of the large bowel, with or without the rectum, is the standard clinical recommendation for individuals found to have multiple adenomas (39). Individuals identified on the basis of mutation analysis as being susceptible to FAP are recommended to undergo surveillance until the development of adenomas, and then have prophylactic surgery to prevent the emergence of cancer. Owing to heterogeneity, clinical recommendations for surgery should be based on estimates of individual risk (40).

One cost analysis of two different strategies for preventing cancer in FAP pedigrees has been published (41). This analysis, conducted from a payer perspective, compares the costs of surveillance of family members with the cost of molecular tests for family members followed by surveillance of individuals identified as carrying a mutation. In each case, surveillance is by flexible sigmoidoscopy until the age of 50 or the emergence of adenomas. The conclusion is that for a test cost below $833, genetic testing is less expensive than conventional surveillance. Because health outcomes were not measured, the report is not a cost-effectiveness analysis.

The FAP cost analysis has several limitations. First, it assumes 100% adherence. This is unlikely for either genetic testing or colonoscopy. Second, the results are sensitive to assumptions about cost. The baseline estimate for the cost of a test for mutations on the APC gene is $750, which appears low. The analysis does not include the cost of genetic counseling. Alternative strategies for testing family members are not addressed, such as haplotype analysis in place of DNA analysis (42). Hence, the study may not offer sufficient information for a full policy analysis of genetic testing of FAP family members.

Several prevention-effectiveness studies address HNPCC, much more common than FAP as a cause of colorectal cancer. Missense mutations on four DNA repair genes have been found in at least 70% of HNPCC-affected families, most of which are mutations on the hMSH2 and hMLH1 genes. Penetrance for colorectal cancer among individuals with HNPCC genotypes is between 80% and 90%, based on data from highly affected HNPCC kindreds, and the age of onset appears to be an average of 45 years. However, HNPCC is not limited to colorectal cancer; endometrial, ovarian, urinary tract, and stomach cancers are also common (43,44). Expert opinion is that members of HNPCC-affected families should receive routine colonoscopy every 1 to 3 years from age 25, along with endometrial cancer screening in women, unless they are known to not be mutation carriers (45). Prophylactic surgery is also an option, but is not generally recommended.

Two decision analyses of case management of HNPCC mutation carriers have been published (46,47). One, by Vasen et al., is a cost-effectiveness analysis of colonoscopic surveillance every 3 years beginning at age 25 compared to no surveillance (46). The health outcome is life expectancy. No analytic perspective is specified, but the stated uses include influencing legislation and health benefits packages. Only medical costs are included, with no indication of the methods by which costs were computed or derived. The analysis concludes that surveillance of carriers is cost-saving. Because colonoscopic surveillance is already the standard of care for HNPCC carriers, it is not clear that this a policy-relevant study question. A more sophisticated decision analysis by Syngal et al. evaluates a dozen strategies for a hypothetical 25-year-old female mutation carrier, including surgery, colonoscopic surveillance every 3 years, and no surveillance (47). Health outcomes include both life expectancy and quality-adjusted life-years. The intended audience consists of patients and health care providers, which is appropriate given the study design, which excludes costs and addresses only individual harms and benefits.

The assumptions and results of the two decision analyses are summarized in Table 18.3. The two analyses conclude that colonoscopic surveillance can raise life expectancy by 7 years (46) and 13.5 years (47). The marked difference in projected gains in life expectancy from colonoscopy reflects differences in three assumptions, for each of which the second study makes assumptions that are more favorable to screening. The lifetime risk of developing colorectal cancer (CRC) is assumed to be 80% in Vasen et al. (46) and 88% in Syngal et al. (47). The higher the cumulative risk, the greater the benefit of prevention. Similarly, the worse the prognosis is following diagnosis of cancer, the greater is the benefit of prevention. Syngal et al. (47) assume a poor prognosis for HNPCC carriers with CRC, the same as for noncarriers. However, another study reports HNPCC carriers who develop CRC are more likely to have localized disease, a relatively favorable prognosis, and higher age- and stage-specific survival rates than other CRC patients (48). Finally, the greater is the efficacy of colonoscopy, the greater is the benefit of surveillance. Both studies (46,47) cite the same article (49) as the source of their divergent estimates. A sensitivity analysis in Vasen et al. (46) indicates that assuming a 62% efficacy, as in Syngal et al. (47), adds less than an additional year of life to the

Table 18.3 Assumptions and Results of Analyses of Surveillance of 25-Year-Old HNPCC Mutation Carriers

	Vasen et al. (46)	Syngal et al. (47)
Lifetime risk of CRC	80%	88%
Prognosis of CRC in carriers relative to sporadic CRC cases	Lower	Same
Efficacy of colonoscopy	44%	62%
Gain in life expectancy	7.0 years	13.5 years

CRC, colorectal cancer.

projected gain from surveillance, indicating that this accounts for relatively little of the difference in results.

Both studies exclude from consideration extracolonic malignancies. The lifetime risks for HNPCC mutation carriers are reported to be 43% for endometrial cancer (in women) and 9% to 19% for gastric, biliary tract, urinary tract, and ovarian cancers (43). As carriers are at elevated risk of other cancers, it is incorrect to assume that preventing CRC leads to normal life expectancy. The assumption is particularly problematic for the study by Syngal et al. (47), owing to the high rate of endometrial cancer in female HNPCC mutation carriers. Indeed, in a population-based study, the risk of endometrial cancer in female HNPCC carriers was found to exceed that of colorectal cancer (44). Syngal et al. acknowledge the high mortality risk from other cancers and the impact that excluding this factor from their model has on their results.

The second study models the harms and benefits of preventive options (47). Quality-of-life weights are calculated from a panel of ten physicians. Two different prophylactic surgeries are modeled, proctocolectomy with an assumed 100% efficacy, and subtotal colectomy with an assumed 80% efficacy. Besides immediate surgery for a 25-year-old mutation carrier, various delays in surgery are modeled, but the results indicate little gain in life expectancy. As shown in Table 18.4, if life expectancy is the outcome, immediate prophylactic surgery is preferred to surveillance. In contrast, QALYs are higher for the surveillance option. Syngal et al. conclude that providers should be very cautious in recommending prophylactic surgery for high-risk patients, and that surveillance may be a more attractive option.

Syngal et al. (47) correctly interpret the sensitivity of their results to variation in utility weights. Of ten individual physicians who provided weights, QALYs would be maximized by the surveillance strategy for only five. Total colectomy would maximize expected utility for almost as many, four, and only one would maximize expected utility by choosing subtotal colectomy. The results are also sensitive to small variations in epidemiologic parameters whose magnitudes are not well established. For example, if colonoscopy is less than 57% effective (compared to a baseline estimate of 62% effectiveness),

Table 18.4 Expected Outcomes of Surgery Versus Surveillance of 25-Year Old HNPCC Mutation Carrier*

	Life-years	*QALYs*
Immediate proctocolectomy	2.1	−3.1
Immediate subtotal colectomy	1.8	−0.3

* As reported in reference 47.

surveillance no longer maximizes QALYs at mean utility weights. The main conclusion of the study is that no global generalization can be made as to which option is optimal. An individualized assessment is needed that incorporates personal preferences.

Finally, one analysis has evaluated the potential cost-effectiveness of population-based carrier screening for HNPCC (50). One attractive feature of this analysis is its candid approach to dealing with uncertainty. Rather than specify a best estimate of the prevalence of the condition, the investisators use a very wide range of prevalences, from 1 to 50 per 10,000 population. To favor screening for the sake of argument, it was assumed that surveillance would prevent all CRC mortality, that survival of HNPCC carriers with CRC is no better than for other CRC patients, and that no carriers die from extracolonic malignancies. Also, the assumed penetrance for CRC of 80% is based on classical HNPCC kindreds, and CRC penetrance among mutation carriers in the general population is lower, reportedly 56% (44). The conclusion is that screening is unlikely to be cost-effective unless there is a very high prevalence of the mutation in the population (above 23 per 10,000). The investisators also point out that if realistic assumptions had been made, the case for population-based screening would appear even less promising.

Inherited Breast and Ovarian Cancer Syndrome

Germline mutations on the BRCA1 and BRCA2 genes are autosomal dominant mutations that lead to elevated risks of breast and ovarian cancer. The prevalence of BRCA1 and BRCA2 mutation carriers is 1 to 2 per 1000 in the general population. Perhaps 5% of breast cancers and up to 10% of ovarian cancers are attributable to these mutations (51). The exact penetrance of BRCA1 and BRCA2 mutations is unclear. In high-risk families, the probability of developing breast cancer by age 70 is 84% to 85% (52,53). The risk of ovarian cancer to age 70 is more variable. The best estimate of this risk for BRCA1 carriers in high-risk families is 44%, allowing for variation among alleles (52). If no allowance is made for heterogeneity, the estimated risk is 63%, but this estimate is biased because of the selection criteria for recruitment of families. The risk for BRCA2 mutation carriers is lower, 27% on average (53). Penetrance may be lower for mutation carriers in the general population. Two studies conducted among individuals not recruited from high-risk families report cumulative risks of 56% and 68% for breast cancer and 16% and 21% for ovarian cancer, respectively (54,55). A BRCA2 mutation common in Iceland is reported to pose a cumulative risk for breast cancer to age 70 of only 37% (56).

Prevention-effectiveness methods applied to BRCA1 and BRCA2 mutations address two questions. Should an individual seek genetic testing? If a susceptibility genotype is found, is preventive action beneficial? Because the benefits of genetic testing depend on an affirmative response to the second question, we first address the efficacy of prophylactic treatment.

Four published decision analyses model the benefits of prophylactic surgeries for BRCA1 and BRCA2 mutation carriers (57–60). The studies calculate results for a range of penetrance estimates. Estimates of penetrance among members of high-risk families are used to define "high" risk. A study of Ashkenazi Jewish volunteers is used to define a "medium" or "average" risk in three of the studies (57–59). In the first two of these studies "low" risk is defined on the basis of the lower bounds of the 95% confidence intervals. The choice of labels and risk groups is arbitrary; it may be that the "medium" risk parameter reflects relatively low risk.

Two of the studies share an author and epidemiologic assumptions but differ by focusing, respectively, on "average"-risk (59) or "high"-risk women (60). Both also model the decision to be tested. Both studies conclude that the benefit of being tested is also a function of the probability of being a mutation carrier and the probabilities of accepting prophylactic surgery with and without the test results.

The published decision models share several features. Each uses Markov models and age-specific cancer incidence rates. Each assumes that prophylactic oophorectomy is accompanied by hormone replacement therapy (HRT), at least until age 50. Finally, the analyses assume that BRCA2 carriers have the same risks for breast and ovarian cancer as do BRCA1 carriers. The assumption that ovarian cancer risk is the same for BRCA1 and BRCA2 mutation carriers likely overstates the benefits of prophylactic removal of the ovaries.

Other assumptions differ among the models, associated with marked differences in outcomes. Table 18.5 lays out the differences in key assumptions for scenarios involving a hypothetical 30-year-old female mutation carrier. One key parameter is the risk of ovarian cancer in high-risk mutation carriers. Schrag et al. (57) used the 44% estimate from Easton et al. (52) in place of the 63% estimate. The latter estimate ignores variability in risk across mutations and may overstate the benefits of oophorectomy.

Another key parameter is the prognosis of ovarian cancer in mutation carriers. Grann et al. (58) assume the same grim prognosis observed in most women with ovarian cancer, whereas the other three studies all base their models on a finding from one study that the 5-year survival rate from ovarian cancer is several times higher for BRCA1 mutation carriers (61). The better the prognosis, the smaller the potential benefit from prophylactic oophorectomy. One study has reported that the efficacy of prophylactic oophorectomy in preventing ovarian or peritoneal cancer is 50% (62), and two of the decision analyses use this number (57,58). The other studies rely on an expert panel to come up with a 78% efficacy estimate (59,60). Finally, these last two studies

Table 18.5 Assumptions of Decision Analyses of Prophylactic Surgeries for BRCA1/BRCA2 Mutation Carriers

	Schrag et al. (57)	Grann et al. (58)	Tengs et al. (59)	Berry and Parmigiani (60)
Risk of breast cancer— "high" by type of carrier "medium"	85% 60%	85% 56%	NA 56%	85% NA
Risk of ovarian cancer— "high" by type of carrier "medium"	40% 20%	63% 16%	NA 16%	63% NA
Prognosis in ovarian cancer compared to noncarriers	Much better	Same (very poor)	Much better	Much better
Efficacy of prophylactic mastectomy	85%	90%	92%	86%
Efficacy of prophylactic oophorectomy	50%	50%	77%–91%	78%
Efficacy of oophorectomy in preventing breast cancer	0%	0%	9%–25%	11%

NA, not applicable.

Table 18.6 Expected Outcomes of Prophylactic Surgeries for 30-Year Old BRCA1/BRCA2 Mutation Carriers from High-Risk Families, Compared to No Prophylaxis

	Schrag et al. (57)	Grann et al. (58)	Berry and Parmigiani (60)
Immediate prophylactic mastectomy	5.3 years	2.8 years	2.4 QALYs
Immediate prophylactic oophorectomy	1.7 years	2.6 years 0.5 QALYs	6.7 QALYs
Immediate mastectomy and oophorectomy	7.6 years	6.0 years 1.9 QALYs	11.9 QALYs
Mastectomy and 10-year delay in oophorectomy	7.2 years		

assume that oophorectomy reduces the risk of breast cancer, and HRT reduces but does not eliminate this benefit.

In line with varying assumptions, the studies yield varying results, reported in life-years and QALYs in Table 18.6. For high-risk women, it is only possible to make pairwise comparisons. Table 18.6 gives results for the options of immediate prophylactic surgery for a hypothetical 30-year-old high-risk female mutation carrier.

The greater projected gain in life expectancy from oophorectomy in Grann et al. (58) compared to Schrag et al. (57) is due to the assumptions of higher penetrance and worse prognosis from cancer by Grann et al. compared to

Schrag et al. The same difference in assumptions has the effect of reducing the expected benefit of prophylactic mastectomy in Grann et al. compared to the Schrag et al. study. This is because mastectomy without oophorectomy is of lesser benefit if a mutation carrier has a very high risk of dying from ovarian cancer. For this reason, the projected gain in life expectancy with the combination of the two surgeries differs by much less across the studies than the relative gains from the individual surgeries. Compared with the same QALYs metric used in Grann et al., Berry and Parmigiani (60) project much greater benefit from oophorectomy, attributable to a much higher assumed efficacy of prophylactic oophorectomy in preventing both ovarian and breast cancer (Table 18.6).

The question of whether a 30-year-old mutation carrier should delay ovarian surgery has been addressed in two studies, with opposing results. Schrag et al. (57) report that delaying prophylactic oophorectomy by 10 years would have almost no effect on life expectancy (−0.4 years in high-risk carriers). In contrast, Tengs et al. (59) conclude that delaying oophorectomy "is never optimal," but they model only a 20-year delay versus no delay. Schrag et al. (57) assume that virtually no cases of ovarian cancer in high-risk carriers occur before age 40. This assumption is based on data for "average"-risk women (54) and is inconsistent with data on age of onset of ovarian cancer in BRCA1 carriers (61) as well as expert opinion recommending that women from high-risk families consider surgery by age 35 (63).

The impact of surgery on quality of life has been modeled in three studies. Grann et al. (58) calculate QALYs based on a time–trade-off survey of 54 women and mean expected utilities. There was a wide range of responses, and one-quarter of the women surveyed considered there to be no loss of quality of life from prophylactic surgery. Using mean values of the responses, the investigators report that the negative effects of surgery offset most of the gain in expected years of life for high-risk carriers and result in negative net effects on QALYs for medium-risk carriers. The other two studies report QALYs calculated using arbitrary utility weights selected for expository purposes (59,60). The researchers assume that oophorectomy would lower quality of life by only 1%, compared to an average reduction of 9% in the Grann et al. (58) study.

Grann and Colleagues also address cost-effectiveness (58). The analytic perspective is not stated, although one audience mentioned is health insurance companies. In the base analysis, health care costs are based on Medicare payments, which are lower than costs faced by private insurers. Nonmedical costs are excluded, which means that the societal perspective, essential for drawing policy conclusions about cost-effectiveness, is not followed. The discount rate is 3%, appropriate for a health system perspective but less so from a payer's perspective. In the base analysis, prophylactic oophorectomy and the combination of oophorectomy and mastectomy are reported to be cost-saving, and on this basis the authors recommend that insurance companies cover these procedures in BRCA1 and BRCA2 mutation carriers. This conclusion is premature for at least three reasons. First, the parameters are not defined from the perspective of health insurers. Second, with QALYs, net health effects are negative for medium-risk carriers. This disqualifies the interventions as cost saving for that group of patients. Third, the model assumes that all women receive surveillance recommended for high-risk female patients, including ultrasound every 6 months for ovarian cancer surveillance. If all mutation carriers are not already receiving this expensive procedure, any cost savings to payers may not be realizable.

Conclusions

The application of prevention-effectiveness methods to genetic-related diseases or conditions has received increasing attention. The opportunity of identifying individuals in a preclinical state and initiating preventive therapy promises benefits in averting disease treatment costs and suffering. However, results from quantitative prevention-effectiveness models to date are difficult to apply to public policy decisions regarding genetic testing or prevention strategies. This is due only in part to limitations in the application of prevention-effectiveness methods. Typically, the epidemiologic data are too incomplete to reach firm conclusions about the long-term health benefits of screening or testing.

Even if the epidemiologic data were stronger, published standards for conducting economic evaluations of health interventions (1,5–9) have not generally been followed. For example, few cost-effectiveness studies use the societal perspective, as is recommended for any study addressing public health policies. Most analyses only include medical costs. Few studies report multivariate sensitivity analysis (5). Relatively few studies have used population-based data on health preferences to analyze quality-of-life considerations in assessing the harms and benefits of interventions.

Reliable cost data are generally lacking. For most of the conditions reviewed here, no empirical data on the cost of screening is available. For cystic fibrosis, although cost estimates are available from operational screening programs, data on the costs of providing health services to screened and unscreened infants are lacking. Studies of genetic testing for autosomal recessive disorders may fail to take into account genetic counseling and other costs associated with identifying unaffected mutation carriers (10). Finally, even if cost data and assumptions are unassailable, cost-effectiveness is not by itself a sufficient basis for policy decisions. A full policy analysis must address potential ethical and social harms, distributional issues, and broader societal and political ramifications.

The most important contribution of prevention-effectiveness research to public health genetics to date is in providing a framework for understanding complex policy decisions. Clear-cut issues do not require mathematical models to resolve. When there are major harms or uncertainty about benefits, a decision analysis can shed new light. Prevention-effectiveness studies help to identify data needs, facilitate understanding of uncertainty, and focus discussion on critical issues. For example, adverse effects of prophylactic surgery have been shown to be influential in deciding on optimal strategies for carriers of autosomal dominant cancer-susceptibility genes. Use of the societal perspective favors screening strategies that minimize the number of follow-up visits and invasive tests, since costs to individuals and families are important factors to consider when formulating public health policies.

Another issue identified as important in cost-effectiveness studies of genetic testing is the cost of DNA mutation analyses. As technology evolves, the costs of tests for multiple mutations are expected to decline and the cost-effectiveness of screening strategies that incorporate DNA tests should become more favorable relative to other approaches. For this reason, it is important to retain flexibility in modeling as new data emerge rather than to regard a particular set of results as definitive.

References

1. Haddix AH, Teutsch SM, Shaffer PA, Dunet DO (eds). Prevention effectiveness: a guide to decision analysis and economic evaluation. New York: Oxford University Press, 1996.

2. Khoury MJ and the Genetics Working Group. From genes to public health: applications of genetics in disease prevention. Am J Public Health 1996;86:1717–1722.

3. Zweifel P, Breyer F. Health economics. New York: Oxford University Press, 1997.

4. Sonnenberg FA, Beck JR. Markov models in medical decision making: a practical guide. Med Decis Making 1993;13:322–338.

5. Drummond MF, O'Brien B, Stoddart GL, Torrance GW. Methods for the economic evaluation of health care programmes (2nd ed). Oxford: Oxford University Press, 1997.

6. Gold MR, Siegel JE, Russell LB, Weinstein MC (eds). Cost-effectiveness in health and medicine. New York: Oxford University Press, 1996.

7. Drummond MF, Richardson WS, O'Brien BJ, et al. User's guides to the medical literature: XIII. How to use an article on economic analysis of clinical practice. Are the results of the study valid? JAMA 1997;277:1552–1557.

8. Gessner BD, Teutsch SM, Shaffer P. A cost-effectiveness evaluation of newborn hemoglobinopathy screening from the perspective of state health care systems. Early Hum Dev 1996;45:257–275.

9. Provenzale D, Lipscomb J. A reader's guide to economic analysis in the GI literature. Am J Gastroenterol 1996;91:2461–2470.

10. Drummond MF, Jefferson TO. Guidelines for authors and peer reviewers of economic submissions to the BMJ. The BMJ Economic Evaluation Working Party. BMJ 1996;313:275–283.

11. Lieu T, Watson S, Washington AE. Cost-effectiveness of prenatal carrier screening for cystic fibrosis. Presentation to NIH Consensus Development Conference on Genetic Testing for Cystic Fibrosis, Bethesda, MD, April 14–16, 1997.

12. Teutsch SM. A framework for assessing the effectiveness of disease and injury prevention. MMWR 1992;41 (No. RR-3).

13. Barber JA, Thompson G. Analysis and interpretation of cost data in randomized controlled trials: review of published studies. BMJ 1998;317:1195–1200.

14. Holtzman NA, Watson MS. Promoting safe and effective genetic testing in the United States: final report of the Task Force on Genetic Testing. Baltimore: Johns Hopkins University Press, 1998.

15. Cutting GR. Genetic epidemiology and genotype/phenotype correlations. National Institutes of Health. Program and Abstracts. NIH Consensus Development Conference on Genetic Testing for Cystic Fibrosis, Bethesda, MD, April 14–16, 1997.

16. Dankert-Roelse JE, te Meerman GJ. Long-term prognosis of patients with cystic fibrosis in relation to early detection by neonatal screening and treatment in a cystic fibrosis centre. Thorax 1995;50:712–718.

17. Farrell PM, Kosorok MR, Laxova A, et al. Nutritional benefits of neonatal screening for cystic fibrosis. N Engl J Med 1997;337:963–969.

18. Wald NJ, Morris JK. Neonatal screening for cystic fibrosis: no evidence yet of any benefit. BMJ 1998;316:404–405.

19. Centers for Disease Control and Prevention. Newborn screening for cystic fibrosis: a paradigm for public health genetics policy development—proceedings of a 1997 workshop. MMWR 1997;46 (No. RR-16).

20. National Institutes of Health. Program and Abstracts. NIH Consensus Development Conference on Genetic Testing for Cystic Fibrosis, Bethesda, MD, April 14–16, 1997.

21. Wilcken B, Wiley V, Sherry G, Bayliss U. Neonatal screening for cystic fibrosis: a comparison of two strategies for case detection in 1.2 million babies. J Pediatr 1995;127:965–970.

22. Gregg RG, Wilfond BS, Farrell PM, et al. Application of DNA analysis in a population-screening program for neonatal diagnosis of cystic fibrosis (CF): comparison of screening protocols. Am J Hum Gen 1993;52:616–626.

23. Qualls NL, Cono J, Kelly AE, Khoury MJ. The economic impact of population-based newborn screening for cystic fibrosis. MMWR 1997;46 (No. RR-16):14–15.

24. Grosse SD, Webster D, Hannon WH. Cost comparison of IRT and IRT/DNA screening of newborns for cystic fibrosis in New Zealand. Presentation to Thirteenth National Neonatal Screening Symposium, San Diego, March 2, 1998.

25. Burke W, Press N, McDonnell SM, et al. Hemochromatosis: genetics helps to define a multifactorial disease. Clin enet 1998;54:1–9.

26. Niederau C, Fischer R, Purschel A, et al. Long-term survival in patients with hereditary hemochromatosis. Gastroenterology 1996;110:1107–1119.

27. Burke W, Thomson E, Khoury MJ, et al. Hereditary hemochromatosis: gene discovery and its implications for population-based screening. JAMA 1998;280:172–178.

28. Adams PC, Kertesz AE, Valberg LS. Screening for hemochromatosis in children of homozygotes: prevalence and cost-effectiveness. Hepatology 1995;22:1720–1727.

29. Adams PC, Gregor JC, Kertesz AE, Valberg LS. Screening blood donors for hereditary hemochromatosis: decision analysis model based on a 30-year database. Gastroenterology 1995;109:177–188.

30. Balan V, Baldus W, Fairbanks V, et al. Screening for hemochromatosis: a cost-effectiveness study based on 12,258 patients. Gastroenterology 1994;107:453–459.

31. Buffone GJ, Beck JR. Cost-effectiveness analysis for evaluation of screening programs: hereditary hemochromatosis. Clin Chem 1994;40:1631–1636.

32. Phatak PD, Guzman G, Woll JE, et al. Cost-effectiveness of screening for hereditary hemochromatosis. Arch Intern Med 1994;154:769–776.

33. Baer DM, Simons JL, Staples RL, et al. Hemochromatosis screening in asymptomatic ambulatory men 30 years of age and older. Am J Med 1995;98:464–468.

34. Merryweather-Clarke AT, Pointon JJ, Shearman JD, Robson KJ. Global prevalence of putative haemochromatosis mutations. J Med Genet 1997;34:275–278.

35. Adams PC, Valberg LS. Screening blood donors for hereditary hemochromatosis: decision analysis model comparing genotyping to phenotyping. Am J Med Genet 1997;17:A1207.

36. Bassett ML, Leggett BA, Halliday JW. Analysis of the cost of population screening for haemochromatosis using biochemical and genetic markers. J Hepatol 1997; 27:517–524.

37. McDonnell SM, Witte DL, Cogswell ME, et al. Strategies to increase detection of hemochromatosis. Ann Intern Med 1998;129:980–986.

38. Lynch HT, Lynch JF. Genetics of colonic cancer. Digestion 1998;59:481–492.

39. Ambroze WL Jr, Orangio GR, Lucas G. Surgical options for familial adenomatous polyposis. Semin Surg Oncol 1995;11:423–427.

40. Lynch HT, Smyrk TC. Classification of familial adenomatous polyposis: a diagnostic nightmare. Am J Hum Genet 1998;62:1288–1289.

41. Cromwell DM, Moore RD, Brensinger JD, et al. Cost analysis of alternative approaches to colorectal screening in familial adenomatous polyposis. Gastroenterology 1998;114:893–901.

42. Gazzoli I, De Andreis C, Sirchia SM, et al. Molecular screening of families affected by familial adenomatous polyposis (FAP). J Med Screen 1996;3:195–199.

43. Aarnio M, Mecklin JP, Aaltonen LA, et al. Life-time risk of different cancers in hereditary non-polyposis colorectal cancer (HNPCC) syndrome. Int J Cancer 1995; 64:430–433.

44. Dunlop MG, Farrington SM, Carothers AD, et al. Cancer risk associated with germline DNA mismatch repair gene mutations. Hum Mol Genet 1997;6:105–110.

45. Burke W, Petersen G, Lynch P, et al. Recommendations for follow-up care of individuals with an inherited predisposition to cancer: I. Hereditary nonpolyposis colon cancer. Cancer Genetics Studies Consortium. JAMA 1997;277:915–919.

46. Vasen HF, van Ballegooijen M, Buskens E, et al. A cost-effectiveness analysis of colorectal screening of hereditary nonpolyposis colorectal carcinoma gene carriers. Cancer 1998;82:1632–1637.

47. Syngal S, Weeks JC, Schrag D, et al. Benefits of colonoscopic surveillance and prophylactic colectomy in mutation carriers for hereditary nonpolyposis colorectal cancer. Ann Intern Med 1998;129:787–796.

48. Watson P, Lin KM, Rodriguez-Bigas MA, et al. Colorectal cancer survival among hereditary nonpolyposis colorectal cancer family members. Cancer 1998;83:259–266.

49. Jarvinen HJ, Mecklin JP, Sistonen P. Screening reduces colorectal cancer rate in families with hereditary nonpolyposis colorectal cancer. Gastroenterology 1995; 108:1405–1411.

50. Brown ML, Kessler LG. The use of gene tests to detect hereditary predisposition to cancer: economic considerations. J Natl Cancer Inst 1995;87:1131–1136.

51. Parmigiani G, Berry D, Aguilar O. Determining carrier probabilities for breast cancer-susceptibility genes BRCA1 and BRCA2. Am J Hum Genet 1998;62:145–158.

52. Easton DF, Ford D, Bishop DT. Breast and ovarian cancer incidence in BRCA1-mutation carriers. Breast Cancer Linkage Consortium. Am J Hum Genet 1995; 56:265–271.

53. Ford D, Easton DF, Stratton M, et al. Genetic heterogeneity and penetrance analysis of the BRCA1 and BRCA2 genes in breast cancer families. The Breast Cancer Linkage Consortium. Am J Hum Genet 1998;62:676–689.

54. Struewing JP, Hartge P, Wacholder S, et al. The risk of cancer associated with specific mutations of BRCA1 and BRCA2 among Ashkenazi Jews. N Engl J Med 1997;336:1401–1408.

55. Whittemore AS, Gong G, Itnyre J. Prevalence and contribution of BRCA1 mutations in breast cancer and ovarian cancer: results from three U.S. population-based case-control studies of ovarian cancer. Am J Hum Genet 1997;60:496–504.

56. Thorlacius S, Struewing JP, Hartge P, et al. Population-based study of risk of breast cancer in carriers of BRCA2 mutation. Lancet 1998;352:1337–1339.

57. Schrag D, Kuntz KM, Garber JE, Weeks JC. Decision analysis—effects of prophylactic mastectomy and oophorectomy on life expectancy among women with BRCA1 or BRCA2 mutations. N Engl J Med 1997;336:1465–1471.

58. Grann VR, Panageas KS, Whang W, et al. Decision analysis of prophylactic mastectomy and oophorectomy in BRCA1-positive or BRCA2-positive patients. J Clin Oncol 1998;16:979–985.

59. Tengs TO, Winer EP, Paddock S, et al. Testing for the BRCA1 and BRCA2 breast-ovarian cancer susceptibility genes: a decision analysis. Med Decis Making 1998; 18:365–375.

60. Berry DA, Parmigiani G. Assessing the benefits of testing for breast cancer susceptibility genes: a decision analysis. Breast Dis 1998;10:115–125.

61. Rubin SC, Benjamin I, Behbakht K, et al. Clinical and pathological features of ovarian cancer in women with germ-line mutations of BRCA1. N Engl J Med 1996; 335:1413–1416.

62. Struewing JP, Watson P, Easton DF, et al. Prophylactic oophorectomy in inherited breast/ovarian cancer families. J Natl Cancer Inst Monogr 1995;17:33–35.

63. Burke W, Daly M, Garber J, et al. Recommendations for follow-up care of individuals with an inherited predisposition to cancer: II. BRCA1 and BRCA2. Cancer Genetics Studies Consortium. JAMA 1997;277:997–1003.

19

Impact of genetic information and genetic counseling on public health

Judith L. Benkendorf, Beth N. Peshkin,
and Caryn Lerman

In this chapter we will review the evolution of the genetic counseling process as an integral part of genetic health and medical care. We will discuss the settings in which genetic counseling presently occurs and who provides these services. This discussion will include the role of genetic counseling as an adjunct to testing in preconception and prenatal care, as well as in general medicine. In addition, we will review literature on the impact of various genetic counseling and testing programs on patients' quality of life and health-related behaviors. We will conclude with a discussion of the current role of genetic counseling in public health and an examination of the advantages and disadvantages of a model that addresses and integrates the goals of both fields while maximizing the strengths of each.

Genetic Counseling

Definition and History
The term *genetic counseling* was introduced by Sheldon Reed in 1947 (1). Working at the University of Minnesota's Dight Institute, Reed found himself providing support and genetic information—often recurrence risk information—to an increasing number of families. Believing that the scope of this activity reached beyond genetic social work, he introduced the expression "genetic counseling."

The roots of the contemporary genetic counseling movement can be traced to departments of medicine and pediatrics in academic centers, as physician and PhD medical geneticists evaluated individuals with mental retardation, birth defects, and conditions believed to be inherited. Their consultation included: diagnostic workups; medical management; information about the etiology of a condition, including its modes of inheritance, and the risks for that condition occurring among family members or future offspring; and support for patients and their families. With the introduction of mid-trimester amniocentesis and sonography to geneticists' prenatal diagnostic tools, genetic counseling services were established in departments of obstetrics and gynecology. An overview of the current practice of prenatal genetic counseling can be found later in this chapter.

In 1969, Sarah Lawrence College, in Bronxville, New York established the first graduate program for the preparation of master's level genetic counselors. Graduates of that program, trained in the science of medical genetics and the art of counseling, went on to become full-fledged members of health care teams, responsible for serving as liaisons between medical geneticists, laboratories, and families. From this point forward, the term *genetic counseling* referred to both a distinct profession and to an activity performed by an array of genetics specialists. Throughout this chapter, "genetic counseling" will be used to refer to this broader activity.

The widely accepted definition, developed in 1975 by an ad hoc Committee on Genetic Counseling of the American Society of Human Genetics, describes the work of genetic counseling professionals.

> *Genetic counseling is a communication process which deals with the human problems associated with the occurrence, or the risk of occurrence, of a genetic disorder in a family. This process involves an attempt by one or more appropriately trained persons to help the individual or family to: 1) comprehend the medical facts, including the diagnosis, probable course of the disorder, and the available management; 2) appreciate the way heredity contributes to the disorder, and the risk of recurrence in specified relatives; 3) understand the alternatives for dealing with the risk of recurrence; 4) choose the course of action which seems to them appropriate in view of their risk, their family goals, and their ethical and religious standards, and to act in accordance with that decision; and 5) to make the best possible adjustment to the disorder in an affected family member and/or to the risk of recurrence of that disorder (2).*

The values that distinguish genetic counseling from more traditional forms of medical consultation and counseling are spelled out in the Code of Ethics of the National Society of Genetic Counselors (NSGC) (3). The second section of the code describes the relationship of genetic counseling professionals with their clients and encourages them to strive to "respect clients' cultural traditions, circumstances, and feelings," and to "enable clients to make informed, independent decisions, free of coercion, by providing or illuminating necessary facts and clarifying alternative and anticipated consequences" (3). In the final section of this chapter, as we discuss the adaptation of current genetic counseling models to a public health model, we will examine the implications of the guidelines set forth in the NSGC Code of Ethics for the responsibilities that genetic counseling professionals have to society.

The Genetic Pedigree: A Personalized Risk-Assessment and Screening Tool

It is standard practice for genetics professionals to construct a genetic pedigree, or family tree, during encounters with patients seeking genetic services. During this process, a structured interview is used to gather information about the health histories of family members in multiple generations; standardized symbols (4) depict family relationships and the pattern of transmission of genetic conditions in the family. Accurate pedigrees provide the basis for assessing people's risks for both single-gene and multifactorial conditions and for making formal genetics referrals.

Patients who do not have genetic counseling at the time of prenatal diagnosis (or other genetic testing) miss the opportunity to have their pedigree analyzed by a genetics professional. In addition to their use in assessing reproductive risk factors (e.g., family history of mental retardation, birth defects, single gene disorders), pedigrees can provide a great deal of information about common adult-onset conditions. A number of these conditions may have a genetic basis, and in some cases it is possible to identify those individuals at highest risk and to modify personal risk by increased surveillance or by changes in lifestyle or health behaviors. Not only do pedigrees provide a basis for determining who should be offered genetic testing and surveillance and prevention opportunities, but they also allow for the identification of eligibility for genetic research studies. A carefully constructed and analyzed pedigree can sometimes even help allay patients' fears and save health care dollars by reducing the number of unnecessary genetic tests performed. It also can uncover critical information that can improve the accuracy of genetic counseling.

The multiple advantages of replacing conventional medical history-taking with the genetic pedigree-taking process, despite the labor-intensiveness of the latter, are listed in Table 19.1 (5).

Role of Genetic Counseling in Reproductive Health

Genetic testing provides prospective parents opportunities to obtain two distinct types of genetic information, each of which could influence their reproductive decisions. Information about the parents' carrier status for common autosomal recessive disorders can be obtained through heterozygote screening which is usually performed selectively on the basis of patients' ethnic backgrounds. Information about a developing fetus's health, well-being, and genetic status can be gleaned from prenatal screening tests such as sonography and

Table 19.1 Impact of the Genetic Pedigree on Medical Care

As a diagnostic and screening tool, the pedigree
1. Identifies genetic conditions in a family
2. Provides a basis for clinical diagnosis
3. Elucidates modes of inheritance
4. Allows for accurate genetic risk assessment and counseling
5. Documents complex family relationships pictorially
6. Identifies family members "at risk"
7. Is critical for genetic testing by linkage analysis
8. Facilitates referrals to genetics professionals and research protocols
9. Is easily stored and updated in the medical record
10. Promotes communication between medical team members.

---

maternal serum-marker screening, and from prenatal diagnostic procedures such as amniocentesis and chorionic villus sampling (CVS).

Prenatal Diagnosis Modalities

Maternal serum-marker screening is performed on a blood sample taken from a pregnant woman to identify those at increased risk of having a baby with certain birth defects, including spina bifida, anencephaly, Down syndrome, and trisomy 18. The patient's prenatal care provider usually educates the patient and elicits consent; the blood sample is then drawn during the 15th through 20th week of pregnancy. It is analyzed most commonly for concentrations of three chemicals found in women's blood during pregnancy: alpha-fetoprotein (AFP), beta human chorionic gonadotropin (hCG), and unconjugated estriol (uE3). Hence, this test is also referred to as a "triple screen." The concentrations of these three chemicals continue to change during pregnancy, but certain pregnancy complications and birth defects are known to produce specific changes, or patterns, in their concentrations. Maternal serum-marker screening is not diagnostic; it merely identifies women who are at increased statistical risk for having a child with certain birth defects. Women with abnormal triple screen results are referred for sonography, amniocentesis, and, often, genetic counseling.

A unique, statewide public health program for the dissemination, and subsequent follow-up, of maternal serum marker screening was established in California in 1986 (6). Administered and regulated by the California Department of Health Services, Genetic Disease Branch (GDB), the program is a private/public partnership that was initially authorized by the state legislature in 1985. By law, all pregnant women enrolled in prenatal care before 20 weeks' gestation must be provided a state-prepared patient education brochure describing the risks, benefits, and limitations of screening; women then sign the program's consent/refusal form. Under the strict quality control of the state, the specimens are analyzed by one of eight regionalized private laboratories. Positive test results are electronically transmitted to 14 regional state-approved coordinators located at various publicly and privately funded genetics centers contracted by the state to provide follow-up. In addition, the patient's clinician is notified. Genetic counseling services and any indicated prenatal diagnoses are then offered at one of 29 prenatal diagnosis centers with 90 satellite sites, all meeting state criteria for counseling, ultrasound, amniocentesis, and laboratory services. There is a one-time only, all-inclusive fee to participants of $115, which is billed to the patient or her insurance carrier. The state reports a steady increase in participation, from 41% of eligible women in 1986, to 63% of eligible women in 1994.

Although program officials claim that the "model has achieved its overall objective for providing universal access to low-cost, high-quality screening and follow-up" (6) the social risks of screening for the prevention of birth defects as a public health initiative cannot be ignored. Potentially, such programs run the risk that patients will not perceive the offering of these tests as an option they are free to decline, but rather as a recommendation to which they are expected to consent, even if they do not want to obtain the information to be learned. They may also feel obligated to act on abnormal results in a manner inconsistent with their values. Hence, the critical importance of the public education, genetic counseling, and multiculturally focused components of these programs cannot be overemphasized in order to assure their success in an environment that embraces individual patient autonomy. The burden on public health programs and officials may be even greater than those of private health service providers.

Sonography, also referred to as an "ultrasound examination," is a diagnostic imaging technique that uses ultra-frequency sound waves to visualize a developing fetus. Sonography is used routinely to date a pregnancy, determine the number of fetuses, and confirm the presence of a fetal heartbeat. Obstetricians and radiologists with special expertise in the use of sonography can assess fetal development and well-being and also determine the presence of major malformations or birth defects. Because sonography has no known medical risks to the mother or fetus, it is used widely, most commonly without much discussion about the benefits and risks of having the test. However, sonography can pose certain problems should parents begin learning information about their developing baby that they would rather not have known or are unprepared to handle.

Amniocentesis is a diagnostic prenatal test performed by a skilled obstetrician during the 15th through 18th week of pregnancy. The amniocentesis procedure involves using a needle, passed through a woman's abdomen into the uterus, to remove a small sample of the amniotic fluid in which the fetus is developing. The amniotic fluid contains cells shed by the developing fetus; both the amniotic fluid and the fetal cells can be used to test for biochemical disorders and single-gene conditions for which a DNA-based test exists, and to analyze the fetus's chromosome constitution. The most common reasons for performing amniocentesis include an increased risk for chromosome abnormalities due to advancing maternal age (i.e., greater than 35 years at the time of delivery); a family history of a genetic disorder for which prenatal tests are available; and possible problems detected by an abnormal result on a sonogram or maternal serum-marker screen. Because amniocentesis carries a very small increased risk for miscarriage, it is offered only when there is a sound medical indication.

Chorionic villus sampling (CVS) involves removing a very small sample of the cells in the outer layer of the developing placenta during the 10th through the 12th week of pregnancy. These cells, known as chorionic villi, contain the same genetic information as do the cells of the fetus and therefore can be used to test for chromosome abnormalities and biochemical and single gene disorders. CVS does not, however, provide information about neural tube defects or other anatomic malformations. Because the risk for miscarriage associated with CVS is slightly higher than that associated with amniocentesis and because it is not as widely available, CVS is reserved primarily for those women who will be 35 years or older at the time of delivery and those with a significant family history of a genetic disorder for which prenatal testing is available. In these cases, CVS allows parents to obtain genetic information earlier in pregnancy, and this may make it somewhat easier (at least physically) for an abnormal pregnancy to be terminated.

Genetic Counseling for Prenatal Diagnosis

Both amniocentesis and CVS were introduced in research trials—primarily undertaken at academic medical centers—designed to evaluate their safety and efficacy (7–9). Under these conditions, genetic counseling was an integral component of the testing process (10). Beyond facilitating parental decision making, genetic counseling ensured informed parental consent by delineating the risks, benefits, and limitations of the procedures as described above. Genetics professionals explored how parents would use the information they might learn from prenatal diagnosis. If a genetic abnormality was discovered, follow-up counseling could be provided by the same genetics professional who already had an established relationship with the patient and her partner.

Because CVS continues to be offered primarily within genetics units (either in hospitals or medical centers) and a few free-standing genetics centers, genetic counseling prior to CVS remains fairly standard. Amniocentesis, in contrast, is being performed with increasing frequency in obstetricians' offices. The methods by which patients receive pretest information and counseling are highly variable, ranging from being given a pamphlet or having a brief discussion with their physician, to receiving more formal counseling by a board-certified genetics professional. In the former two situations, if a genetic abnormality is discovered via analysis of the amniotic fluid, the patient's physician will either provide further counseling or refer the patient to a genetics professional. Such patient encounters are often difficult for both counselors and patients because a helping relationship must be built at a time of crisis for the family; counselors may also find themselves providing genetics education to patients who have not fully understood the nuances of the genetic information they could learn from these tests.

If current trends continue to move prenatal testing from the tertiary centers to the community, or primary-care settings, and third-party payers are less inclined to reimburse for patient education, most patients seeking prenatal diagnosis will receive genetic counseling only if an abnormal test result occurs. Pre-amniocentesis and pre-CVS genetic counseling will be provided to the shrinking proportion of patients referred to medical centers or to genetics professionals for their procedures and to those seeking genetics services because of a family history of a genetic condition or an abnormal sonogram (e.g., those other than patients of advancing maternal age or with abnormal maternal serum marker screening results). Although many obstetricians have become quite proficient at performing the prenatal diagnostic procedures, far fewer are proficient at conducting pretest genetic counseling and eliciting informed consent, interpreting complex genetic test results, and providing support during decision making about whether to continue or terminate a pregnancy.

Models for Delivery of Heterozygote Screening

Heterozygote screening refers to voluntary blood tests, generally performed before or during the early part of pregnancy, to identify individuals who carry one copy of an altered gene for a recessive disorder, in which receiving two copies of the altered gene results in an individual affected with the disorder. In other words, if both members of a couple are found to be carriers of the same altered gene, each pregnancy will have a 25% risk to have a child affected with the disease. It is estimated that each person carries 5 to 12 altered genes for recessive conditions. The likelihood that a given individual and his or her partner carry the same recessive gene increases if they share a common ethnic background. In their "Guidelines for Perinatal Care," the American Academy of Pediatrics and the American College of Obstetricians and Gynecologists (ACOG) state that *"Certain autosomal recessive diseases are sufficiently common to warrant screening for heterozygosity. For example, such screening should be offered to those of Jewish ancestry to identify carriers of Tay-Sachs disease; to Blacks, to identify carriers of sickle cell anemia; and to individuals of Italian, Greek and Oriental descent to identify carriers of thalassemia"* (11). The 1998 ACOG recommendation to add Canavan disease to the screening guidelines for Ashkenazi Jewish individuals (12) represents the first expansion to carrier screening protocols in over two decades. This trend is expected to continue, driven by the proliferation of new genetic tests as an outgrowth of the Human Genome Project.

In the United States the vast majority of heterozygote screening is currently provided by professionals rendering prenatal care (obstetrician-gynecologists, nurse-midwives, and family physicians), either preconceptionally or at the time of the first prenatal visit. The amount of patient education provided before-hand is not standardized, but often involves no more than the dissemination of a patient education brochure. Referrals for formal genetic counseling are rarely made unless both members of a couple are identified as carriers of the same recessive gene (13). Historically, sickle cell and Tay-Sachs screening programs have offered some important lessons about the impact of carrier screening on public health and policy, and are discussed in Chapter 4. These are lessons that should still not be forgotten today.

In 1983, the President's Commission for the Study of Ethical Problems in Medicine and Biomedical and Behavioral Research examined the sickle cell and Tay-Sachs screening models retrospectively and outlined the following parameters for heterozygote screening programs: (1) test results should be kept private and confidential; (2) decisions about screening should be made autonomously by the parents to ensure that screening is used for reproductive planning and not specifically to alter the gene pool; (3) pilot studies should be conducted to demonstrate that screening is valuable and can be conducted safely and effectively; (4) laboratory assays should have a high degree of sensitivity in the target population and be inexpensive enough to allow for cost-effective screening; (5) laboratory results should be reproducible; (6) the full range of prescreening and follow-up genetics education and counseling services should be available to the population being screened; and (7) equity of access to screening should be ensured (14). Given the nature of the health care delivery system in the United States, it seems unlikely that a national public health effort to provide heterozygote screening for reproductive risks will occur again; rather, such screening will likely continue to be provided under the purview of primary reproductive health care providers, with sensitivity to the parameters outlined in the President's commission report.

Role of Genetic Counseling in Adult-Onset Disorders

Common adult disorders such as heart disease, diabetes, certain types of mental illness and neurologic conditions, and many cancers have a genetic component that may be inferred from examination of the family history. However, as most of these conditions are multifactorial and only rarely are caused by mutations in a single gene, risk assessment is usually based on empirical data and pedigree analysis. Although genetic test results may provide more precise information for making risk estimates, including the determination of

Table 19.2 Characteristics of Monogenic Versus Complex Conditions of Adulthood

Parameter	Monogenic Conditions	Complex Conditions
Primary indication for genetic counseling/testing	At least one affected first-degree relative with distinct phenotype	Constellation of affected relatives in the same lineage
Goal of gene testing	Presymptomatic diagnosis	Identification of susceptibility
Gene penetrance	Usually very high	Highly variable
Phenotype	Somewhat consistent	Highly variable
Impact of environmental factors on phenotype	Usually minor	Potentially significant

those who are not at high risk, such testing is often not feasible or available. For some diseases, mutations in a single gene (monogenic diseases) appear to account for the majority of the cases. In these scenarios, options for testing and the approaches to counseling are quite different from those that exist for complex conditions, such as polygenic and multifactorial disorders (see Table 19.2). This section will highlight some monogenic and complex conditions of adulthood with particular attention to the utility of testing and the important issues that arise in the context of genetic counseling. A discussion of research on the outcomes of genetic testing for adult onset diseases can be found later in this chapter.

Monogenic Conditions

Monogenic conditions are genetic disorders that appears to involve only one gene. Following are two examples: familial adenomatous polyposis (FAP) and Huntington's disease (HD).

Familial Adenomatous Polyposis. An autosomal dominant condition affecting over 50,000 people in the United States (15), FAP is characterized by the development of hundreds of adenomatous colorectal polyps, which, if left untreated, invariably progress to cancer. The polyps are generally evident by the second or third decade of life but may also occur in early childhood. As more people live longer after being successfully treated for FAP (often by colectomy at a young age), the later manifestations of FAP may become apparent and cause significant morbidity. These later manifestations include gastric polyps and cancers of the thyroid and duodenum. Mutations of the APC gene are detectable in over 85% of patients with classic FAP (15). There is a compelling argument that people with FAP, especially those with an identifiable mutation, should inform their relatives about their risk and the availability of testing. Results of testing could then determine if intensive colon surveillance, which should commence in childhood, must be continued in carriers or eventually discontinued in noncarriers (16). Thus, genetic counseling and testing may help individuals and families obtain important information that can assist in critical medical management decisions.

Huntington's Disease. This condition is caused by mutations in the IT-15 gene on chromosome 4p (17). If people with the altered gene live to old age, they are virtually certain to be affected by an inevitable progression of characteristic neurological and psychiatric symptoms culminating in death. It is estimated that approximately 30,000 Americans have HD and that another 150,000 are at risk for inheriting HD from a parent (18). At present, there is no proven intervention or treatment that can delay or prevent the natural progression of HD. As a result, people considering genetic testing for HD should be informed that if they do carry the IT-15 mutation, learning so will not help them to reduce their risk of developing HD nor will it necessarily have an impact on management of the disease. However, testing may be potentially beneficial for psychological reasons and may aid in reproductive decision making (19,20). The impact of test results on an asymptomatic individual, whether positive or negative, can be substantial, which is why extensive genetic counseling and psychological evaluations are critical (21).

Complex Conditions

Most conditions of adulthood are caused by a complex interplay of multiple genes acting in conjunction with environmental factors. This scenario makes risk assessment particularly challenging. People with one or two affected relatives may be counseled with the use of empirical data, although these data sets have inherent limitations. When pedigree analysis reveals a Mendelian or monogenic pattern of inheritance, genetic testing is more likely to be of value in risk assessment. However, interpretation of results can be complicated by the uninformative nature of some negative test results and the unknown role of modifying factors. The following examples illustrate these points.

Alzheimer's Disease. Alzheimer's disease (AD) is very prevalent, affecting over 4 million Americans, and resulting in more than 100,000 deaths each year (22). Sporadic and familial forms of AD have been noted, and three genes have been associated with early onset forms of AD (22). The 4 allele of the apolipoprotein E (*APOE*) gene has been observed in both sporadic and familial cases of AD and has been associated with as many as half of all AD cases (22). In addition, the gene exhibits a dose-dependent relationship with risk. As is the case with many other genes conferring disease susceptibility, gene penetrance (i.e., the likelihood that a carrier will develop the disease) is not absolute, and the gene expressivity with respect to age of onset and severity is variable. Unlike HD, however, AD may be mitigated by certain medications, although the effectiveness of interventions with these medications is yet unproven (23–25). Thus, the psychological impact of learning that one is susceptible to AD may be less severe given that penetrance is unclear and there are proposed prevention and treatment options.

The strongest arguments supporting *APOE* genotyping relate to its potential usefulness for diagnostic purposes and for targeting individuals who may be good candidates for therapeutic interventions (26,27). Such testing is very controversial and has not been endorsed (26). Nevertheless, there may be valid reasons for offering genetic testing, but it should be offered only after careful discussion of the potential risks as well as the benefits of such testing, especially since positive test results could have negative psychosocial consequences for the person tested, as well as implications for his or her relatives.

Breast Cancer. Breast cancer, the most common malignancy affecting women in the United States (28), is another prevalent disease that can be inherited. Five percent to 10% of breast cancer cases have been attributed to alterations in a single susceptibility gene such as BRCA1 or BRCA2 (29); however, other less common genes also contribute to hereditary breast cancer, such as *p*53, ATM, and other unidentified genes (30). Mutations in the two major "cancer genes," BRCA1 and BRCA2, confer dramatically increased risks for breast cancer (36%–85%) and ovarian cancer (15%–60%), with a significant amount of the risk occurring premenopausally (31–33). In the absence of long-term outcome data or controlled clinical trials of interventions, there are no standard recommendations about ways to reduce these risks, and optimal methods of early detection have not been established; however, increased surveillance and discussion of prophylactic surgery have both been suggested as options for BRCA1/2 carriers (34–36). Heightened screening can be an effective early detection measure for at least some high-risk women. As the effects of reproductive and environmental factors, hormone use, and modifier genes become better characterized, clinicians may be able to tailor risk estimates for specific patients and provide additional options for risk reduction. Counselors should address the uncertainty associated with interpreting test results including issues related to the variable expression and incomplete penetrance of these genes and also discuss the uncertainty of efficacy of measures to reduce risk.

Although BRCA1 and BRCA2 mutations do not appear to be implicated strongly in the development of sporadic breast cancers, an improved understanding of the function of these genes and the development of new screening and prevention methods for carriers may translate into more effective prevention and treatment options for the population at large, thus dramatically affecting public health considerations. Eventually, women in the general population may also benefit from obtaining risk profiles based on genotyping of common low-penetrance genes such as GST and CYP17 (37,38) in combination with an assessment of environmental risk factors. It may then become possible to target interventions such as those involving chemopreventive agents to certain subsets of women on the basis of more precise risk estimates. This approach to identifying women at high risk for breast cancer was used in the NASBP-P1 Breast Cancer Prevention Trial of tamoxifen (39). In this trial, eligible high-risk women were identified on the basis of risk calculations derived from the Gail model, which uses family history, personal breast biopsy history, and reproductive factors to determine level of risk. The trial data indicate that the incidence of breast cancer was 49% lower among women who received tamoxifen. A substudy will determine what proportion of participants were BRCA1/2 carriers and whether the effects of tamoxifen in this population were comparable to the results as a whole. It is important to note that other studies of tamoxifen use by women at high risk for breast cancer did not show a protective effect (40,41).

Counseling Issues

Identifying individuals and families who are most likely to benefit from genetic testing and counseling can be a challenge. The clinician must consider several factors: the likelihood that a test will be informative; the degree of uncertainty associated with interpretation of results; the impact of test results on medical management; the implications of test results for family members; and the potential risks of testing, including insurance discrimination and psychological sequelae. For many monogenic conditions, mutations in the causative genes tend to be highly penetrant, meaning that carriers almost always develop the condition. Although steps may be taken to mitigate the disease course, the disorders are usually not entirely preventable. The interpretation of genetic test results for monogenic conditions can be relatively straightforward and can lead to an improved medical management plan for the individual tested. Because monogenic conditions have low rates of sporadic occurrence, true negative results (i.e., obtained after a mutation is identified in a family) indicate that the person tested is at very low risk for developing the disorder. Thus, the psychological relief from knowing one's genetic status can be substantial.

Genetic counseling and testing for complex disorders requires a broader discussion of the limitations of pedigree analysis and the uncertainties associated with test-result interpretation. Medical management for these types of conditions can be more varied and have differing or even an unknown level of efficacy. Because multifactorial conditions are common, people who test negative for a mutation in their family still need to be aware of general population risks and follow screening guidelines, when applicable.

Genetic Counseling Process

The issues described herein are of sufficient complexity that patients who have suggestive family histories should consider genetic counseling. Where genetic testing is an option, genetic counseling is critical both before and after testing. Counseling for adult-onset disorders is a departure from "traditional" genetic counseling in that the emphasis is not on reproductive risks, but on issues related to an individual's own disease susceptibility and preventive options (42). Typically, an initial genetic counseling session consists of the following: (*1*) a compilation of a detailed, minimum three-generation pedigree, with documentation of diagnoses where possible; (*2*) a review of the patient's medical history, with added attention to lifestyle habits, exposures, and current medical management; (*3*) a risk assessment based on pedigree analysis and empiric data, where applicable, including notification of anyone else who might be at increased risk for the condition in question; (*4*) a review of the potential benefits, limitations, and risks of genetic testing; (*5*) a discussion of medical management options, including uncertainties about efficacy; (*6*) consideration of the patient's and his or her family's coping mechanisms and their likely emotional response to risk assessment or genetic-testing results; and (*7*) provision of referrals and follow-up plan (43).

If an individual chooses to undergo genetic testing, post-test counseling is critical. In many cases, counseling at this time may focus less on the medical implications of the test results and more on the psychological integration of risk notification and issues in family communication. Thus, genetic testing and counseling should remain intrinsically linked. Such counseling maximizes the likelihood that people will better understand the meaning and interpretation of their test results and will obtain the greatest benefit from testing while minimizing the potential for adverse consequences.

Because of the nature of the conditions discussed in this chapter, individuals who might benefit from genetic counseling are most likely to be identified by physicians in disciplines such as internal medicine/primary care, gynecology, and oncology. These providers need to elicit and recognize suggestive family histories and to make referrals for genetic counseling when needed. Still today, much of the genetic counseling for adult-onset conditions is provided by genetic specialists who often work in university hospitals or tertiary-care centers. In fact, much of the early presymptomatic genetic testing occurs within the context of research protocols, which include institutional review board approval, genetic education and counseling, and informed consent. The comprehensive model of cancer-risk counseling may be useful in developing testing protocols for other conditions because it involves both pre- and post-test counseling, integrates epidemiologic data into risk assessment, and is often performed in a multidisciplinary setting (43,44). However, as new genetic technologies move into the primary-care arena, physicians in those settings may become increasingly responsible for providing pre-test education and counseling (45). In this situation, patients may be referred to a genetics specialist only in the event of a positive, uninterpretable or uninformative test result, an unusual family history, or other complex or unanticipated outcomes.

Implications

In examining the leading medical causes of death in the United States in 1997 (28), over half the conditions may have arisen from an inherited predisposition. Heart disease, cancer, and diabetes all develop as a result of combinations of exogenous and genetic factors. Genetic testing may have broad public health implications in that it may allow improved identification of those at increased risk for these and other illnesses; however, the full potential benefits of such testing are not likely to be obtained without concomitant genetic education and counseling (45), the realization of interventions to reduce risk, and widespread access to these services. A model that will likely develop to deal with common chronic adult-onset conditions will include risk assessment and management plans based upon genetic and environmental variables that will need to be tailored to each individual (46). Data obtained from epidemiologic studies and public health research will likely be used to develop the models. At this time, it is vital to educate people about the importance of knowing one's own family history, adhering to age-appropriate screening, and adopting healthy lifestyles and behaviors.

Outcomes of Genetic Counseling

In this section we review both the literature on outcomes of genetic testing and individual factors that may modify outcomes in different population groups.

Reproductive Intentions and Behaviors

Although change in reproductive behavior is not considered a primary outcome of genetic testing and counseling, preliminary data suggest that such testing may have an impact on reproductive choices. For disorders that are not preventable or successfully treated, carrier testing and subsequent prenatal diagnosis may provide an option for those who wish to have children and avoid having an affected child. In a screening program to detect carriers for hemoglobinopathies, Rowley et al. (47) reported that 55% of pregnant women identified as carriers suggested testing to their partners; however, only one-half of partners were actually tested. Among pregnant couples found to be at one-in-four risk to have an affected child, 47% accepted prenatal testing; however, the pregnancies were continued in all but one case (in which the woman was herself affected).

Similar outcomes were observed in screening programs for cystic fibrosis (CF). In one CF screening program in the United Kingdom, 57 of 100 identified carriers suggested testing to their partners, and 87% of those 57 partners were subsequently tested (48). Of those who participated in genetic counseling, 36% said that they would consider terminating an affected pregnancy, whereas 20% of those not receiving genetic counseling said they would. Similarly, Loader and colleagues (49) found that avoiding having an affected child was a primary motivation for accepting CF screening in a primary-care setting. People who agreed to undergo CF screening were more likely to report prior to screening that they would consider terminating a pregnancy if the fetus was affected. However, data on actual reproductive decisions by carrier couples are not available.

In a review of the literature on predictive testing programs for Huntington's disease, researchers indicated that childbearing decisions were reported as a primary motivation for testing by 20% to 60% of study participants (50). In an another study, three-fourths of participants reported that they would terminate a pregnancy if the fetus was found to have the HD gene (51). As yet, however, data on actual use and the outcomes of prenatal testing for HD have not been reported.

Behavior Modification and Personal Risk Reduction

Even though no interventions have been proven to reduce risk in carriers of BRCA1 and BRCA2 mutations, data from surveys of individuals at risk have suggested that behavior modification is a primary motivation for genetic testing. For example, in a study of first-degree relatives of breast cancer patients, 80% of respondents reported that obtaining more frequent screening tests was an important motivation for pursuing BRCA1 testing (52). In a study of hereditary breast–ovarian cancer families, 93% of women reported that they wished to obtain genetic testing in order to increase the frequency of cancer screening, and 85% were motivated by the desire to obtain information to make decisions about surgical prevention (53).

Although outcome data from genetic testing programs for most complex diseases are not yet available, preliminary data on genetic testing for cancer-predisposing genes suggest that these reported motivations may not translate into actual behavior changes (53). Among those aged 35 and older who were due for an annual mammogram, only 61% had a mammogram within 6 months after testing. Furthermore, only 6% adhered to the recommendations for biannual ovarian cancer screening tests. Such low percentages of women who followed recommended cancer screening practices following BRCA1/2 testing may be attributable at least in part to the limited data available on the efficacy of cancer screening among younger women at increased risk for cancer. However, even if efficacy was proven, some women still might not adhere to recommendations.

Reports documenting a lack of behavioral change among people found to be at genetic risk for lung cancer are particularly striking (54,55). Smokers who received genetic test results indicating a two- to four–fold increased risk for lung cancer associated with smoking reported short-term increases in their motivation to quit smoking and made more attempts to quit. However, they were no more likely to quit smoking than were smokers receiving standard counseling without genetic test results. Moreover, smokers found to be at increased risk reported short-term increases in depression symptoms; however, these symptoms returned to baseline 12 months later. Thus, even when there is an unequivocally beneficial action for reducing risk, genetic testing may not lead to the hoped for changes in health practices.

Quality of Life

Despite the potential medical benefits of genetic testing, there are concerns that disclosure of genetic information may create a significant emotional burden. Research on the psychological effects of prenatal and carrier testing was reviewed recently by Croyle and Lerman (56). This review, and a review of studies focused on HD (50), concluded that testing may lead to short-term increases in emotional distress but that most participants suffer no significant longer-term effects on their quality of life.

More recent reports extend these findings to other adult-onset diseases. For example, in the study of hereditary breast–ovarian cancer families noted above, people found to carry mutations in the BRCA1 or BRCA2 genes exhibited little change in depression symptoms or functional health status from their pre-test assessment to 6 months after the test (57). Prior to testing, their levels of distress were not different from those in the general population. Noncarriers of mutations experienced a significant improvement in mood during the month following testing, but their scores on this measure returned to baseline levels 6 months later. People who declined to be tested reported the highest levels of distress, but these levels were not significantly different from those of carriers or noncarriers; all scores before and after testing were well within the normal ranges. Interestingly, these results mirror the findings of Wiggins and colleagues (58), who studied people offered predictive testing for HD.

Although individuals found to carry disease-predisposing genes may not experience significant adverse psychological effects, there is evidence that testing may have more subtle influences on their quality of life. For example, Croyle and colleagues found evidence of short-term increases (1 to 2 weeks) in cancer-related distress among women identified as BRCA1 carriers who had not had a prior diagnosis of cancer or preventive surgery (59). Marteau and colleagues studied emotional responses following carrier testing for CF (60). Although they found that clinical levels of anxiety were not observed during the 3-year follow-up period, carriers and noncarriers differed significantly in more subtle cognitive and emotional responses (e.g., having troubling thoughts about the test results). Similarly, Tibben and colleagues (61) found that carriers of HD gene mutations experienced a variety of stress symptoms involving intrusive thoughts and avoidance of HD-related situations. However, they suggested that this pattern reflects a healthy coping response required to process the significance of subjects' test results. In general, the partners of carriers showed patterns of stress symptoms similar to those of tested individuals.

Individual Differences

Observing the lack of significant adverse psychological effects that genetic testing had on patients' overall quality of life, researchers have sought to determine whether particular subgroups of patients may be more psychologically vulnerable. A recent report found that precounseling levels of cancer-related stress may be a useful predictor of quality-of-life outcomes among individuals undergoing BRCA1/2 testing (57). However, contrary to expectations, people with high precounseling distress levels who declined to be tested were at greatest risk for subsequent psychological morbidity. A post hoc analysis indicated that this subgroup of patients had strong motivations to be tested yet were concerned about their ability to cope with the information and had some fear of discrimination.

In the HD testing arena, research has also begun to identify subgroups of patients who may be more vulnerable to the negative emotional effects of genetic information. Similar to the study of hereditary breast and ovarian cancer families noted above, Tibben et al. found that precounseling levels of HD-related distress predicted poorer psychological adjustment. However, in this study, the carriers and not the decliners, were more prone to adverse effects (62). In another prospective study of HD testing, mutation carriers who were closer in age to the estimated onset of HD in their family were significantly more distressed than were other carriers (63).

Other studies have focused on sociodemographic factors that might influence responses to genetic information. In their study of HD testing, Codori et al. found that marital status modified the psychological impact of testing (63). However, contrary to predictions, married carriers of HD mutations were found to be less well adjusted than were unmarried carriers. Among people tested for CF, women were found to respond more positively than men when informed that they were noncarriers and less positively when informed that they were carriers (60). Investigators suggest that these differences may be attributable to different appraisals of threats to reproduction among men and women.

In a randomized trial, ethnic differences were observed in the responses of women with a family history of breast cancer to two alternate BRCA1 pre-test education strategies: a standard education model and an education plus counseling model (64). Among black women, those who received education plus counseling were more likely to plan to be tested and to provide a blood sample for genetic testing than were those who received education only. They were also marginally more likely to report cancer-specific distress. Among white women, there were no differential effects of the interventions on these outcomes.

Other studies suggest that people also differ in their preferences for providers of genetic counseling. For example, in a study of healthy women with a strong family history of breast cancer, 42% preferred that pre-test education for BRCA1/2 testing be delivered by a genetic counselor, whereas 22% preferred an oncologist (65). For post-test counseling, 38% preferred an oncologist, while only 20% preferred a genetic counselor. However, women who desired supportive counseling during this session were significantly more likely to prefer a genetic counselor to an oncologist.

These studies provide important insights needed to begin to understand patients' preferences for different modes of genetic counseling and to identify patients who may be more psychologically vulnerable to the effects of genetic testing. The results of such research can be used to develop counseling approaches that can be tailored to an individual's informational and psychological needs and sociodemographic background.

The Future of Genetic Counseling and Public Health

Can the current genetic counseling model be applied to a population-based, public health approach to genetic screening and predisposition testing? The present-day genetic counseling model focuses on helping individuals and their families make informed, autonomous decisions rather than on motivating individuals to change their health behaviors to improve the health of society. Lessons learned from counseling individuals and families may be helpful in developing genetic testing for subsets of the population deemed to be at risk. Experiences with sickle cell and Tay-Sachs screening should have sensitized both health professionals and consumers to social issues that can arise when a specific racial or ethnic group is targeted for genetic screening and research. For example, concerns about stigmatization and discrimination associated with predisposition testing resurfaced recently when investigators revealed not only specific genetic mutations in BRCA1 and BRCA2 in the Ashkenazi Jewish community (66), but also specific genetic mutations for colon cancer and deafness in the same population.

Genetics professionals are committed to participating in activities that promote the well-being of individuals and society, as delineated in Section IV of the Code of Ethics of the National Society of Genetic Counselors (3). This includes keeping abreast of societal developments that may endanger the physical and psychological health of individuals, serving as sources of reliable information for policymakers and public officials, and keeping the public informed and educated about the impact on society of new technological and scientific advances. It is here that partnerships between genetics and public health professionals the begin, with the goal of improving the health of society without losing sight of the needs and experiences of individual patients and

Table 19.3 Board-Certified Genetics Professionals as of 9/99*

Genetics Specialty	Number of Diplomates with Certificates
Genetic counselors	1410
M.D. clinical geneticists	1006
Ph.D. medical geneticists	150
Clinical cytogeneticists	522
Clinical biochemical geneticists	180
Clinical biochemical/molecular geneticists (combined exam given in 1990 only)	49
Clinical molecular geneticists	284

*This table represents 3601 certificates, held by 3269 individuals.
(Information provided by Sharon Robinson, Administrator to the American Board of Medical Genetics and the American Board of Genetic Counseling; personal communication).

their families. The challenge of the new millennium will be for genetics professionals to maintain a balance between their duties to patients and families and their commitment to addressing and advancing public health interests. The addition of public health professionals to the genetics team and the addition of genetics professionals to the public health team is therefore critical to fulfilling these goals and responding to the profound limits of our nation's pool of genetics professionals, as illustrated in Table 19.3.

Public Health Professionals and Genetics Professionals: A Critical Partnership

Genetics services will increasingly become an integral component of health care, especially as genetic risk factors become better understood and interventions to reduce risk become available. Public health professionals will provide leadership in designing programs that target specific populations and assure that these programs are readily accessible to all segments of society, including minority and underserved groups.

Public health professionals can have a role in assuring that genetics education is incorporated into all levels of public and professional education. They will also be pivotal to the development of general and specific education materials regarding the risks, benefits, and limitations of genetic tests and interventions to reduce risk. These materials might take the form of printed media, interactive videos, CD-ROMs, and even public service announcements that will supplement the activities of genetics professionals in this realm, and make this information more accessible than it is today. It will be vital for these genetics educational materials to provide more than the facts. They should also challenge the public to engage in values clarification strategies that would allow them to think about whether they would consider genetic testing and assess how they might personally use the information gleaned from genetic tests.

Just as important is the growing need for public health professionals to work with the genetics community in responding to new and rapid scientific breakthroughs that can engender a great deal of public and professional misinterpretation and misunderstanding. As information about genetic advances and new genetic tests becomes available to the public through the media and the Internet, such publicity is likely to generate more widespread interest in genetic counseling and testing. Thus, public health professionals must be equipped to respond to new advances, and subsequent public reactions, by specifically targeting education programs to populations for whom genetic counseling and testing may not be appropriate, and the number of genetics specialists too constrained to address and allay each individual's concerns and fears.

As genetics permeates all medical and health care, public health professionals will be called upon to serve as critical links for case finding, referral, and follow-up. This approach will have the power to combine the skills and expertise of the genetics specialists, especially in working with complicated family situations, genealogies, and very rare conditions, with the long-standing relationship among public health professionals, individuals, and society.

Finally, because rapid advances in genetics are expected to continue into the foreseeable future and the time from gene discovery to test development and clinical application will continue to become more compressed, ongoing professional education of the existing workforce is just as critical as the training of new professionals and informing the public. Genetics and public health professionals will share roles as consultants and partners in both public and professional education, with the ultimate goals of optimizing health care and the appropriate utilization of services. Such educational efforts will help ensure that individuals considering genetic testing will have an opportunity to make informed decisions and will be less likely to experience adverse or unanticipated consequences as a result of those decisions.

References

1. Reed SC. A short history of genetic counseling. Soc Biol 1994;21:332–339.

2. American Society of Human Genetics. Report of the Ad Hoc Committee on Genetic Counseling of the American Society of Human Genetics. Am J Hum Genet 1975;27:240–242.

3. National Society of Genetic Counselors, Inc. National Society of Genetic Counselors Code of Ethics. J Genet Counsel 1992;1:41–43.

4. Bennett RL, Steinhaus KA, Uhrich SB, et al. Recommendations for standardized human pedigree nomenclature. Am J Hum Genet 1995;56:745–752.

5. Benkendorf JL, Fine BA. Improving medical communication using the tools of the genetic pedigree: toward a family-centered understanding. Abstract/poster presentation at the Oxford Conference on Teaching about Communication in Medicine, St. Catherine's College, Oxford, England, July 24–26, 1996.

6. Cunningham GC, Tompkinson DG. Cost and effectiveness of the California triple marker prenatal screening program. Genetics in Medicine 1999;1:199–206.

7. NICHD National Registry for Amniocentesis Study Group. Midtrimester amniocentesis for prenatal diagnosis: safety and accuracy. JAMA 1976;236:1471–1477.

8. National Institutes of Health. Antenatal diagnosis. Report of a Consensus Development Conference (NIH Publication No. 79-1973). Bethesda, MD: 1973.

9. Rhoads GC, Jackson LG, Schlesselman SE, et al. The safety and efficacy of chorionic villus sampling for early prenatal diagnosis of cytogenetic abnormalities. N Engl J Med 1989;320:609–617.

10. Powledge TM, Fletcher J. Guidelines for the ethical, social and legal issues in prenatal diagnosis: a report from the genetics research group of the Hastings Center, Institute of Society, Ethics and the Life Sciences. N Engl J Med 1979;300:168–172.

11. American Academy of Pediatrics and American College of Obstetricians and Gynecologists. Guidelines for perinatal care, (3rd ed). Elk Grove Village, IL: American Academy of Pediatrics, 1992, p. 56.

12. American College of Obstetricians and Gynecologists, Committee on Genetics. Screening for Canavan disease. Committee Opinion 212: Washington, DC, 1998.

13. U.S. Congress, Office of Technology Assessment. Cystic Fibrosis and DNA Tests: Implications of Carrier Screening, OTA-BA-532. Washington, DC: U.S. Government Printing Office, 1992. Appendix B, Case studies of other carrier screening programs. Q54-270.

14. President's Commission for the Study of Ethical Problems in Medicine and Biomedical and Behavioral Research. Screening and counseling for genetic conditions. Washington, DC: U.S. Government Printing Office, 1983.

15. Powell SM, Peterson GM, Krush AJ, et al. Molecular diagnosis of familial adenomatous polyposis. N Engl J Med 1993;329:1982–1987.

16. Petersen GM, Brensinger JD. Genetic testing and counseling in familial adenomatous polyposis. Oncology 1996;10:89–94.

17. The Huntington's Disease Collaborative Research Group. A novel gene containing a trinucleotide repeat that is expanded and unstable on Huntington's disease chromosomes. Cell 1993;72:971–983.

18. Huntington's Disease Society of America. Huntington's disease. http://neuro-www2.mgh.harvard.edu/. . .ingtonsdisease.nclk#factsataglance1998.

19. Wiggins S, Whyte P, Huggins M, et al. The psychological consequences of predictive testing for Huntington's disease. N Engl J Med 1992;327:1401–1405.

20. Holloway S, Mennie M, Crosbie A, et al. Predictive testing for Huntington disease: social characteristics and knowledge of applicants, attitudes to the test procedure and decisions made after testing. Clin Genet (Denmark) 1994;46:175–180.

21. Quaid KA. Presymptomatic testing for Huntington disease: recommendations for counseling. J Genet Counsel 1992;1:277–302.

22. Lendon CL, Ashall F, Goate AM. Exploring the etiology of Alzheimer disease using molecular genetics. JAMA 1997;277:825–831.

23. Sano M, Ernesto C, Thomas RG, et al. A controlled trial of selegiline, alphatocopherol, or both as treatment for Alzheimer's disease. N Engl J Med 1997;336:1216–1222.

24. Stewart WF, Kawas C, Corrada M, Metter EJ. Risk of Alzheimer's disease and duration of NSAID use. Neurology 1997;48:626–632.

25. Yaffe K, Sawaya G, Lieberburg I, Grady D. Estrogen therapy in postmenopausal women. JAMA 1998;279:688–695.

26. Post SG, Whitehouse PJ, Binstock RH, et al. The clinical introduction of genetic testing for Alzheimer disease. JAMA 1997;277:832–836.

27. Mayeux R, Saunders AM, Shea S, et al. Utility of the apolipoprotein E genotype in the diagnosis of Alzheimer's disease. N Engl J Med 1998;338:506–511.

28. Landis SH, Murray T, Bolden S, Wingo PA. Cancer statistics, 1998. CA Cancer J Clin 1998;48:6–29.

29. Claus EB, Schildkraut JM, Thompson WD, Risch NJ. The genetic attributable risk of breast and ovarian cancer. Cancer 1996;77:2318–2324.

30. Greene MH. Genetics of breast cancer. Mayo Clin Proc 1997;72:54–65.

31. Struewing JP, Hartge P, Wacholder S, et al. The risk of cancer associated with specific mutations of BRCA1 and BRCA2 among Ashkenazi Jews. N Engl J Med 1997;336:1401–1408.

32. Ford D, Easton DF, Stratton M, et al. Genetic heterogeneity and penetrance analysis of the BRCA1 and BRCA2 genes in breast cancer families. Am J Hum Genet 1998;62:676–689.

33. Easton DF, Ford D, Bishop DT, et al. Breast and ovarian cancer incidence in BRCA1-mutation carriers. Am J Hum Genet 1995;56:265–271.

34. Burke W, Daly M, Garber J, et al. Recommendations for follow-up care of individuals with an inherited predisposition to cancer: II. BRCA1 and BRCA2. JAMA 1997;277:997–1003.

35. Piver MS, Jishi MF, Tsukada Y, Nava G. Primary peritoneal carcinoma after prophylactic oophorectomy in women with a family history of ovarian cancer. Cancer 1993;71:2751–2755.

36. Hartmann L, Schaid DJ, Woods JE, et al. Efficacy of bilateral prophylactic mastectomy in women with a family history of breast cancer. N Engl J Med 1999;340:77–84.

37. Helzlsouer KJ, Selmin O, Huang H, et al. Association between glutathione-S-transferase M1, P1, and T1 genetic polymorphisms and development of breast cancer. J Natl Cancer Inst 1998;90:512–518.

38. Feigelson HS, Coetzee GA, Kolonel LN, Ross RK, Henderson BE. A polymorphism in the CYP17 gene increases the risk of breast cancer. Cancer Res 1997;57:1063–1065.

39. Fisher B, Costantino JP, Wickerham DL, et al. Tamoxifen for prevention of breast cancer: report of the National Surgical Adjuvant Breast and Bowel Project P-1 study. J Natl Cancer Inst 1998;90:1371–1388.

40. Powles T, Eeles R, Ashley S, et al. Interim analysis of the incidence of breast cancer in the Royal Marsden Hospital Tamoxifen Randomised Chemoprevention Trial. Lancet 1998;352:98–101.

41. Veronesi U, Maisonneuve P, Costa A, et al. Prevention of breast cancer with tamoxifen: preliminary findings from the Italian randomised trial among hysterectomised women. Lancet 1998;352:93–97.

42. Lerman C, Croyle R. Psychological issues in genetic testing for breast cancer susceptibility. Arch Intern Med 1994;154:609–616.

43. Biesecker BB, Boehnke M, Calzone K, et al. Genetic susceptibility for families with inherited susceptibility to breast and ovarian cancer. JAMA 1993;269:1970–1974.

44. Schneider KA, Marnane D. Cancer risk counseling: how is it different? J Genet Counsel 1997;6:97–109.

45. Pyeritz RE. Family history and genetic risk factors: forward to the future. JAMA 1997;278:1284–1285.

46. White, R. Excess risk of colon cancer associated with a polymorphism of the APC gene? Cancer Res 1998;58:4038–4039.

47. Rowley PT, Loader S, Sutera CJ, Walden M, Kozyra A. Prenatal screening for hemoglobinopathies: I. A prospective regional trial. Am J Hum Genet 1991;48:439–446.

48. Watson EK, Mayall ES, Lamb J, Chapple J, Williamson R. Psychological and

social consequences of community carrier screening programme for cystic fibrosis. Lancet 1992;340:217–220.

49. Loader S, Caldwell P, Kozyra A, et al. Cystic fibrosis carrier population screening in the primary care setting. Am J Hum Genet 1996;59:234–247.

50. Van't Spijker A, ten Kroode HFJ. Psychological aspects of genetic counseling: a review of the experience with Huntington's disease. Patient Educa Counsel 1997; 32:33–40.

51. Bloch M, Fahy M, Fox S, Hayden MR. Predictive testing for Huntington disease: II. Demographic characteristics, life-style patterns, attitudes, and psychosocial assessments of the first fifty-one test candidates. Am J Med Genet 1989;32:217–224.

52. Lerman C, Seay J, Balshem A, Audrain J. Interest in genetic testing among first-degree relatives of breast cancer patients. Am J Med Genet 1995;57:385–392.

53. Lerman C, Narod S, Schulman K, et al. BRCA1 testing in families with hereditary breast-ovarian cancer. JAMA 1996;275:1885–1892.

54. Lerman C, Gold K, Audrain J, et al. Incorporating biomarkers of exposure and genetic susceptibility into smoking cessation treatment: effects on smoking-related cognitions, emotions, and behavior change. Health Psychol 1997;16:87–99.

55. Audrain J, Boyd NR, Roth J, Main D, Caporaso NE, Lerman C. Genetic susceptibility testing in smoking-cessation treatment: one-year outcomes of a randomized trial. Addict Behav 1997;22:741–751.

56. Croyle RT, Lerman C. Psychological impact of genetic testing. In: Croyle RT (ed). Psychosocial effects of screening for disease prevention and detection. New York: Oxford University Press,1995, pp. 11–38.

57. Lerman C, Hughes C, Lemon SJ, et al. What you don't know can hurt you: adverse psychologic effects in members of BRCA1-linked and BRCA2-linked families who decline genetic testing. J Clin Oncol 1998;16:1650–1654.

58. Wiggins S, Whyte P, Huggins M, et al. The psychological consequences of predictive testing for Huntington's disease. N Engl J Med 1992;327:1401–1405.

59. Croyle RT, Smith KR, Botkin JR, Baty B, Nash J. Psychological responses to BRCA1 mutation testing: preliminary findings. Health Psychol 1997;16:63–72.

60. Marteau TM, Dundas R, Axworthy D. Long-term cognitive and emotional impact of genetic testing for carriers of cystic fibrosis: the effects of test result and gender. Health Psychol 1997;16:51–62.

61. Tibben A, Timman R, Bannink EC, Duivenvoorden HJ. Three-year follow-up after presymptomatic testing for Huntington's disease in tested individuals and partners. Health Psychol 1997;16:20–35.

62. Tibben A, Duivenvoorden HJ, Vegter-van der Vlis M, et al. Presymptomatic DNA testing for Huntington disease: identifying the need for psychological intervention. Am J Med Genet 1993;48:137–144.

63. Codori A, Slavney PR, Young C, Miglioretti DL, Brandt J. Predictors of psychological adjustment to genetic testing for Huntington's disease. Health Psychol 1997;16:36–50.

64. Lerman C, Hughes C, Benkendorf JL, et al. Racial differences in testing motivation and psychological distress following pretest education for BRCA1 gene testing. Cancer Epidemiol Biomarkers Prev 1999;8:361–367.

65. Audrain J, Rimer B, Cella D, et al. Genetic counseling and testing for breast–ovarian cancer susceptibility: what do women want? J Clin Oncol 1998; 16:133–138.

66. Weiss R. Discovery of Jewish cancer gene raises fears of more than disease. Washington Post, Sept. 3, 1997, p. A3.

20

Lessons learned from newborn screening for phenylketonuria

Kenneth A. Pass

Newborn screening began in the United States in 1957. In that year California initiated screening for phenylketonuria (PKU) in some of its health clinics, using ferric chloride to test the urine in infant's wet diapers for phenylpyruvic acid. Over the next 5 years, 65,000 infants were tested by this procedure, and two newborns were identified with PKU (1). Recognizing the potential importance of this method to identify infants with PKU, the Children's Bureau (now the Maternal and Child Health Bureau, Genetics Services Branch, Federal Health Resources and Services Administration) sponsored a multistate urine screening program. The intent of the study was to determine the prevalence of PKU in the U.S. population. Although investigators had a test that could detect PKU and a system for recruiting subjects at random, they had not accounted for the fastidiousness of new mothers, who felt it inappropriate to bring their new child in for examination with a wet diaper, and, in many cases, refreshed the diaper just before the clinic appointment. Thus, the number of untested infants was quite large (up to 30%), and the tidiness of these new mothers introduced a bias for which the statisticians could not correct (2). Subsequent studies revealed that the ferric chloride diaper test used primarily in physicians' offices sometimes gave false-positive readings, depending on the brand of the disposable diaper used (3).

In retrospect, several lessons can be learned from these early attempts at newborn screening: (*1*) Specimen collection and delivery are very important; (*2*) newborn screening is more than a laboratory analytical procedure; (*3*) an untested infant is just that: untested; (*4*) follow-up and education are vital parts of every newborn screening program; and (*5*) a wet diaper probably is not the specimen of choice for population-based screening programs.

Ever since its beginning in California, newborn screening has expanded and advanced in ways and to levels never envisioned by those early investigators. Today a single drop of blood is not only sufficient for eight to ten assays of metabolic disease indicators, but also provides generous amounts of specimen for alternative tests; molecular techniques reveal the genetic instructions behind inborn metabolic defects; information on the infant's mother (genetic and infectious) is gleaned from the infant's drop of blood; data about the perinatal environment of the mother–fetus are transmitted via the blood collection form to the public health agency for use in perinatal health programs; and assessment of epidemics in the general population is accomplished from the newborn's specimen and used to manage mammoth public health intervention programs. As suggested by Clayton in her article, "These are heady times for newborn screening" (4).

It has been a long but exciting trip from the wet diaper to today's regional laboratory, which processes thousands of specimens daily. Researchers have learned much along the way that can, and should, serve future public health practitioners.

Lesson 1: Careful Planning Is Requisite for Success or, "Bob was lucky"

There are many reasons why Robert Guthrie, MD, PhD, acknowledged as the father of newborn screening, chose to direct his attention first to phenylketonuria (PKU). He discusses his reasons in the opening pages of the journal *Screening* (5). In addition, Jean Koch, in her wonderful book *Robert Guthrie— The PKU Story* (Hope Publishing House, 1997), also addresses the reasons for Guthrie's interest in PKU. Still, we should acknowledge that Guthrie's decision, although not a calculated one, was indeed fortuitous.

The incidence of PKU in the American population is about 1:16,000, sufficiently high that routine testing of any general population would quickly detect a positive finding. The major (classic) form of PKU is easily detected by the BIA (bacterial inhibition assay) developed by Guthrie. Although there are variant forms of PKU, some benign and others not, they will all appear as a positive result in the BIA, even though it is not a quantitative test. Only a few substances cause a false-positive or false-negative result in the BIA. The test is easy to perform, inexpensive, reliable, and works quite well with the newborn heel-stick blood specimen dried onto a special paper used by newborn screening programs (the Guthrie spot), without any extraction or pretreatment of the blood specimen. When he began testing for PKU, Guthrie chose a procedure he was then using in his cancer work rather than more sophisticated techniques such as chromatography; consequently, today we have the simple, elegant BIA.

Had Guthrie chosen first to develop a test for homocystinuria (as he did later in his career), undoubtedly he would have been successful with that assay, but he probably would not have established newborn screening. We know today that the Guthrie BIA will identify infants with some forms of homocystinuria, even though it is really a test for hypermethionenemia (6). We also know there are problems with the test's sensitivity and specificity, causing a large number of false results that must be followed to diagnosis. We know that homocystinuria is extremely rare, with fewer than one case identified per year among New York's 280,000 newborns. Thus, had Guthrie chosen to launch the ship of newborn screening on the ocean of homocystinuria, almost certainly he would have failed. The early trials demonstrating the efficacy of using the dried blood spot to identify PKU infants at 1 week of age would have had few positives had the testing been for hypermethionenemia.

Additionally, the tests would have failed to identify a group of infants clinically affected with homocystinuria; thus, the trials almost certainly would have been declared a failure for use as a public health program. And as we know all too well, once an idea is proven useless, it is very difficult for the researcher to find support necessary for continued investigation. Newborn screening would have lost its advocate, and the development of screening programs in the United States and around the world would certainly have been delayed. As others have recently pointed out, Bob Guthrie was, indeed, "fortunate" in the inborn condition he chose to study—and we are equally fortunate to have had him as a pioneer in the field of newborn screening (7).

Guthrie was also lucky in his timing. In the early 1960s, *Camelot*, the magical 1000 days of President John F. Kennedy's tenure, was in session. The President had a personal interest in mental retardation, and the country was willing and able to support that interest. Consequently, federal programs to reduce mental retardation were well funded (8). A decade earlier or later, the effort to establish newborn screening programs would likely have fared quite differently.

The lesson then is that we should be careful and deliberate when seeking to expand newborn screening profiles, for newborn screening has had its "dole of luck." Careful attention should be given to any assay proposed for a new disease addition: The test should be accurate, specific, and sensitive for the disease being sought; it should utilize the existing newborn specimen, the Guthrie spot; it should integrate into existing newborn screening programs, both in its analytical performance and in its time of expression of metabolic signal; it should have a prevalence in the population sufficient to warrant public health attention and population-wide testing; it should be affordable; and it should provide measurable benefits to the newborn being tested (i.e., there should be a therapy available). Many of these precepts are difficult to attain when the various agents or forces target newborn screening for reform.

Lesson 2: Newborn Screening Expansion or, "Acorns fall everywhere"

Initial newborn screening programs tested infants only for PKU. (Even today, universal testing in the United States includes only PKU and hypothyroidism [9].) As programs were started in the 1960s, and systems for specimen collection, testing, reporting, and follow-up were designed, all components were optimized for detection of PKU. Because detection of PKU by the Guthrie test required several protein feedings (or so it was thought then), and because new mothers routinely stayed in the hospital for up to a week following delivery, collection of the infant's heel-stick specimen during the first 3 to 5 days after delivery was easy to accomplish. The Guthrie test had sufficient sensitivity and specificity that the number of false-positive test results was kept to a minimum. Pediatricians were known to the family and hospital staff prior to discharge of the mother and infant, making follow-up easy. The newness of the programs stimulated the interests of medical staff and parents alike and increased the efforts of both parties to become more educated on the subject.

Subsequent additions to the screening profile, such as maple syrup urine disease (MSUD) and homocystinuria, required little, if any, effort on the part of the screening programs, as they required only implementation of another BIA. Adding other disorders, such as galactosemia, tyrosinemia, and sickle cell disease, brought additional problems such as timing for therapy options and carrier detection, but none that could not be resolved by existing procedures and policies. Testing for hypothyroidism introduced radioactive markers into the newborn screening laboratory and necessitated more stringent quality-control measures, which were provided by timely intervention of the Centers for Disease Control (CDC) through provision of a national quality-assurance program for newborn screening (10). The introduction of testing for biotinidase deficiency (11), although not without some controversy (even still, 12), presented no great difficulties for most U.S. newborn screening programs (13).

However, these were the last of the "acorns to fall near the tree." With the demonstration that antibodies to HIV-1, conveyed to the infant by an HIV-infected mother, could be detected by analysis of the Guthrie spot (14), newborn screening changed forever. During 1987 and 1988, newborn screening programs across the United States were recruited by the CDC to perform assays for HIV-1 antibodies on "blinded" specimens, i.e., on specimens left over after the traditional newborn testing that had been completely stripped of linkable identifiers (15). Results of these HIV assays proved valuable in charting the course of the HIV epidemic in the United States (16). One noteworthy example is that of New York State: Since November 1987, all infants born in the state have been tested for HIV antibodies at birth using blinded residual specimens, rather than a statistical sampling as was done in other states (17,18). Today with newborn HIV testing unblinded in New York and results reported for every infant born in New York (19), newly available therapies can be applied quickly and with promising results (20). Other states are considering this unblinding step.

The basic premise that newborn screening should benefit the newborn whose blood is being tested was not readily apparent in the blinded HIV seroprevalence studies described above. Some would argue that benefits are still insufficient to outweigh the risks, even now with reporting of newborn HIV test results (21). However, none can make a viable argument for benefit to the child whose newborn specimen is tested for Duchenne muscular dystrophy (DMD). There is no medical intervention for that child; the outcome is determined at birth. Yet DMD is a part of one newborn screening program in the United States and of several in Europe (22). The justification that has been advanced is that identifying affected infants as early as possible rather than waiting for symptoms of the disease to appear provides the family with an opportunity for counseling regarding future pregnancies (22).

With the addition of testing for hemoglobinopathies by many screening programs in the late 1980s, the issue of identification of carrier status first became real. The tests used to detect hemoglobin S and other abnormal hemoglobins also identify infants with the heterozygous or carrier condition (23). These children face no immediate medical crisis; indeed, they are free of symptoms throughout their life. Nevertheless, their carrier status warrants attention of geneticists for two reasons: It is indicative of the presence of the S mutation in the parents and other family members and is information that may be of value to them later in life during their reproductive years. (See Chapter 22 by Richard Olney.) The Sickle Cell, Thalassemia, and Other Hemoglobin Variants Committee of the Council of Regional Networks for Genetic Services (CORN) has addressed this issue recently and issued guidelines for follow-up of these infants (24).

Assays for apolipoprotein (25), glucose-6-phosphate dehydrogenase deficiency (26), and alpha-1-antitrypsin deficiency (27) using the Guthrie spot have been described. These assays are used to identify asymptomatic infants who, years hence, may develop clinical manifestations that could have been prevented by earlier therapy or lifestyle changes. Whereas the decision to screen a newborn population for alpha-1-antitrypsin might be justified on the basis of preventing severe liver disease, in other instances such decisions can be difficult, when the benefit of knowing remains unproven (28).

Testing for toxoplasmosis has been part of a major U.S. newborn screening program for several years, but has not migrated to other programs (29). A possible explanation for why it has not been included in other programs lies in two areas: analytical procedures and therapeutic intervention. The newborn assay for toxoplasmosis is not available commercially and, thus, must be

produced by the testing laboratory. Although many screening laboratories are
at ease producing components for the Guthrie BIA, the development and
routine production of immunoassay reagents present difficulties best not
brought into these high-volume laboratories. In addition, the medical intervention prescribed for infants infected with toxoplasmosis is itself risky and
not completely effective (30). These factors, coupled with the very low prevalence of toxoplasmosis outside certain ethnic groups, argue against inclusion
of toxoplasmosis screening in most American programs.

The lesson here states that rapid, unlimited expansion of newborn screening programs beyond their intended function can bring stress on the system
and untoward effects. Testing for HIV in Guthrie spots has illuminated
newborn screening, a public health program that, like water purification, had
operated in the background, usually out of public view. Prior to the introduction of HIV antibody testing, only a small segment of the medical community
and an even smaller part of the general population knew, in any detail, the
functions of newborn screening programs. Some programs even operated on
a "no news is good news" premise: the understanding that if the parents
weren't contacted with "bad news," then everything was okay, at least for PKU
and hypothyroidism. Admittedly, that may have been a bad policy, and is no
longer operative in most screening programs, which have extensive and effective educational and follow-up programs.

Still, to illuminate the public health operations of newborn screening and
simultaneously to associate them with the HIV epidemic has caused some
problems with their universal acceptance as beneficent operations. Concerns
were raised, sometimes strenuously, regarding confidentiality and privacy of
results, lack of informed consent for testing, completeness of blinding practices before commencing HIV tests, and ownership of the residual newborn
specimen (22). A sufficient amount of time has not passed to determine
whether the public health benefit accomplished through HIV seroprevalence
studies will outweigh the harm done to newborn screening.

Lesson 3: Newborn Screening Is More Than a Laboratory Function, or, "It takes a system to help a child"

The laboratory analysis of the Guthrie spot is perhaps the simplest and most
routine part of newborn screening. Bob Guthrie traveled to all parts of the
world teaching medical professionals to use his BIA. Today's automated analytical procedures, while introducing a level of complexity quite beyond that
of the BIA, are nevertheless routine procedures found in laboratories everywhere. If newborn screening were only a laboratory function, then it would
probably be introduced at the hospital of birth, or maybe even at the bedside
of the new mother, using recently developed point-of-care testing procedures
(31).

But newborn screening is much more than a laboratory test. As described in the CORN Guidelines for newborn screening (32), it is a system comprised of many professionals with expertise in many different areas of medical care: phlebotomist, laboratory technician, social worker, nurse, pediatrician, obstetrician, medical geneticist, and genetic counselor. Because of the infrequent occurrence of some of the conditions in newborn screening profiles, some as low as 1:250,000 births, it is possible for a laboratory to go long periods without detecting a true-positive infant. This infrequency can lead to disruption of quality-control parameters and needless anxiety on the part of laboratory staff in looking for a "problem" within the assay, when there really is none. Even in a program as large as New York's, there are years where there are no true positives for some of the eight conditions in the screening profile. For a laboratory testing 10,000 to 20,000 specimens annually, only a single PKU child might be expected each year, with some years having none. Because of the potential infrequency of positive results over a protracted period, experts recommend that a laboratory should process no fewer than 50,000 newborns each year (33) and argue against numerous small laboratories operating within a region.

In the only in-depth study of missed cases in newborn screening programs, Holtzman and Colleagues (34) reported a rate of less that two missed hypothyroid cases per million infants screened and one missed PKU for every 70 detected. Nearly half of these missed cases (43%) were attributable to laboratory procedures. Laboratory size was an associated factor, with laboratories processing fewer than 10,000 specimens each year having an error rate of 3.71 per 100,000 specimens tested, and laboratories processing 150,000 to 250,000 specimens annually having an error rate of 0.3 per 10,000 specimens tested. Ever since that report, over a decade ago, the CDC's intense quality-assurance programs have had a great impact on such procedures.

Without diminishing the importance of the laboratory, a major part of a newborn screening program consists of pre- and postanalytic components integrated with the laboratory analysis. The importance of specimen collection cannot be overemphasized; receipt of a poor specimen (either inadequate or somehow compromised) at the laboratory negates any analytical efforts that the laboratory might utilize. There are no reliable results obtainable from a poor specimen. Education of hospital staff both on proper specimen collection and on the impact of inadequate specimens is the tool that screening programs use to address the problem of poor specimen collection. When newborn screening is performed as part of a public health program, the program can bring the power of the public health agency to discussions regarding the collection of poor specimens by a hospital or other birthing facility.

Other preanalytical components of newborn screening include transportation of the specimen to the laboratory; provision of educational materials to parents about the tests and the importance of getting test results on their new infant; provision of specimen collection forms for hospitals; and consultation on questions of appropriateness of testing in unusual situations, such as cases where infants have been transfused or may not have a heel available for specimen collection. These activities normally are not viewed as laboratory functions, but are integral and routine for all public health-based newborn screening programs.

Postanalytic functions in a newborn screening program include much more than the reporting of the test results. In many cases, the results are reported to more than one health care provider: the infant's pediatrician, a staff physician at the hospital of birth, and a follow-up specialty care center that may be certified as such by the state health department. Reporting test results is the initial step in locating the child for confirmation of the screening results. Follow-up by program staff to ensure that the child and family receive appropriate medical care and all benefits made available through state-sponsored programs is one of the most important aspects of a complete newborn screening program. For any infant whose initial specimen is of such poor quality that it could not be tested, the screening program initiates a sequence of events to ensure that a second specimen is collected as quickly as possible. Additionally, many programs in the United States are now developing electronic linkages between the birth record and the newborn specimen. This technology helps to quickly identify infants from whom a specimen has not been obtained, or whose specimen has been lost in transit to the laboratory.

Because of the lifelong nature of the conditions detected by newborn screening profiles, it is not uncommon for the staff of a screening program to develop personal relationships with families of infants detected by the program. Several screening programs hold a "birthday" celebration each year during which parents can meet the individuals on the staff, whose efforts they have applauded (35). The support of parents and their interaction with the program staff are viewed by all involved parties as a positive aspect of newborn screening programs.

Lesson three, then, is that a laboratory alone does not constitute a newborn screening program. Numerous components are vital to a screening program's effectiveness, many of which cannot be provided by other than a public-sponsored program.

Lesson 4: Expanding the Scope of Newborn Screening, or, "Semper fidelis"

Newborn screening can trace its noble beginnings to a case in which a mother simply would not accept the notion that the illness in two of her children could not be defined. Inspired by these children, Asborn Fölling embarked on a series of experiments that defined the youngsters' disorder as PKU, a heretofore-unrecognized biochemical cause of mental retardation (36). Other pioneers in the field of newborn screening include Horst Bickel, who worked many long hours conceptualizing and then developing a diet that reduces the offending phenylalanine while supplying necessary amounts of other essential amino acids so as to prevent the damaging effects of PKU (37); Robert Guthrie (38), who, while developing not only the BIA but also the dried-blood specimen (for which he often expressed a desire to be remembered), refused to reap a profit (which would have occurred had he patented his process for testing newborns); Hirosi Naruse, who sought only to make newborn screening an integral part of Japanese medicine and public health, rather than to establish a national testing institute (39); Harvey Levy, who provided clear evidence of the benefits of early detection of these metabolic defects, and who, with Dick Koch, helped to expand the impact of newborn screening through elucidation of the syndrome of maternal PKU (40,41); and, Ed McCabe, who led newborn screening into the molecular age with demonstration of the utility of the Guthrie spot for analysis of DNA (42). These, our past and present leaders in newborn screening, and the many others too numerous to mention, have seen newborn screening as a supremely effective public health program, providing incalculable good for a minimum expenditure of the public's dollar.

Coincident with expansion of managed care in the United States has come the commercialization of newborn screening. Beginning with the assessment of fees by existing state programs, continuing with the subsequent augmentation of these fees to support other programs within the public health laboratory, and now culminating in the privatization of laboratory analysis of newborn specimens, the noble beginnings of newborn screening appear almost as relics rather than as examples to follow. This is not to say that laboratories outside of public health departments cannot provide quality testing, but as pointed out earlier in this chapter, the laboratory test is a single component of what needs to be a comprehensive program of care.

Partly because of the use of the newborn specimen for HIV antibody detection and partly because of the application of molecular techniques for the detection of DNA within the specimen, newborn screening programs have been subjected to criticisms in recent years, which had rarely been raised in the preceding decades of their operation. These criticisms relate mostly to collection of the specimen without written consent from the newborn's mother (43).

While one can make plausible arguments for requiring informed consent for any medical procedure or test, and perhaps most especially for genetic tests—of which newborn screening certainly qualifies (44)—pragmatists believe that full informed consent is precluded. Because newborn screening test profiles in most states now consist of several congenital conditions in addition to PKU and hypothyroidism, a fair and complete informed consent would require discussion of all of the quite complicated conditions that are tested for (eight in New York), the possible implications of positive (or negative) results, the risks of the specimen collection procedure (small but measurable), and the risks to the child if no testing is done. The ability to perform this educational process in a manner that is truly understandable to the average parent during a short, busy, and usually intense hospital period surrounding labor, delivery, and postpartum is questionable. Conversely, trying to move the consent process outside the birth arena quickly entangles the entire system with trails of paper and lost consent forms. Although most programs provide for refusal by the mother on religious grounds, this infers knowledge by the mother of this option; thus its designation as "informed dissent." Nevertheless, the criticisms continue, with only two viable solutions evident: continuation of the present system, in which efforts are made by screening programs to provide educational materials prenatally and at the first postpartum visit, or termination of programs except where informed consent can be documented prior to collection of the specimen. I see no middle ground that would allow for only token education and the extraction of "informed" consent from a frequently preoccupied, sometimes overwhelmed, woman immediately postpartum.

The Guthrie spot has proven to be almost a wonder of science. When dried into the special cotton fibers, enzymes are immobilized, proteins stabilized, amino acids fixed for easy retrieval, and DNA made virtually immortal (45). Bob Guthrie was truly ahead of his time! Today a casual search of medical literature will reveal literally thousands of citations using the Guthrie spot for applications far removed from newborn screening (46).

However, this same versatility could add to the problems of newborn screening programs by encouraging development of assays that might have little proven benefit to the child or family. Merely to develop an analytical result and report it—because it is there—is not necessarily helpful in the medical management of the child. Tandem mass spectrometry (MS-MS) has been cited as an example of this type of application in analyzing Guthrie spots. Although the technique is elegant by any scientific measure, it provides in an instant many potential metabolic anomalies. Incorporation of this methodology—or any other—must be accompanied by a proper understanding of the relationship between newborn screening and the benefit of disease detection in the newborn period. To use the instrument without such appropriate control would overwhelm any existing newborn screening follow-up system and perhaps lead to unnecessary anxiety and medical intervention. However, when used with thoughtful control, MS-MS has the capability of providing the same analytical precision while reducing the number of false-positive results (e.g., as occurred in screening for PKU) (47).

Levy has recently noted that MS-MS offers the solution to a long sought goal in newborn screening: the ability to perform multiple analyses on a single aliquot of the Guthrie spot (48). This characteristic of the procedure, which it shares with other techniques such as high pressure liquid chromatography (HPLC) (49), makes it very attractive and possibly an alternative to the sequential, multioperational procedures presently in use. Following proper validation and outcome studies, MS-MS could revolutionize the practice of newborn screening. Use of this emerging technology is presently the subject of much debate in the field of newborn screening. A HRSA conference held in May 1999 addressed the issue in detail and sought to provide guidance for its utilization in newborn screening.

It would be wrong not to mention here the successful use of the much-maligned urine specimen. Programs in Japan today use urine specimens to screen for neuroblastoma, a cancer found in children (50). The efficacy of this screening has been questioned by the results of a large multicenter collaborative study in North America (51). For many years, Quebec, Massachusetts, and New South Wales, Australia, used a urine specimen, in addition to the Guthrie spot, to screen for inborn errors not detectable in blood, such as hyperglycemia, methylmalonic acidemia, and cystinuria (52). The screening program in Quebec continues to perform such screening and, in 1988, reported its experience in screening over a million infants using urine specimens (53). New South Wales, in contrast, discontinued urine screening because of an experience considered less beneficial than required for its continuation (54). It seems safe to say urine screening is not an integral part of newborn screening, and that this is unlikely to change.

Lesson four, then, is that newborn screening has an admirable history, with mentors of whom we can be proud. As programs acquire new aspects, whether disease coverage, specimen type, test methodology, or funding source, we should consider our heritage and maintain the integrity of our actions.

Lesson 5: Importance of Staying Focused, or, "*Titanic*'s creed: Women and children first"

No one would question the fact that newborn screening started as a program to help newborn infants, its basic premise being that by early detection of elevated phenylalanine levels, important and effective therapeutic measures could be taken. Through the years, improvements have been made in infants' diets, and ongoing discussions debate the merits of dietary maintenance beyond early childhood (55). Because of the successful management of children with PKU, the little girls grew up to become young women who started families of their own, and a new term was coined: *maternal PKU*. This term was applied to women with PKU who were no longer being treated for their

PKU and who gave birth to children who had been damaged by their mother's disorder. Astute observations of Dick Koch and Harvey Levy quickly led to descriptions of this iatrogenic condition and to an effective treatment (56). Now, the monitoring of girls with PKU into adulthood is part of most newborn screening programs, and educational efforts have extended these findings to the obstetrical and gynecological communities.

Recent studies indicate that attention deficit hyperactivity disorder (ADHD) may be more common among individuals with PKU, further emphasizing the need to maintain contact with families identified by newborn screening programs (57). This lesson of extended follow-up has been learned quickly and now is being applied to long-term studies of children with hypothyroidism (58) and biotinidase deficiency (59). Will other unexpected and long-term sequelae associated with conditions in today's screening profiles surface? Newborn screening has become a truly intergenerational program.

Discussion elsewhere has addressed the use of newborn specimens for detection of conditions in the infant's mother. Similarly, the newborn screening specimen form itself has become a convenient vehicle for transferring medical data of various sorts. Information regarding the infant's feeding and transfusion status, treatment with antibiotics, birth weight, and sex is provided on many newborn screening forms. This information is used by the laboratory in evaluating results of tests whose interpretation is dependent on one or more of these factors. As part of the effort to ensure a complete vaccination series for every infant, the newborn screening form would be a logical initiator of a medical record for children. In New York and other states, information on the mother's hepatitis status is recorded on the newborn's specimen form. This information is used to monitor hospital performance of required hepatitis testing on all pregnant women prior to delivery so that treatment of an exposed infant can be achieved quickly postpartum. However, collection of other information, such as hearing test results and hospital payment status, causes one to question the use of newborn specimen forms as a convenient data-transfer system.

Many states have a duly constituted advisory board that regularly meets to oversee activities in the newborn screening program. Such a board can be very helpful by deflecting some of the outside influences (political and commercial) that seek to alter functions of a program. A board can also provide a strong advocacy when needed resources are lacking.

Lesson five reminds us that when newborn screening programs attempt to expand their activities beyond the immediate care of the newborn and mother, oftentimes the program becomes muddled and ineffective. The charge to newborn screening is first to provide a firm footing for the newly delivered life, and then provide continued follow-up of that individual so as to provide the same assurance for the next generation.

Lesson 6: Continuing Challenges, or, "The details bring out the Devil"

The function of a newborn screening program can be expressed very simply: to identify all newborns at risk for a defined set of disorders. Translating that function into practice exposes the extensive infrastructure necessary for successful operation of a newborn screening program. Although technological innovations have markedly altered the analytical procedures used by the program's testing laboratory, specimen collection has remained virtually unchanged. Inherent in specimen collection is proper identification of the infant whose blood is being taken. Some might consider this a simple matter; however, mistakes occur frequently. Usually errors become apparent when results on a repeat (confirmatory) specimen contradict the original findings. The program must then assume that two different infants provided the blood specimens, and that the initial infant remains outside the screening program's care. Prior to development of DNA identity testing, such a situation could only be resolved by retesting all infants resident in the nursery at the time of the original specimen collection, a process causing much disruption in the lives of both the parents and hospital staff. Now, a DNA identity test can indicate definitively if more than one infant is involved. This test can be performed on the Guthrie spot with results available in under 2 days (60).

As noted earlier, not all specimens received by the program's laboratory are of sufficient quality to enter into the testing procedures. Generally, these specimens are not tested, and a request for another specimen is immediately sent to the responsible party. The difficulty arises when some of the requested second collections are not made, thereby potentially denying some newborns the important medical interventions provided by the state. Education is the primary tool used by screening programs to reduce the number of invalid specimens, but the number never reaches zero (61).

More troublesome is the fact that some hospitals, for a number of reasons, never have a specimen collected for submission to the screening program. Among the causes are the presence of life-threatening illnesses in infants, which distract care providers from providing this testing, inter- or intrahospital transfers, birth outside a traditional medical facility, objection to the testing by parents or caregiver, and error in protocols at the birth facility. No matter the reason, when a specimen does not arrive at the screening laboratory, the event usually goes unnoted. As mentioned earlier, efforts to link birth records with newborn screening records will help to overcome this problem.

Still another issue that is important in specimen collection is that of timing. As mentioned previously, newborn screening protocols evolved when postpartum hospital stays were typically 5 to 7 days, and specimen collection was recommended when the infant was 3 days of age. As this postpartum hospitalization time shortened, so did the interval between birth and specimen collection, until, in 1993, a crisis was reached when infants less than 24 hours of age were being discharged from hospitals, and the collection of the newborn screening specimen took place during that short period after birth. Specimens collected from an infant so young do not give reliable test results for a number of conditions in the screening profiles, including PKU (62). A national conference in 1995 addressed these concerns and issued guidelines for newborn specimen collection (63). Fortunately for women, their newborns, and the screening programs, this "drive-thru" delivery process attracted such national attention that many states, and subsequently, the federal government, adopted legislation designed to prevent this from occurring.

Even with the apparent resolution of the "early discharge" dilemma, discussions regarding proper interpretation of screening results for thyroid disease still persist. The thyroid axis is in flux during gestation and immediately following birth (64); thus, the timing of specimen collection, coupled with the maturity of the newborn, can have profound effects on interpretation of the neonatal tests for hypothyroidism. Some programs have adopted a graded interpretation system (65) to account for these variables; others have instituted a two-specimen system, in which all infants are retested at about 14 days of age (66).

Despite the fact that most screening program regulations are quite specific concerning the conditions for which the laboratory is to test, frequently other related medical conditions will be determined, such as discovering hyperphenylalanenemia when testing for classical PKU. Screening programs generally report these mild elevations of phenylalanine, most often with no formalized follow-up procedures. Techniques using HPLC as a supplemental test on these specimens prior to notification of physician and family can greatly reduce the number of these false-positive results (67,68). Recent evidence indicates these elevations in phenylalanine may not be benign as had been previously thought, and that programs may need to institute rigorous follow-up efforts in cases where elevations are revealed (69). Similarly, programs screening for sickle cell disease identify many more infants with the heterozygous carrier condition than with true sickle cell disease. No consensus has yet been reached by the screening community regarding how best to deal with this situation (70), although CORN (Council of Regional Networks) has recently issued guidelines for carrier follow-up, which will help (24).

Lesson six informs us that the infrastructure of newborn screening programs is large and complex. Constant attention to all aspects of the program is necessary to ensure optimum performance. As many of the events that can impact on the program are extramural, it is important that the program speak with the authority of a public health department.

Lesson 7: We Must Learn from Our History, or "The more things change, the more they remain the same"

Even with such advances in testing technology as electronic reporting of test results, or electronic matching of databases to ensure that every infant is tested, if an infant is 12 days of age when the first specimen is obtained for newborn screening, irrecoverable time has been lost. Ideally, testing (and reporting) should take place within the first week following birth. If the infant's medical condition is less than ideal, the attending physician should be aware that the "safety net" of newborn screening is not in place and that all conditions in the screening profile should be a part of the differential diagnosis of a sick child. A major focus of newborn screening programs is to emphasize to the provider population that with a screening program, any result, whether positive or negative, should be considered tentative until a complete diagnostic evaluation has been done (71).

Only tests that provide a reliable, accurate result are useful. The CDC has been instrumental in providing materials to the screening laboratory for daily quality control of newborn screening tests and periodic evaluations of test performance though the provision of unknown specimens for testing by the screening laboratory. This support has greatly improved the performance of screening laboratories across the United States and in other parts of the world (72), a decade before CLIA '88 (federal legislation regulating clinical laboratory operations enacted in 1988) addressed similar issues of quality testing in clinical laboratories. Laboratories have become aware of the need for constant monitoring of test performance, and manufacturers have responded with controls and standards to facilitate this process.

The NCCLS (National Center for Clinical Laboratory Standards) has addressed newborn screening in several monographs, most recently describing again the proper method for collecting a newborn specimen (73). Although almost all newborn screening programs specify that the specimen be collected by heel-stick, the contention still persists that alternative methods are better (74). It is unlikely that this controversy will disappear, and, in fact, it serves a useful purpose in continuing to remind program personnel and clinicians of the need for a reliable, testable newborn specimen.

Paramount in all newborn screening programs is the recognition by program staff that each infant gets only a single chance for effective screening. The window within which the program operates is tiny and affords little room for error. Unlike diagnostic laboratories in which a specific result is sought and expected, and a repeat specimen is usually available, screening programs cannot anticipate a positive result and often cannot obtain a second specimen. Thus, technicians must be mindful that every specimen should be afforded special care, and that the very life of an infant could depend on the accuracy of their work. Laboratory testing in newborn screening can be boring and routine—but very important. Technical staff understand this, and they bring care and caring to each day's work.

Lesson seven reminds us that the basic tenets from the early studies of Bob Guthrie still apply to newborn screening programs today: Newborn population screening takes place one infant at a time. Both speed and extreme care are necessary components of the screening program.

In summary, from 35 years of screening experience in the United States, we have learned that newborn screening is, conceptually, a simple public health program, with well-defined goals. And yet, implementation of a successful program requires many components outside the testing laboratory, extensive expertise in areas ranging from phlebotomy to genetic counseling, attention to innumerable details, and, above all, dedication by all staff involved. In terms of public health impact, newborn screening touches more lives daily than perhaps any other public health program, and its influence now extends far beyond the perinatal period. As a lightening rod for public health debate on genetic testing, newborn screening has provided stimulus for a number of conferences and scientific deliberations, some casting it in an unfavorable light. Yet, thankfully, the debates continue. Each day in the United States, more than 15,000 newborns are tested for PKU, hypothyroidism, and several other congenital conditions and inborn errors of metabolism; each day, 14 newborns are referred for expert medical care for these conditions; and each day these programs improve the health of those children and this nation.

References

1. Pook BD. Testing for phenylketonuria. J Pediatr 1963;62:955–957.

2. Hormuth R. Personal communication.

3. Kishel M, Lightly P. Some diaper brands give false-positive test for PKU. N Engl J Med 1979;300:200.

4. Clayton EW. Issues in state newborn screening program. Pediatrics 1997;90: 641–645.

5. Guthrie R. The origin of newborn screening. Screening 1992;1:5–15.

6. Levy HL. Newborn and metabolic screening: past and present. N Engl J Med 1975;293:824–825.

7. Allen DB, Farrell PM. Newborn screening: principles and practice. Adv Pediatr 1996;43:231–270.

8. Hormuth R. Newborn screening systems. Proceedings of the 10th National Neonatal Screening Symposium, Seattle, WA, 1994, pp. 1–6.

9. Newborn Screening Committee. The Council of Regional Networks for Genetic Services (CORN), National Newborn Screening Report—1993. CORN, Atlanta, GA, January 1998.

10. Hannon WH, Slazyk WE. Quality control of newborn screening for inborn metabolic errors. In: Advances in neonatal screening. Proceedings of the 6th Neonatal Screening Symposium. New York: Elsevier Science, 1987.

11. Dove Pettit DA, Amador PS, Wolf B. The quantitation of biotinidase activity in dried blood spots using microtiter transfer plates: identification of biotinidase-deficient and heterozygous individuals. Anal Biochem 1989;179:371–374.

12. Warner-Rogers J, Wassbren SE, Levy HL. Cognitive function in early treated biotinidase deficiency: follow-up of children detected by newborn screening. Screening 1995;4:125–130.

13. Wolf B. Worldwide survey of neonatal screening for biotinidase deficiency. J Inherit Metabol Dis 1991;14:923–931.

14. Hoff R, Berardi VP, Weiblen BJ, Mahoney-Trout L, Mitchell ML, Grady GF. Seroprevalence of human immunodeficiency virus among childbearing women: estimation by testing samples of blood from newborns. New Engl J Med 1988;318:525–530.

15. Pass KA, Schedlbauer LM, Berns DS. Utilization of newborn screening specimens for HIV seroprevalence studies. In: Bellisario R, Mizejewski G (eds). Placental-mediated disorders: detection, treatment and management. New York: Alan R. Liss, 1989.

16. Novick LF, Berns D, Stricof R, Stevens R, Pass K, Wethers J. HIV seroprevalence in newborns in New York State. JAMA 1989;261:1745–1750.

17. Pass KA, Schedlbauer LM, MacCubbin PA, Glebatis DM. Comparison of newborn screening records and birth certificates to estimate bias in newborn HIV sero-surveys. Am J Public Health 1991;81(Suppl):22–24.

18. Hoxie NJ, Bergeront JM, Pfister JR, Hoffman G, Markwardt PA, Davis JP. HIV among childbearing women and newborns in Wisconsin. Wis Med J 1990;89: 627–631.

19. Pass KA. Newborn testing for HIV in New York. Proceedings of the 13th National Neonatal Screening Symposium, San Diego, CA, 1998.

20. Pass KA. Mandatory HIV testing: the New York experience. Proceedings of the 13th Annual Human Retrovirus Testing Conference, San Diego, CA, 1998.

21. Rips J, Powderly K. Mandatory HIV testing of newborns as public policy: the New York experience. 125th Meeting of the American Public Health Association, Indianapolis, IN, 1997.

22. Naylor EW, Hoffman J, Paulus-Thomas HB, Wessel KS, Reid BM, Schmidt BJ. Neonatal screening for Duchenne/Becker muscular dystrophy: reconsideration based on molecular diagnosis and potential therapeutics. Screening 1992;1:99–114.

23. Schedlbauer LM, Pass KA. Importance of multiple testing methods in hemoglobin screening. Proceedings of the 8th National Neonatal Screening Symposium, Saratoga Springs, NY, 1991, pp. 120–123.

24. Guidelines for Follow-up of Carriers of Hemoglobin Variants Detected by Newborn Screening. Council of Regional Networks, 1997.

25. Ohta T, Migita M, Yasutake T, Matsuda I. Enzyme-linked immunosorbent assay for apolipoprotein on dried blood spots derived from newborn infants: its application to neonatal mass screening for hypercholestrolemia. J Pediatr Gastroenterol Nutr 1988;7:524–531.

26. Missiou-Tsagaraki S. Screening for glucose-6-phosphate dehydrogenase deficiency as a preventive measure: prevalence among 1,286,000 Greek newborn infants. J Pediatr 1991;119:293–299.

27. Spence WC, Morris JE, Pass KA, Murphy PD. Molecular confirmation of alpha-1-antitrypsin genotypes in newborn dried blood specimens. Biochem Med Metabol Biol 1993;50:233–240.

28. Hitzeroth HW. Familial hypercholesterolemia in South Africa: to screen or not to screen? A national perspective. Screening 1996;4:233–246.

29. Hoff R, Weiblen BJ, Readon LA, Maguire JH. Screening for congenital toxo-

plasma infection. In: Bellisario R, Mizejewski G (eds). Placental-mediated disorders: detection, treatment, and management. New York: Alan R. Liss, 1989.

30. Wilson CB, Remington JS, Stagno S, Reynolds W. Development of adverse sequalae in children born with subclinical congenital toxoplasma infection. Pediatrics 1980;66:767–774.

31. Pass KA. Newborn screening in the next millennium. Seventh Internationl Congress of Inborn Errors of Metabolism, Vienna, 1997.

32. Therrell BL, Panny SR, Davidson A, et al. U.S. newborn screening system guidelines: statement of the Council of Regional Networks for Genetic Services. Screening 1992;1:135–148.

33. Andrews LB (ed). Legal liability and quality assurance in newborn screening. Am Bar Foundation (Chicago) 1985;54.

34. Holtzman C, Slazyk WE, Cordero JF, Hannon WH. Descriptive epidemiology of missed cases of phenylketonuria and congenital hypothyroidism. Pediatrics 1986; 78:553–558.

35. Andrews WC, Mitchell P. Celebration of life: Virginia statewide PKU party. Proceedings of the 8th National Neonatal Screening Symposium, Saratoga Springs, NY, 1991.

36. Folling A. Uber ausscheidung von phenylbrenztraubensaure in den harn als stoffwechselanomalie in verbindung mit imbezilliat. Hoppe Seyler a Physiol Chem 1934;227:169–176.

37. Bickel H, Gerrard J, Hickmans EM. Influence of phenylalanine intake on phenylketonuria. Lancet 1953;2:812–813.

38. Personal communication.

39. Personal communication, Robert Guthrie.

40. Levy HL. Maternal PKU: Control of an emerging problem. Am J Public Health 1982;72:1320–1321.

41. Koch R, Friedman EG, Azen C, et al. The North American Maternal PKU Collaborative Study. In: Wilcken B, Webster D (eds). Neonatal screening in the nineties. New South Wales, Australia: Kelvin Press, 1991, pp. 320–322.

42. McCabe ERB, Huang SZ, Seltzer WK, Law ML. DNA microextraction from dried blood spots on filter paper blotters: potential applications to newborn screening. Hum Genet 1987;75:213–216.

43. Ibid. (14).

44. Holtzman NA, Watson MS (eds). Promoting safe and effective genetic testing in the United States. Final report of the Task Force on Genetic Testing. NIH-DOE Worker, Group on Ethical, Legal, and Social Implications of Human Genuine Research, 1997.

45. Levy HL, Simmon JR, MacCready RA. Stability of amino acids and galactose in newborn screening filter paper blood specimens. J Pediatr 1985;107:757–760.

46. Pass KA. Use of dried blood specimens in clinical chemistry. Symposium. CliniChem 93. Albany, NY, 1993.

47. Reilly AA, Bellisario R, Pass KA. Multivariant discrimination for phenylketonuria (PKU) and non-PKU hyperphenylalaninemia after analysis of newborns' dried blood spot specimen for six amino acids by ion-exchange chromatography. Clin Chem 1998;44:317–326.

48. Levy HL. Newborn screening by tandem mass spectrometry: a new era. Clin Chem 1998;44:2401–2403.

49. Ibid (43A).

50. Nishi M, Miyake H, Takeda T, Takasagi N, Sato Y, Hanai J. Effects of the mass

screenings for neuroblastoma in Japan: a study of 68 cases. Eur J Pediatr 1988;147:308–311.

51. Parker L. Newborn screening for neuroblastoma. Curr Opin Pediatr 1997;9:70–73.

52. Levy HL, Madigan PM, Shih VE. Massachusetts metabolic disorders screening program: techniques and results of urine screening. Pediatrics 1972;49:825–836.

53. Lemieux B, Avray-Blais C, Giguere R, Shapcott D, Scriver CR. Newborn urine screening experience with over one million infants in the Quebec Network of Genetic Medicine. J Inherit Metab Dis 1988;11:45–55.

54. Wilken B, Smith A, Brown DA. Urine screening for aminoacidopathies: is it beneficial? Pediatrics 1980;97:492–497.

55. Legido A, Tonyes L, Carter D, Schoemaker A, DiGeorge A, Grover WD. Treatment variables and intellectual outcome in children with classic phenylketonuria. Clin Pediatr 1993;32:417–425.

56. Koch R, Levy HL, Matalon R, Rouse B, Hanley W, Agen C. The North American collaborative study of maternal phenylketonuria: status report 1993. Am J Dis Child 1993;147:1224–1230.

57. Weglage J, Peitsch M, Fundas B, Koch GH, Ulrick K. Deficits in selective and sustained attention processes in early treated children with phenylketonuria—result of impaired frontal lobe formation? Eur J Pediatr 1996;155:200–204.

58. Hunter MK, Mandel SH, Sesser DE, et al. Follow-up of newborns with low thyroxine and non-elevated thyroid stimulating hormone screening concentrations: results of the 20-year experience in the Northwest Regional Newborn Screening Program. J Pediatr 1998;132:70–74.

59. Ibid (14).

60. Pass KA, Anyane-Yeboa K, Sansaricq C, Schedlbauer L, Stevens C, Flaherty L. Use of DNA identity analysis in search of a potentially "missing" PKU infant. Proceedings of the 13th National Newborn Screening Symposium, San Diego, CA, 1998.

61. Tuerck JM. Introduction to screening practice issues. Proceedings of the 10th National Newborn Screening Symposium, Seattle, WA, 1994.

62. McCabe ERB, McCabe L, Mosher GA, Allen RJ, Berman JL. Newborn screening for phenylketonuria: predictive validity as a function of age. Pediatrics 1983; 72:390–398.

63. Pass KA, Levy HL (eds). Early hospital discharge: impact on newborn Proceedings screening. CORN, Washington, 1995.

64. Fisher DA, Klein AH. Thyroid development and disorders of thyroid function in the newborn. N Engl J Med 1981;304:702–712.

65. Allen DB, Seiger JE, Litsheim T, et al. Age-adjusted thyrotropin criteria for neonatal screening for hypothyroidism. J Pediatr 1990;117:309–312.

66. LaFranchi SH, Hanna CD, Krainz PL, et al. Screening for congenital hypothyroidism with specimen collection at two time periods: results of the Northwest Regional Screening Program. Pediatrics 1985;76:734–740.

67. Ou Y, Miller JB, Slocum RH, Shapira E. Rapid automated quantitation of isoleucine, leucine, tyrosine and phenylalanine from dried blood filter paper specimens. Clinica Chemica 1991;203:191–198.

68. Reilly AA, Bellisario R, Pass KA. Multivariate discrimination for phenylketonuria (PKU) and non-PKU hyperphenylalaninemia after analysis of newborns' dried blood spot specimens for six amino acids by ion-exchange chromatography. Clin Chem 1998;44:317–326.

69. Diamond A. Phenylalanine levels of 6–10 mg/dl may not be as benign as once thought. Acta Pediatr 1994;(Suppl):407:89–91.

70. Laird L, Dezateux C, Anionwu EN. Neonatal screening for sickle cell disorders: what about the carrier infant's? BMJ 1996;313:407–411.

71. Ibid (53).

72. Hearn T, Hannon WH. Interlaboratory surveys of the quantitation of thyroxine and thyrotropin in dried blood spot specimens. Clin Chem 1982;28:2022–2025.

73. NCCLS. Blood collection on filter paper for neonatal screening programs: approved standard (3rd ed). NCCLS document LA4-A3, Wayne, PA, 1997.

74. Larsson BA, Tannfeldt G, Lagercrantz H, Olsson GL. Venipuncture is more effective and less painful than heel lancing for blood tests in neonates. Pediatrics 1998;101:882–885.

21

Newborn screening for cystic fibrosis: A paradigm for public health genetics policy development

Philip M. Farrell, Michael R. Kosorok, Michael J. Rock,
Anita Laxova, Lan Zeng, Gary Hoffman,
Ronald H. Laessig, Mark L. Splaingard, and
the Wisconsin Cystic Fibrosis Neonatal
Screening Study Group

The overall purpose of this chapter is to illustrate how scientific studies can be used to facilitate public health policy decisions, particularly those concerned with newborn screening programs. More specifically, we wish to review the autosomal recessive hereditary disorder cystic fibrosis (CF) and describe how it has become a model disease for policy development in the application of molecular genetics testing to newborn screening (1). The chapter includes a summary of the salient characteristics of CF, with particular emphasis on epidemiologic and diagnostic considerations (2); a brief overview of the immunoreactive trypsinogen (IRT) and IRT/DNA tests used to facilitate CF diagnosis in the newborn period through screening; and detailed information on the unique features and results of the Wisconsin CF Neonatal Screening Project, including how and why it was planned, organized, and conducted to access the benefits, risks, and costs of CF neonatal screening (3).

This project was designed in 1983/84, implemented with randomized screening in April 1985, and completed with respect to patient accrual in April 1998; randomization was terminated in July 1994 when compelling evidence of nutritional benefits (4) meeting predetermined criteria (5) led the Wisconsin Division of Health to continue CF neonatal screening as a pilot program offered routinely to all newborns (6). Evaluation of study populations continues from both the randomized screening period (4/15/85–6/30/94) and the

In addition to the authors listed above, the following faculty members have participated in the Wisconsin Cystic Fibrosis Neonatal Screening Group: Norman Fost, M.D., M.P.H., Christopher Green, M.D., Ronald G. Gregg, Ph.D., Mari Palta, Ph.D., L.J. Wei, Ph.D., and Benjamin Wilfond, M.D., University of Wisconsin–Madison Medical School; W. Theodore Bruns, M.D., William Gershan, M.D., Elaine H. Mischler, M.D., and Lee Rusakow, M.D., Medical College of Wisconsin–Milwaukee.

extension phase (7/1/94–present). Stronger evidence in support of screening has accumulated since patient accrual was completed and is described herein as part of a summary of benefits. More information is available in various reviews (2,3,6) and in a Centers for Disease Control and Prevention (CDC) Workshop Report (1) of December 1997. This workshop, the first involving a national review of neonatal screening, could have a seminal influence on future screening practices. Consequently, we have included several statements verbatim from the CDC report (1).

Since 1985, the Wisconsin Cystic Fibrosis Neonatal Screening Project has screened nearly a million Wisconsin infants for CF and has become the largest prospective pediatric research project since the polio vaccine field trials of 1954. It is the only randomized, controlled study of any newborn screening test and was designed after we resolved various ethical concerns that are described in this chapter (7). Because the relationship of benefits and risks is so pivotal in the current debate about nationwide CF neonatal screening, we present extensive information on the nutritional benefits of early diagnosis, along with an overview on other potential benefits that are currently being investigated, such as pulmonary outcomes, genetic counseling, quality of life, cognitive function, and cost of health care.

We also provide an assessment of the risks associated with this screening and compare these risks with the benefits of screening. Experience with the Wisconsin randomized clinical trial has clearly shown why carefully designed, rigorously controlled investigations of screening with a comprehensive scope of inquiry are invaluable in efforts to apply advances in human genetics to public health action plans and to determine whether such screening should be part of public health policy. The intuitive expectation that early diagnosis through neonatal screening will have a favorable benefit/risk relationship should be confirmed whenever possible with comprehensive research before such programs are implemented permanently as routine clinical services. As stated in the CDC Workshop report, "Direct benefits to the CF-affected child should be the prerequisite for newborn screening programs" (1). This principle should be applied whenever a neonatal screening program is being contemplated for any congenital abnormality. Unfortunately, experience shows that it is rarely the guiding force in public health policy decisions of state screening organizations.

The Evolution and Current Status of Neonatal Screening Programs

Newborn screening has been defined as a "population-based public health program applying preventive medicine in defined regions to reduce newborn morbidity and mortality from certain biochemical and genetic disorders by using presymptomatic detection/diagnosis with dried blood specimens analyzed in central laboratories that generally employ automated procedures linked to clinical follow-up systems" (6). Hennekens and Buring (8) define "screening" as "the application of a test to people who are yet asymptomatic for the purpose of classifying them with respect to their likelihood of having a particular disease." They also point out that "the screening procedure itself does not diagnose illness" and that "those who test positive are sent on for further evaluation by a subsequent diagnostic test or procedure to determine whether they do, in fact, have the disease."

The first neonatal screening programs were developed in the mid-1960s to diagnose phenylketonuria (PKU) before brain damage occurred in affected infants (9). Most newborn screening tests have traditionally used biochemical or microbiological assay methods, but more recently, molecular techniques have been applied (10). As a consequence of the use of molecular techniques, two powerful secondary advances have emerged in this decade: (*1*) genetic carriers are being identified for disorders such as CF and sickle cell disease ("trait detection"); and (*2*) current screening tests can actually diagnose diseases rapidly and accurately under circumstances in which the test detects abnormal gene products (e.g., hemoglobins) or two mutant alleles in an autosomal recessive disease (e.g., the ΔF508/ΔF508 CF genotype).

Many problems occurred after PKU testing was implemented, and difficulties intensified when screening for hemoglobinopathies began. Many of the problems are attributable to the tests being implemented without sufficient research, health policy analysis, or planning. Efforts within individual regions and states have sometimes been driven by either the simple availability of a new technology or entrepreneurial financial considerations, rather than by critical analysis of tests, benefits and risks, or its cost-effectiveness. Often, boundaries have not been maintained between research and clinical practice. Furthermore, new screening tests of all types have often been implemented in some regions of the United States without systematic planning (11).

Cystic Fibrosis: A Great Diagnostic and Therapeutic Challenge

Cystic fibrosis is a life-threatening, autosomal recessive disease that occurs in approximately one out of every 4000 North American live births (2,3,12). Molecular genetics research in the past decade, reviewed by Welsh et al. (2), has demonstrated that the pathogenesis of CF can be attributed to a variety of mutations in a gene located on the long arm of chromosome 7 that encodes the cystic fibrosis transmembrane regulatory protein (CFTR). These mutations alter the functioning of the chloride channel on the apical membrane of epithelial cells. As a result, ion transport is altered at the apical surface of various epithelial cells of the sweat gland ductules, pancreatic ducts, and respiratory tract. This physiologic disturbance leads to high salt concentrations in sweat—which serves as the basis of the traditional diagnostic test. The major clinical problems in patients with CF are intestinal malabsorption, leading to malnutrition, and chronic obstructive pulmonary disease with recurrent infections.

Both the onset and the severity of these abnormalities vary greatly. Pancreatic insufficiency is often present prenatally and can lead to fetal intestinal obstruction in about 20% of patients, followed by neonatal blockage of the terminal ileum and colon—a condition known as *meconium ileus*. In contrast, another 10% to 20% of children with CF have pancreatic sufficiency and an inherently better prognosis with minimal risk for malnutrition (2). Interestingly, the lungs of children with CF are histologically normal at birth, but functional disturbances are demonstrable by 2 to 3 months (13).

Cystic fibrosis is a model disease for public health genetics-policy development because it illustrates all the issues that must be addressed in applying molecular diagnostic and therapeutic strategies. The use of DNA analysis to detect the ΔF508 allele and other mutations through newborn screening programs (14,15) and to detect adult CF heterozygotes (2,16) has truly placed this disease at the heart of controversies related to genetics and public health policy. Its relatively high incidence compared with other life-threatening inborn errors of metabolism, the severe malnutrition and pulmonary disease that often develops in children with CF, the disease's genetic complexity, and the difficulties involved in diagnosis and treatment all combine to make CF a most challenging disease.

The genetic aspects of CF are particularly complicated and interesting. The historical origin of CF in the Middle East and its apparent translocation first to Northern Europe and then to North America provide a fascinating story of evolutionary migration (17,18). The most common mutation is a three-base pair deletion at codon-508, known as the ΔF508 allele, but there are over 800 other mutations now recognized, most of which are "private" (one person only) mutations, and more are being discovered each year (2). Although there must be an advantage for CF heterozygote carriers, the nature of this advantage remains uncertain, despite much speculation (19,20). Table 21.1 lists the most frequent mutations among CF patients in the United States. The predominance of the ΔF508 mutation, which accounts for over 70% of mutant CFTR chromosomes, is the factor that made it possible to introduce DNA testing in CF neonatal screening programs (15,21–23). In most states, approximately 90% or more of CF patients have at least one ΔF508 allele. Because about half the CF patients in North America are homozygous for ΔF508, detection of two such mutant alleles in the dried blood specimen allows *diagnosis* to occur routinely with the IRT/DNA (ΔF508) screening test.

Conversely, our research in association with the CF Foundation on CFTR

Table 21.1 The Most Common CFTR Mutations in the United States based on DNA Analysis of 13,080 Genotyped CF Patients (26,160 alleles) Reported to the CF Foundation Registry* in 1998

	N	Percent
ΔF508	19,730	75.4
G542X	673	2.6
G551D	642	2.4
W1282X	414	1.6
N1303K	357	1.4
R553X	257	1.0
Other	524	2.0
Unidentified	3,563	13.6

* Data from Cystic Fibrosis Registry, 1998 Annual Report. Note that 52.2% of the genotyped patients are homozygous for the Δf508 allele and one other mutation, and 11.4% have two mutations other than ΔF508.

mutations in U.S. patients has shown that some states have atypical genotype profiles (Fig. 21.1). For instance, compared with Wisconsin and the United States as a whole, New York and New Jersey appear to have lower prevalences of ΔF508/Δ508 (38% and 34%, respectively). These differences may be attributable to racial/ethnic variations. The CFTR mutations of special interest include W1282X, which accounts for more than half the mutations in Ashkenazi Jews (2), and $3120 + 1G \rightarrow A$, which is commonly found in African Americans (24). Another interesting mutation is R117H because it has been associated with normal sweat electrolyte levels and with atypical lung disease (2). Interesting genotype-phenotype correlations are reviewed by Welsh et al. (2). There has also been a clear association between certain genotypes and pancreatic sufficiency, but no CFTR mutation patterns are evident that relate to pulmonary disease or its severity.

Unfortunately, despite CF's presence from birth and its serious consequences, the diagnosis of CF is often delayed. As shown in Figure 21.2, in 1996 the average age of CF diagnosis among 900 CF patients was 4.8 years, with a median of 0.5 years. Similar figures have been published for the past decade (3) indicating that there has been no improvement in the diagnosis of CF in the United States despite so many other advances in health care. Bar graphs like Figure 21.2, which show the cumulative percentage of new diagnoses, underscore the diagnostic challenge but are sometimes misconstrued in an overly optimistic fashion. For instance, although 64% of CF patients had CF diagnosed during their first year, more than half of these (35.7%) had either meconium ileus (20.1%) or a positive family history for CF (15.6%) and were readily detectable shortly after birth. Any delay in diagnosis is potentially associated with increased morbidity (2,4) and also with some mortality due to

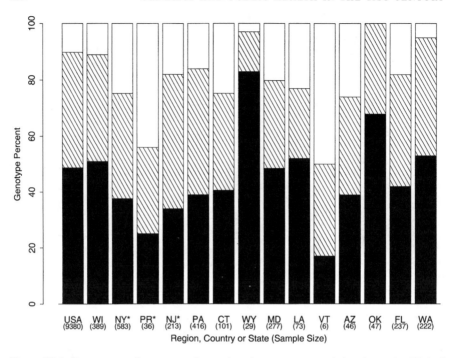

Figure 21.1 Percentage of genotypes by region (state or country) for the entire United States, for Wisconsin, and for states (plus Puerto Rico) for which the chi-square p-value indicates significantly different from Wisconsin (at the 0.05 level), ranging from the most significant (New York) to least significant (Washington). Asterisks indicate states that remain significantly different after adjustments were made from multiple comparisons. The number in parentheses is the sample size for the given region. The bottom black segment of each bar is the percent homozygous for ΔF508, the middle crosshatched segment is the percentage heterozygous for ΔF508, and the top white segment is the percentage of other genotypes (which is zero in the case of Oklahoma). Data analyzed were from the 1995 CF Patient Registry, courtesy of Dr. Stacy FitzSimmons, Cystic Fibrosis Foundation.

hyponatremic dehydration, acute kwashiorkor, or pulmonary disease (25). By evaluating the 1993 National CF Patient Registry data, Lai et al. (26) showed that signs of severe malnutrition (height or weight for age less than the 5th percentile) were present in 44% of patients with newly diagnosed CF; this analysis included 790 diagnosed patients less than 10 years old who were identified at an average age of 1.41 years (median, 0.50 years). In addition, symptoms and signs of respiratory tract abnormalities are common among CF patients diagnosed after infancy (27,28). The general experience of U.S. CF centers (27) and specific evidence generated in the Wisconsin CF Neonatal Screening Project indicate that many patients have already developed obstructive lung disease or show recurrent respiratory infections when their CF is first recognized by a sweat test.

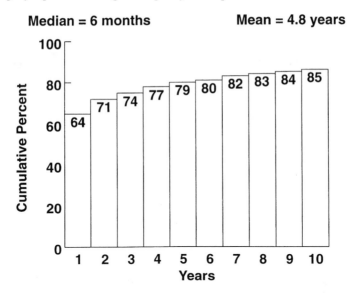

Figure 21.2 Age of diagnosis for CF patients identified in the CFF Patient Registry during 1996.

Other pulmonary morbidity associated with delayed diagnosis includes segmental or lobar atelectasis, spontaneous pneumothorax, life-threatening bacterial pneumonias (usually associated with *Staphylococcus aureus*), and rarely even *cor pulmonale*. It is not clear how many infants and children with CF die without their CF being diagnosed, but some estimates are alarming (29). Not only does delayed diagnosis increase the morbidity and mortality risk for CF patients, but it can also lead to significant psychological trauma among parents whose children have obvious but explained steatorrhea, malnutrition, or lung disease. Often, parents will take their child from doctor to doctor attempting to obtain an answer to their questions about these symptoms. Therefore, it is obvious that significant problems are associated with the common delay in diagnosing CF.

The Rationale and Plan for CF Neonatal Screening Research

In view of the problems associated with delayed diagnosis, it is not surprising that newborn screening for CF was suggested as long ago as 1970 (30). Indeed, an underlying principle of medical practice is that a physician has an ethical duty to diagnose promptly and accurately when effective treatments are available. Excellent nutritional management methods for CF have been available for decades, and respiratory care has improved significantly since the 1970s

Table 21.2 Recommendations by the Cystic Fibrosis Foundation Task Force on Neonatal Screening*

Further study the reliability and validity of the IRT (immunoreactive trypsinogen) method.
Develop better standardization of reagents.
Further study the time-related decline of IRT levels.
Perform sweat tests on all infants testing positive on initial IRT tests.
Determine the cost-benefit relationship of screening.
Study the value of early treatment related to prognosis.
Evaluate the psychosocial benefits and risks of early detection.

---

*Data from Ad Hoc Committee Task Force on Neonatal Screening, Cystic Fibrosis Foundation. See reference 33.

(2). Early screening attempts involved an analysis of meconium to detect the high level of albumin characteristic of newborns with CF (31).

A more attractive method based on analysis of dried neonatal blood specimens became possible in 1979 when researchers (32) reported the use of trypsinogen determinations using radioimmunoassay methods. Many questions arose, however, about trypsinogen tests and their efficacy. Consequently, the United States Cystic Fibrosis Foundation urged caution and recommended more research (33). The seven recommendations listed in Table 21.2 were published after we had already initiated planning in Wisconsin for a comprehensive, controlled investigation of the benefits and risks of IRT tests for the routine detection of CF in early infancy. It was clear that an opportunity had become available that should not be missed, and that investment in a randomized clinical trial could pay dividends. Therefore, after securing funding, we began a controlled, comprehensive study on April 15, 1985. After 4 years of randomized screening with IRT analyses, and at a time when the trypsinogen single-tier test appeared discouraging, collaborating investigators in Toronto and Michigan (34) identified the principal CFTR mutation and made it possible to develop a two-tiered method of neonatal screening initially recommended by Rock et al. (35). In 1991, after several months of developing methods and securing approvals following another ethical review, we began using the trypsinogen/DNA (ΔF508) method to make early diagnoses of CF and thereby generate an expanded population of study patients in the screened group. Our plan included a randomization phase, a surveillance method for complete patient accrual, and a long term follow-up, evaluation phase.

Although the original newborn screening test for CF using meconium had to be abandoned owing to its deficiencies (36), the use of dried blood specimens for analysis of trypsinogen has proven to be of great value. The original discovery of trypsinogen testing occurred in Auckland, New Zealand, when IRT measurements were applied retrospectively on stored Guthrie cards (32). Subsequent prospective studies (15,22,37–39) have led to four methods that use trypsinogen testing, and more are likely to follow. The four methods can be summarized as follows: (*1*) single IRT test (35); (*2*) IRT tests on the initial blood sample followed by repeat testing typically at 4 to 6 weeks of age ("recall method") when the trypsinogen level is above a predetermined cutoff point (38); (*3*) trypsinogen testing as a prescreening procedure followed by DNA extraction and analysis for the ΔF508 mutation (15,21); and (*4*) another version of the two-tiered testing system, with trypsinogen prescreening followed by CFTR multimutation analysis (39) using a variety of analytical methods.

All of these options have excellent specificity and positive predictive values. Indeed, the positive predictive value of CF neonatal screening by any of the four methods greatly exceeds that of other newborn screening tests (5,6). In contrast, the sensitivity of these four methods varies and depends, of course, on the cutoff point selected and particularly on the discrimination level set for trypsinogen values. In reported studies, the sensitivity has been as low as 85% for the IRT or IRT/IRT testing methods (22,35). The IRT/DNA methods with a lower cutoff point for trypsinogen level have shown increased sensitivity; in fact, a sensitivity level as high as 100% has been reported for the IRT/DNA (ΔF508) method (39), although in general it is likely to be 90% to 95% in most large populations.

Analysis of Potential Benefits and Hypothetical Risks of CF Neonatal Screening

When the Wisconsin CF Neonatal Screening Project was designed in 1983/84, we decided to perform a comprehensive investigation to determine the relative benefit/risk relationship of CF neonatal screening after accumulating scientific evidence. This conclusion was based on an underlying principle of medical practice, namely that *diagnostic or therapeutic interventions should occur only when the anticipated benefits outweigh the potential risks.* When the randomized screening trial actually began in April 1985, short-term observational (uncontrolled) studies had already indicated some benefits from CF neonatal screening (40,41), but there was also a prevailing concern about psychosocial risks and some reservations about potential medical harm (33). Therefore, we initially designed this project to examine the following categories of potential benefits: nutritional, pulmonary, and psychosocial. Later, we also began studying a potential genetic counseling benefit (42) when the screening procedure changed to the two-tiered IRT/DNA method (39).

Similarly, we added quality-of-life and cognitive function to our study of potential benefits after accumulated data demonstrated significant nutritional advantages of screening, including a larger head circumference in the early diagnosis group (4). Among the potential risks we have investigated are "missed diagnoses," laboratory errors, pulmonary problems (especially increased risk for early acquisition and infection with *Pseudomonas aeruginosa*), insurance discrimination, and psychosocial disturbances. We also have been investigating the costs of diagnosis and health care in both the screened and control groups. We did not consider the mortality rate in the screened group compared with that in the control group to be a realistic outcome measure based on projections in 1983/84; this was subsequently confirmed in an analysis published in the CDC Workshop Report by Cono and Khoury (1).

Design and Execution of the Wisconsin CF Neonatal Screening Trial

The Wisconsin CF Neonatal Screening Project was originally designed as a randomized clinical trial whose highest priority was to assess both the benefits and risks of neonatal screening. We later began studying screening tests and their costs to arrive at a comprehensive assessment of benefits and risks. This investigation has many distinctive features and has dealt successfully with numerous ethical and logistical issues, as described in detail elsewhere (7). The critical research question has focused on the age of CF patients at diagnosis to determine whether delayed recognition alters the outcome of these patients. The overall hypothesis of the project has been that "Early diagnosis of CF through neonatal screening will be medically beneficial without major risks."

All infants born in Wisconsin, beginning on April 15, 1985, and ending on June 30, 1994, were randomized to either the screened (early diagnosis) or control (standard diagnosis) group. The infants were determined to have CF if they tested positive on a sweat chloride test after screening with either a single immunoreactive trypsinogen (IRT) or two-tiered IRT/DNA assay (35,39). The case definition established in 1983/84 required a sweat chloride level of 60 mEq/L or greater. Infants were referred for sweat tests to either the Madison or Milwaukee CF centers. Positive test results on infants randomized to the screened group were reported to the parents by primary-care physicians. The parents were then urged to obtain a sweat test promptly for confirmation so that active clinical follow-up and treatment (43,44) could be initiated (unless the sweat test was nonconfirmatory or negative). An evaluation and treatment protocol was used by both centers.

For those infants randomized to the control group, the results of the initial IRT or IRT/DNA assay were computer-stored and not reported to either the family or physicians unless they requested a report. After the child's fourth birthday, as long as a diagnosis of CF did not occur through other means, positive screening test results were generated from computer data and were reported to the parents through their primary-care physician, and a request was made to perform a sweat test. This strategy—the key to avoiding selection bias (45)—has been referred to as "unblinding" (4,7) and could conceivably be used in other neonatal screening research programs. Using the "unblinding" method and an active surveillance system, we were able to study benefits and risks to determine whether CF neonatal screening led to more good than harm (46). Assessment of adverse impact included examining the control population for confusion and stigmatization (47), monitoring for toxic effects of early antibiotic therapy (48), and evaluating the cost of care.

In calculating the benefits of screening, the primary nutritional outcomes we used were age-adjusted height and weight, and the Shwachman–Kulczycki score (49), and our pulmonary outcomes of interest were Brasfield (50) and Wisconsin (51) chest radiograph scores, forced expiratory volume in 1 second (FEV_1) expressed relative to forced vital capacity (FVC), and residual lung volume over total lung volume (RV/TLV). We then stratified these outcomes by the subject's sex, meconium ileus (MI) status, pancreatic functional status, genotype (homozygous or heterozygous for $\Delta F508$ or other), age, and center (Madison or Milwaukee). At each interim analysis, this procedure is essentially an analysis of covariance (ANCOVA) for repeated measures with treatment group as the main effect of interest and the stratification variables as covariates, except that boys and girls were for some time analyzed separately. We used the method of Wei et al., (52) to assess the effect of screening while adjusting for stratification variables and multiple interim analyses.

Because of unexpectedly slow data accrual, we have made some adjustments to the initially proposed alpha levels and timing of interim analyses. This can be justified by the methodology of Lan and DeMets (53), which allows for the alpha levels for each interim analysis to be determined by the amount of data accrued (see, for example, Gange and DeMets [54]), provided that this determination is not inappropriately influenced by observed treatment differences. The original plan was to use alpha levels of 0.005, 0.005, 0.01, 0.01, and 0.15 in 1991, 1992, 1993, 1994, and 1995, respectively. Instead, because we had more than 90 patients without meconium ileus, we elected to "spend the alpha" in 1996 and complete the analysis of nutritional outcomes. Using the method of Slud and Wei (55) to construct group sequential boundaries, we ensured that an alpha level of 0.05 was maintained across all analysis times.

Evidence of Nutritional Benefits

The Wisconsin CF Neonatal Screening Project thus far has concentrated on potential nutritional benefits with emphasis on biochemical and anthropometric indices that can be measured with high precision. Our results (56) indicate that biochemical evidence of inadequate nutrition is common at diagnosis among infants who are screened for CF as newborns (i.e., the screened group) and among those diagnosed as having CF on the basis of signs and symptoms (i.e., the control group). Nutritional intervention therapy, however, corrected low levels of serum albumin and fat-soluble vitamins identified at the time of diagnosis. Data demonstrating nutritional advantages based on anthropometric indices in the screening group were published (4) after a primary statistical analysis was performed on data accumulated through October 15, 1996. Assessment of nutritional status has been ongoing, and another analysis of data accumulated through April 15, 1998, demonstrates even greater nutritional benefit, as summarized below and shown in accompanying graphs.

Between April 15, 1985, and June 30, 1994, a total of 650,341 infants were screened for CF in the first 28 days of life. This led to an early CF diagnosis for 54 infants. In addition, 15 infants in the early diagnosis group had meconium ileus, and five others were identified because of either a family history (two infants) or symptoms of cystic fibrosis (three infants) even though they had false-negative screening tests. Thus, a total of 74 CF patients were identified from the screening arm of the randomization protocol. The control group included 75 infants or children, 18 of whom had meconium ileus and 15 of whom had abnormal ($\geq 60\,mEq/L$) results on sweat tests performed when they were 4 years old because computer-stored neonatal IRT or trypsinogen/DNA results showed that they had tested positive for CF. It is noteworthy that 20% (15/75) of the control patients were only known because of the "unblinding" procedures and vigorous surveillance methods. Because the presence of meconium ileus routinely led to an early diagnosis in both groups and because (as described earlier) screening involves the use of a test to identify people who are still asymptomatic (8), our nutritional outcome assessment has focused on CF patients without meconium ileus. The data presented below are for 57 patients assigned to the early diagnosis group and 51 control subjects.

The demographic and genetic characteristics of the two groups of patients without meconium ileus are presented in Table 21.3. A significant difference existed in the age at diagnosis, with a mean of 13 weeks in the screened group compared with 107 weeks in the control group ($p < 0.001$). The age at the time of diagnosis among the control patients did not differ significantly from that of patients diagnosed at the Madison CF center prior to 1985 (4,28), and the distribution of their ages at diagnoses was similar to national data (26). Although no significant differences occurred in sex or center distribution between the screened and control groups, more patients in the screened group had the ΔF508 mutation and more had pancreatic insufficiency. Thus, by chance the control group had better pancreatic function status and genotype profiles. This is significant because the control group had a higher proportion of patients with pancreatic sufficiency and "milder genotypes" and therefore an inherently lower risk of malnutrition, lung disease, and death in childhood (2).

Table 21.3 Demographic, Nutritional, and Clinical Characteristics at the Time of Diagnosis of Cystic Fibrosis in Patients Without Meconium Ileus

Characteristic	Screened Group (n = 57)	Control Group (n = 51)	p Value
Age at diagnosis—week			<0.001
Mean (SD)	13 (36)	107 (118)	
Median (range)	7 (4–281)	30 (3–372)	
Sex—no. (%)			0.844
Male	36 (63)	31 (61)	
Female	21 (37)	20 (39)	
Genotype—no. (%)			<0.001
ΔF508/ΔF508	33 (58)	22 (44)	
ΔF508/other	24 (42)	19 (38)	
Other/other	0	9 (18)	
Pancreatic status—no. (%)			<0.001
Sufficiency (probable or established)	5 (9)	15 (33)	
Insufficiency (probable or established)	49 (91)	31 (67)	
Length or height			
Percentile (SD)	44 (28)	25 (27)	<0.001
z score (SD)	−0.21 (1.0)	−1.0 (1.3)	<0.001
Weight			
Percentile (SD)	35 (28)	24 (26)	0.018
z score (SD)	−0.5 (1.1)	−1.1 (1.1)	0.018
Head circumference			
Percentile	52 (28)	32 (24)	0.003
Shwachman-Kulczycki score*			
Activity (SD)	24 (1.9)	24 (1.5)	0.707
Physical examination (SD)	23 (3.6)	22 (3.9)	0.511
Growth and nutrition (SD)	22 (4.5)	20 (4.5)	0.084
Chest film (SD)	23 (2.7)	22 (3.4)	0.224
Total (SD)	91 (10)	89 (10)	0.069
Mean (SD) age-adjusted score	87 (1.6)	92 (1.5)	0.006
Plasma vitamin A—μg/d (SD)	28 (16)	36 (20)	0.023
Plasma vitamin B—μg/d (SD)	471 (375)	512 (450)	0.715

*Age-dependent variable.

At the time of diagnosis, the length/height, weight, and head circumference percentiles in the early diagnosis group were significantly higher than in the control group (Table 21.3). Although the Schwachman-Kulczycki score (49) was higher in the screened patients when first analyzed (4), the two groups were similar after "unblinding." Information from the 12-year follow-up period is provided in Figure 21.3. Overall, our longitudinal assessment revealed that average weight and height were significantly higher in the early diagnosis group than in the control group. Statistical analyses indicated that the height-for-age and weight-for-age percentiles were significantly higher in the early diagnosis group, as were the z scores (4). When we used height or weight below the 5th or 10th percentile as an index of severe malnutrition

Weight-for-Age Percentile versus Age by Group

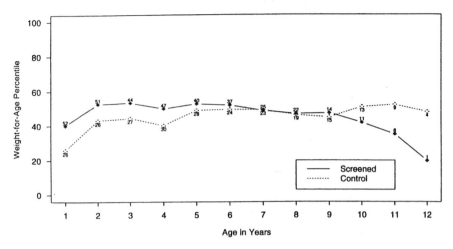

Height-for-Age Percentile versus Age by Group

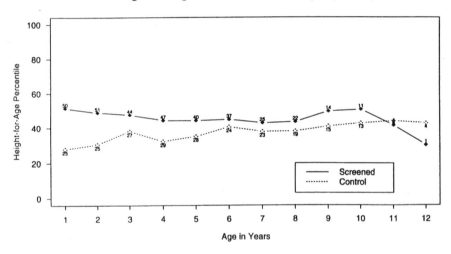

Figure 21.3 Anthropometric indexes in relation to age in the early-diagnosis and control groups, standardized according to percentiles for weight (p = 0.07) and height (p = 0.01).

(26), the outcome was also significantly better in the early diagnosis group. Patients in the control group were 4.23 times more likely than those in the early diagnosis group to be below the 10th percentile in weight and 4.58 times more likely to be in the lowest 10th percentile for height (95% CI = 1.69–10.63 and 1.67–12.59, respectively). As shown in Figures 21.3 and 21.4, the most striking differences were in height. Neonatal screening reduced a child's risk of being below the 10th percentile in height throughout the first 11 years of life, with no overlap in values between the two groups.

Proportion of Patients with Weight-for-age below the 10th Percentile

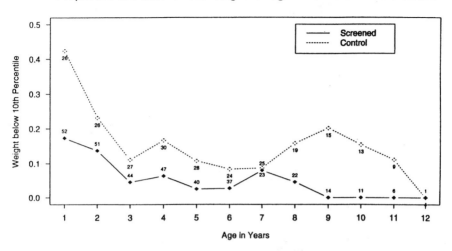

Proportion of Patients with Height-for-age below the 10th Percentile

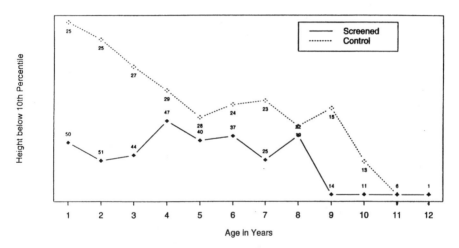

Figure 21.4 Proportions of patients in the early-diagnosis and control groups whose weight (p = 0.002) or height (p = 0.003) were below the 10th percentile at the annual assessment.

To address the issue of selection bias, particularly with 20% of the control patients identified by "unblinding" at 4 years of age, we performed other statistical analyses. Specifically, once the control patients were completely identified by the "unblinding" process, we obtained their anthropometric indices of nutritional status from birth forward by reviewing records, and then we incorporated these indices into a "What if?" analysis (i.e., a statistical analysis to determine how the total control group would have compared with the screened group had all patients been identified from birth). This expanded database showed that the growth of control patients remained significantly less than that of the screened group (i.e., no conclusions changed).

Thus, we found that patients in whom CF was detected by screening were heavier and longer and had a larger head circumference than did those in whom the disorder was diagnosed on the basis of a positive family history, illness, or sweat testing at 4 years of age because of a high trypsinogen concentration at birth. Differences associated with screening were especially marked in subgroups of CF patients who had pancreatic insufficiency or the ΔF508/ΔF508 genotype (4); such patients are known to have the most severe disease (2,57). We conclude, therefore, that age at time of diagnosis is an important factor in the nutritional status of CF patients and that identification through neonatal screening provides an ideal opportunity to prevent malnutrition.

Evidence of Pulmonary Benefits

Whether a CF patient has pulmonary disease is the usual critical determinant of long-term prognosis and greatly influences that patient's quality of life and need for hospitalization. Some observations indicate no relationship between age of diagnosis and the prognosis (58), but others (59), especially newborn screening studies, suggest that early diagnosis leads to significantly better outcomes. Unfortunately, in the Wisconsin project, we have had much more difficulty obtaining high-quality data on pulmonary outcomes than on nutritional outcomes because of deficiencies in chest radiograph scoring methods (49–51) and limitations in pulmonary function testing of young children.

Conversely, we did identify a potentially reduced risk for infection with *Pseudomonas aeruginosa* among screened patients while studying patients followed at the Madison and Milwaukee CF centers (60,61). In addition, observational studies elsewhere have generated evidence of better respiratory disease status among patients identified by screening than among those in various cohorts identified with standard diagnostic methods. In particular, the results of three nonrandomized screening investigations presented at the 1997 CDC Workshop provided strong evidence of such superior respiratory disease status (1). These studies include observations in (*1*) northeastern Italy, where screening began in 1973 and 16 years of assessment revealed delayed Pseudomonas colonization, less "lung damage," and lower mortality associated with early diagnosis; (*2*) the Netherlands, where a screened cohort born between 1973 and 1979 showed better pulmonary function and life expectancy; and (*3*) Australia, where New South Wales has screened with IRT and IRT/DNA methods for almost 20 years and found improved nutritional and pulmonary outcomes, as well as less hospitalization, in association with early diagnosis through neonatal screening.

Recently, the complete data analysis from the observational study in New South Wales, Australia, has been published, including both nutritional and pulmonary outcome measures over 10 years of follow-up evaluation (62). The growth of the early diagnosis group (median age at diagnosis, 1.8 months) was significantly greater than a nonscreened birth cohort from the previous 3 years (1978 to 1981) who were diagnosed at a median age of 6.2 months (excluding meconium ileus patients). The screened subjects also had better pulmonary function than did the historical controls, with significantly higher FEV_1 and FVC data at 5 and 10 years of age. The chest X-ray scores were not different using the Shwachman-Kulczycki method (49), which has limited sensitivity (51). Although these results demonstrate more favorable outcomes associated with screening, various limitations are related to the design. These are discussed by the authors (62) and include variations in demographics and changes in therapeutic methods after 1981 that could have differentially benefited the screened group.

The CDC Workshop report (1) also summarized recent investigations with the following statements: Observational studies suggest an association between poor growth and more severe lung disease in populations of CF-affected patients investigated in recent epidemiologic studies. Observational studies also have demonstrated that infants who are diagnosed as having CF as newborns through screening have pulmonary function that is similar to or better than those who are diagnosed later.

Other research findings that are relevant include an investigation in Great Britain (63) where a reduced number of hospital admissions was recognized in the screened group (usually for intensive respiratory therapy), and results in Colorado where patients diagnosed through CF neonatal screening showed an early onset of pulmonary disease (13) and nutritional deficits (64).

Benefit/Risk Relationship

The two most significant benefits of CF neonatal screening are prevention of malnutrition and prevention or alleviation of chronic lung disease. Early diagnosis also allows health care providers to prevent salt loss, which can lead to fatal hyponatremic dehydration. In contrast, the only adverse impact of screening identified thus far relates to short-term psychological risks, namely the parental stress associated with a child testing false-positive (which applies for any newborn screening test and not just for the cystic fibrosis test) and the parental trauma associated with the early diagnosis of an infant with a life-threatening disease.

The risk assessment component of the Wisconsin Neonatal Screening Project has included a variety of psychosocial and communication issues. Our observations indicate that short-term anxiety and/or anger can occur in families of infants testing false-positive for CF and that communication methods are extremely important in preventing persistent problems. An associated study (65) of parenting stress among mothers whose infants had either false-positive screening tests or CF diagnoses revealed that they had less stress but greater defensiveness than did comparison families whose infants were healthy.

Additionally, we have also studied the impact of newborn screening on the reproductive decision making of parents with a child identified as having CF and the implications of identifying carriers of the CF gene with the IRT/DNA approach (42); these studies suggest a potential genetic counseling benefit for many families. The major medical risk we have studied relates to the acquisition of *P. aeruginosa* by young children with CF. Overall, there were no differences in acquisition of respiratory pathogens between the screened and control groups (58). We did find, however, that screened patients followed at old clinics of one CF center acquired *P. aeruginosa* significantly earlier than did those followed at the other CF center. Further analysis of these results suggests that clinic exposures and/or aerosol therapy may predispose CF patients to pseudomonas infections and that segregated clinics may be appropriate for young children diagnosed through screening (58,59).

Public Health Policy Considerations

The processes by which newborn-screening policy decisions are made vary from state to state; consequently, the United States lacks consistency in the implementation of neonatal screening tests. To obtain systematic information on this issue, investigators (11) conducted a nationwide survey of newborn screening programs and determined that a marked variation exists in the use of tests, and various approaches are being used for policy development. In fact, some states have no predetermined procedure for adding or deleting tests. There is also marked variation in the analytical biochemistry techniques used in newborn screening programs. The information obtained in the Stoddard and Farrell survey (11) underscores the diversity of methods used to decide whether to add or delete newborn screening tests from the panel. Their observations also support the views of Wilfond and Nolan (66), who describe two models of health policy development (namely the extemporaneous model and the evidentiary model). Newborn screening tests have generally followed the extemporaneous models, but testing for CF is a singular exception because of the Wisconsin randomized trial and the studies conducted longitudinally in the Netherlands, northeastern Italy, and Australia.

In 1993, Wisconsin began a process of establishing criteria for adding or deleting of newborn screening tests when a proposal was presented to add screening for congenital adrenal hyperplasia (CAH). Health policy decision

Table 21.4 Wisconsin Addition and Deletion Criteria for Newborn Screening Tests*

---

1. *Incidence:* The identification of 1 case per 100,000 births should be the minimum number for any specific disorder. With an annual birth rate of 70,000 to 75,000, Wisconsin should expect to identify approximately 1 case each year.

2. *Morbidity and mortality:* Scientific evidence should show that the benefits of identification in the neonatal period will outweigh the adverse consequences (treatment effective only when started before the age at which a clinical diagnosis is usually made).

3. *Potential for successful treatment:* There should be evidence that effective management can be implemented to benefit infants and their families; diagnosis without effective treatment is inappropriate.

4. *Cost:* Laboratory costs of any test to be added should be comparable with the cost of well-established tests such as that for phenylketonuria.

5. *Laboratory feasibility:* The test must be adaptable to a mass screening program. At this time, both the health care system and the laboratory technology limit tests to those that use blood specimens.

---

*These criteria were developed in 1992 by the Newborn Screening Advisory Group, which was appointed by the Wisconsin Division of Health, Department of Health and Social Services. The group also issued the following statement: "In general, screening should not take place unless the disorder is recognized as an important public health problem for which there will be a commitment of financial support. Benefits to identified infants should outweigh the costs of the screening program."

making was facilitated by employing addition and deletion criteria that were first developed and approved before a decision was made to add CAH screening (6). One year later, following the determination that significant nutritional benefits occurred with neonatal screening for cystic fibrosis, Wisconsin public health officials decided to add trypsinogen/DNA (ΔF508) testing to the panel. In essence, they determined that CF fit the criteria described in Table 21.4. In the case of both CAH and CF, however, a 5-year "sunset clause" was incorporated into the plan; thus, these two tests were added as pilot programs with a requirement that rigorous analysis of outcomes be performed during the fourth year of statewide screening. This assessment is currently under way in Wisconsin.

The evidentiary model, therefore, was used in Wisconsin before routine screening occurred after discontinuation of the randomization strategy employed in the clinical trial. Our overall conclusion is even stronger in 1998/99 because it has clearly been shown that significant benefits occur with CF screening, whereas no long-term risks of any significance have been identified despite intensive efforts to uncover them. We have now reached the conviction that "the burden of proof is on those who argue against neonatal screening for cystic fibrosis" (23).

In contrast, opposing opinions have been expressed in the United States and various countries. Only Australia thus far, evolving in a region-by-region fashion as evidence accumulated, has proceeded to universal CF neonatal screening. Most counteropinions are based on concerns about demonstrating long-term pulmonary benefits and cost-effectiveness. Although the Wisconsin CF Neonatal Project has not yet demonstrated long-term pulmonary benefits associated with screening, that aspect of the investigation continues, and there is no evidence that patients in the screened group are at greater risk for pulmonary disease because their CF was diagnosed early. Furthermore, the long-term observational study in Australia (63) did reveal better pulmonary outcomes in screened patients. In responding to this increasingly favorable evidence on the benefit/risk relationship, both the CDC (1) and the Cystic Fibrosis Foundation have issued statements encouraging more states to introduce pilot programs.

Implications for Other States and Regions and for the United States as a Whole

As George Santayana stated at the beginning of the 20th century, "Those who cannot remember the past are condemned to repeat it." The lessons of history are clear with respect to neonatal screening in general and CF screening in particular. Both the potential good and the possible harm of such programs have become obvious. In a larger sense, the scope and magnitude of neonatal screening programs compel public health advocates to enhance both decision-making processes and routine procedures so that better outcomes can be ensured in the future.

With approximately 4 million births annually in the United States, we estimate that approximately 20 million newborn screening tests are performed each year—translating to about 100,000 interpersonal diagnostic encounters when one takes into account recall tests for infants testing false positive and the diagnostic interaction with true positives (67). Such a situation requires continuous quality improvement attitudes, effective mechanisms for positive change in all the states, and, ideally, more national guidelines to promote consistently excellent and appropriate service. There is a relatively urgent need to devote more attention to these concerns, particularly with a likely proliferation of molecular tests as a by-product of the Human Genome Project (9). It is especially important to devote more attention to improving communication methods for false-positive families as the greatest psychosocial toxicity probably occurs in this population and has largely been ignored despite strong evidence of adverse impact. In general, genetic counseling needs to be addressed and improved by research linked to newborn screening programs aimed at enhancing all aspects of risk communication.

The following is a summary of six key lessons we learned from CF neonatal screening in Wisconsin and their implications for future programs:

(*1*) Comprehensive study is needed in neonatal screening research to assess both benefits and the risks. This is the only approach that will allow researchers to determine whether screening does "more harm than good" (46). (*2*) Properly designed research with a randomized clinical trial is clearly feasible for newborn screening issues, allowing the evidentiary model to be used for decision making. To achieve success, however, investigators must have a combination of patience and tenacity as well as a willingness to address ethical and legal obstacles. (*3*) Newborn screening research requires multicenter or even multistate studies with excellent organization and communication. Such studies may need to be conducted over a longer term than most randomized clinical trials. (*4*) Accurate information about the incidence of a hereditary disorder is essential for planning both neonatal screening research and clinical services. This is readily available for CF now as a result of studies in Wisconsin (12). When more states embark on neonatal screening, however, they should be aware not only of the CF incidence but also of CF genotype profiles, especially when the IRT/DNA method is used or if CFTR multimutation analyses are performed. (*5*) The well-organized network of CF centers in the United States will facilitate screening, but cooperation is essential to optimize procedures and results. As stated in the CDC Workshop report (1), "The development of CF screening programs for newborns will lead to unique challenges for almost all states. Patients' access to CF centers must be ensured, and screening laboratories must have good rapport and effective collaboration." (*6*) Enhanced development of risk communication methods is essential. Risk should be communicated both through traditional genetic counseling techniques and through other approaches. Because the number of trained genetic counselors is so limited (66), it is clear that physicians and nurses will have to assume much of the responsibility for risk communication in newborn screening programs.

Finally, taking into account the lessons learned in Wisconsin, we recommend that a cautious approach be followed in considering decisions to add future newborn screening tests. Mistakes have been made in the past (e.g., maple syrup urine disease [5]) and others are on the horizon (possibly the case with medium-chain acyl-CoA dehydrogenase deficiency). The temptation should be resisted to proceed with neonatal screening just because a test is available and intuition suggests that it will benefit children. The scientific method can clearly be used to arrive at better public health policy decisions. The desirability of using science rather than intuition led the Cystic Fibrosis Foundation to urge research in 1983 (Table 21.2) and the Wisconsin Cystic Fibrosis Neonatal Screening Group to embark on a controlled investigation that has obviously made a difference. We hope that investigators concerned about other diseases amenable to screening take advantage of the scientific method.

Acknowledgments

We are grateful to all members of the Wisconsin Cystic Fibrosis Neonatal Research Group. This project could not have been implemented successfully and sustained without an extremely talented, dedicated group of nurses, physicians, biostatisticians, genetic counselors, and laboratory personnel. We especially want to thank three individuals who were essential in the design and initiation of this project: Mari Palta, Ph.D. (who completed an important analysis of data available in 1984 and performed statistical projections of sample size); Norman Fost, M.D., M.P.H. (who performed an analysis of the ethical issues and suggested that our assessment include genetic counseling and reproductive behavior); and David Hassemer, M.S. (who served as leader of the Wisconsin Newborn Screening Program for the State Laboratory of Hygiene). In addition, we thank David DeMets, Ph.D., who has advised us on statistical and data management throughout this study. Five CF center directors have supported and contributed to this project and are greatly appreciated for their efforts, namely Drs. Elaine Mischler, Christopher Green, and Michael, Rock in Madison, and Drs. W. Theodore Bruns and Mark Splaingard in Milwaukee. Research nurses have included Miriam Block, Holly Colby, Lynn Feenan, Mary Ellen Freeman, Catherine McCarthy, and Audry Tluczek—all of whom have been outstanding. We also thank our sweat test technician and research assistant, Linda Makholm, and the excellent genetic counselors associated with this project since the IRT/DNA test was introduced, namely Margaret K. (Peggy) Modaff, Catherine A. Reiser, and Christine Sauer.

References

1. Centers for Disease Control and Prevention. Newborn screening for cystic fibrosis: a paradigm for public health genetics policy development. MMWR Morbi Mortal Wkly Rep 1997;46(RR-16):1–24.

2. Welsh MJ, Tsui L, Boat TF, et al. The metabolic and molecular bases of inherited disease (17th ed). In: Shriver CR, Baudet AL, Sly WS, Valle D (eds). Cystic fibrosis. New York: McGraw-Hill, 1995, pp. 3799–3876.

3. Farrell PM, Mischler EH. Newborn screening for cystic fibrosis. Adv Pediatr 1992;39:31–64.

4. Farrell PM, Kosorok MR, Laxova A, et al. Nutritional benefits of newborn screening for cystic fibrosis. N Engl J Med 1997;337:963–969.

5. Allen DB, Farrell PM. Newborn screening. Adv Pediatr 1996;43:231–270.

6. Farrell PM, Aronson RA, Hoffman GL, et al. Newborn screening for cystic fibrosis in Wisconsin: first application of population-based molecular genetics testing. Wis Med J 1994;93:415–421.

7. Fost NC, Farrell PM. A prospective randomized trial of early diagnosis and treatment of cystic fibrosis: a unique ethical dilemma. Clin Res 1989;37:495–500.

8. Hennekens CH, Buring JE. Epidemiology in medicine. Boston/Toronto: Little, Brown, 1987.

9. Guthrie R. The origin of newborn screening. Screening 1992;1:5–15.

10. Khoury MJ. From genes to public health: the applications of genetic technology in disease prevention. Am J Public Health 1996;86:1717–1722.

11. Stoddard JF, Farrell PM. State-to-state variations in newborn screening policies. Arch Pediatr Adolesc Med 1997;151:561–564.

12. Kosorok MR, Wei W-H, Farrell PM. The incidence of cystic fibrosis. Stat Med 1996;15:449–462.

13. Mohon RT, Wagener JS, Abman SH, et al. Relationship of genotype to early pulmonary function in infants with cystic fibrosis identified through neonatal screening. J Pediatr 1993;122:550–555.

14. Farrell PM, Mischler EH, Fost NC, et al. Current issues in neonatal screening for cystic fibrosis and implications of the CF gene discovery. Pediatr Pulmonal Suppl 1991;7:11–18.

15. Gregg RC, Wilfond BS, Farrell PM, et al. The application of DNA analysis in a population screening program for neonatal diagnosis of cystic fibrosis: comparison of screening protocols. Am J Hum Genet 1993;52:616–626.

16. Genetic testing for cystic fibrosis NIH Concensus Statement. 1997 Apr 14–16; 15:1–37.

17. Morral N, Bertranpetit J, Estivill X, et al. The origin of the major cystic fibrosis mutation (ΔF508) in European populations. Nat Genet 1994;5:169–175.

18. Serre JL, Bimon-Bouy B, Mornet E, et al. Studies of RFLP closely linked to the cystic fibrosis locus throughout Europe lead to new considerations in population genetics. Hum Genet 1990;84:449–454.

19. Schroeder SCA, Gaughan DM, Swift M. Protection against bronchial asthma by CFTR ΔF508 mutation: a heterozygote advantage in cystic fibrosis. Nat Med 1995;1:703–705.

20. Abraham EH, Vos P, Kahn J, et al. Cystic fibrosis hetero- and homozygosity is associated with inhibition of breast cancer growth. Nat Med 1996;2:593–596.

21. Ranieri E, Lewis BD, Gerace RL, et al. Neonatal screening for cystic fibrosis using immunoreactive trypsinogen and direct gene analysis: four years' experience. BMJ 1994;127:965–970.

22. Wilcken B. Newborn screening for cystic fibrosis: its evolution and a review of the current situation. Screening 1993;2:43–62.

23. Farrell PM, Kosorok MR, Rock MJ, Laxova A, Zeng L, Hoffman G, et al. Assessment of the benefits, risks and costs of cystic fibrosis screening in Wisconsin, USA. *In*: Travert G and Wursteisen B (eds). *Neonatal Screening for Cystic Fibrosis*. Presses Universitaires de Caen, pp. 239–253, 1999.

24. Macek M, Mackova A, Hamosh A, et al. Identification of common cystic fibrosis mutations in African-Americans with cystic fibrosis increases the detection rate to 75%. Am J Hum Genet 1997;60:1122–1127.

25. Farrell PM, Gilbert-Barness E, Bell J, et al. Progressive malnutrition, severe anemia, hepatic dysfunction, and respiratory failure in a three-month-old white girl. Am J Med Genet 1993;45:725–738.

26. Lai HC, Kosorok MR, Sondel SA, et al. Growth status in children with cystic fibrosis based on the National Cystic Fibrosis Patient Registry data: evaluation of various criteria used to identify malnutrition. J Pediatr 1998;132:478–485.

27. Rosenstein BJ, Langbaum TS, Metz SJ. Cystic fibrosis: diagnostic considerations. Johns Hopkins Med J 1982;150:113–120.

28. Blythe SA, Farrell PM. Advances in the diagnosis and management of cystic fibrosis. Clin Biochem 1984;17:277–283.

29. Warwick WJ. Undiagnosed patients with cystic fibrosis. J Chron Dis 1979;33:685–696.

30. Shwachman H, Redmond A, Khaw KT. Studies in cystic fibrosis: report of 130 patients diagnosed under 3 months of age over a 20-year period. Pediatrics 1970;46: 335–343.

31. Stephan U, Busch EW, Kollberg H, et al. Cystic fibrosis detection by means of a test strip. Pediatrics 1975;55:35–38.

32. Crossley JR, Elliott RB, Smith PA. Dried-blood spot screening for cystic fibrosis in the newborn. Lancet 1979;1:742–744.

33. AD Hoc Committee Task Force on Neonatal Screening, Cystic Fibrosis Foundation. Neonatal screening for cystic fibrosis: position paper. Pediatrics 1983;72:741–745.

34. Kerem B, Rommens JM, Buchanan JA, et al. Identification of the cystic fibrosis gene: genetic analysis. Science 1989;245:1073–1080.

35. Rock MJ, Mischler EH, Farrell PM, et al. Newborn screening for cystic fibrosis is complicated by age-related decline in immunoreactive trypsinogen levels. Pediatrics 1990;85:1001–1007.

36. Bruns WT, Connell TR, Lacey JA, et al. Test-strip meconium screening for cystic fibrosis. Am J Dis Child 1977;131:71–73.

37. Wilcken D, Wiley V, Sherry G, et al. Neonatal screening for cystic fibrosis: a comparison of two strategies for case detection in 1.2 million babies. J Pediatr 1995;127:965–970.

38. Hammond KB, Abman SH, Sokol RJ, et al. Efficacy of statewide neonatal screening for cystic fibrosis by assay of trypsinogen concentrations. N Engl J Med 1991; 325:769–774.

39. Gregg RG, Simantel A, Farrell PM, et al. Newborn screening for cystic fibrosis in Wisconsin: comparison of biochemical and molecular methods. Pediatrics 1997; 99:819–824.

40. Wilcken B, Chalmers G. Reduced morbidity in cystic fibrosis patients detected by newborn screening. Lancet 1985;ii:1319–1321.

41. Farrell PM. Early diagnosis of cystic fibrosis: to screen or not to screen—an important question. Pediatrics 1984;73:115–117.

42. Mischler EH, Wilfond BS, Fost N, et al. Cystic fibrosis newborn screening: impact on reproductive behavior and implications for genetic counseling. Pediatrics 1998; 102:44–52.

43. Ramsey BW, Farrell PM, Pencharz P. The Consensus Committee. Nutritional assessment and management in cystic fibrosis; a consensus report. Am J Clin Nutr 1992;55:108–116.

44. Mischler EH. Treatment of pulmonary disease in cystic fibrosis. Sem Resp Med 1985;6:271–284.

45. Wald NJ, Morris JK. Neonatal screening for cystic fibrosis. BMJ 1998;316: 404–405.

46. Cadman D, Chambers L, Feldman W, et al. Assessing the effectiveness of community screening programs. JAMA 1984;251:1580–1585.

47. Green M, Solnit AJ. Reactions to the threatened loss of a child: vulnerable child syndrome. Pediatrics 1964;34:58–66.

48. Loening-Bauche VA, Mischler EH, Myers MG. A placebo-controlled trial of cephalexin therapy in the ambulatory management of patients with cystic fibrosis. J Pediatr 1979;95:630–637.

49. Shwachman H, Kulczycki LL. Long-term study of one hundred five patients with cystic fibrosis. Am J Dis Child 1958;96:6–15.

50. Brasfield D, Hicks G, Soong S, Tiller RE. The chest roentgenogram in cystic fibrosis: a new scoring system. Pediatrics 1979;63:24–29.

51. Weatherly MR, Palmer CGS, Peters ME, et al. Wisconsin cystic fibrosis chest radiograph scoring system. Pediatrics 1993;91:488–495.

52. Wei LJ, Su JQ, Lachin JM. Interim analyses with repeated measurements in a sequential clinical trial. Biometrika 1990;77:359–364.

53. Lan KKG, DeMets DL. Discrete sequential boundaries for clinical trials. Biometrika 1983;70:659–663.

54. Gange SJ, DeMets DL. Sequential monitoring of clinical trials with correlated responses. Biometrika 1996;83:157–167.

55. Slud EV, Wei LJ. Two-sample repeated significance tests based on the modified Wilcoxon statistic. J Am Stat Assoc 1982;77:862–868.

56. Marcus MS, Sondel SA, Farrell PM, et al. Nutritional status of infants with cystic fibrosis associated with early diagnosis and intervention. Am J Clin Nutr 1991;54: 578–585.

57. Wood RE. Prognosis. In: Verlag GT, (ed). Cystic fibrosis. New York: Thieme-Stratton, 1984, pp. 434–460.

58. Kerem E, Corey M, Kerem B, et al. The relation between genotype and phenotype in cystic fibrosis—analysis of the most common mutation (ΔF508). N Engl J Med 1990;323:1517–1522.

59. Orenstein DM, Boat TF, Stem RC, et al. The effect of early diagnosis and treatment of cystic fibrosis. Am J Dis Child 1977;131:973–977.

60. Farrell PM, Shen G, Splaingard M, et al. Acquisition of Pseudomonas aeruginosa in children with cystic fibrosis. Pediatrics 1997;100:1–9.

61. Kosorok MR, Jalaluddin M, Farrell PM, et al. Comprehensive analysis of risk factors for acquisition of *Pseudomonas aeruginosa* in young children with cystic fibrosis. Pediatr Pulmonol 1998;26:81–88.

62. Waters DL, Wilcken B, Irwig L, et al. Clinical outcomes of newborn screening for cystic fibrosis. Arch Dis Child Fetal Neonatal Ed 1999;80:F1–F7.

63. Chatfield S, Owen G, Ryley HC, et al. Neonatal screening for cystic fibrosis in Wales and the West Midlands: clinical assessment after five years of screening. Arch Dis Child 1991:66:29–33.

64. Sokol RJ, Reardon MC, Accurso FJ, et al. Fat-soluble-vitamin status during the first year of life in infants with cystic fibrosis identified by screening of newborns. Am J Clin Nutr 1989;50:1064–1071.

65. Baroni MA, Anderson YE, Mischler EH. Cystic fibrosis newborn screening: impact early screening results on parenting stress. J Pediatr Nurs 1997;23:143–151.

66. Wilfond BS, Nolan K. National policy development for the clinical application of genetic diagnostic technologies: lessons from cystic fibrosis. JAMA 1993;270: 2948–2954.

67. Kwon C, Farrell PM. The magnitude and challenge of false-positive newborn screening test results. Arch Pediatr Adoles Med (in press).

22

Newborn screening for sickle cell disease: Public health impact and evaluation

The most common abnormal hemoglobin detected by newborn screening programs in the United States is *S*, or sickle hemoglobin, the defining characteristic for sickle cell disease. Hemoglobin S is produced by a mutated gene coding for one of the blood proteins. Homozygous sickle cell (hemoglobin SS) disease results when the sickle gene mutation is inherited from each parent. Sickle cell disease also occurs when the sickle mutation is inherited from one parent, and one of several other mutations is inherited from the other parent: the most common resulting conditions are sickle cell–hemoglobin C disease and the sickle beta-thalassemia syndromes. Childhood manifestations of these conditions may include susceptibility to serious infections, life-threatening splenic sequestration, and severe anemia, stroke, episodes of severe pain, or events of respiratory compromise known as the "acute chest syndrome." Newborn screening allows for enrollment in comprehensive specialty care programs, early institution of prophylactic therapies, and parental education to recognize these serious complications.

Many details about basic scientific, clinical, and general preventive aspects of sickle cell disease are beyond the scope of this chapter, but several review articles pertinent to these topics have been published recently (1–7). Three recent sickle cell or newborn screening textbooks include chapters on newborn hemoglobinopathy screening with details about laboratory aspects and programmatic issues, and a supplemental issue of the journal *Pediatrics* published in 1989 was devoted to experiences of individual states' with hemoglobinopathy screening and other perspectives (8–11). This chapter provides a broad overview of public health aspects of newborn hemoglobinopathy screening in the United States, with special emphasis on epidemiologic efforts to evaluate pediatric outcomes after newborn screening.

Establishment of Newborn Screening Programs

Research programs directed at screening large numbers of cord blood specimens for hemoglobinopathies were done in the 1960s, but local pilot programs with clinical follow-up were not initiated by hematologists until the early 1970s, and the first statewide newborn screening program was not implemented until 1975 (Table 22.1) (12–14). In 1972, the 92nd Congress of the United States passed the National Sickle Cell Anemia Control Act, which called for grant support for screening programs, "first to those persons who are entering their child-producing years, and secondly to children under the age of 7" (15). After passage of this and other legislation at the federal and state level, many state health departments received funding and mandates to expand their newborn screening programs to include hemoglobinopathies.

Table 22.1 Selected States with Newborn Hemoglobinopathy Screening Programs, by Year Started and Number of Infants Screened in 1993 (excludes states with incomplete reporting, limited screening, or no screening program)

Year Started	State	Number of Infants Screened, 1993	Total Live Births, 1993
1975	New York	282,978	283,328
1980	Georgia	83,284*	111,318
1983	Texas	(estimated) 319,742	326,267
1985	Maryland	69,293	69,494
1985	Indiana	83,387	83,622
1987	North Carolina	36,404*	101,663
1987	South Carolina	52,314	52,110
1987	Iowa	37,865	38,113
1988	Florida	193,032	193,035
1988	Louisiana	105,030**	69,474**
1988	Arkansas	33,738	33,173
1988	Minnesota	65,900	64,517
1989	Virginia	96,667	92,499
1989	Connecticut	47,496	46,756
1989	Wisconsin	68,532	68,917
1989	Illinois	190,500	187,461
1990	New Jersey	113,928	114,501
1990	Pennsylvania	155,657	161,493
1990	California	578,820	585,564
1991	Tennessee	76,988	77,534
1991	Oklahoma	50,763	45,351
1991	Mississippi	41,639	41,639
1991	Washington	72,983	77,182
1992	Kansas	45,341	35,850
	Total, 24 states	(estimated) 2,902,281	2,960,861
	U.S. totals	(estimated) 3,660,355	4,068,211

Source: Council of Regional Networks for Genetic Services (14).

*Targeted screening in 1993.

**1992: 70,245 hemoglobin results reported, 70,902 total births (33).

However, widespread acceptance and implementation of newborn hemoglobinopathy screening were hampered by several factors. Doubts about one of these issues, the effectiveness of early treatment, were greatly relieved after the results of a randomized trial published in 1986 showed the efficacy of daily oral penicillin prophylaxis in preventing infection among young children with sickle cell disease (16,17).

The results of prophylactic penicillin trials in the United States and Jamaica led to scientific consensus about the need for screening and subsequently widespread adoption of newborn hemoglobinopathy screening programs. Details of these events provide an unusual example of the results of well-designed epidemiologic studies driving newborn screening policy; newborn screening for other conditions in the United States has not often been preceded by such rigorous studies of efficacy and safety (18).

In these studies, penicillin was prescribed for daily oral use in the United States and monthly home intramuscular injections in Jamaica (17,19). All but one of the treated children in both countries were younger than 36 months of age at study entry, but only some were identified at birth by newborn screening. In the United States, 105 children with hemoglobin SS were randomized to receive penicillin, and there were 143 Jamaican children in the penicillin group. Among Jamaican children younger than age 36 months, no pneumococci were isolated from the blood or spinal fluid of these youngsters while they were receiving penicillin, whereas two pneumococcal organisms were isolated in the group not treated with penicillin; no deaths occurred in either group among children younger than age 36 months (the age when penicillin prophylaxis was terminated). In the United States, the rate of pneumococcal septicemia or meningitis was 1.9% among the children treated with penicillin compared with 7.9% in the control group, and there were no deaths in the penicillin group compared with three in the control group.

The Jamaican results were not statistically significant, and few deaths occurred even among children in the control groups of the two studies. However, the paucity of serious pneumococcal infections in children treated with penicillin was compelling. In 1987, after publication of the U.S. study, two federal agencies, the National Institutes of Health and the Health Resources and Services Administration, sponsored a Consensus Development Conference on Newborn Screening for Sickle Cell Disease and Other Hemoglobinopathies. Published recommendations from this conference cited the U.S. trial and called for universal hemoglobinopathy screening of newborns in most states, and a similar recommendation was made in 1993 by an expert panel convened at the federal level by the Agency for Health Care Policy and Research (AHCPR) (20,21). Statewide newborn screening programs covering the majority of children born in the United States began after the 1987 Consensus Conference (Table 22.1). In 1993, of approximately 4 million newborns in the United States, more than 3.6 million were screened for hemoglobinopathies (Table 22.1) (14). In 1996, recognizing that a few state health departments (e.g., in the Rocky Mountains) had chosen not to develop any hemoglobinopathy screening program, the American Academy of Pediatrics recommended that pediatric practitioners in these areas screen "at-risk" newborns (22,23).

Targeted Versus Universal Screening

Definition of the "screened population" has been a controversial topic in hemoglobinopathy screening. The practice of selecting certain infants for hemoglobinopathy testing on the basis of race and ethnicity is commonly known as *targeted screening*. As noted above, the American Academy of Pediatrics has recommended targeted screening of certain infants younger than 2 months of age when newborn screening is not done through a state program "in addition to African-Americans, Hispanics from Panama, South America, and the Caribbean and those whose ancestors are from the Mediterranean, India, or the Near East" (22). Until 1998, targeted screening was done statewide in Georgia among a larger group of infants of specified heritages: African, Arabian, Central American, Greek, Maltese, Hispanic, Indian, Portuguese, Puerto Rican, Sardinian, Sicilian, South American, and Southern Asian (24). Georgia investigators compared the number of black newborns screened for hemoglobinopathies between 1981 and 1985 with black natality figures for the same period and estimated that approximately 20% of black newborns were not screened (24). This figure has been widely quoted to illustrate the deficiencies of a targeted approach. Results of a study of universal screening in the multiethnic California population also indicated that an approach of targeting certain groups in that state would have missed at least 10% of those whose sickle cell disease was actually diagnosed at birth (25). Critics of the targeted approach have also raised the issue of the cost of determining race and ethnicity in the newborn nursery (26).

The costs of various screening approaches are logical issues for public policy discussion as newborn screening has been in the province of U.S. public health departments. Although all cost-effectiveness investigators have conceded the value of newborn screening in certain populations, they differ as to whether universal screening in certain areas of the United States is a rational policy (26–29). Some investigators analyzing cost-effectiveness data have discussed the financial advantages of using multistate laboratory consortiums and suggested that this approach would justify universal screening (29). Multistate consortiums have actually been used in a few geographic areas, and virtually all state health departments with hemoglobinopathy screening programs (including Georgia) have now adopted the universal approach.

Public Health Importance of Hemoglobinopathy Screening

Any screening program should be justified not only by demonstrated efficacy of early treatment, as was shown by the penicillin trials for sickle cell disease, but also first by the public health importance and prevalence of the screened condition and second by the broad effectiveness of these interventions in large populations (actual outcomes) (30,31). Population-based outcome studies are a major focus of the rest of this chapter, but the prevalence issue must first be addressed by examining well-established population-based data.

Rates of sickle cell disease by race and ethnicity are often cited in discussions about the population to be screened. Table 22.2 shows abbreviated results of a meta-analysis of newborn screening and other data published by the AHCPR (Agency for Health Care Policy and Research) Sickle Cell Disease Guideline Panel in 1993. Although sickle cell disease is most prevalent among African Americans, in certain states Hispanic infants constitute a substantial percentage of those identified by newborn screening, and other races are also affected. In California, in the early to mid-1990s approximately 45% of newborns were classified as Hispanic, 35% white (not Hispanic), 10% Asian, and 7% black, and the rate of sickle cell disease at birth in the entire population was 1 per every 4417 births (6% of infants with sickle cell disease were reportedly Hispanic and not black) (32). This figure is similar to the rate of congenital hypothyroidism, the most prevalent condition of U.S. newborn screening programs (23). In states such as New York and those in the American Southeast with a higher percentage of black births, the rate of sickle cell disease in the entire birth population would be even higher than the California

Table 22.2 Prevalence of Sickle Cell Disease (Hb SS, sickle cell–hemoglobin C disease and sickle–beta-thalassemia syndromes) by Racial or Ethnic Group, per 100,000 Live Births, United States, 1990 and Unspecified Years*

Racial or Ethnic Group	Mean Prevalence	95% CI
White	1.72	1.06–2.66
Black	289.00	277–300
Hispanic, total	5.28	2.60–9.61
Hispanic, Eastern states	89.80	27.0–190.0
Hispanic, Western states	3.14	1.19–6.86
Asian	7.61	1.85–57.20
Native American	36.20	0.04–182.0

* Abbreviated and modified from results of Bayesian meta-analysis, published by Sickle Cell Disease Guideline Panel, 1993 (20).

figures. With these rates of sickle cell disease, at birth more than 2000 infants are identified annually with sickle cell disease in the United States, and at least 50,000 Americans are estimated to be currently affected (14,20,33). World-wide, birth prevalence figures have been calculated from trait frequencies in different continents since newborn screening is not widely done; an esti-mated 120,000 to 250,000 affected infants are born annually across the globe (7,34).

Other hemoglobinopathies found particularly among people of Asian and Mediterranean descent, such as beta-thalassemia major, are also detected by hemoglobinopathy screening. Identification and counseling of families with sickle cell and other hemoglobinopathy traits is a natural by-product of these newborn screening programs. Some public health advocates point to counsel-ing of carriers as a positive benefit; as an example of this "benefit beyond the target," these investigators discuss the opportunity that trait counseling pro-vides for offering prenatal diagnosis in subsequent pregnancies (35). Parents with sickle cell disease who were unaware of their diagnosis have also been identified when their newborns were screened. In contrast, other researchers have presented arguments against carrier identification and counseling by state-sponsored newborn screening programs, citing a number of issues: ethical concerns about government involvement in this issue, insurance and employ-ment discrimination as a consequence of carrier identification, and the potential for the "vulnerable child syndrome" scenario in affected families (28). Nevertheless, national newborn screening guidelines advanced by the U.S. Council of Regional Networks for Genetic Services strongly advocate resource allocation for carrier counseling (with particular reference to hemo-globinopathy screening) (36).

Evaluation of Outcomes After Newborn Screening

As noted above, while the efficacy of prophylactic penicillin was demonstrated by randomized trials, the true measure of effectiveness of the combination of newborn screening and early preventive measures is actual outcomes in large populations. The distinction between efficacy and effectiveness is that efficacy is often a research demonstration of a therapy under ideal conditions, whereas the effectiveness of a prevention strategy should be measured in community settings (37). Stated another way, in the public health arena, research must be translated into practice, and newborn screening follow-up studies are neces-sary to evaluate fully these programs—a key step in applying genetic tech-nology to disease prevention (30).

Mortality Studies
One traditional epidemiologic approach to population-based studies is to use large, public, electronic databases. The major strengths of this approach are

that it is truly population-based, often has sufficient power to answer epidemiologic questions because large numbers of records can be analyzed, and does not usually suffer from questions of representativeness or selection bias as the entire U.S. or other population can be analyzed. Disadvantages of using large databases to measure clinical outcomes include systematic problems with coding that may be magnified if the study period is long or if the study area is large; inadequate sensitivity caused by missing data, as such databases are usually not exclusively designed to examine specific diseases; and inability to analyze health outcomes associated with risk factors other than those provided by the basic demographic information (e.g., race, sex, age) contained in many such databases.

One of the most easily quantifiable outcomes available in the United States is mortality since the National Center for Health Statistics compiles death certificates from each state in the Multiple Cause Mortality Files. Investigators have analyzed sickle cell-coded death certificates to examine age-specific death rates, temporal trends, and geographic variation in recent U.S. mortality (38–41). A problem with examining temporal trends in rates of sickle cell disease relates to the coding scheme for these records: From 1968 until 1979, the International Classification of Diseases lumped sickle cell trait with sickle disease, and even after 1978 the coding system lumped sickle–beta-thalassemia syndromes with thalassemia major rather than with the category for hemoglobin SS disease and sickle cell–hemoglobin C disease. As a result, some investigators have excluded pre-1979 records or children with sickle–beta-thalassemia syndromes from their analyses, making the results of various death certificate studies not completely comparable with each other or with results from published cohort studies. Nevertheless, results of these studies have consistently demonstrated a decline in mortality among children with sickle cell disease in recent years.

The study by Davis et al. (38) provided the most published details of pediatric mortality trends based on death certificates. Mortality rates during the years 1968 through 1992 declined in three different pediatric age groups (infants were excluded from the analysis), although the steepest declines occurred among young children born before 1980, when most newborn screening programs had not been established (Table 22.1). In a separate analysis of the same data, these investigators also concluded that individual states had statistically significant differences in pediatric mortality rates and identified a handful of states with particularly high or low mortality rates relative to the entire United States (39). However, in that analysis, Davis and colleagues did not attempt to isolate any influence that newborn screening may have had on mortality rates by, for example, analyzing data before and after statewide screening programs started or comparing mortality rates in states with targeted screening versus those in states with universal screening during certain time periods.

Results of clinic-based cohort studies have also provided data addressing mortality after newborn screening. Two studies warrant special discussion because of their size and ongoing influence on screening policy: the U.S. Cooperative Study of Sickle Cell Disease (CSSCD) and a large Jamaican cohort study. The prophylactic penicillin studies discussed above both included children from these studies, but published mortality and morbidity data include data from a much larger pool of children followed in the same centers. The comprehensive care provided by these specialty centers, generally large academic hospitals, represents the "gold standard" of prophylactic and acute medical care for children with sickle cell disease.

Enrollment of children in the CSSCD began in 1979, and Leikin et al. (42) first published mortality data in 1989. The CSSCD was not purely a follow-up study of a cohort of children identified as newborns: of 2824 youngsters who enrolled in the study, only 640 entered the study before 6 months of age. Among this group of children identified in early infancy, those with hemoglobin SS disease had a mortality rate before age 3 years ranging from 5.08 deaths per 100 person-years among those entering in 1980 to 0.69 deaths per 100 person-years among those entering in 1983. The overall rates of mortality during the entire study period (1979 to 1987) were 0.81 deaths per 100 person-years for infants and 1.66 per 100 person-years for children age 1 to 3 years. In an updated report on the cohort of infants from the CSSCD, Gill et al. (43) calculated a rate of 1.1 deaths per 100 person-years with a mean follow-up period of 4.2 years, with the highest rate among children between 6 months and 3 years of age. Davis et al. (38) also estimated person-year mortality rates in their study of national death certificates and found rates comparable with those of the CSSCD for children in three different age groups.

In their discussion of the mortality data, Leikin and colleagues (42) point out the difficulty of comparing the CSSCD with earlier studies with different methodologies, but nevertheless cite higher rates of person-year mortality among children born before the CSSCD and attribute improvements to the increased use of antibiotics for febrile episodes. In contrast, Davis et al. (38) suggest that improved survival from 1968 through 1992 was due to multiple factors, including the establishment of newborn screening programs, more comprehensive medical care, widespread acceptance of penicillin prophylaxis, and new vaccinations.

The Jamaican study provides another perspective on the effect of newborn screening and early intervention on sickle cell-related mortality rates (44). Children with hemoglobin SS disease were identified after 100,000 consecutive deliveries from 1973 through 1981 at the main hospital in Kingston. The mortality rates among children born later in the study period were significantly lower than those among youngsters born earlier, in particular mortality rates from pneumococcal infections and splenic sequestration. Jamaican investigators attributed these changes partly to improved pneumococcal prophylaxis and parental education programs to recognize splenic sequestration.

In a separate Jamaican study of splenic sequestration, investigators analyzed morbidity from these events among children identified by newborn screening before and after an education program about splenic palpation was instituted (45). They found that the rate of sequestration increased but that the fatality rate from this event fell, suggesting that increased early detection by parents after education led to a decline in mortality rates. The Jamaican studies provide direct evidence that recent reductions in pediatric mortality rates are not due solely to newborn screening per se, as the trends were seen among children who were all identified as having sickle cell disease at birth. However, early diagnosis provided the opportunity to institute public health programs that would not have affected survival so dramatically if not directed toward infants and their parents.

In the United States, investigators have also studied outcomes in cohorts of children identified with sickle cell disease shortly after birth. In northern California, newborn screening was done in a limited number of hospitals between 1975 and 1985, which allowed investigators to study two cohorts of children followed at a comprehensive sickle cell center: a group diagnosed shortly after birth and a group diagnosed at a mean age of 21 months (46). The overall mortality rate in the newborn screening group after approximately 7 years of follow-up was 1.8%, compared with 8% in the group diagnosed later and followed for a mean of approximately 9 years. As in Jamaica, parents of infants screened at birth were offered an extensive education program, although most of the children were born before the widespread use of prophylactic penicillin and some new vaccinations. The authors of the above study (46) noted that life-threatening events did not occur less frequently in the group screened at birth but suggested that early recognition of these complications by parents and tertiary-care providers resulted in improved survival rates.

Several state newborn screening programs have also been conducting follow-up studies to evaluate outcomes among children they have identified with sickle cell disease. Some of the states with large and well-established newborn screening programs actively involved with such studies include California, Georgia, Illinois, Louisiana, Maryland, Mississippi, New Jersey, New York, and Texas. Types of follow-up efforts include periodic or one-time physician surveys, parent interviews, medical record abstraction, and analysis of vital records. Some states such as California, Illinois, and New York have collaborated and pooled their data for publication of large outcome studies (47). These collaborative efforts have been particularly useful for mortality studies in this era of markedly improved survival.

In California, Illinois, and New York, investigators used identifying variables from state sickle cell databases for children born 1990 through 1994 and compared these with state death certificate files. Some additional follow-up information was available through physician surveys and reports from public health nurses about details of deaths. During the 5-year period, 2487 children with sickle cell disease were identified by the three newborn screening programs. Among the children with hemoglobin SS disease with follow-up information through age 3 years, 1.0% died of sickle cell-related causes. This mortality rate was equivalent to 0.35 per 100 person-years, less than the lowest mortality rate in the 1989 report of the Cooperative Study of Sickle Cell Disease discussed above. Similarly low mortality rates have been reported by other state newborn screening programs in recent years (47).

Morbidity Studies

The low mortality rates of the 1990s, which now approach expected infant mortality rates for the general population, have focused public health efforts on reducing other serious complications of sickle cell disease following newborn screening. Improved preventive strategies such as pneumococcal vaccines for infants may also reduce the burden of sickle cell-related hospitalizations in the future, as may new therapeutic strategies such as outpatient treatment of febrile children with sickle cell disease and outpatient transfusion therapy (6,48). Morbidity in the early childhood years (the immediate focus of newborn screening programs) focuses on the effects of the disease on three organs: the brain, spleen, and lungs, including infections that involve these organs (1). As with mortality data, epidemiologic studies of these complications include large studies of state or national databases, clinically based cohort studies, and population-based follow-up studies (43,47,49–51).

Two examples of large electronic databases amenable to sickle cell studies are the National Hospital Discharge Survey and state hospital discharge tapes. A recent publication containing data from the National Hospital Discharge Survey reported no detailed information about causes of morbidity but did provide information about the annual numbers of hospitalization, the costs of these hospitalizations, and the sources of payment including government programs (49). In this study of U.S. hospitalizations from 1989 to 1993, children under the age of 20 years accounted for more than half of the estimated 75,000 annual hospitalizations for people with sickle cell disease. Results of a study of state hospital discharge data showed more than 3000 pediatric hospitalizations in California for hemoglobinopathies in 1991, with a mean charge of $7000 per hospitalization (50). The California data also contained detailed information about discharge diagnoses (not published because sickle cell was not the focus of the article), which showed that the predominant reasons for hospitalization among children under the age of 3 years were bacterial and pulmonary infections, and other suspected infections. This type of data can be used to follow temporal trends in the types, volume, and costs of hospitalization and the age-distribution of patients hospitalized. Indeed, as part of the follow-up study in Illinois discussed above (47), investigators have examined state hospital discharge records.

The Cooperative Study of Sickle Cell Disease has provided volumes of epidemiological data relating to pediatric morbidity, although as with the mortality studies mentioned earlier, these investigators have not focused exclusively on outcomes after newborn screening. However, for the most part the outcomes of 703 infants who were enrolled in the study at less than 6 months of age (mean 3 months) reflect the experience of those identified through newborn screening, as most adverse events begin later in infancy (43,51). As noted above, because these children were offered the "gold standard" of medical care, their outcomes might be expected to reflect the best possible scenario, but the strength of this data is the clinical detail, specificity, and prospective nature of data collection.

In general, children with sickle cell–hemoglobin C disease had fewer episodes of sepsis, splenic sequestration, stroke, and other events compared with children with hemoglobin SS disease. In children with hemoglobin SS, the peak age for bacteremia was the second 6 months of infancy; splenic sequestration occurred most frequently among 1-year-olds; and stroke did not occur among infants but occurred at the highest rate (2.1 events per 100 person-years) among 6-year-olds. There was a suggestion of a decreased rate of pneumococcal infections after 1986 when penicillin prophylaxis became routine, although the decrease was not statistically significant. An ongoing extension study should provide more information about temporal trends in the rates of these pediatric complications among children born in the 1990s with an opportunity to benefit from new vaccines and therapies and more widespread use of prophylactic penicillin.

State newborn screening programs doing follow-up studies of morbidity have focused on such endpoints as hospitalizations, emergency room visits, and developmental status. Many of these studies, such as those in Georgia, Illinois, Louisiana, Maryland, Mississippi, New Jersey, and New York, are ongoing, with observations currently unpublished or in abstract or health department report form (47,52–54). The Maryland health department is particularly interested in preventable hospitalizations related to sickle cell disease and is attempting to correlate factors such as use of penicillin (ascertained from Medicaid claims) with these outcomes. In the California, Illinois, and New York studies, researchers have collected information such as children's demographic characteristics, antibiotic use, immunization status, and genetic subtypes, as well as parental sickle cell knowledge, and insurance status to analyze the association of these variables with outcomes.

Importance of Follow-up Studies for Newborns: Future Directions

Data collected by evaluating the community effectiveness of trial-proven strategies such as penicillin prophylaxis have an obvious value in academic studies such as cost-effectiveness analyses. However, they also have considerable practical uses. For example, state health departments could potentially use collected data to improve procedures for enrolling children in comprehensive care if delays in initiation of prophylaxis are found in certain cities, or to target high-risk populations that continue to experience excess morbidity. There is also evidence of a need for ongoing surveillance of outcomes even when proven prevention strategies have been implemented. For example, the emergence of penicillin-resistant organisms and evident problems with youngsters not receiving their prescribed penicillin daily have raised concerns and provided further impetus for trials of new pneumococcal vaccines for infants (55–57).

As state health departments have become more involved with diagnosis of genetic disease through their state laboratories, many have become obligated to adopt regulations to control the content and quantity of services provided for children they have identified after diagnosis. For example, in funding Illinois hematologists, the Department of Public Health has included provisions that require penicillin prophylaxis for young children identified by the state screening program (58). Some state health departments such as California's are involved with certifying sickle cell counselors; this type of regulation ensures the quality of genetic education at the provider level, but the proof of the efficacy of these policies is the actual knowledge taken home by parents (59). The ongoing California and Illinois follow-up studies include a parental questionnaire that theoretically can ascertain the type and quality of services parents are receiving from regulated providers; this type of data has been difficult to collect retrospectively, and in future studies the data might be more easily collected through a questionnaire regularly administered as the services are provided.

Public interest in sickle cell disease has been piqued by well-publicized studies in which researchers have attempted to cure sickle cell disease through bone marrow transplantation or gene therapy (60,61). Although it is safe to say that these efforts are currently in early stages and have had little public health impact to date, when they become more widespread they will lead to dilemmas such as the selection of ideal candidates and the timing for such therapy. Population-based outcome studies will provide further data with which to identify children at particularly high risk for morbidity and mortality.

Conclusions

Despite controversies about cost-effectiveness and ethical quandaries of carrier identification and targeted versus universal approaches, newborn screening programs for hemoglobinopathies in the United States are firmly entrenched, at least in part because of strong epidemiological data suggesting that early identification of affected newborns is a rational policy. As prevention-oriented policies are directed toward large populations and manifestations of disease complications change, however, ongoing data collection is needed to ensure the effectiveness of these strategies at the community level. Funding for follow-up studies is as important as funding for studies at the basic science level to understand and even cure the underlying disease. Sickle cell disease is an example of a common genetic condition for which preventive strategies have been particularly effective at reducing rates of complications, and the historical precedents of sickle cell newborn screening and treatment may serve as a public health model for other conditions considered for population screening in the future.

References

1. Lane PA. Sickle cell disease. Pediatr Clin North Am 1996;43:639–664.

2. Bunn HF. Pathogenesis and treatment of sickle cell disease. N Engl J Med 1997;337:762–769.

3. Rodgers GP. Overview of pathophysiology and rationale for treatment of sickle cell anemia. Semin Hematol 1997;34(3 Suppl 3):2–7.

4. Davies SC, Oni L. Management of patients with sickle cell disease. BMJ 1997;315:656–660.

5. Olney RS. Preventing morbidity and mortality from sickle cell disease: a public health perspective. Am J Prev Med 1999;16:116–121.

6. Serjeant GR. The role of preventive medicine in sickle cell disease. The Watson Smith lecture. J R Coll Physicians Lond 1996;30:37–41.

7. Serjeant GR. Sickle-cell disease. Lancet 1997;350:725–730.

8. Eckman JR. Neonatal screening. In: Embury SH, Hebbel RP, Mohandas N, Steinberg MH (eds). Sickle cell disease: basic principles and clinical practice. New York: Raven Press, 1994, pp. 509–515.

9. Serjeant GR. Sickle cell disease (2nd ed). New York: Oxford University Press, 1992, pp. 39–53.

10. Therrell BL, Pass KA. Hemoglobinopathy screening laboratory techniques for newborns. In: Therrell BL (ed). Laboratory methods for neonatal screening. Washington, DC: American Public Health Association, 1993, pp. 169–189.

11. Wethers D, Pearson H, Gaston M, et al. Newborn screening for sickle cell disease and other hemoglobinopathies. Pediatrics 1989;83(5 Pt 2):813–914.

12. Pearson HA. Neonatal testing for sickle cell diseases—a historical and personal review. Pediatrics 1989;83(5 Pt 2):815–818.

13. Grover R. Newborn screening in New York City. Pediatrics 1989;83(5 Pt 2):819–822.

14. Newborn Screening Committee. The Council of Regional Networks for Genetic Services (CORN). National Newborn Screening Report—1993. Atlanta, GA: CORN, 1998:16,156–160,169.

15. National Sickle Cell Anemia Control Act. Pub. L. No. 92-294, 86 Stat. 138 (May 16, 1972).

16. Wethers D, Pearson H, Gaston M. Newborn screening for sickle cell disease and other hemoglobinopathies. Pediatrics 1989;83(5 Pt 2):813–814.

17. Gaston MH, Verter JI, Woods G, et al. Prophylaxis with oral penicillin in children with sickle cell anemia: a randomized trial. N Engl J Med 1986;314:1593–1599.

18. Andrews LB, Fullarton JE, Holtzman NA, Motulsky AG (eds). Assessing genetic risks: implication for health and social policy. Washington, DC: National Academy Press, 1994, p. 40.

19. John AB, Ramlal A, Jackson H, Maude GH, Waight Sharma A, Serjeant GR. Prevention of pneumococcal infection in children with homozygous sickle cell disease. BMJ 1984;288:1567–1570.

20. Sickle Cell Disease Guideline Panel. Sickle cell disease: screening, diagnosis, management, and counseling in newborns and infants. Clinical practice guideline no. 6. Rockville, MD: Agency for Health Care Policy and Research, Public Health Service, U.S. Department of Health and Human Services, 1993 (AHCPR publication no. 93-0562).

21. Consensus conference. Newborn screening for sickle cell disease and other hemoglobinopathies. JAMA 1987;258:1205–1209.

22. American Academy of Pediatrics Committee on Genetics. Health supervision for children with sickle cell diseases and their families. Pediatrics 1996;98:467–472.

23. American Academy of Pediatrics Committee on Genetics. Newborn screening fact sheets. Pediatrics 1996;98:473–501.

24. Harris MS, Eckman JR. Georgia's experience with newborn screening: 1981 to 1985. Pediatrics 1989;83(5 Pt 2):858–860.

25. Shafer FE, Lorey F, Cunningham GC, Klumpp C, Vichinsky E, Lubin B. Newborn screening for sickle cell disease: 4 years of experience from California's newborn screening program. J Pediatr Hematol Oncol 1996;18:36–41.

26. Lane PA, Eckman JR. Cost-effectiveness of neonatal screening for sickle cell disease. J Pediatr 1992;120:162–163.

27. Tsevat J, Wong JB, Pauker SG, Steinberg MH. Neonatal screening for sickle cell disease: a cost-effectiveness analysis. J Pediatr 1991;118(4 Pt 1):546–554.

28. Gessner BD, Teutsch SM, Shaffer PA. A cost-effectiveness evaluation of newborn hemoglobinopathy screening from the perspective of state health care systems. Early Hum Dev 1996;45:257–275.

29. Sprinkle RH, Hynes DM, Konrad TR. Is universal hemoglobinopathy screening cost-effective? Arch Pediatr Adolesc Med 1994;148:461–469.

30. Khoury MJ, Genetics Working Group. From genes to public health: the applications of genetic technology in disease prevention. Am J Public Health 1996;86:1717–1722.

31. Gordis L. The scope of screening. J Med Screen 1994;1:98–100.

32. Lorey FW, Arnopp J, Cunningham GC. Distribution of hemoglobinopathy variants by ethnicity in a multiethnic state. Genet Epidemiol 1996;13:501–512.

33. Newborn Screening Committee. The Council of Regional Networks for Genetic Services (CORN). National Newborn Screening Report—1992. Atlanta, GA: CORN, 1995:100.

34. WHO Working Group. Community control of hereditary anaemias: memorandum from a WHO meeting. Bull World Health Organ 1983;61:63–80.

35. Grover R, Newman S, Wethers D, Anyane-Yeboa K, Pass K. Newborn screening for hemoglobinopathies: the benefit beyond the target. Am J Public Health 1986;76:1236–1237.

36. Therrell BL, Panny SR, Davidson A, et al. U.S. newborn screening system guide-

lines: statement of the Council of Regional Networks for Genetic Services. Screening 1992;1:135–147.

37. Haddix AC, Teutsch SM, Shaffer PA (eds). Prevention effectiveness: a guide to decision analysis and economic evaluation. New York: Oxford University Press, 1996, pp. 4–5.

38. Davis H, Schoendorf KC, Gergen PJ, Moore RM Jr. National trends in the mortality of children with sickle cell disease, 1968 through 1992. Am J Public Health 1997;87:1317–1322.

39. Davis H, Gergen PJ, Moore RM Jr. Geographic differences in mortality of young children with sickle cell disease in the United States. Public Health Rep 1997;112:52–58.

40. Yang Q, Khoury MJ, Mannino D. Trends and patterns of mortality associated with birth defects and genetic diseases in the United States, 1979–1992: an analysis of multiple-cause mortality data. Genet Epidemiol 1997;14:493–505.

41. Cono J, Yang Q, Olney RS, Khoury MJ. Trends in sickle cell disease mortality among African-Americans, United States, 1979–1992: an analysis using multiple-cause mortality data. Proceedings of the 3rd Joint Clinical Genetics Meeting, Mar 11–14; 1996, San Antonio, TX, p. 140.

42. Leikin SL, Gallagher D, Kinney TR, Sloane D, Klug P, Rida W. Mortality in children and adolescents with sickle cell disease. Cooperative Study of Sickle Cell Disease. Pediatrics 1989;84:500–508.

43. Gill FM, Sleeper LA, Weiner SJ, et al. Clinical events in the first decade in a cohort of infants with sickle cell disease. Blood 1995;86:776–783.

44. Lee A, Thomas P, Cupidore L, Serjeant B, Serjeant G. Improved survival in homozygous sickle cell disease: lessons from a cohort study. BMJ 1995;311:1600–1602.

45. Emond AM, Collis R, Darvill D, Higgs DR, Maude GH, Serjeant GR. Acute splenic sequestration in homozygous sickle cell disease: natural history and management. J Pediatr 1985;107:201–206.

46. Vichinsky E, Hurst D, Earles A, Kleman K, Lubin B. Newborn screening for sickle cell disease: effect on mortality. Pediatrics 1988;81:749–755.

47. Centers for Disease Control and Prevention. Mortality among children with sickle cell disease identified by newborn screening during 1990–1994—California, Illinois, and New York. MMWR 1998;47:169–172.

48. Wilimas JA, Flynn PM, Harris S, et al. A randomized study of outpatient treatment with ceftriaxone for selected febrile children with sickle cell disease. N Engl J Med 1993;329:472–476.

49. Davis H, Moore RM Jr., Gergen PJ. Cost of hospitalizations associated with sickle cell disease in the United States. Public Health Rep 1997;112:40–43.

50. Yoon PW, Olney RS, Khoury MJ, Sappenfield WM, Chavez GF, Taylor D. Contribution of birth defects and genetic diseases to pediatric hospitalizations: a population-based study. Arch Pediatr Adolesc Med 1997;151:1096–1103.

51. Gill FM, Brown A, Gallagher D, et al. Newborn experience in the Cooperative Study of Sickle Cell Disease. Pediatrics 1989;83(5 Pt 2):827–829.

52. Panny S. Utilization of surveillance data and programs for services, education, and outreach. Proceedings of the 1st Annual National Birth Defects Prevention Workshop, December 7–8, 1997, Atlanta, GA.

53. New Jersey Department of Health and Senior Services. Long-term tracking of children with sickle cell disease and other hemoglobinopathies. Trenton: New Jersey Department of Health and Senior Services, Division of Family Health Services, Special Child and Adult Health Services, 1997.

54. Eckman J. Newborn screening for sickle cell anemia in region IV. SERGG Newsletter, June 1997:5.

55. Steele RW, Warrier R, Unkel PJ, et al. Colonization with antibiotic-resistant Streptococcus pneumoniae in children with sickle cell disease. J Pediatr 1996; 128:531–535.

56. Teach SJ, Lillis KA, Grossi M. Compliance with penicillin prophylaxis in patients with sickle cell disease. Arch Pediatr Adolesc Med 1998;152:274–278.

57. Centers for Disease Control and Prevention. Defining the public health impact of drug-resistant *Streptococcus pneumoniae*: report of a working group. MMWR 1996;45(No. RR-1):1–20.

58. Illinois Administrative Code. Title 77, Chapter 1, Subchapter i, Section 661.50 (1995).

59. Cunningham G, Kohatsu N, Stratton N, Neutra R. Meeting the challenge of genetics and public health: state perspectives on program activities (California). Proceedings of the 1st Annual Conference on Genetics and Public Health, May 13–15, 1998, Atlanta, GA, pp. 50–51.

60. Platt OS, Guinan EC. Bone marrow transplantation in sickle cell anemia—the dilemma of choice. N Engl J Med 1996;335:426–428.

61. Schechter AN, Rodgers GP. Sickle cell anemia—basic research reaches the clinic. N Engl J Med 1995;332:1372–1374.

23

Public health strategies to prevent the complications of hemochromatosis

Wylie Burke, Mary E. Cogswell, Sharon M. McDonnell, and Adele Franks

Hemochromatosis is a treatable, adult-onset genetic disorder for which screening tests are available. These characteristics make hemochromatosis an important model for public health to explore as it begins to address genetic contributions to adult disease. Whereas newborn screening programs are motivated by the need to provide early treatment of genetic conditions like phenylketonuria (PKU), this urgency does not apply to adult-onset disorders like hemochromatosis. Conversely, other adult onset disorders for which genetic testing is available, such as hereditary breast/ovarian cancer and Alzheimer disease, are not readily treatable. As our knowledge of genetic susceptibility to chronic diseases grows, the issues raised in the public health approach to hemochromatosis are likely to be relevant to many future efforts in genetics and public health.

Hemochromatosis results in the accumulation of excess iron stores over time. Complications occur when iron overload is sufficient to cause organ damage; these complications include cirrhosis, primary liver cancer, cardiomyopathy, arthritis, and diabetes (1–3). Current therapy for hemochromatosis starts with a "de-ironing" procedure at diagnosis, also called *quantitative phlebotomy*. This procedure consists of the removal of multiple units of blood, often over a period of several months. After the initial therapy, a maintenance program of periodic blood drawing is instituted to prevent reaccumulation of iron stores (1–3). This therapy prolongs survival in symptomatic individuals and appears to normalize life expectancy if begun early in the course of the disease (4).

Accordingly, early diagnosis of hemochromatosis can be expected to reduce the burden of the disease. A decrease in the proportion of affected people with late-stage disease has already been seen in recently reported clinical cohorts, compared with those reported two or three decades ago (3–5). This shift

447

reflects changing criteria for diagnosis and, in particular, increased use of abnormal serum iron measures such as elevated transferrin saturation or serum ferritin to detect those with iron overload (3,5). Even in these recent reports, however, a significant number of affected people had diabetes, heart disease, or cirrhosis at the time of diagnosis (3,5). Increasing physician awareness of the need for early diagnosis and treatment of hemochromatosis could result in further reductions in late-stage complications. We call this approach to the prevention of iron overload disease *enhanced case finding*.

Another strategy for reducing disease burden is *universal screening*. Serum iron measures—in particular transferrin saturation (TS = serum iron/total iron binding capacity × 100)—can be used to identify asymptomatic individuals with iron overload (6). The DNA-based tests for mutations in the *HFE* gene also provide a means to detect asymptomatic persons (7). Cost analyses suggest that the cost of TS screening is offset by savings from reduced end-stage complications of hemochromatosis (8–10). Also, DNA-based screening could be cost-effective were the sensitivity of the test high and the cost of testing reduced to a level similar to TS testing (11).

An elevated TS value or a positive result on a genetic test, however, does not predict certain progression to symptoms or serious complications of hemochromatosis. It is not known what proportion of those with a positive screening test will remain healthy without treatment. Nor is it known whether the full benefits of treatment require detection at an asymptomatic stage, as opposed to detection at the time of early signs or symptoms. Thus, calculations of the cost-effectiveness of screening for hemochromatosis are to some degree speculative. In addition, little attention has been given to the resources required to implement and maintain hemochromatosis screening programs, or to the social or economic effects of screening. Whether these uncertainties provide a substantive rationale against screening has been the subject of debate (12).

Enhanced case finding can be seen as the first stage in a public health response, when evidence for an effective early treatment of a disorder has emerged. In contrast, universal screening generally calls for more stringent evidence of benefit than case finding, because screening involves the testing and treatment of healthy people who are without medical complaints. In this chapter we review current knowledge about the natural history and genetics of hemochromatosis, and we consider the implications for public health policy of a transition from enhanced case finding to universal screening.

Uncertainties About the Natural History and Disease Burden of Hemochromatosis

For both enhanced case finding and universal screening, a reliable means of diagnosing hemochromatosis at an early stage is needed. Persistently elevated

TS—defined as an elevated TS value on both a random blood draw and a follow-up fasting sample—is an indicator of possible hemochromatosis. The serum ferritin level can also be used to detect affected persons in an asymptomatic stage. However, the serum ferritin level is less sensitive than TS, because it usually rises later in the disease process, and is also less specific because it is elevated in other common conditions, such as infection and inflammation (6). Some experts recommend using elevated serum ferritin as an indicator for liver biopsy, to determine whether cirrhosis is present or not, after a persistently elevated TS has been documented (3,6).

Transferrin saturation screening studies have used thresholds ranging from 45% to 70% to define an elevated TS value (12–15). The percentage of the Caucasian population in the United States with an elevated random TS ranges from 1% to 6%, depending on both the threshold used and the population tested (10,13–16); of these, 10% to 35% will have a persistently elevated TS value on a follow-up fasting test (13–15). Among those with persistently elevated TS levels, 40% to 75% will have evidence of iron overload by liver biopsy or quantitative phlebotomy (13–15); the remainder are likely to include some affected persons in the early stages of iron accumulation. Estimates of the prevalence of hemochromatosis derived from TS screening studies range from 2 to 8 per 1000 population (8–11,12–15).

Yet rates of documented hospitalizations, outpatient visits, and mortality attributed to hemochromatosis are much lower than predicted by TS screening studies (12,17). This discrepancy suggests that hemochromatosis is underdiagnosed, or that the risk of morbidity and mortality among individuals identified through TS screening is low, or both (12). Several factors might contribute to underdiagnosis of hemochromatosis. Methods of documentation may contribute; for example, some data sources (such as Medicaid data) are limited to one diagnosis. If a complication of hemochromatosis is the primary reason for a visit (e.g., diabetes mellitus, chronic liver disease, or arthritis), hemochromatosis is unlikely to be documented. Failure to recognize hemochromatosis may also contribute to underdiagnosis. Until recently, the diagnosis of hemochromatosis relied on late-stage symptoms. One patient survey indicated that many affected persons experience a long delay between the onset of symptoms and the diagnosis of hemochromatosis, even when medical consultation is sought repeatedly (18). Screening studies among those with chronic disease such as arthritis and diabetes also suggest that when hemochromatosis is the underlying cause of the disease it is often unrecognized (12,19–21).

Although failure to diagnose hemochromatosis is a likely contributor to the low rate of documented cases, lack of disease progression among individuals who would be identified in screening programs also seems likely. In large population screening studies, only 45% of men and 43% of women aged >40 years with iron overload exhibited one or more clinical manifestations of hemochromatosis (22). These percentages are high enough to predict many more cases of iron overload than are seen in clinical data sources. The clinical manifestations assessed in these large screening studies, however, included both the severe complications of hemochromatosis (such as liver disease, diabetes, and cardiomyopathy) and the more nonspecific symptoms seen early in the course of the disease (arthropathy, fatigue, weight loss, abdominal pain, and impotence) (22). Because the nonspecific symptoms are relatively common among persons without hemochromatosis, some of the morbidity attributed to hemochromatosis in screening studies could be due to other causes. It is thus possible that only a subset of those detected in screening programs would develop disorders attributable to iron overload.

No screening studies have reported longitudinal follow-up. The current standard of care for those with persistently elevated TS (in the absence of other causes) is to proceed to quantitative phlebotomy, both for confirmation of the diagnosis and to initiate therapy. In addition, serum ferritin and liver function tests are usually done, and a liver biopsy recommended if the results of these tests are significantly elevated. Ongoing blood removal is recommended if quantitative phlebotomy or liver biopsy indicates iron overload (1,3). Because TS screening leads to treatment, prospective follow-up in itself cannot be used to determine the proportion of individuals testing positive who would remain healthy over time if untreated.

Contribution of Genetic Testing to the Diagnosis of Hemochromatosis

The discovery of the gene for hemochromatosis, *HFE* (23,24), was expected to provide a clearer approach to diagnosis. Genetic testing, however, has turned out to involve uncertainties similar to those posed by TS testing. Two *HFE* mutations have been defined, C282Y and H63D (23). In control populations, carriers of the H63D mutation are more common than C282Y carriers (23,25–33). In genotype studies of patients with hemochromatosis, however, most of those affected are homozygous for the C282Y mutation (60%–100%) (23,25–33). A small proportion are compound heterozygotes (C282Y/H63D) (0%–7%) or H63D homozygotes (0%–4%) (23,25–33). Some individuals with iron overload are heterozygous for one of the mutations (0%–15%) or have no identifiable *HFE* mutation (0%–21%), suggesting that as yet unidentified mutations may contribute to the etiology of hemochromatosis (23,25–33).

These data indicate that the C282Y mutation is associated with a higher risk of iron overload than the H63D mutation, a conclusion supported by a pooled analysis of case-control studies reporting *HFE* genotype data (34) and by functional studies of the *HFE* protein (35–37). The pooled analysis indicated a gra-

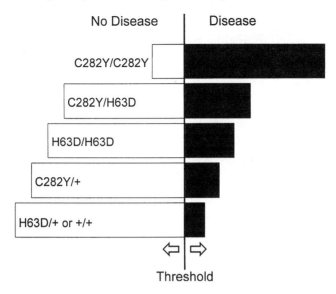

Figure 23.1 The likelihood of developing overt hemochromatosis is shown as a function of the HFE genotype. The C282Y homozygotes have the highest risk, with risk declining progressively for compound heterozygotes, H63D homozygotes, and C282Y heterozgotes. The H63D heterozygotes are assumed to have the same minimal degree of risk as do individuals without identifiable mutations; in this category, the risk reflects the small possibility of carrying mutations not currently identifiable. For all genotypes, the risk of disease increases or decreases according to the presence of modifying factors such as gender, alcohol use, and iron intake.

dient of risk for iron overload according to *HFE* genotype: Risk was much higher in C282Y homozygotes than in persons with other *HFE* genotypes, and was progressively lower for C282Y/H63D, H63D/H63D, and C282Y heterozygosity (34,38). A model for this gradient of risk is illustrated in Figure 23.1. Taken together, the genetic data indicate that DNA-based testing cannot provide a simple positive test result for hemochromatosis, but instead identifies many persons with a low or intermediate risk of iron overload. Even among C282Y homozygotes, risk of future disease is uncertain. Case reports have documented elderly individuals with this genotype who are without evidence of significant disease; some have no evidence of iron overload (3,31,39).

Risk Modifiers

Interacting with the susceptibility conferred by *HFE* mutations are modifiers that contribute to the risk of iron overload, such as gender and physiologic and pathologic factors. Several observations suggest that women have a lower risk of clinical complications of hemochromatosis than do men. These observations include the finding of fewer women than men among those diagnosed with hemochromatosis on the basis of either clinical symptoms (4,40) or TS screening (8,10,15). In addition, lower concentrations of hepatic iron and fewer cases of cirrhosis are seen in women with hemochromatosis, both among siblings identified by family-based HLA screening (41) and among those diagnosed on the basis of clinical symptoms (42). This gender difference is presumed to be due to the protective effect of iron loss during menstruation and pregnancy.

Physiologic and pathologic factors that influence iron stores also affect the likelihood of symptoms for iron overload. Increased dietary iron or vitamin C, an enhancer of iron absorption, may increase iron overload (43), whereas conditions that result in loss of iron, such as chronic gastrointestinal blood loss due to peptic ulcer disease or helminth infection, may ameliorate iron overload (43). Liver toxins can influence the course of disease; for example, alcohol abuse increases the likelihood of liver disease and is associated with decreased survival among individuals with hemochromatosis (33,44,45). Chronic hepatitis may also be a contributor to liver disease in hemochromatosis (33). In addition to increased absorption of iron, increased absorption of zinc and lead has been observed in patients with hemochromatosis (46,47) and may contribute to end-stage organ damage.

What Meaning Should Be Applied to a Diagnosis of Hemochromatosis?

Several methods are available for identifying those in the early stages of hemochromatosis, as summarized in Table 23.1. For each method, choices must be made concerning the cutoffs used to define a positive test result. All methods potentially generate false-positive and false-negative results, but the sensitivity, specificity, and predictive value of any given method can be calculated only after agreement exists about the best-case definition. The lack of a single accepted case definition for early-stage hemochromatosis represents the major difficulty in evaluating methods for early detection.

In considering what should constitute a diagnosis of hemochromatosis, the meaning applied to the diagnosis must be taken into account. Should hemochromatosis be considered a risk state, akin to hypertension or hypercholesterolemia? Or is it more accurately classified as a genetic disease with delayed but potentially severe complications, like PKU? In the usual sense of the term, a genetic disease carries with it the implication that all or most individuals carrying the disease-associated genotype will be clinically affected. In this context, a genetic test is assumed to be highly predictive of future disease. The differential risk of disease seen with different *HFE* genotypes, including

Table 23.1 Potential Case Definitions for the Early Diagnosis of Hemochromatosis

---

Persistently elevated TS*
Persistently elevated TS* *and* iron overload[†]
Persistently elevated TS* *and* iron overload[†] *and* symptoms or signs of hemochromatosis
Persistently elevated TS* *and* hemochromatosis genotype[‡]
Hemochromatosis genotype[‡]
Hemochromatosis genotype[‡] *and* iron overload[†]
Hemochromatosis genotype[‡] *and* iron overload[†] *and* symptoms or signs of hemochromatosis

---

*Persistently elevated TS = elevated transferrin saturation level on a random blood sample and a follow-up fasting blood sample.
[†]Iron overload = elevated hepatic iron index (>1.9) on tissue sample from liver biopsy, or >4 g or iron removed by quantitative phlebotomy. The latter is a series of blood draws allowing quantification of iron stores. One to two units of blood are drawn each week until serum ferritin is below 100 ng/mL or hematocrit is below normal.
[‡]Hemochromatosis genotype = presence of two *HFE* mutations.

evidence of incomplete penetrance for the genotype conferring the highest risk (3,31,39), makes it difficult to define hemochromatosis as a genetic disease in this traditional sense.

Another approach is to consider hemochromatosis as a genetic susceptibility state rather than as a disease condition. This distinction is more than semantic because it has implications for case definition, for the other diagnoses with which hemochromatosis should be compared, and for patients' and providers' expectations after a diagnosis is made. When hemochromatosis is defined by a simple inclusive criterion—for example, persistently elevated TS, in the absence of other causes—a pool of people with increased risk can be readily identified. Such a definition is comparable to identifying hypertensive or hypercholesterolemic individuals on the basis of blood pressure or serum cholesterol level. Treatment may benefit only a subset of those with persistently elevated TS, but the same is true of mild to moderate hypertension and hypercholesterolemia: The absolute reduction in cardiovascular risk produced by treatment of elevated blood pressure or cholesterol is small (48). Many people are labeled as hypertensive or hypercholesterolemic so that a minority can avoid premature cardiovascular events (48); this is done because there is no method for determining which individuals with elevated blood pressure or high levels of cholesterol will suffer adverse events if untreated. Identification of those with persistently elevated TS, or persistently elevated TS in combination with elevated serum ferritin, may provide a similar benefit.

Enhanced Case Finding

The purpose of enhanced case finding is to reduce the morbidity and mortality of hemochromatosis through early detection and treatment of affected patients in clinical settings. This approach assumes that detecting hemochromatosis at the time symptoms first appear is sufficient to gain the benefits of phlebotomy treatment. Although controlled trials of phlebotomy treatment have not been conducted, observational data provide strong support for its efficacy in reducing mortality. These data include the documentation of an apparently normal life expectancy in individuals treated before the onset of cirrhosis or diabetes (4,49) and a prolongation of survival in patients at all stages of the disease compared with historic controls (4,50). The efficacy of phlebotomy treatment in reducing early symptoms such as fatigue or joint pain is unknown.

The initiation of enhanced case finding would require a concerted educational campaign to increase awareness of hemochromatosis among physicians and health care systems (51). Key educational points to be included in the educational campaign include estimated prevalence of hemochromatosis, the severity of end-stage organ complications, the efficacy of treatment, and the nature of the common nonspecific symptoms seen early in the course of disease. In addition, physicians are likely to benefit from guidance on the use and interpretation of serum iron measures and other diagnostic strategies for hemochromatosis.

Educational efforts are likely to succeed only if they move beyond conventional conference-based continuing medical education to incorporate practice-based interventions (52). Approaches such as adding TS testing to the usual workup of patients with newly diagnosed diabetes, arthritis, and impotence, or of patients with ill-defined abdominal pain or fatigue, could be helpful. In addition to an educational effort for health care providers, this approach may require public education so as to increase the likelihood that complaints consistent with early hemochromatosis are evaluated (51).

A program to increase the use of TS testing would also require efforts to ensure laboratory standardization and quality assurance. Multiple laboratory methods are available for determining serum iron and total iron-binding capacity (the components of a TS measurement); a pilot study of laboratory proficiency found significant variability in these measurements (53). Standardization procedures, including the development of an analytic reference system similar to that implemented for serum cholesterol, may be required to ensure an acceptable level of accuracy for TS measurements (13,53). The same issues of standardization apply to genetic testing as well.

The enhanced case-finding approach has several advantages. Because testing occurs within the usual health care setting, no additional screening infrastructure is required, and follow-up is accessible to those with positive test results. Although a substantial proportion of patients seen in primary-care settings may have complaints that merit consideration of testing for hemochromatosis, the number tested will still be considerably lower than would be the case with universal screening. In addition, testing will be done in the context of an identified health problem. These factors would reduce the number of patients with a false-positive test result. Further, when a diagnosis of hemochromatosis is made, it will occur in the context of a patient seeking care and thus will avoid diagnostic labeling of those who consider themselves to be healthy.

In contrast, several factors might limit the benefits of enhanced case finding. Individuals with early symptoms may not be evaluated or treated, and appropriate treatment might not occur after the diagnosis is made. Lack of adequate follow-up has been documented in other early-detection programs (54,55); any educational efforts or quality-assurance programs developed to increase detection of hemochromatosis should include efforts to monitor the effectiveness of medical follow-up.

The biggest potential drawback to this approach, however, is the possibility that treatment initiated after symptoms occur may be too late to achieve the full benefits of prevention. Even if treatment on the basis of early symptoms is sufficient to prevent premature mortality, patients' quality of life could be diminished if early symptoms are not reversible. These considerations underscore the need for a systematic study of the natural history of hemochromatosis. In addition, data are needed on the efficacy of phlebotomy treatment in reversing early symptoms of hemochromatosis.

Universal Screening

Compared with enhanced case finding, universal screening for hemochromatosis would lead to more testing and more false-positive results, but would also offer the possibility of a greater reduction in the avoidable medical complications of hemochromatosis. The primary assumption underlying universal screening is that hemochromatosis must be detected before symptoms occur to prevent fully the complications of iron overload. Proponents of universal screening also assume that the risks and harms of screening asymptomatic persons are outweighed by the benefits of early detection and treatment.

Implementation of universal screening would require additional resources within the health care system, the nature of which would depend on the strategy chosen to accomplish screening. If screening is proposed as an adjunct to other routine health care—for example, offered at the same time as Pap testing or colorectal cancer screening—the resources required would be related primarily to health provider education, similar to what would be required for enhanced case finding. For men, however, screening in early adulthood might be difficult to accomplish in this way, because fewer men than women are likely to be regular users of preventive health care services between the ages of 20 and 50. If separate screening programs were instituted, resources for a screening infrastructure would be needed, including provisions to ensure follow-up care of those who screen positive. Laboratory standardization issues would be of the same nature as for case finding, but on a larger scale. If screening included genetic testing, current practice standards would also require pre- and posttest genetic counseling.

With the larger number of persons screened and treated, universal screening increases the number of those individuals exposed to the possibility of adverse psychologic, social, or economic consequences of a diagnosis of hemochromatosis. The potential for loss of health insurance and employment after a genetic diagnosis is a concern for both consumers and policymakers (56–59). Legislative efforts to minimize these risks are being implemented (60), but the degree of protection they will provide is unknown. Although adverse outcomes after a diagnosis of hemochromatosis have been reported (18,61), no systematic study has been undertaken to assess them.

Adverse psychologic effects of screening may occur, but the few data available for other conditions are conflicting. Increased absenteeism from work has been seen after a diagnosis of hypertension (62), and perceptions of ill health have been described after a diagnosis of hypercholesterolemia (63). Conversely, a workplace cholesterol screening trial and a primary care-based assessment of cardiovascular risk factors failed to show evidence of adverse psychologic effects by standard measures (64,65). The wide acceptance of these screening strategies implies that many view the benefits of cardiovascular screening as outweighing any psychologic burdens imposed. There may be greater reluctance to proceed with screening for a genetic condition than with screening for nongenetic risk factors, however, because the personal burdens are perceived as being heavier (66). These include the ramifications of identifying a risk that may affect family members and, perhaps more important, the possibility that a genetic diagnosis may be stigmatizing (66). The way in which a disorder is understood might influence the psychological response to a positive screening test (64,67). With hemochromatosis, the psychological burdens of the diagnosis may be reduced by clear communication that it is an indicator of increased susceptibility rather than a prediction of certain future disease, and that treatment can be offered to reduce substantially the risk of developing disease. Whether communication of this kind can change the perception of hemochromatosis from a genetic disease to a risk state, or reduce the likelihood of discrimination, remains to be determined. More research is needed to address these questions.

Conclusions

Enhanced case finding can be justified on the basis of current evidence, because a reasonable likelihood of benefit can be inferred when symptomatic individuals are treated. Thus, efforts to increase public and health care provider awareness of hemochromatosis are merited. The educational programs required to increase the early detection of hemochromatosis could also serve as a preparatory step in the development of universal screening programs.

The strongest argument in favor of universal screening is the possibility that enhanced case finding will fail to detect affected individuals before irreversible complications of hemochromatosis occur. However, reductions in the frequency of late-stage complications of hemochromatosis appear to be occurring already, in the absence of large-scale programs to improve case finding. Thus, more direct evidence for outcome benefit is needed to justify universal screening of healthy persons. This is particularly true given the uncertainty about the number of individuals who might be exposed to unnecessary treatment and the unknown potential for social, psychological, and economic harms, if universal screening were implemented.

The burden of disease associated with hemochromatosis also needs to be considered when addressing the question of universal screening. Although hemochromatosis can be construed as a risk state similar to hypertension and hypercholesterolemia, it is much less common than these diagnoses (approximately 15% of adults are hypertensive (48) and 20% are hypercholesterolemic (68), with the proportion rising with age for both).Hemochromatosis is thus a less common contributor to the disease burden of the population than either hypertension or hypercholesterolemia, and the resources required for universal screening may not be merited on this basis.

In determining the value of universal screening, however, the prevalence of the disorder may be less important than the effectiveness of screening and treatment. The two conditions for which newborn screening is mandated throughout the United States—PKU and congenital hypothyroidism—occur in about 1 in 12,000 and 1 in 3600 newborns, respectively (48). Universal newborn screening is recommended, despite the low prevalence of these conditions, because of the effectiveness of screening and subsequent treatment in preventing mental retardation and other neurological complications in affected infants (48). These examples highlight timing of treatment as an important factor in determining the need for screening—that is, whether therapy must be initiated before symptoms occur to provide benefit. For PKU or neonatal hypothyroidism, treatment of asymptomatic infants is essential if complications are to be avoided. In contrast, when a mildly symptomatic latency period occurs—as in adult-onset hypothyroidism, for example—efforts to increase case finding are likely to be more efficient for improving health outcome than a policy of universal screening.

The data critical to a consideration of universal screening for hemochromatosis thus include a full description of the symptoms associated with the early stages of the disease, their reversibility, and the degree to which other complications are prevented when treatment is initiated early. In addition, more information is needed on the potential for personal and economic harms resulting from a diagnosis of hemochromatosis and the measures available to reduce or prevent such risks. One important way to minimize the risk of adverse labeling is to limit the diagnosis of hemochromatosis to those most likely to benefit from treatment. Better information about the natural history of hemochromatosis is needed to accomplish this goal.

If hemochromatosis is underdiagnosed, as current estimates of prevalence suggest, much of the data needed on the natural history of the disease may be obtainable with well-designed case-control and cross-sectional studies that include an adequate sample of older persons. Such research should be able to define the disease status by age of those who carry *HFE* mutations or have biochemical evidence of iron overload, and should allow a better estimation of the proportion of young asymptomatic individuals likely to benefit from therapy. If these data supported screening, pilot studies that include assessment of the psychosocial outcomes of screening would be merited. As a matter of policy, it is important to ensure that evidence of this kind is generated before screening options are evaluated further. Without such data, the added benefit provided by universal screening cannot be determined.

The issues raised in the consideration of universal screening for hemochromatosis are likely to be relevant to future discussions of genetics and public health. Many new genetic tests emerging from current research are related to diseases of adult onset, and most identify an increased probability of disease, rather than a certainty. Because future disease is not certain, the effect of interventions designed to reduce risk may be difficult to measure. Yet the value of testing can be determined only by weighing the effectiveness of screening and treatment against potential psychological, social, and economic risks. As the hemochromatosis example illustrates, these questions constitute a research agenda.

In the translation of genetic advances into effective public health action, research strategies that address the multiple aspects of genetic susceptibility are needed. As other tests to identify genetically susceptible persons are developed, targeted interventions to reduce risk must be developed and assessed. This effort will require knowledge about the natural history of the genetic condition, including the gene–environment interactions that influence disease risk and response to treatment. Evaluation of the outcomes of genetic testing will also require an assessment of the psychosocial consequences of testing and treatment. Hemochromatosis provides an early and instructive example of the interdependence of these important questions.

References

1. Bothwell TH, Charlton RW, Motulsky AG. Hemochromatosis. In: Scriver CR, Beaudet AL, Sly WS, Valle D (eds). The metabolic and molecular bases of inherited disease (7th ed). New York: McGraw-Hill, 1995.

2. Motulsky AG, Wolff RK. Update on hemochromatosis, addendum to chapter 69. In: Scriver CR, Beaudet AL, Sly WS, Valle D (eds). The metabolic and molecular bases of inherited disease [book in CD-ROM]. New York: McGraw-Hill, 1997.

3. Bacon BR. Diagnosis and management of hemochromatosis. Gastroenterology 1997;113:995–999.

4. Niederau C, Fischer R, Purschel A, et al. Long-term survival in patients with hereditary hemochromatosis. Gastroenterology 1996;110:1107–1119.

5. Adams PC, Valberg LS. Evolving expression of hereditary hemochromatosis. Semin Liver Dis 1996;16:47–54.

6. Witte DL, Crosby WH, Edwards CQ, Fairbanks VF, Mitros FA. Practice guideline development task force of the College of American Pathologists: hereditary hemochromatosis. Clin Chim Acta 1996;245:139–200.

7. Burke W, Thomson E, Khoury MJ, et al. Hereditary hemochromatosis: gene discovery and its implications for population-based screening. JAMA 1998;280:172–178.

8. Balan V, Baldus W, Fairbanks V, Michels V, Burritt M, Klee G. Screening for hemochromatosis: cost-effectiveness study based on 12,258 patients. Gastroenterology 1994;107:453–459.

9. Phatak PD, Guzman G, Woll JE, et al. Cost-effectiveness of screening for hereditary hemochromatosis. Arch Intern Med 1994;154:769–776.

10. Edwards CQ, Griffen LM, Goldgar D, et al. Prevalence of hemochromatosis among 11,065 presumably healthy blood donors. N Engl J Med 1988;318:1355–1362.

11. Adams PC, Valberg LS. Screening blood donors for hemochromatosis: decision analysis model comparing genotyping to phenotyping. Am J Gastroenterol 1999;94:1593–1600.

12. Cogswell ME, McDonnell SM, Khoury MJ, Franks AL, Burke W, Brittenham G. Iron overload, public health and genetics: evaluating the evidence for hemochromatosis screening. Ann Intern Med 1998;129:971–979.

13. McDonnell SM, Phatak PD, Felitti V, Hover A, McLaren GD. Screening for hemochromatosis in primary care. Ann Intern Med 1998;129:962–970.

14. Adams PC, Gregor JC, Kertesz AE, Valberg LS. Screening blood donors for hereditary hemochromatosis: decision analysis model based on a 30-year database. Gastroenterology 1995;109:177–186.

15. Phatak PD, Sham RL, Raubertas RF, et al. Prevalence of hereditary hemochromatosis in a sample of 16,031 primary care patients. Ann Intern Med 1998;129:954–961.

16. Looker AC, Johnson CL. Prevalence of elevated serum transferrin saturation in adults in the United States. Ann Intern Med 1998;129:940–945.

17. Yang Q, McDonnell SM, Khoury MJ, Cono J, Parrish RG. Hemochromatosis-associated mortality in the United States from 1979 to 1992: an analysis of multiple-cause mortality data. Ann Intern Med 1998;129:946–953.

18. McDonnell SM, Preston BL, Jewell SA, et al. A survey of 2851 patients with hemochromatosis: symptoms and response to treatment. Am J Med 1999;106:619–624.

19. Conte D, Manachino D, Colli A, et al. Prevalence of genetic hemochromatosis in a cohort of Italian patients with diabetes mellitus. Ann Intern Med 1998;128:370–373.

20. Olynyk J, Hall P, Ahern M, Kwiatek R, Mackinnon M. Screening for genetic haemochromatosis in a rheumatology clinic. Aust N Z J Med 1994;24:588–589.

21. George DK, Evans RM, Crofton RW, Gunn IR. Testing for haemochromatosis in the diabetic clinic. Ann Clin Biochem 1995;32:521–526.

22. Bradley LA, Haddow JE, Palomaki GE. Population screening for haemochromatosis: a unifying analysis of published intervention trials. J Med Screen 1996;3:178–184.

23. Feder JN, Gnirke A, Thomas W, et al. A novel MHC class I-like gene is mutated in patients with hereditary haemochromatosis. Nat Genet 1996;13:399–408.

24. Mercier B, Mura C, Ferec C, et al., on behalf of the WHO Nomenclature Committee for Factors of the HLA System. Putting a hold on "HLA-H." Nat Genet 1997;15:234.

25. Beutler E, Gelbart T, West C, et al. Mutation analysis in hereditary hemochromatosis. Blood Cells Mol Dis 1996;22:187–194.

26. Barton JC, Shih WWH, Sawada-Hirai R, et al. Genetic and clinical description of hemochromatosis probands and heterozygotes: evidence that multiple genes linked to the major histocompatibility complex are responsible for hemochromatosis. Blood Cells Mol Dis 1997;23:135–145.

27. Carella M, D'Ambrosio L, Totaro A, et al. Mutation analysis of the HFE gene in Italian hemochromatosis patients. Am J Hum Genet 1997;60:828–832.

28. Jazwinska EC, Cullen LM, Busfield F, et al. Hemochromatosis and HLA-H. Nat Genet 1996;14:249–251.

29. Jouanolle AM, Gandon G, Jezequel P, et al. Hemochromatosis and HLA-H. Nat Genet 1996;14:251–252.

30. Borot N, Roth M-P, Malfroy L, et al. Mutations in the MHC class 1-like candidate gene for hemochromatosis in French patients. Immunogenetics 1997;45:320–324.

31. Adams PC, Chakrabarti S. Genotypic/phenotypic correlations in genetic hemochromatosis: evolution of diagnostic criteria. Gastroenterology 1998;114:319–323.

32. UK Haemochromatosis Consortium. A simple genetic test identifies 90 percent of UK patients with haemochromatosis. Gut 1997;41:841–844.

33. Piperno A, Sampietro M, Pietrangelo A, et al. Heterogeneity of hemochromatosis in Italy. Gastroenterology 1998;114:996–1002.

34. Burke W, McDonnell SM, Khoury MK. Contribution of different genotypes in the HFE gene to the etiology of hemochromatosis: a pooled analysis. Presented at the 13th National Conference on Chronic Disease Prevention and Control, Atlanta, GA, December 8, 1998.

35. Feder JN, Tsuchiihashi Z, Irrinki A, et al. The hemochromatosis founder mutation in HLA-H disrupts β_2-macroglobulin interaction and cell surface expression. J Biol Chem 1997;272:14025–14028.

36. Waheed A, Parkkila S, Zhou XY, et al. Hereditary hemochromatosis: effects of C282Y and H63D mutations on association with β_2-macroglobulin, intracellular processing, and cell surface expression of the HFE protein in COS-7 cells. Proc Natl Acad Sci U S A 1997;94:12384–12389.

37. Feder JN, Penny DM, Irrinki A, et al. The hemochromatosis gene product complexes with the transferrin receptor and lowers its affinity for ligand binding. Proc Natl Acad Sci U S A 1998;95:1472–1477.

38. Burke W, Press N, McDonnell SM. Hemochromatosis: genetics helps to define a multifactorial disease. Clin Genet 1998;54:1–9.

39. Adams PC, Campion ML, Gardon G, et al. Clinical and family studies in genetics hemochromatosis: microsatellite and HFE studies in five atypical families. Hepatology 1997;26:991–995.

40. Adams PC, Deugnier Y, Moirand R, Brissot P. The relationship between iron overload, clinical symptoms and age in 410 hemochromatosis patients. Hepatology 1997;25:162–166.

41. Edwards CQ, Griffen LM, Kushner JP. The morbidity of hemochromatosis among clinically unselected homozygotes: preliminary report. Adv Exp Med Biol 1994;356:303–308.

42. Moirand R, Adams PC, Bicheler V, Brissot P, Deugnier Y. Clinical features of genetic hemochromatosis in women compared to men. Ann Intern Med 1997;127: 105–110.

43. Powell LW, Burt MJ, Halliday JW, Jazwinska EC. Hemochromatosis: genetics and pathogenesis. Semin Liver Dis 1996;16:55–63.

44. Adams PC, Agnew S. Alcoholism in hereditary hemochromatosis revisited: prevalence and clinical consequences amongst homozygous siblings. Hepatology 1996;23:724–727.

45. Loreal O, Duegnier Y, Morand R, et al. Liver fibrosis in genetic hemochromatosis: respective roles of iron and non–iron-related factors in 127 homozygous patients. J Hepatol 1992;16:122–127.

46. Adams PC, Bradley C, Frei JV. Hepatic zinc in hemochromatosis. Clin Invest Med 1991;141:16–20.

47. Barton JC, Patton MA, Edwards CQ, et al. Blood lead concentrations in hereditary hemochromatosis. J Lab Clin Med 1994;124:193–198.

48. US Preventive Service Task Force. Guide to clinical preventive services (2nd ed). Baltimore: Williams & Wilkins, 1996.

49. Adams PC, Speechley M, Kertesz AE. Long-term survival analysis in hereditary hemochromatosis. Gastroenterology 1991;101:368–372.

50. Bomford A, Williams R. Long-term results of venesection therapy in idiopathic hemochromatosis. Q J Med 1976;45:611–623.

51. NcDonnell SM, Witte DL, Cogswell ME, McIntyre R. Strategies to increase detection of hemochromatosis. Ann Intern Med 1998;129:987–992.

52. Davis DA, Thomson MA, Oxman AD, Haynes RB. Changing physician performance. JAMA 1995;274:700–705.

53. Elaine Gunter, personal communication, 1998.

54. Bonelli L, Branca M, Ferreri M, et al. Attitude of women toward early cancer detection and estimation of compliance to a screening program for cervix and breast cancer. Cancer Detect Prev 1996;20:342–352.

55. Paskett ED, McMahon K, Tatum C, et al. Clinic-based interventions to promote breast and cervical cancer screening. Prev Med 1998;27:120–128.

56. Hudson KL, Rothenberg KH, Andrews LB, Kahn MJE, Collins FS. Genetic discrimination and health insurance: an urgent need for reform. Science 1995;270:391–393.

57. Lapham EV, Kozma C, Weiss JO. Genetic discrimination: perspectives of consumers. Science 1996;274:621–624.

58. Rothenberg K, Fuller B, Rothstien M, et al. Genetic information and the workplace: legislative approaches and policy challenges. Science 1997;275:1755–1757.

59. Task Force on Genetic Testing. Promoting safe and effective genetic testing in the United States: final Report, 1997 (in press).

60. Rothenberg KH. Genetic information and health insurance: state legislative approaches. J Law Med Ethics 1995;23:312–319.

61. Alper JS, Geller LN, Barash CI, et al. Genetic discrimination and screening for hemochromatosis. J Public Health Policy 1994;15:345–358.

62. Haynes RB, Sackett DL, Taylor DW, Gibson ES, Johnson AL. Increased absenteeism after detection and labelling of hypertensive patients. N Engl J Med 1978;299:741–744.

63. Brett AS. Psychologic effects of the diagnosis and treatment of hypercholesterolemia: lessons from case studies. Am J Med 1992;91:842–847.

64. Irvine MJ, Logan AG. Is knowing your cholesterol number harmful? J Clin Epidemiol 1994;47:131–145.

65. Marteau TM, Kinmouth AL, Thompson S, Pyke S. The psychological impact of cardiovascular screening and intervention in primary care: a problem of false reassurance? Br J Gen Practice 1996;46:577–582.

66. Markel H. The stigma of disease: implications of genetic screening. Am J Med 1992;93:209–215.

67. Millar MG, Millar K. Negative affective consequences of thinking about disease-detection behaviors. Health Psychol 1995;14:141–146.

68. Sempos CT, Cleeman JI, Carroll MD, et al. Prevalence of high blood cholesterol among US adults. JAMA 1993;269:3009–3014.

24

Applying genetic strategies to prevent atherosclerosis

Roger R. Williams, Paul N. Hopkins, Lily L. Wu, and Steven C. Hunt

Atherosclerotic disease of coronary and cerebral arteries accounts for almost half of all deaths in the United States each year. Heart attacks and strokes are often attributable to inherited predisposition, especially when they occur at a relatively early age. Researchers are accumulating information regarding the role of genetics in influencing the risk factors for atherosclerosis in several major categories, including lipids and lipoproteins (LDL, HDL, and VLDL cholesterol; Lp(a); triglycerides; apo AI, AII, and B; apo E genotypes); glucose and insulin metabolism (diabetes, glucose intolerance, and insulin resistance); prothrombotic factors (fibrinogen, plasminogen activator inhibitor-1, factor VII coagulant activity, homocysteine); and hypertension, just to mention a few of about 300 risk factors identified in published medical literature. In addition, other forms of heart disease can occur in individuals with genetic susceptibility, including arrhythmic disorders (atrial fibrillation, long QT sudden arrhythmic death syndrome, Wolff-Parkinson-White syndrome), congenital heart disease (disorders of valves, great vessels, septal defects, and hypoplastic syndromes), myocardiopathies (primary muscle disorders, assymetrical hypertrophy), and valvular diseases (rheumatic, mitral valve prolapse).

Although this chapter will not focus on these other forms of heart disease, the basic approaches discussed for evaluating and addressing heritable factors for atherosclerosis will also serve as a paradigm for these other familial cardiovascular syndromes. We are currently witnessing a great increase in the understanding of how genetic factors promote or prevent atherosclerosis (1). In light of this new knowledge, we should soon see changes in the approaches taken to prevent atherosclerosis. Presently, we stand at the intersection of discovery and application. This chapter will help us consider how to apply the growing knowledge of genetics toward the preventive medicine of the future.

Practical Differences Between Monogenic and Polygenic Factors

Genetic influences on phenotypes can be classified as *monogenic* or *polygenic*. Both mechanisms can contribute to a person's susceptibility or resistance to atherosclerosis, as illustrated in Figure 24.1. Polygenic traits (like the LDL cholesterol in most of us) show a continuous blending effect. Offspring generally have a polygenically determined cholesterol level approximately halfway between the levels of the two parents when values are measured at about the same age for both generations. Classic polygenic traits lead to sibling similarity. If we find a patient with a polygenically high cholesterol level, all siblings will usually have a similarly elevated cholesterol level, as shown for one sibship in Figure 24.2. This finding leads to a practical application: When a patient meets the criteria for treatment of a polygenically elevated LDL cholesterol level (the most common cause), we should routinely arrange for siblings, who will generally also have elevated levels, to be tested so as to identify those who also need treatment (2). Also, HDL cholesterol, blood pressure, and weight are examples of other common risk factors showing strong polygenic effects.

Monogenic traits such as heterozygous familial hypercholesterolemia (FH)

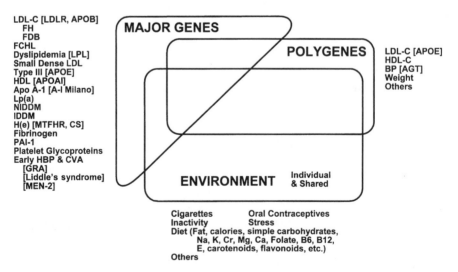

Figure 24.1 Overlapping domains represent combined (additive or multiplicative) effects of monogenic, polygenic, and environmental factors promoting atherosclerosis.

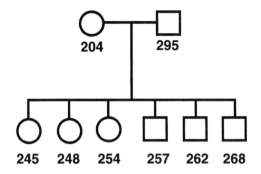

Figure 24.2 Sibship illustrating common polygenic hypercholesterolemia.

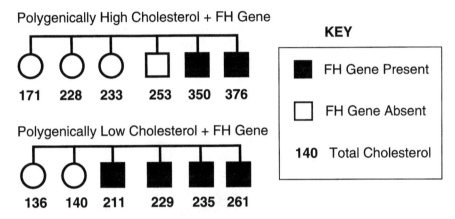

Figure 24.3 Two FH sibships demonstrate monogenic bimodality (from LDL receptor defect) and polygenic effects shifting the entire sibship toward higher cholesterol levels in the upper sibship and toward lower levels in the bottom sibship.

have mendelian inheritance (dominant for FH heterozygotes). If one parent carries a dominant gene, on average, half of the offspring will receive the gene and half will not, causing segregation or bimodal separation of the offspring into two groups: those with twofold elevated LDL cholesterol levels and those with normal LDL cholesterol levels (3). Monogenic separation is very evident in the two sibships shown in Figure 24.3 from families with heterozygous FH. The DNA markers for the receptor locus on the short arm of chromosome 19 were used to diagnose genetically the presence or absence of FH in these two sibships, as indicated. In the upper sibship of Figure 24.3, siblings, sorted in order of increasing cholesterol level, show an increase of almost 100 mg/dL (2.6 mmol/L) between the sibling with the highest normal reading and the sibling with the lowest reading and the gene. In the second FH sibship, shown at the bottom of Figure 24.3, a similar large gap of 71 mg/dL, or 1.8 mmol/L, distinguishes FH gene carriers from noncarriers. Separation into distinct groups ("bimodality") is characteristic of a monogenic trait. These

Table 24.1 Criteria for Diagnosing Heterozygous Familial Hypercholesterolemia

	Age	LDL-C Cutpoints, mg/dL (mmol/L)*	
		Index Case	Relative
INDIVIDUAL CRITERIA			
1. Very high LDL cholesterol	40+	260 (6.7)	205 (5.3)
	30s	240 (6.2)	190 (4.9)
	20s	220 (5.4)	170 (4.4)
	<20	200 (5.2)	160 (4.1)
2. No secondary cause (nephrosis, pregnancy, etc.)			
FAMILY CRITERIA			
3. Tendon xanthoma or youth >LDL criteria			
4. Bimodal LDL cholesterol (70–100 mg/dL gap)			

*Because of higher a priori probability of having FH, relatives of an FH index case can be diagnosed with FH using lower LDL cholesterol criteria than individuals evaluated as new index cases not known to be part of a family with FH (ref. 4).

principles have been summarized into diagnostic criteria for FH (4) in Table 24.1.

The left side of Figure 24.1 lists other monogenic risk factors for atherosclerosis including familial defective apolipoprotein (apo) B (FDB); high Lp(a); dominant and recessive variants of apo E causing type III hyperlipidemia; and three dominant hypertension syndromes, glucocorticoid remediable aldosteronism (GRA), Liddle's syndrome, and multiple endocrine neoplasia type II (MEN-II) (5–7). Other single-gene loci being studied for potential atherogenic effects include heterozygous lipoprotein lipase deficiency (LPL) and homozygous deficiency of methylene tetrahydrofolate reductase (hyperhomocysteinemia), the latter of which interacts with intake of folate and B vitamins to elevate plasma homocysteine levels. There are also some genetic loci with variants that seem to be antiatherogenic, including CETP deficiency with very high HDL (8), apo A-I Milano with apparent facilitated reverse cholesterol transport (9), and hypobetalipoproteinemia with very low apo B and LDL cholesterol (10).

Diabetes, familial combined hyperlipidemia (FCHL), and low HDL cholesterol are clinical atherogenic syndromes that exhibit some of the characteristics of major gene traits (bimodality and vertical transmission in multigenerational pedigrees). However, genetic studies of these traits suggest that they result from more than one gene, and are sometimes referred to as *oligogenetic traits* (i.e., traits involving a few genes). Table 24.2 presents a large number of candidate gene loci that are under investigation for their possible connections to atherogenesis. Some are known sequences with a physiological effect suspected of being related to atherogenesis. Others are loci suggested

Table 24.2 Candidate Genes for Atherosclerosis Risk Factors

LIPIDS AND LIPOPROTEINS
    AI-CIII-AIV apolipoprotein group
    Apo B (FDB, HypoBeta)
    Apo E
    Cholesterol ester transfer protein (CETP)
    Cholesterol-7-alpha hydroxylase (CYP7)
    Apo CII
    Fatty acid binding protein (FABP3)
    HMG Co-A reductase (HMGCR)
    Hepatic triglyceride lipase (LIPC)
    Lecithin cholesterol acetyl transferase (LCAT)
    LDL receptor
    Lp(a)
    Lipoprotein lipase (LPL)
    Scavenger receptor (HDL receptor)
    VLDL receptor
    Paraoxonase (PON1,2,3)
    PPAR$_\gamma$ (PPARG)
    Microsomal triglyceride transfer protein (MTP)
    Hormone sensitive lipase (LIPE)

THROMBOGENIC FACTORS
    Antithrombin III
    Factor V Leiden (venous thrombosis)
    Factor VII
    Fibrinogen (FGA, FGG, FGB, HAEIII and beta-854)
    PAI-1
    PDGF
    Platelet IIIa/IIb glycoprotein receptor
    Platelet activating factor receptor (PTAFR)
    TGF$_\gamma$
    Thrombomodulin (THBD)
    Thromboxane A$_2$ receptor (TBXA2R)

OBESITY
    Leptin receptor
    Leptin/OB
    TNF (tumor necrosis factor)
    Uncoupling protein (UCP2)
    Melanocortin receptors (MC3R,4R,5R)
    Agouti signaling protein (ASIP)
    Beta-3 adrenergic receptor

DIABETES AND INSULIN RESISTANCE
    Glucagon receptor
    Glucokinase
    Glycogen synthase
    NIDDM1
    Sulfonurea receptor (SUR)
    Insulin

ADHESION MOLECULES
    Endothelial leukocyte adhesion molecule (ELAM1)
    Vascular cell adhesion molecule-1 (VCAM1)
    Intracellular adhesion molecule-1 (ICAM1)

(continued)

Table 24.2 *(Cont.)*

ANTIOXIDANTS
  PAF acetylhydrolase
  Bilirubin

HOMOCYSTEINE
  Methylenetetrahydrofolate reductase
  Cystathionine β-synthase
  Methionine synthase

HYPERTENSION: RENIN ANGIOTENSIN SYSTEM
  Angiotensinogen (AGT)
  Angiotensin-converting enzyme (ACE)
  Renin (REN)
  Renin binding protein (RBP)
  Angiotensin II receptor type-1 (AT1R1)

HYPERTENSION: KALLIKREIN SYSTEM
  Kallikrein (KLK1)
  Kininogen (KNG)
  Bradykinin receptor B2 (BDKRB2)

HYPERTENSION: NITRIC OXIDE SYSTEM
  Endothelial NO synthase (NOS3)
  Inducible NO synthase (NOS2A)
  Neuronal NO synthase in brain (NOS1)
  Guanylyl cyclase NOS receptors (GUCY1A3,GUCY1B3)

HYPERTENSION: ION TRANSPORT AND ION
  CHANNELS
  Adducin
  Epithelial Na channel (Liddle's locus)
  Na-H antiporter (NHE3)
  Anion exchanger 3 (SLC4A3)
  Glucocorticoid receptor
  Na-K-ATPase transporter

HYPERTENSION: OTHER CANDIDATES
  Aldosterone synthase (CYP11B2)
  Mineralocorticoid receptor
  Alpha 1,2 and beta 1,2 adrenergic receptors
    (ADRA1,ADRA2,ADRB1,ADRB2)
  Near LPL locus (8p22)
  Endothelin 1 (EDN1)
  Endothelin receptor (EDNRA)

---

to be genetically linked or associated with either atherosclerosis or a risk factor for atherosclerosis. Recently, some of these have not shown any linkage or association, making them more questionable as candidates (11).

Polygenic background influences phenotypic expression of a major gene. The pedigrees shown in Figure 24.3, illustrate this effect with two FH families. Polygenic influence has shifted the entire upper sibship toward higher background cholesterol and the entire lower sibship toward lower cholesterol without confounding the major gene effects between the non-FH and FH siblings. This interesting result illustrates how overlap can occur between the cholesterol values of carriers and noncarriers in the general population. In these two sibships, carriers of the FH gene in the lower sibship have lower cholesterol levels than do the noncarriers in the upper sibship. Recognizing bimodality in sibships establishes a cutpoint between gene carriers and noncarriers in families with monogenic traits like FH. Applying this practical knowledge to the two sibships in Figure 24.3 helps us correctly infer that the 29-year-old man in the top sibship with a cholesterol of 253 does not carry the gene for FH, whereas the 16-year-old male in the bottom sibship with a cholesterol of 211 does carry the gene for FH.

Interaction Between Genes and Environment

Environmental risk factors can have an exaggerated adverse effect in patients with genetic susceptibility (12), as illustrated in Figure 24.4. Among persons aged 30 to 49 years, cigarette smoking shows a multiplicative interaction with genetic predisposition, detected in this case using family history of early coronary heart disease (CHD). A CHD relative risk of 4 for smokers with a strong positive family history (+FHx) compares to the usual relative risk of 2 for smokers with a negative family history (–FHx). (This difference in risk translates into a 10-to-14-year life span increase in those who quit smoking and

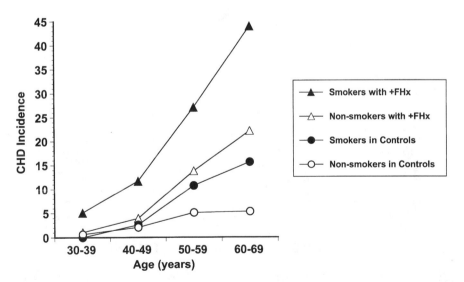

Figure 24.4 Coronary heart disease (CHD) incidence rates by family history and smoking status illustrate a multiplicative interaction, especially in the two younger age groups.

have genes like FH, compared to about 2 to 4 years of added longevity for those in the general population who quit.) Understanding interactions between genes and the environment should lead to practical applications. In this case, vigorous smoking avoidance and smoking cessation projects should be especially beneficial when offered to genetically susceptible individuals such as those with familial lipid disorders or diabetes, because these people can benefit even more than the average person from risk reduction.

Some genetic factors may be hidden unless there is exposure to necessary environmental factors. Homocysteine levels above 13 to 19 μmol/L seem to promote coronary atherosclerosis (13), as illustrated in Figure 24.5. The level of homocysteine can be affected by a common heat labile mutation of the gene for methylene tetrahydrofolate reductase (MTHFR), as well as by dietary intake of a common vitamin, folic acid. Individuals who were homozygous for the MTHFR heat labile mutation and had low folic acid intake (as reflected in serum levels) had greatly elevated homocysteine levels (14). The data in Figure 24.6 suggest that neither low folate intake nor homozygous MTHFR

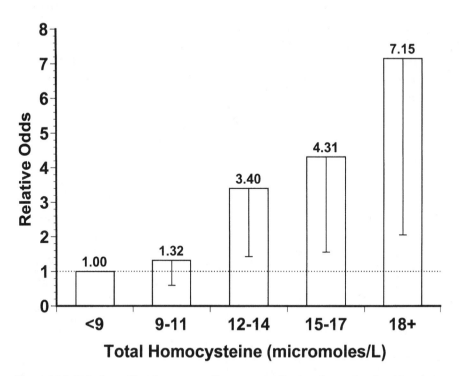

Figure 24.5 Relative odds of coronary disease according to plasma levels of homocysteine in 162 men and women with early coronary heart disease compared to 155 age-sex matched controls without coronary heart disease (ref. 13). Increased risk of CHD is prominent for persons with homocysteine levels above 13 μmol/L.

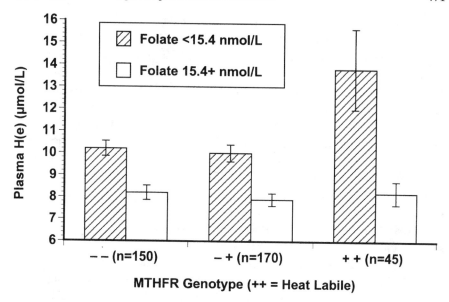

Figure 24.6 Plasma homocysteine levels (mean H(e) + SEM), according to presence (+) or absence (−) of the MTHFR mutation and folate intake levels (ref. 14). Levels associated with substantially increased risk for CHD (i.e., above 13 μmol/L) are limited to those with both homozygous MTHFR deficiency and low folate intake.

mutation status alone would confer the strong risk of hyperhomocysteinemia and early CHD, but that both genetic and environmental exposures are required for an increased risk of CHD in this example.

Meaningful synergy has been suggested for selected environmental factors with other inherited atherogenic syndromes. Restricting saturated fat and cholesterol helps lower cholesterol for those with FH, while restricting calories or simple carbohydrates is not particularly helpful. Physical activity, weight reduction, and a diet similar to that recommended for diabetics seem to be especially beneficial for people with familial combined hyperlipidemia (FCHL). Recent studies also indicate that the angiotensinogen gene variant promoting hypertension identifies a subset of people in whom sodium restriction may be especially beneficial (i.e., salt-sensitive hypertension) (15). A generous intake of B vitamins and folate seems particularly important for those carrying genes that promote hyperhomocysteinemia. Thus, genetic testing should lead to more effective risk reduction by identifying interventions that focus on specific environmental factors found to have strong interaction with each person's particular genetic makeup.

Environment

Strict compliance with a diet very low in fat and cholesterol can reduce serum cholesterol about 20% to 30% in people strictly following the Pritikin (16) and Ornish (17) diets. If we assume a "normal" cholesterol level to be about 200 mg/dL (about 5 mmol/L), then the maximum effect of a high-fat diet would elevate cholesterol about 20% to 30% to about 240 to 260 mg/dL, or about 6.0 to 6.5 mmol/L. Thus, most people who have a cholesterol level above 240 to 260 mg/dL or 6.0 to 6.5 mmol/L need treatment as their cholesterol level is more likely to be influenced by important genetic effects beyond the effects of a high-fat diet. This observation leads to several important conclusions. First, individuals with cholesterol levels high enough to meet National Cholesterol Education Committee (NCEP) guidelines for drug therapy are not just reckless eaters; they are "genetically challenged" and deserve our sympathy and help. Second, whether their underlying genetic cause is monogenic, or polygenic, most have siblings who are likely to need screening and treatment. In other words, the most serious cholesterol patients are also probands for family screening.

Obesity, particularly fat distribution, is another prominent factor in atherosclerosis. While diet and exercise obviously play an important role, genes also play a strong role, especially for those who are extremely obese. Major research efforts are currently underway to map and understand genes for obesity. Future medications will likely include drugs to normalize weight for morbidly obese patients just as potent statins now help patients with FH to normalize their cholesterol levels. These developments illustrate another practical benefit from applying genetics to disease prevention and control. The ongoing discovery of genes that promote disease is leading medical professionals to new and better diagnostic and therapeutic approaches.

Sample Application of Lipid Genetics

Case History

A 45-year-old man has a fasting total cholesterol of 310 mg/dL, normal triglycerides (125 mg/dL), low HDL cholesterol (33 mg/dL), and high calculated LDL cholesterol (252 mg/dL). He has no secondary causes of hyperlipidemia such as hypothyroidism or nephrosis. His father and brother both had myocardial infarctions before age 55. The lipid levels in relatives are not known.

Questions regarding this lipid patient include:

1. Is this patient's high LDL cholesterol most likely due to genes or environment or both?
   Answer: The magnitude of this cholesterol elevation (55% above the median for his age) strongly suggests an underlying genetic factor.

2. What would be the differential diagnosis?

Answer: Heterozygous familial hypercholesterolemia (FH), familial combined hyperlipidemia (FCHL), and polygenic hypercholesterolemia (PH) are all possibilities. Both FH and PH are more likely than FCHL, because individuals with PH and FH usually have normal triglycerides. Although 75% of affected persons in families with FCHL have high triglycerides, about 25% will have high LDL and normal triglycerides. The LDL cholesterol levels are not normally this high in families with FCHL.

3. What would be required to determine the exact genetic diagnosis?

Answer: The patient should be examined for tendon xanthoma, which would establish the diagnosis of FH. In the absence of tendon xanthoma, lipid levels should be obtained in siblings, children, aunts and uncles, nieces and nephews to help distinguish the diagnosis. Collecting a lipid family history, as illustrated in Figure 24.7, is a key tool for diagnosing both familial lipid disorders and for finding affected relatives who need treatment. High triglyceride levels, as well as high cholesterol levels in siblings, support the diagnosis of familial combined hyperlipidemia (FCHL). Bimodal distribution of LDL cholesterol, and very high LDL cholesterol in children, indicate FH. A blending effect that produces similar cholesterol elevations in siblings and an absence of severe pediatric hypercholesterolemia support PH.

4. Should medication for this patient's cholesterol be prescribed regardless of the genetic causes? If so, are there any important practical reasons for making the genetic diagnosis?

Answer: An LDL cholesterol level of 252 mg/dL will usually not drop below 200 mg/dL even with a superb diet. This 45-year-old man with low HDL and a positive family history for coronary heart disease meets NCEP guidelines for medication. The goal should be to reduce the LDL cholesterol level to about 130 mg/dL.

Drug therapy will be indicated regardless of whether the diagnosis is FH, PH, or FCHL. However, distinguishing among FH, PH, or FCHL can lead to different tailored approaches to relative screening, cardiology workup, exercise recommendations, and dietary prescription. (Perhaps only the choice of medication, often a potent statin, may be the same regardless of diagnosis.) If we extend cardiovascular disease prevention and control beyond isolated drug therapy to a more comprehensive approach, then the correct diagnosis does make a difference, in the following ways:

a. Screening relatives based on genetic diagnosis

Screening of lipid levels in relatives is necessary to help make the diagnosis. At the same time, it will identify other persons requiring

Medical Family History

This section is important. Please complete it as accurately as possible

List all relatives, not just those with problems. Please make an effort to obtain as much information as possible. **Give approximate age for first occurrence or diagnosis for each disease or problem listed.** See the example provided. **You may need to call your relatives for missing information. Circle either Bro / Sis, Son / Dau, A / U for gender.**

RELATIONSHIP	First Name	Living (L) or Dead (D)	Age (now or at death)	CAUSE OF DEATH IF DECEASED	HEART ATTACK	CORONARY BYPASS SURGERY	CORONARY ANGIOPLASTY (PTCA)	STROKE	HIGH BLOOD PRESSURE (treated)	DIABETES	CIGARETTES (C)urrent (F)ormer (N)ever	WEIGHT (A)verage (O)verweight 50+ lbs	Total Cholesterol	Triglycerides	HDL Cholesterol
Example	John	D	70	Heart Attack	50	52			40		C	A	255	140	35
You															
Father															
Mother															
Bro / Sis															
Bro / Sis															
Bro / Sis															
Bro / Sis															
Bro / Sis															
Spouse															
Son / Dau															
Son / Dau															
Son / Dau															
Son / Dau															
Pat GF															
Pat GM															
Pat A / U															
Pat A / U															
Pat A / U															
Pat A / U															
Pat A / U															
Mat GF															
Mat GM															
Mat A / U															
Mat A / U															
Mat A / U															
Mat A / U															
Mat A / U															

BLOOD LEVELS: List the worst levels known - highest serum cholesterol, triglycerides. Approximate levels may be listed. Phone calls may be necessary to verify.

Pat = paternal, Mat = maternal, GF = grandfather, GM = grandmother, A = aunt, U = uncle

If cholesterol is OVER 320 and triglycerides under 320, call **MedPed toll free at 1-888-2Hi-CHOL** for free help.

Figure 24.7 A questionnaire for obtaining a detailed "Lipid Family History." It may often take about 6 months of writing letters and making phone calls to collect all of this information from the relatives listed. Once collected, this information usually leads to a specific diagnosis and also identifies affected relatives needing treatment (a basic tool of the MED PED project).

treatment for FH, PH, or FCHL. Extended relative screening is not recommended for PH, but is recommended for FH and FCHL. If this patient has FH, screening should extend to third-degree relatives, including children, because this major gene is easy to trace in extended relatives. For PH, only siblings and adult children need screening. In FCHL families, extended adult relatives have been found to need treatment.

b. Workup for cardiovascular disease

Some FH experts recommend a treadmill test, as well as other tests, for FH men in their 40s, even in the absence of symptoms, because a significant number have been found to have lesions suggesting bypass surgery or angioplasty. A newly diagnosed, untreated 45-year-old male with heterozygous FH has a high risk of current silent coronary atherosclerosis and myocardial infarction (MI) in the near future. It is important to remember that his very high cholesterol level has been present for over four decades, in contrast to men the same age with PH or FCHL whose cholesterol levels may have been this high for only one or two decades.

c. Exercise prescription tailored to a genetic diagnosis

Beginning a new jogging routine without safety testing by a treadmill could be dangerous for a man with FH: Many FH men in their 40s have died during vigorous physical exercise. The benefit of jogging is also limited for the FH patient because exercise does not help LDL receptor defects or lower LDL cholesterol in those with FH. Perhaps walking would be a more prudent form of exercise than jogging for this man. Exercise poses less risk and offers more benefit for FCHL men in their 40s than for men with FH. Therefore, jogging should be encouraged if the patient has FCHL and passes a treadmill ECG. The FCHL patients who do regular aerobic exercise will often see improvement in conditions such as hyperinsulinemia, obesity, high triglycerides, low HDL, and high blood pressure. Jogging is less dangerous, and more beneficial, for those with PH than for individuals with FH. It is less dramatically beneficial for individuals with PH compared to those with FCHL.

d. Genetically based dietary prescription

Dietary prescriptions can also be tailored to a specific genetic diagnosis. Patients with FCHL often need a diet like that prescribed for diabetics: low in calories, limited quantities of simple carbohydrates, and fat. The FH patients do not need to limit calories or simple carbohydrates, as neither has an effect on LDL receptor defects that cause their high LDL cholesterol. The recommended diet for an FH man is one that is low in both fat and cholesterol. For patients with polygenic hypercholesterolemia, a diet similar to the one for FH is recommended.

Monogenic Hypertension Syndromes

Two severe dominant forms of hypertension, GRA and Liddle's syndrome, lead to severe hypertension and strokes. Because of our new understanding of these disorders, we can perform informative diagnostic tests and prescribe effective therapy that is tailored to the specific pathophysiology. In the past, many patients died from early strokes in the fourth decade of life because they remained undiagnosed, severely hypertensive, and unresponsive to ineffective ordinary therapy.

Glucocorticoid remediable aldosteronism (GRA) results from a dominant "gain of function" mutation on chromosome 8. The mutation induces high levels of abnormal adrenal steroids, 18-hydroxycortisol, and 18-oxocortisol (5). This unusual chimeric mutation derives from the combination of fragments of two genes, the aldosterone synthase gene and the steroid 11-beta-hydroxylase gene. The DNA sequences of these two genes are 95% identical, the genes have identical intron-exon boundaries, and the genes are located next to each other on chromosome 8. During recombination, unequal crossing over has occurred, producing the mutant gene with the sequences and functions of both genes combined into the variant. Administration of exogenous glucocorticoids (like dexamethasone) can often suppress aldosterone, abnormal steroids, and severe blood pressure elevations. Individuals with the gene for GRA have reported having early severe hypertension and having close relatives die from cerebral hemorrhage in their 40s. Also, GRA is reported to fail to respond to ordinary antihypertensive medications but can respond to prednisone (which will suppress hormone production), spironolactone (which will competitively inhibit the aldosterone receptor), or amiloride (which will inhibit distal renal epithelial sodium channel response to mineralocorticoid action).

Liddle's syndrome results from dominant mutations at a locus coding for the beta-subunit of the epithelial sodium channel on chromosome 16p. A genetically activated channel cannot be maintained in a properly closed state (6). A low plasma renin activity and variable hypokalemia are seen in this syndrome as in GRA. However, Liddle's syndrome also causes suppressed aldosterone secretion in contrast to the hyperaldosteronism seen in GRA. Excessive reabsorption of sodium and exchange for potassium in the distal nephron probably account for the hypertension and hypokalemia. Both of these features of Liddle's syndrome are responsive to triamterene or amiloride, both of which specifically inhibit the epithelial sodium channel. Unlike GRA, this syndrome is not responsive to spironolactone, which inhibits the mineralocorticoid receptor. Kidney transplant also seems to eliminate the problem.

Angiotensinogen: A Common Gene for "Salt-Sensitive"
Hypertension?

Commonly occurring hypertension is also thought to result from milder effects of multiple genes in combination with environmental factors. Major studies that are currently underway in several countries are likely to produce a list of several common genes contributing to hypertension. Variants of the gene for angiotensinogen (AGT) on chromosome 1 seem to promote hypertension in a manner consistent with several theories of "salt-sensitive" hypertension. The angiotensinogen gene (AGT) has been genetically linked to essential hypertension in several diverse populations (18,19), and genetically associated with both essential hypertension and pre-eclampsia in several, but not all, populations (18,20–22). Higher levels by genotype suggest a pathophysiologic mechanism involving increased production of the substrate angiotensinogen.

Homozygous carriers of this AGT variant show blunting of renal response to infusion of angiotensin II (thought by some to be a sign of "salt-sensitive" hypertension) (23). In the Trials of Hypertension Prevention (TOHP), 378 middle-aged adults with diastolic blood pressure between 83–89 mm Hg were randomly assigned to sodium-reduced diets (average 25% reduction at 36 months) and were then compared to 384 similar participants assigned to usual care (24). New hypertension occurred in 34% of the sodium-reduction group compared to 39% of the usual-care group ($p = 0.09$) (24). However, when these participants were subdivided according to their angiotensinogen genotype (15), those with the most salt-sensitive genotype (–6 AA) had the most hypertension in the usual-care group (45%) and the least hypertension in the sodium-reduction group (28%). An additional insight is suggested for population differences in the frequency of hypertension when one considers that the most sodium-sensitive genotype is found in about 20% of Caucasians and 75% of African Americans.

Future Application of Genes for Sodium Sensitivity

Researchers are currently trying to confirm the findings of the TOHP study and extend data on salt-sensitivity associated with other genes to better predict individual responses to salt-lowering diets. Currently, with the high percentage of daily salt intake coming from prepackaged foods as opposed to discretionary salt use, low-salt diets are very difficult to maintain. In the future, management of patients with moderate hypertension may be directed by tests for genotypes at the angiotensinogen gene and other genes, that together may define the probability of success with a reduced-sodium diet.

Applying Hypertension Genetics to Management

Case History

A 40-year-old man has a resting blood pressure of 210/135 mm Hg that has not responded to diuretics, beta-blockers, ACE inhibitors, or calcium channel blockers. The patient has normal renal function and no evidence of renal artery stenosis. His older brother died of a stroke when the brother was 45 years of age. The patient has a 16-year-old daughter with a blood pressure of 160/95. Practical questions regarding a severe hypertensive patient include:

1. What possible genetic diagnoses should be considered?

    Answer: Glucocorticoid remediable aldosteronism (GRA) and Liddle's syndrome are both dominant hypertension syndromes that lead to early severe hypertension and stroke. Both are unresponsive to the ordinary antihypertensive medications listed above.

2. What could be done to establish or rule out one of the dominant hypertension syndromes?

    Answer: Often, GRA responds to a trial with spironolactone or dexamethasone, both of which address the two problems of abnormal steroids: hyperaldosteronism and severe hypertension. Severe hypertension with Liddle's syndrome responds to amiloride or triamterene. If there are clinical reasons to suspect a dominant hypertension syndrome, specific diagnoses may be made by testing blood and urine for the endocrine abnormalities described above. Also, DNA testing can often identify a specific causal mutation for these disorders.

3. How could screening relatives help prevent early strokes? Which relatives should be screened?

    Answer: All first- and second-degree relatives should be screened for hypertension or diagnostic endocrine abnormalities. If specific mutations are known for a given family, other relatives can be sequentially screened and given a definitive result (gene present or absent) from a single blood sample. It is important to make the diagnosis and institute effective treatment as early as possible. If hypertension is undiagnosed and untreated for too long it generates vessel and renal changes that may cause irreversible hypertension, even with proper medication.

    Tracing families with GRA and Liddle's syndrome can save relatives from early strokes and premature death. All easily found relatives on the affected side of the family, including siblings, offspring, parents, aunts and uncles, should be screened. If affected second-degree relatives are found, their offspring should also be screened.

4. How specifically should the medications be tailored to genetic diagnoses for these dominant hypertension syndromes?

    Answer: Both GRA and Liddle's syndrome are two excellent examples of clinical settings in which very specific medications can be chosen to match a specific genetic mechanism. Steroids or spironolactone are specific for GRA. Specific treatments for Liddle's syndrome include triamterene, amiloride, and renal transplantation.

A Genetically Oriented Public Health Approach to Detecting High Risk Individuals

Unfortunately, even well-understood and very treatable dominant disorders like FH are not diagnosed or treated in most gene carriers (25). For relatively uncommon gene traits like FH, FDB (familial defective apolipoprotein B),

GRA, and Liddle's syndrome, additional cases can be found efficiently by screening relatives of known probands. Because treatment can normalize levels and prevent or delay early CHD or stroke deaths, a vigorous effort to find and help individuals in these high-risk pedigrees is justified. The MED PED (Make Early Diagnoses to Prevent Early Deaths in MEDical PEDigrees) project is a nonprofit humanitarian effort that attempts to answer that need. Currently organized in 38 collaborating countries, MED PED registries try to collect all known index cases with FH or FDB, to facilitate investigators' efforts to contact relatives for screening and treatment in both close and distant MEDical PEDigrees.

From one index case, 5 to 15 new FH cases can often be found among "close relatives" (siblings, parents, offspring, aunt, uncles, nieces, nephews, first cousins, and their offspring) (26). In some families, hundreds of FH cases have been found by extending screening to "distant relatives" (second, third, and fourth cousins and their offspring). At the present time, MED PED collaborators are setting an example of case detection through relative screening. Collecting detailed medical family histories and screening relatives in high-risk pedigrees (like these with FH, FDB, GRA, and Liddle's syndrome) should become a routine activity for genetically oriented prevention and disease control. The MED PED effort is supported by humanitarian funding to demonstrate the need and feasibility of this approach and to justify future support by government and health insurance agencies. (Health care providers can obtain free help tracing undiagnosed relatives of patients with FH [see criteria in Table 24.1], GRA, or Liddle's syndrome by calling a toll-free number: 1-888-2Hi-CHOL.) The MED PED collaborators in 38 countries have collectively identified over 18,000 patients with FH (27). By educating patients and their personal physicians and by helping them get additional aid from referral specialists, the MED PED effort has made it possible for many FH patients to experience dramatic (40%–50%) reductions in cholesterol levels (unpublished data).

In addition, annual follow-up contacts and involvement in FH support groups and lay organizations help address the most important challenge to lifelong medication: long-term compliance. Because relatives in high-risk families often have different health plans and HMOs and sometimes live in different states, or even different countries, it would seem most appropriate for MED PED efforts to be coordinated nationally or even internationally by the World Health Organization (WHO). These efforts could include coordinated relative tracing, registration of severe gene carriers, education of personal physicians, and long-term follow-up to prevent the discontinuation of life-saving medications, with appropriate attention to privacy, confidentiality, and the voluntary nature of participation in the program (see discussion of informed consent below). The World Health Organization has convened two meetings devoted to FH and the MED PED concept and has published a

Table 24.3 Treatable Dominant Cardiovascular Diseases

Genetic Trait	Description	Clinical Diagnosis	Genetic Diagnosis	Treatment or Prevention
Familial hypercholesterolemia (FH)	High LDL cholesterol and very early heart attack deaths	LDL cholesterol and xanthoma; quite reliable	LDL receptor gene tests (>600 causal mutations)	Drugs reduce cholesterol, and likely extend life 10–30 years
Familial defective apo B (FDB)	High apolipoprotein B and cholesterol with early heart attack deaths	High cholesterol can mimic FH, but some levels are lower than FH	Two specific causal mutations	Same as for FH for those with very high cholesterol
Dominant type III hyperlipidemia	Very high beta-VLDL cholesterol with early heart attack deaths	High triglyceride and abnormal Trig/VLDL ratio	Several specific causal mutations	Specific medications can often normalize levels and prolong life
Long QT syndrome	High risk for sudden arrhythmic death in youth and young adults	Long duration of QT interval on electrocardiogram	Linkage found and mutations being sought	Medication can lower risk of sudden death and prolong life
GRA hypertension	Severe high blood pressure and early stroke	Abnormal steroid hormones; blood pressure normal after dexamethasone	Several specific causal mutations	Suppress abnormal steroids with hormones like dexamethasone
Liddle's syndrome	Severe high blood pressure and early stroke	Selective blood pressure response to amiloride and triamterene	Causal mutations	Amiloride or triamterene
MEN-II	Pheochromocytoma and other endocrine neoplasia	MRI and CT scans for tumors	Causal mutations	Surgical removal of endocrine tumors

report with practical recommendations for this approach (28). This same approach could work for similar diseases as long as they meet the criteria listed below. Several other single-gene disorders that fit these criteria are presented in Table 24.3.

1. A single dominant gene causes preventable serious illness.
2. Validated diagnostic tests are available (gene test or clinical test).
3. Treatment or prevention is available and has been shown to be effective.

Social Issues: Cost and Informed Consent

The cost-effectiveness of drug therapy for FH has been rigorously analyzed and documented (27,29). Daily treatment of FH patients with a low dose of lovastatin was projected to save money as well as lives. Higher-dose therapy was associated with an acceptable cost per year of life saved in one conservative analysis (29), and it was more cost-effective than secondary prevention in FH men from the 4S study (30). Some social scientists have raised concerns that projects like MED PED might cause psychological stress by contacting relatives to talk about their family history. The dramatic occurrence of very early heart attack deaths in FH families is usually well known to relatives. Whether they know their cholesterol level or not, many relatives in FH pedigrees already worry about having an early heart attack death, long before being contacted by MED PED. The MED PED collaborators in several countries report a large preponderance of positive reactions from relatives contacted in FH families. Over 80% of relatives agreed with the statement, "I'm satisfied to know that I have heterozygous FH" (27). Over 80% disagreed with the statement, "I wish I didn't know that I have heterozygous FH." Because of MED PED, thousands of relatives have been screened and found to have normal cholesterol and reassured that their fear of early death from a heart attack due to FH was not warranted. Others found to have very high cholesterol levels have learned something very few of them knew before MED PED: Their very high cholesterol levels can be dramatically reduced and early heart attack deaths can be prevented. Similar observations are likely to be found in the dominant hypertension families.

Informed consent is always obtained from every individual participating in MED PED activities. As each proband is identified, he or she provides consent to the investigator along with the proband's cholesterol level and other medical data. The proband is asked if he or she would provide the names of close relatives who could be contacted for cholesterol screening. Those relatives are contacted by letter or phone and provided with a description of the study and the name of the relative who referred them. Each relative is asked whether he or she is interested in participating and, if so, to provide informed consent.

Gene Therapy for Future Prevention and Disease Control

Today we take air travel for granted as a part of daily life, but it was not always that way. The Wright brothers traveled a very short distance in a very crude airplane. But their flight marked the beginning of something big. Gene therapy is already beyond its historic first flight. For atherosclerotic diseases, the first short flight was launched in 1992 for a person with homozygous FH (31). To replace the genetically absent LDL receptors, doctors surgically removed some of his liver cells, infected them with a virus containing the human gene sequence for normal LDL receptors, and returned them to his liver. To produce a perceptible drop in serum cholesterol, this procedure required statin drug stimulation of the few newly acquired LDL receptors. The effect was too small to have a meaningful clinical result. But, like the first airplane flight at Kitty Hawk, the first gene therapy for FH got off the ground. At this beginning stage, some scientists probably view gene therapy as a last-chance hope for rare FH homozygotes. But gene therapy offers the potential of a permanent cure for 10 million FH heterozygotes. We have drugs that help many FH heterozygotes now, but noncompliance deprives many of them of the full benefit of therapy. A recipient of successful gene therapy will not need to remember to take the next dose.

Basic technical challenges of gene therapy include obtaining a gene sequence with beneficial effects when expressed in the appropriate tissue, attaching the therapeutic DNA to a vehicle like a virus, and delivering the DNA in large numbers to cells where its effect is needed. These are not trivial tasks, but solutions to technical challenges often require time before ingenious minds can forge the path from first flight to jet flight. Gene therapy has potential beyond replacing defective genes. It can override the effects of existing genes. It can carry the benefits of antiatherogenic genes from naturally protected humans to others born without this good fortune.

Citing some current gene therapy research projects illustrates progress well underway. In Rochester, Minnesota, the endothelial nitric oxide synthase gene (NOS3) is being studied because nitric oxide is a potent vasodilator that might also inhibit platelet aggregation and smooth muscle cell proliferation. An adenoviral vector encoding cDNA for NOS3 was generated by homologous recombination and applied in vitro to porcine coronary smooth muscle cells, achieving increased levels of nitrate and cGMP and diminished cell proliferation (32).

In Milan, Italy, apo-E–deficient mice were given intramuscular injections of naked supercoiled plasmids containing complete human apo-E cDNA. The injected DNA was maintained in an episomal, circular form and did not replicate. But transgene persistence has been demonstrated up to 19 months. In these apo-E–deficient mice, average total cholesterol levels were significantly decreased from the first week after plasmid injection and achieved a drop from 441 mg/dL to 273 mg/dL by the eighth week (33).

In Houston, Texas, synthetic DNA complexes have been constructed that are as efficient vectors as viruses, but lack the immunological limitations. Furthermore, specific high-level expression of these exogenous genes was achieved by receptor-mediated delivery of synthetic DNA vectors, coated, condensed, and targeted by lipophilic nonexchangeable derivatives of apolipoprotein E-3 peptides, which are high-affinity ligands for the LDL and VLDL receptors. This method is being used to identify and modify the barriers to targeted delivery to hepatocytes in vivo (34).

In Parma, Italy, a molecular variant called apo A-I Milano is being studied because it seems to protect against coronary disease (despite causing a low

HDL cholesterol level). In transgenic mice, it seems to promote more efficient cholesterol efflux from cells (reverse cholesterol transport) (35).

Within two decades, we may well be writing prescriptions for genes rather than for medications. With gene therapy, compliance will be complete and automatic. High-risk genes that now cause tragedy in some families will be conquered, and protective genes that now prevent atherosclerosis in a few lucky families may be shared with everyone who needs them. The technology seems likely to succeed. Access to health services and costs of gene therapy may be the rate-limiting steps in applying this new science to individuals.

References

1. Hopkins PN, Williams RR. Human genetics and coronary heart disease: a public health perspective. Annu Rev Nutr 1989;9:303–345.

2. Williams RR, Hopkins PN, Wu LL, Hunt SC. Diagnosing and treating severe familial lipid disorders. Prim Cardiol 1995;21:47–53.

3. Hobbs HH, Brown MS, Goldstein JL. Molecular genetics of the LDL receptor gene in familial hypercholesterolemia. Hum Mutat 1992;1:445–466.

4. Williams RR, Hunt SC, Schumacher MC, et al. Diagnosing heterozygous familial hypercholesterolemia using new practical criteria validated by molecular genetics. Am J Cardiol 1993;72:171–176.

5. Lifton RP, Dluhy RG, Powers M, et al. A chimaeric 11β-hydroxylase/aldosterone synthase gene causes glucocorticoid-remediable aldosteronism and human hypertension. Nature 1992;355:262–265.

6. Shimkets RA, Warnock DG, Bositis CM, et al. Liddle's syndrome: heritable human hypertension caused by mutations in the β-subunit of the epithelial sodium channel. Cell 1994;79:407–414.

7. Neumann HPH, Eng C, Mulligan LM, et al. Consequences of direct genetic testing for germline mutations in the clinical management of families with multiple endocrine neoplasia, type II. JAMA 1995;274:1149–1151.

8. Inazu A, Brown ML, Hesler CB, et al. Increased high-density lipoprotein levels caused by a common cholesteryl-ester transfer protein gene mutation. N Engl J Med 1990;323:1234–1238.

9. Sirtori CR, Franceschini G. Hypoalphalipoproteinemia: from a mutation to drug development. In: Woodford FP, Davignon, Sniderman A (eds). Atherosclerosis X. Amsterdam: Elsevier, 1995, pp. 50–55.

10. Pullinger CR, Hillas E, Hardman DA, et al. Two apolipoprotein B gene defects in a kindred with hypobetalipoproteinemia, one of which results in a truncated variant, apoB-61, in VLDL and LDL. J Lipid Res 1992;33:699–710.

11. Hunt SC, Hopkins PN, Williams RR. Hypertension: genetics and mechanisms. In: Fuster V, Ross R, Topol EJ (eds). Atherosclerosis and coronary artery disease. Philadelphia: Lippincott-Raven, 1996, pp. 209–235.

12. Hopkins PN, Williams RR, Hunt SC. Magnified risks from cigarette smoking for coronary-prone families in Utah. West J Med 1984;141:196–202.

13. Hopkins PN, Wu LL, Wu J, et al. Higher plasma homocyst(e)ine and increased susceptibility to adverse effects of low folate in early familial coronary artery disease. Arterioscler Thromb Vasc Biol 1995;15:1314–1320.

14. Jacques PF, Bostom AG, Williams RR, et al. Relation between folate status, a common mutation in methylenetetrahydrofolate reductase, and plasma homocysteine concentrations. Circulation 1996;93:7–9.

15. Hunt SC, Cook NR, Oberman A, et al. Angiotensinogen genotype, sodium reduction, weight loss, and the prevention of hypertension: trials of hypertension prevention, phase II. Hypertension 1998;32:393–401.

16. Barnard RJ. Effects of life-style modification on serum lipids. Arch Intern Med 1991;151:1389–1394.

17. Ornish D, Brown SE, Scherwitz LW, et al. Can lifestyle changes reverse coronary heart disease? The Lifestyle Heart Trial. Lancet 1990;336:129–133.

18. Jeunemaitre X, Soubrier F, Kotelevtsev Y, et al. Molecular basis of human hypertension: role of angiotensinogen. Cell 1992;71:169–180.

19. Caulfield M, Lavender P, Farrall M, et al. Linkage of the angiotensinogen gene to essential hypertension. N Engl J Med 1994;330:1629–1633.

20. Hata A, Namikawa C, Sasaki M, et al. Angiotensinogen as a risk factor for essential hypertension in Japan. Clin Invest 1994;93:1285–1287.

21. Ward K, Hata A, Jeunemaitre X, et al. A molecular variant of angiotensinogen associated with preeclampsia. Nat Genet 1993;4:59–61.

22. Fornage M, Turner ST, Sing CF, Boerwinkle E. Variation at the M235T locus of the angiotensinogen gene and essential hypertension: a population-based case-control study from Rochester, Minnesota. Hum Genet 1995;96:295–300.

23. Hopkins PN, Lifton RP, Hollenberg NK, et al. Blunted renal vascular response to angiotensin II is associated with a common variant of angiotensinogen gene and obesity. J Hypertens 1996;14:199–207.

24. The Trials of Hypertension Prevention Collaborative Research Group. Effects of weight loss and sodium reduction intervention on blood pressure and hypertension incidence in overweight people with high-normal blood pressure: the trials of hypertension prevention, phase II. Arch Intern Med 1997;157:657–667.

25. Williams RR, Schumacher MC, Barlow GK, et al. Documented need for more effective diagnosis and treatment of familial hypercholesterolemia according to data from 502 heterozygotes in Utah. Am J Cardiol 1993;72:18D–24D.

26. Williams RR, Schumacher MC, Hopkins PN, et al. Practical approaches for finding and helping coronary-prone families with special reference to familial hypercholesterolaemia. In: Goldbourt U, de Faire U, Berg K (eds). Genetic factors in coronary heart disease. Lancaster, UK: Kluwer Academic Publishers, 1995.

27. Williams RR, Hamilton-Craig I, Kostner GM, et al. MED-PED: an integrated genetic strategy for preventing early deaths. In: Berg K, Boulyjenkov V, Christen Y (eds). Genetic approaches to noncommunicable diseases. Berlin, Heidelberg: Springer-Verlag, 1996, pp. 35–45.

28. World Health Organization. Familial hypercholesterolaemia (FH). Report of a WHO consultation. WHO, 1998.

29. Goldman L, Goldman PA, Williams LW, Weinstein MC. Cost-effectiveness considerations in the treatment of heterozygous familial hypercholesterolemia with medications. Am J Cardiol 1993;72:75D–79D.

30. Jonsson B, Johannesson M, Kjekshus J, Olsson AG, Pedersen TR, Wedel H. Cost-effectiveness of cholesterol lowering: results from the Scandinavian Simvastatin Survival Study (4S). Eur Heart J 1996;17:1001–1007.

31. Grossman M, Raper SE, Kozarsky K, et al. Successful ex vivo gene therapy directed to the liver in a patient with familial hypercholesterolemia. Nat Genet 1994;6:335–341.

32. Kullo IJ, Mozes G, Schwartz RS, et al. Adventitial gene transfer of recombinant endothelial nitric oxide synthase to rabbit carotid arteries alters vascular reactivity. Circulation 1997;96:2254–2261.

33. Fazio VM, Rinaldi M, Ciafre SA, et al. Functional chronic correction of dyslipidemia in apo E-deficient mice by direct intramuscular injection of naked plasmid DNA. Abstract Book, 66th Congress of the European Atherosclerosis Society, Florence, Italy, July 13–17, 1996, p. 28. Published by the Giovanni Lorenzini Medical Foundation, Milan, Italy.

34. Gottschalk S, Sparrow JT, Hauer J, et al. A novel DNA–peptide complex for efficient gene transfer and expression in mammalian cells. Gene Ther 1996;3:48–57.

35. Chiesa G, Stoltzfus LJ, Michelagnoli S, et al. Elevated triglycerides and low HDL cholesterol in transgenic mice expressing human apolipoprotein A-I (Milano). Atherosclerosis 1998;136:139–146.

V

GENETICS AND PUBLIC HEALTH: ETHICAL, LEGAL, AND SOCIAL ISSUES

25

Genetics, public health, and the law

Ellen Wright Clayton

For many people, it is difficult to imagine how genetics and public health can intersect. We repeatedly hear that genetic information is individual, intensely private—indeed, more private than almost any other kind of information, and in today's environment potentially hazardous to one's access to employment and insurance. One person's genetic makeup rarely presents a risk to the health of others; a woman who has a mutation in the BRCA1 gene and so is more susceptible to breast cancer cannot transmit the disease or even the mutation to her best friend. At the same time, most people think of public health in terms of the interventions that public health agencies impose on large groups of people to improve health, ranging from fluoridation of water to immunization or, in extreme cases, quarantine. Thinking about the conjunction of private concerns and public actions makes it difficult even to consider genetics and public health at the same time.

A committee of the national Institute of Medicine recently defined "the mission of public health as fulfilling society's interest in assuring conditions in which people can be healthy" (1). Viewed in terms of this sweeping mission statement, mutations that contribute to health problems could be seen simply as factors to be ameliorated or eliminated, as with polluted air or water or infectious diseases such as measles. Further, the public's health can be promoted through the actions of numerous institutions throughout society that function outside, but often in coordination with, the traditional public health sector. The private health care sector is perhaps the most obvious example of an institution that affects the public health, but others include housing agencies, water departments, and sewage disposal systems. Indeed, the Institute of Medicine committee concluded that the core functions of governmental entities in public health are "assessment, policy development, and assurance" (1), rather than direct provision of services. Yet the government's role necessarily extends beyond surveillance, planning, and assurance because it is the only institution in society that is empowered to alter behaviors that affect health. The government's authority to promote the public health, however, is not unlimited, but rather is both based upon and limited by the law (2–4). The goal of this chapter is to discuss the legally defined scope of the government's powers to use genetic information to improve the public health. I begin by discussing public health law more generally before turning to the particular challenges raised by genetics.

The General Power to Protect the Public Health

Understanding where the government's power to protect the public health comes from is the first step in understanding what the government is and is not permitted to do in pursuit of this goal. Some modern political philosophers argue for a number of reasons that protection of the public health is an inherent function of the government (5). One set of arguments is that without healthy citizens, there can be no state, and that the community is harmed when some of its members are not well. Some argue, in fact, that the primary justification for government is its use of the so-called "police power" to promote the common good, including public health. Legal historians have demonstrated that protection of the public health has always been important in our country's governance and that the government has often acted quite broadly in pursuit of this goal (6–8). Many efforts of the current regulatory state, ranging from the provision of clean water to safety requirements for motor vehicles, are designed to protect individuals and are imposed without regard to whether a particular person wants these protections or not. These commentators urge that an examination of both history and practice reveals that the government has extremely broad powers to promote health.

A separate function of the government, but one that often overlaps to a significant degree with the exercise of the police power, is to protect individuals who cannot protect themselves in the state's role as *parens patriae* (3,4). Examples of individuals who are subject to this sort of protection include the mentally ill, who are unable to provide for their own needs, and young children who are abandoned, neglected, or abused by their parents. An important limitation of the *parens patriae* power is that it is almost never invoked to protect competent adults.

A critical issue in the federal system is the allocation of authority among governments. The power to promote the public health was reserved to the states under the Tenth Amendment to the United States Constitution. On those rare occasions when the United States Supreme Court has addressed public health issues, the justices have stated that the states' powers in this area are very far-reaching. States, in turn, often delegate some of their authority to local governments. In the 20th century, the federal government has played an increasingly important and even dominant role in promoting the public health, acting primarily through its imposing conditions on the provision of funds to state and local agencies as well as its authority to regulate interstate commerce (9). Nonetheless, as a result of the limited powers of the federal government as defined in the Constitution and of the recent reconsideration of the reach of its authority under the Constitution's Commerce Clause, the federal government's power to affect matters related to public health is more limited than that of the states. The result is a complex interplay among the different levels of government that changes over time (10).

The constraints of federalism are not the only limits on governmental actions undertaken to promote the public health. Efforts in this area can be pursued only if authorized by statutes and regulations (2). Put another way, there is no "common law" of public health, so that judges may not uphold a public health activity in the absence of an authorizing statute or regulation. This means that all public health actions must survive the public scrutiny that accompanies the political process. The fact that growing and selling tobacco is still permitted and even subsidized in the face of overwhelming evidence of the adverse health consequences of this product is evidence of the impact of political considerations on the government's actions in the public health arena.

Although the government's policy powers are broad, several constitutionally protected individual rights have emerged as increasingly important restraints on governmental efforts to protect the public health (4). The *right to privacy*, a term that actually encompasses a number of different claims of the individual against the government, is the newest and the most ill-defined of these rights, being derived generally from the "penumbra" of various amendments to the Constitution. The first, and more widely discussed, aspect of the right to privacy is the right of the individual to make some decisions about certain important matters free from governmental interference; at least at the level of the United States Supreme Court, this principle has been analyzed in the context of decisions about whether to bear children and about refusing life-sustaining medical treatment (11–15). Another aspect of the right to privacy is the "right to avoid disclosure of personal matters" by the government (16). The right to privacy, broadly viewed, also overlaps with other freedoms, such as the right to refuse "unreasonable searches and seizures."

The requirement of *due process* means that procedural protections must be in place to prevent inappropriate governmental interference with individuals. The specific procedures required vary directly with the importance of the individual interest that is being invaded. Thus, when the government is searching for evidence of a crime, it must obtain a search warrant before entering a person's house but not before watching that same person walk down a public street, a distinction justified because the home is more private than the street.

Finally, the provision ensuring individuals *equal protection* of the laws means both that the state may not make distinctions that have no basis in fact (17) and that the state may not categorize individuals using certain suspect classifications, such as race and ethnicity, without compelling justification. To demonstrate both aspects of equal protection, the government could not permissibly mandate immunizations only for blacks and Hispanics, while exempting whites. There is no evidence that whites are already immune to vaccine-preventable diseases, and requiring only blacks and Hispanics to be immunized burdens and discriminates against those groups in ways that could promote unfounded negative stereotypes.

To summarize, the government inherently has broad powers to protect the public health that necessarily entail imposing some limitations on individual actions. These powers, however, are not unlimited but rather are subject to numerous constraints, ranging from the mandates of federalism and the requirement of specific legislative or regulatory authorization for public health activities, to the protection of individual liberties under the Constitution. The result is authority whose allocation among different levels of government and whose contours change over time in response to many pressures. With this complex and varying structure in mind, we can turn to what the law does and can say about how genetics should be incorporated within the primary functions of public health agencies as identified by the Institute of Medicine.

Genetics and Public Health

The Federal Role

Surveillance, Policy Development, and Assessment. Congress created the Public Health Service (PHS) at the turn of the 20th century. Its functions now include research and surveillance (performed both by an array of PHS agencies such as the Centers for Disease Control and Prevention and the National Institutes of Health as well as by state agencies and private entities), funding of hospital construction and of undergraduate and graduate medical education, and direct provision of health services (18). Within this extremely broad and complex mandate that spans volumes of the federal statutes, Congress has said almost nothing specifically about genetics. In 1978, Congress directed the secretary of what is now the Department of Health and Human Services (hereafter "Secretary") to use "an identifiable administrative unit" to

> (1) conduct epidemiological assessments and surveillance of genetic diseases to define the scope and extent of such [genetic] diseases and the need

for programs for the diagnosis, treatment, and control of such diseases, screening for such diseases, and the counseling of persons with such diseases;

(2) on the basis of the assessments and surveillance described in paragraph (1), develop for use by the States programs which combine in an effective manner diagnosis, treatment, and control of such diseases, screening for such diseases, and counseling of persons with such diseases; and

(3) on the basis of the assessments and surveillance described in paragraph (1), provide technical assistance to States to implement the programs developed under paragraph (2) and train appropriate personnel for such programs. (19)

It appears, however, that the Secretary explicitly relied on this statutory authority to define the impact of genetic diseases only to permit the Centers for Disease Control and Prevention (CDC) to enter into cooperative agreements with the International Centre for Birth Defects, reasoning that "the scientific knowledge gained will . . . yield important data to strengthen the scientific basis in the United States' quest for the prevention of genetic disease" (20).

At present, no systematic national system of surveillance for genetic diseases exists in the United States, although the CDC in its recent strategic plan called for more efforts in this area (21). In this regard, the statute appears to authorize the federal government not only to create a specific system to determine the frequency of genetic disease but also to use existing data and samples, such as those found in tumor and birth defects registries, for this sort of examination. President Clinton's 1998 order that federal governmental agencies comply with the Health Care Consumer Bill of Rights and Responsibilities (22) appeared to require changes in current approaches to surveillance. That document provides, inter alia, that

disclosure of individually identifiable health care information without written consent should be permitted in very limited circumstances where there is a clear legal basis for doing so. Such reasons include: medical or health care research for which an institutional review board has determined anonymous records will not suffice, investigation of health care fraud, and public health reporting. *To the maximum feasible extent in all situations, nonidentifiable health care information should be used unless the individual has consented to the disclosure of individually identifiable information* [italics added]. When disclosure is required, no greater amount of information should be disclosed than is necessary to achieve the specific purpose of the disclosure. (23)

The recently proposed Standards for Privacy of Individually Identifiable Health Information (24), by contrast, are much more permissive about release of patient data for public health and other purposes. Whether these standards will remain unchanged following public comment, whether they will preempt or supersede the President's earlier order, and whether Congress will choose to intervene are all matters that remain to be seen. In the meantime, states remain largely free to provide greater protection of patient information, and many have chosen to do so (25).

Given the current understanding of the contributions of genetic factors to disease, at least some of the activities that will be undertaken by federal agencies will likely be more in the nature of research rather than surveillance. Determining which type of activity is being undertaken in any particular case requires analysis of the agency's intentions, the methodology used, and the state of scientific knowledge. The distinction between surveillance and research is important because to the extent that the CDC and other governmental agencies engage in the latter, their actions will be governed by the regulations for the protection of human subjects, which require at least review by an institutional review board and in many cases consent of the individuals being studied (26).

Parts of the federal government have made efforts to develop policy recommendations for the use of screening and diagnostic techniques for genetic diseases, evidently relying on the broad authority of the Public Health Act. Examples include a consensus conference convened by the National Institutes of Health (NIH) to decide how broadly carrier testing for cystic fibrosis (CF) ought to be offered (27) and a conference sponsored by the CDC to consider the appropriateness of newborn screening for CF (28). More broadly, a task force put together by the NIH-DOE (Department of Energy) ELSI Working Group (29) recently promulgated sweeping recommendations for assessing when and how diagnostic genetics tests are appropriately incorporated into medical practice, an effort that the CDC will play a major role in implementing (21).

The CDC itself has set forth a far-reaching agenda for the development of policy regarding public health and genetics. Significantly, in its planning document, the CDC set forth its fundamental assumption that "the use of genetic information in public health is appropriate in promoting health and in diagnosing, treating, and preventing disease, disability, and death among people who inherit specific genotypes. Such prevention concerns the use of medical, behavioral, and environmental interventions to reduce the risk for disease among people susceptible because of their genetic makeup. It does not include efforts to prevent the birth of infants with specific genotypes" (21), thereby indicating its view that reproductive genetic testing is a matter for individuals and not for public health policy.

A critical part of policy development is the assessment of the capacity for delivery of needed health care services. Although such an assessment is inherently within the scope of the statute described above, data are incomplete. The ten regional genetics networks and their governing Council of Regional Networks (CORN) for Genetics Services, funded in part by the Maternal and

Child Health Bureau, attempted for more than a decade to collect uniform information about types and quality of genetic services delivered in this country (30,31). These efforts were tabled by CORN in 1997, reportedly due to difficulties in data collection (32). This project, even had it been successful, would have painted an incomplete picture of the impact of genetic medicine given the increasing frequency with which nongenetics professionals are and will be providing genetics services.

Delivery of Services Using Federal Funds. Although the primary goals of public health today are surveillance, policy development, and assessment, the public health sector has for years been a direct provider of services for certain segments of the population. In 1976, as part of the National Sickle Cell Anemia, Cooley's Anemia, Tay-Sachs, and Genetic Diseases Act, Congress directed the Secretary of Health, Education, and Welfare to "establish a program within the [Public Health] Service to provide voluntary testing, diagnosis, counseling, and treatment of individuals respecting genetic diseases" (33). In 1978, the Senate Human Resources Committee stated that these services were to include: "1. Early detection of disease: (a) Newborn screening, (b) Prenatal screening, (c) Prenatal diagnosis; (d) Screening at later ages; 2. Carrier detection; 3. Counseling; 4. Diagnosis and monitoring of effectiveness of treatment; and 5. Information and education" (34), requirements that were embodied in 42 CFR Part 51f (35). At the same time, Congress provided that "[t]he participation by any individual in any program or portion thereof under this part [addressing genetic diseases] shall be wholly voluntary and shall not be a prerequisite to eligibility for or receipt of any other service or assistance from, or to participation in, any other program" (36).

In 1981, these programs were rolled into block grants administered by the Maternal and Child Health Bureau (MCHB); the grants provide funding only for "special projects of regional and national significance, research, and training (37)." For instance, the MCHB currently funds "demonstration projects to provide counseling for individuals and families affected by thalassemia; [and to] enhance utilization of genetic services by Southeast Asian refugees" (38). Broadly based services for the general population are not funded. The provision for voluntary participation by patients was left in place during the consolidation of the block grants. At that time, however, the types of services that could be provided by genetics programs receiving federal funds were seriously limited because Congress mandated that abortion could be provided only when the life of the pregnant woman was in danger or when the pregnancy was the result of rape or incest, conditions rarely met by women seeking genetic services (39).

The State Role
The states play a major role in providing genetic services and in establishing policy. All states have established programs to screen newborns for a number

of diseases, many of which are caused by single-gene mutations, such as phenylketonuria (PKU) and sickle cell disease (40). These programs have become well established because the affected children they identify can benefit greatly from early intervention. The programs nonetheless raise a number of concerns, some of which revolve around decisions regarding which diseases are incorporated into the testing panel and the mandatory nature of the testing. In addition, although universal screening is the norm, a few states have chosen to screen only a subset of neonates for hemoglobinopathies, such as sickle cell disease. Although the strategies of these few states vary, in general, children identified as Caucasian are not tested. To date, few concerns have been expressed that this sort of targeting of non-Caucasians inappropriately stigmatizes those populations who are being tested, a result that is somewhat surprising in light of the history of carrier screening for sickle cell disease in this country.

Many states also provide therapy for individuals who have genetic disorders, such as the special foods required for a child with PKU or the factor VIII required by a child with hemophilia A. These activities fit comfortably within the public health safety net, which ensures medically necessary services to at least some people who otherwise would go without.

The states' role in shaping the delivery of reproductive genetic services, such as prenatal diagnosis and carrier screening, tends to be more complex and contradictory, reflecting ambivalence about the appropriateness of averting the birth of children with serious genetic disorders (41,42). Only some states provide these services, and their ability to do so has been limited by the federal requirement that its funds may not be used for abortions, a restriction that increasingly is interpreted to preclude prenatal diagnosis for disorders that cannot be treated in utero as well. Many state legislatures have also chosen to impose similar limitations on the use of their own funds to pay for abortions.

At the same time and despite the general absence of explicit statutory mandates that they do so, state newborn screening programs generally strive to provide genetic counseling to parents whose children are found in the state-run newborn screening programs to have genetic diseases or to be carriers of these diseases (40). These efforts to provide counseling are usually justified on the ground that these couples should have the opportunity to make informed reproductive decisions. Some state officials acknowledge, however, that another goal of this type of counseling is to decrease the number of affected children. Public health officials may also be influenced by the large number of lawsuits that have been filed against private practitioners who fail to provide genetic information even though state entities are governed by different liability rules and are entitled in many instances to immunity.

The states also send differing messages about the provision of these services in the private sector. A review of state statutes conducted in the early 1990s revealed that four states required insurers to pay for prenatal diagnostic tests

(42). For years, California has required clinicians to offer maternal serum alpha-feto protein screening, a test to detect neural tube defects as well as a number of chromosome anomalies, to pregnant women (43), with the explicit goal of decreasing the number of children born with these disorders (44).

A far more important force promoting the delivery of reproductive genetic testing by private clinicians is the steady stream of lawsuits in which couples who have a child with a genetic disorder allege that they were negligently denied accurate information about that possibility. The overwhelming majority of state courts permit at least some measure of damages to be awarded to parents who can demonstrate that they would have avoided having such a child had they been appropriately informed. Most clinicians have responded by incorporating these diagnostic tests into their practices, and many women have chosen to terminate their pregnancies after serious disorders or anomalies were detected. A few state courts, however, ban such claims, and a small number of legislatures have enacted laws eliminating some or all of such causes of action (42).

The Impact of Politics and History

The federal and state policies discussed above, particularly those regarding reproductive genetic testing, have been influenced by a number of forces. The impact of abortion politics on the development of policy regarding the use of genetic information at both the federal and state levels cannot be underestimated. Another important factor in the current debate is the effort to ensure the protection and inclusion of individuals with disabilities in mainstream society, evidenced most dramatically by the enactment of the Americans with Disabilities Act (45).

Many disability-rights advocates have conveyed serious reservations about the often unexpressed values that underlie the use of reproductive genetic testing and selective abortion of affected fetuses (46). Beyond the context of childbearing, people are fearful that genetic information will be used to deny them and their relatives access to health insurance and employment, worries that have only partially been addressed by such laws as the Health Insurance Portability and Accessibility Act (47). Some relatively well-defined ethnic groups, such as American Indians and Ashkenazi Jews, have also expressed concern that genetic research and testing will cause them to be perceived to be unusually unhealthy and, therefore, burdens on society (48).

Less often mentioned than these current, often heated, public debates but probably no less important for the future of efforts to integrate public health and genetics is the history of eugenics in this country, which during the first half of the 20th century led not only to the state-mandated sterilization of thousands of individuals but also to wholesale stigmatization of numerous groups, resulting in, among other things, extremely restrictive immigration laws (49,50). The government used, with the full approval of the courts, what was then asserted to be scientific information about the heritability of human traits to exclude and harm large numbers of individuals in ways that are now deemed to be unacceptable. Subsequently, in the 1970s, many states enacted laws requiring the testing of blacks for sickle cell trait. Although the motives of many of the legislators who passed these laws were beneficent, the lack of counseling, the absence of confidentiality, and the general misunderstanding of the difference between sickle cell disease and sickle cell trait led to widespread discrimination against blacks in employment and insurability. Cries of genocide and eugenics were raised because the inability at that time to perform prenatal diagnosis for sickle cell disease meant that couples at risk had only two choices: avoiding procreation altogether or simply hoping for the best (51). During that same period, Congress passed several laws, culminating in the one quoted earlier, that made provisions for the "control" of genetic disease, language that seems to suggest a desire to rid society of individuals with these disorders (19). This complex history, combined with the worries about discrimination, casts a shadow over current public health activities in genetics that must be confronted directly (52).

Where Are the Gaps?

The most noticeable gap is that public health policymakers are only beginning to discuss the appropriate role of genetic testing for identification of personal risk in the adult population. Guidelines, for example, regarding the use of testing for mutations in the BRCA and HNPCC genes are coming almost exclusively from professional societies (53) and groups of investigators (54,55), not from the public health sector. One notable exception is the recent conference convened by the CDC and National Human Genome Research Institute to decide whether to screen individuals for hereditary hemochromatosis (56). Despite the fact that this disorder may well represent one of the best cases for widespread genetic screening among adults—the disease is easily treated if detected before end organ damage occurs—this group of professionals appropriately concluded that, if screening is to be done at this time, periodic assessment of iron saturation, a phenotypic test, is the preferred approach. The group decided not to endorse widespread screening for the known mutations that predispose individuals to develop this disease, reasoning that too little is known about the penetrance of the mutation (although it is undoubtedly much less than 100%) and the timing of the onset of the disorder and that too many concerns exist about the effects of knowing that one has the mutation long before intervention may be warranted. This group's well-founded reluctance to recommend the use of genetic tests to screen for hemochromatosis is particularly notable because members were considering only what advice to give to clinicians about the preventive care of their patients and not whether to recommend a state-run program.

Looking more generally, the more complex subject of widespread, government-sponsored genetic screening of adults is rarely considered. The possibility that the government or a third party might limit the activities or even require treatment of adults who have specific mutations is barely even mentioned. It may be that once the clinical implications of mutations are actually understood, clinicians will use tests appropriately and people will alter their behavior and use medical care in ways that improve their health. Difficult questions will arise, however, if the public or regulators perceive that the medical system is providing too much or too little genetic testing or that individuals are not acting to avert illness in themselves.

Legislators to date have said almost nothing about how and when tests for mutations that predispose individuals to develop diseases that become symptomatic only after infancy should be incorporated into clinical and public health practice. They have, however, become quite concerned that information about genetic risk factors will be used to interfere with individuals' access to employment and health insurance. In response, Congress and a growing number of state legislatures have passed laws that seek to limit or prevent these sorts of adverse consequences (47,57). Although driven primarily by the concern that this sort of discrimination is "unfair" in some way, legislators are also motivated to pass these laws by the fear that individuals at risk will be deterred from having beneficial tests and engaging in health-promoting behavior. Failing to strike down barriers to the appropriate use of testing and care poses risks to the health of the individual and in turn to the well-being of the public at large.

What Role Will the Law Play in Shaping Our Response to These Dilemmas?

The phenomenon of enthusiasm for new technologies, which may be unwarranted before their role is clearly defined, extends far beyond genetic medicine. An important step in curbing this sort of enthusiasm is educating clinicians about the harm that can be done by adopting new interventions too quickly. In these days of evidence-based medicine and the mandate of the Task Force on Genetic Testing, we can anticipate that government agencies, such as the Agency for Health Care Policy and Research, entities such as the Genetics Advisory Committee to the Secretary of Health and Human Services, and major professional organizations, will develop sound guidelines for the use of genetic tests. State governments could do much to quell the fears of liability that often promote the perhaps premature adoption of new tests by enacting laws that provide that compliance with well-grounded, recognized guidelines is irrebutable proof of compliance with the standard of care.

The problem of too little testing could be addressed most easily by establishing guidelines and imposing civil liability on clinicians who fail to comply. If these steps were inadequate, the next question might be whether a government-sponsored mass screening program would be the right way to respond to the perceived medical system failure, an approach that was taken in the case of newborn screening for PKU. States clearly have the power to establish such programs, particularly if they ensure voluntariness and confidentiality and provide informed consent. Nonetheless, state programs may be seen as more coercive simply because of their origin and may be less able than the private sector to respond in a timely fashion to changes in scientific knowledge.

The most difficult problem may be that presented by adults who are found to be at increased risk of becoming ill and who fail to engage in health-promoting behavior. The issue is whether adults can be given incentives, or even forced, to try to ameliorate their risks. At the limit, such questions would require consideration of the constitutional scope of governmental authority, particularly under the police power, which already justifies such interventions as fluoridation of water, and the constitutionally protected scope of individual freedom, due process, and equal protection. In all likelihood, however, governments will not seek to require people to undergo unwanted testing and treatment. Political forces and the weight of our society's past history of what are now seen as misguided efforts taken in the name of eugenics and genetics will probably lead the government not to test the full extent of its legal power to require compliance with medical recommendations or to force lifestyle changes. Instead, the government will likely devote its efforts to educating clinicians and the public and creating incentives for health care providers to encourage health-promoting behaviors.

Acknowledgments

I would like to thank Marie R. Griffin, M.D., M.P.H., and William O. Cooper, M.D., M.P.H., for their helpful comments on earlier drafts of this chapter. This publication was supported in part by Grant Number 1 R01 HG01974-01 from the National Human Genome Research Institute. Its contents are solely the responsibility of the author and do not necessarily represent the official views of the National Human Genome Research Institute.

References

1. Committee for the Study of the Future of Public Health, Division of Health Care Services, Institute of Medicine. The future of public health. Washington, DC: National Academy Press, 1988, p. 7.

2. Grad FP. The public health law manual (2d ed). Washington, DC: American Public Health Association, 1990.

3. Wing KR. The law and the public's health (4th ed). Ann Arbor, MI: Health Administration Press, 1995.

4. Gostin LO. American public health law. Berkeley, CA: University of California Press (in press).

5. Beauchamp DE. The health of the republic: epidemics, medicine, and moralism as challenges to democracy. Philadelphia: Temple University Press, 1988.

6. Parmet WE. From Slaughter-House to Lochner: the rise and fall of the constitutionalization of public health. Am J Leg Hist 1996;40:476–505.

7. Parmet WE. Health care and the Constitution: public health and the role of the state in the framing era. Hastings Const Law Q 1993;20:267–335.

8. Parmet WE. Public health protection and the privacy of medical records. Harv Civ-Rts-Civ Liberties Law Rev 1981;16:265–304.

9. Medtronic, Inc. v. Lohr, 116 S.Ct. 2240 (1996).

10. Hodge JG Jr. Implementing modern public health goals through government: an examination of new federalism and public health law. J Contemp Health Law Policy 1997;14:93–126.

11. Pierce v. Society of Sisters, 268 U.S. 510 (1925).

12. Griswold v. Connecticut, 381 U.S. 479 (1965).

13. Eisenstadt v. Baird, 405 U.S. 438 (1972).

14. Roe v. Wade, 410 U.S. 113 (1973).

15. Cruzan v. Director, Missouri Dept. Health, 497 U.S. 261 (1990).

16. Whalen v. Roe, 97 S.Ct. 869 (1977).

17. Skinner v. Oklahoma, 315 U.S. 535 (1942).

18. 42 U.S.C.A. §§201–300aaa (1998).

19. 42 U.S.C.A. §300b-6 (1998).

20. 59 Fed. Reg. 28107, May 31, 1994.

21. Centers for Disease Control and Prevention. Translating advances in human genetics into public health action: a strategic plan, October 1, 1997, p. 3.

22. Clinton directs federal agencies to implement patient bill of rights. USLW 1998;66:2554–2555.

23. President's Advisory Commission on Consumer Protection and Quality in the Health Care System. Consumer Bill of Rights and Responsibilities. http://www.hcqualitycommission.gov/CBORR/Consbill.htm.

24. 64 Fed. Res. 59917–59944 (11/3/99).

25. Gostin LO. Health information privacy. Cornell Law Rev 1995;80:451–528.

26. 45 CFR Part 46 (1998).

27. Genetic Testing for Cystic Fibrosis. NIH consensus statement, April 14–16, 1997; 15(4):1–37.

28. Centers for Disease Control and Prevention. Newborn screening for cystic fibrosis: a paradigm for public health genetics policy development—proceedings of a 1997 workshop. MMWR 1997;46(No. RR-16):1–22.

29. Task Force on Genetic Testing, NIH-DOE Working Group on Ethical, Legal, and Social Implications of Human Genome Research. Promoting safe and effective genetic testing in the United States: principles and recommendations. http://www.med.jhu.edu/tfgelsi/promoting.

30. Council of Regional Networks. http://www.emory.edu/PEDIATRICS/corn/corn.htm.

31. Council of Regional Networks for Genetics Services. Supported in part by project MCJ-131006-01 from the Maternal and Child Health Program (Title V, Social

Security Act), Maternal and Child Health Bureau, Health Resources and Services Administration, U.S. Department of Health and Human Services.

32. Letter to Dr. Wertz. http://www.geneletter.org/0897/letter_to_dr._wertz.htm.

33. 42 U.S.C.A. §300b-4 (1998).

34. Senate Report No. 95-860, 95th Congress, 2d Sess., at 33–34 (May 27, 1978), in 1978 U.S. Code Cong. Ad. News 9134, 9166–9167.

35. 42 CFR Part 51f, removed as obsolete, 53 Fed. Reg. 27859 (7/25/88).

36. 42 U.S.C.A. §300b-2 (1998).

37. 42 U.S.C.A. §§701 & 702 (1998).

38. Maternal and Child Health Bureau, Genetic Services Program. Genetics and maternal and child health. http://www.os.dhhs.gov/hrsa/mchb/genetics.htm.

39. 42 CFR Part 51a (1998).

40. Clayton EW. Screening and treatment of newborns. Houston Law Rev 1992;29: 85–148.

41. Clayton EW. What should be the role of public health in newborn screening and prenatal diagnosis? Am J Prev Med 1999;16:111–115.

42. Clayton EW. What the law says about reproductive genetic testing and what it doesn't. In: Rothenberg K, Thomson E (eds). Women and prenatal testing: facing the challenges of genetic technology. Columbus: Ohio State University Press, 1994, pp. 131–178.

43. 17 Cal. Code Reg. §§ 6521 et seq. (1998).

44. Cunningham G. Balancing the individual's rights to privacy against the need for information to protect and advance public health. In: Knoppers BM, Laberge CM (eds). Genetic screening: from newborns to DNA typing. New York: Excerpta Medica, 1990, pp. 239–252.

45. 42 USCA §§ 12101–12213 (1998).

46. Kaplan D. Prenatal screening and diagnosis: the impact on persons with disabilities. In: Rothenberg K, Thomson E (eds). Women and prenatal testing: facing the challenges of genetic technology. Columbus: Ohio State University Press, 1994, pp. 49–61.

47. Rothenberg KH. Genetic discrimination and health insurance: a call for legislative action. J Am Med Womens Assoc 1997;52:43–44.

48. Stolberg SJ. Concern among Jews is heightened as scientists deepen gene studies. New York Times, April 22, 1998, p. A24.

49. Duster T. Backdoor to eugenics. New York: Routledge, 1990.

50. Kevles DJ. In the name of eugenics: genetics and the uses of human heredity. New York: Knopf, 1985.

51. Reilly P. Genetics, law, and social policy. Cambridge, MA: Harvard University Press, 1977.

52. Pernick MS. Eugenics and public health in American history. Am J Public Health 1997;87:1767–1772.

53. American Society for Clinical Oncology. Genetic testing for cancer susceptibility. J Clin Oncol 1996;14:1730–1736.

54. Burke W, Petersen G, Lynch P, et al. Recommendations for follow-up care of individuals with an inherited predisposition to cancer: I. hereditary nonpolyposis colon cancer. Cancer genetics studies consortium. JAMA 1997;277:915–919.

55. Burke W, Daly M, Garber J, et al. Recommendations for the follow-up care of individuals with an inherited predisposition to cancer: II. BRCA1 and BRCA2. Cancer genetics studies consortium. JAMA 1997;277:997–1003.

56. Burke W, Thomson E, Khoury M, et al. Hereditary hemochromatosis: gene discovery and its implications for population-based screening. JAMA 1998;280:172–178.

57. Reilly P. Laws to regulate the use of genetic information. In: Rothstein M (ed). Genetic secrets: protecting privacy and confidentiality in the genetic era. New Haven, CT: Yale University Press, 1997, p. 369.

26

Genetics and public health: Informed consent beyond the clinical encounter

Nancy Press and Ellen Wright Clayton

Placing public health and genetics together would seem to require a robust process of informed consent. There is an historical memory of eugenics (1–5) and many recent disclosures about inadequately protected subjects of human experimentation (6–11). However, currently available genetic technologies are quite different from those images, providing mainly diagnostic information, not new "genetic" treatments. Certainly abuses are possible: Insurance discrimination based on genetics is a commonly cited concern (12–15) and may already have occurred (16,17). The same potential jeopardy exists for individuals involved in research, especially as samples rendered anonymous will leave many forms of epidemiological research unfeasible. The possibility of screening employees for disease susceptibility suggests possible conflicts between the rights of individuals to take risks in pursuit of gainful employment and the rights of employers to be protected from future litigation, and even issues of public safety versus individual privacy (18–22).

In addition, perhaps one of the most worrisome aspects of integrating genetics and public health is that if prenatal diagnostic programs were to be provided primarily in a public health context, it could suggest that it is in the public interest to avoid the birth of babies with disabilities by the use of prenatal diagnosis followed by selective abortion. Yet insurance discrimination and workplace issues are in essence legislative not informed-consent issues. And in present-day America, lack of access to pregnancy termination for women who desire it is far more of a threat than explicit social pressure for abortion. Moreover, some public health geneticists have been explicit about their desire to remove prenatal testing and selective abortion (i.e., genotypic prevention) from the public health genetics arena entirely (see Chapters 1 and 4 of this volume).

Indeed, with the current state of genetics technology, the real issues involved with informed consent are quite the opposite of what might at first appear. Rather than being about protection from dramatic abuses, informed consent is important precisely because genetic technology—which is really a mechanism to gain genetic information—seems so simple. Most provision of genetic information begins with what is often called "just a simple blood test." In some cases, not even a blood draw is required (e.g., buccal swab testing for cystic fibrosis carriers), yet the information that can be provided by genetic testing is powerful. It can disclose potential health risks that may be unalterable and may lead to a process of self-stigmatization (5,23–25). It tells about risks that might not occur for years or decades, if ever; individuals with no current health problems may, upon receiving genetic information, label themselves as somehow ill. It provides information whose psychological safety and medical usefulness depend on the comprehension of probability and risk information. Finally, it gives one person information that may have exactly equal relevance for relatives who did not ask for this information (26–32). One bioethicist claims these familial implications are "a reality [that] haunts genetic medicine" (32). Thus, it is precisely the contradiction between the innocuous way in which genetic information is created and the powerful long-term implications of that information that makes *informed* consent necessary for genetic testing. And because the primary dangers of genetic testing (noninvasive though it may be) all stem from the power and implications of the information received, it is likewise the information provision aspect of informed consent that is of greatest importance.

There is little doubt that informed-consent conversations succeed more in getting consent than in imparting information. This is true in research and in clinical-care settings. Studies have shown that often little information is successfully imparted to patients or research participants and even less is remembered (33–37). Several studies found that many patients did not even read consent forms before signing them (36,38,39); others found that despite not being able to explain to a researcher what was on the form, they nevertheless consented in high numbers to procedures they did not really understand (38,39). Although some researchers and practitioners find this unproblematic (39), the majority are troubled and some have tried to pinpoint specific problems and suggest solutions.

What Are the Barriers to Adequate Informed Consent?

There is a body of literature on the barriers to adequate informed consent in almost any clinical or research setting. At its most pessimistic, certain investigators view informed consent as doomed to fail because the goals are simply unattainable (40). For example, they see the essential problem stemming from the fact that informed-consent conversations center on risks, whereas what patients want is certainty. Others reverse the problem, citing the fact that it is the physician who seeks the certainty of legal protection by informing patients about the potential risks of procedures (41).

Some researchers have laid the blame for lack of adequate informed consent squarely on clinicians and researchers. Andrews, for example, believes that physicians may lack adequate communication skills (42). Others believe that physicians sometimes lack sufficient knowledge about the topic (42–44).

The majority of empirical investigations of informed consent have focused on the consent forms. Many studies have found significant problems with the readability of the forms (37,45–51). The most frequent problem cited is that the language level is far too high for the majority of patients or subjects; this is true even when forms purportedly are written at a high school reading level or below. Jubelirer's (47) work suggests that one problem with level-of-readability scales may be that individuals do not read at the grade level they attained. His survey showed that 30% of patients with a 10th grade education could not read at the 10th grade level. This suggests that individuals with only a high school education could be expected to have trouble with comprehension of consent forms and, indeed, this is the finding of numerous studies in which high level of education is the best predictor of comprehension of consent forms (33–34,52).

All of the above are problems associated with all types of informed consent. There are, however, several problems that are more specific to informed consent for genetic testing or the provision of genetic information. First, there is concern that physicians and other health care providers lack adequate knowledge on the topic about which they are informing patients (44,53). Second, much genetic information is presented in terms of risk and probabilities. Substantial data from social psychology demonstrate the difficulties people of all educational levels have in understanding and/or making use of this sort of information (54–57). That this difficulty may have as much to do with psychological as with cognitive dimensions is suggested by related findings that subtle linguistic differences can have a large effect in patient perceptions (58,59). For example, Bursztajin and colleagues (58) found that results were significantly different when subjects were asked whether they would "accept" or "risk" a certain medication side effect.

Solutions to these problems have proven difficult. This seems unsurprising as uncertainty may be inherent in many medical procedures, difficulty with probability concepts and linguistic framing may be a normal part of species functioning, and patient education and reading levels cannot be changed by those writing informed-consent forms. One interesting finding, however, was from research by White et al. (60), who investigated the readability of a variety of research consent forms submitted to institutional review boards by medical researchers. They looked at compliance of the forms with federal requirements *and* also measured the level of readability of the forms. Their conclusion was that "designing a consent form to meet all of the federal requirements while maintaining a level of reading comprehension suitable for the general population is a difficult task for investigators" (60). Yet it is interesting how thoroughly the emphasis of this research is on the consent form (cf. 52,61,62 for exceptions). The findings by White et al. suggest one way in which legal requirements for informed *consent* may actually impede informed patient decision making (60).

In line with this thinking, Lidz et al. (41) created the useful distinction between an *event model* of informed consent, which stresses signing of the consent form, and a *process model*, which takes into account the changing needs of the patient at various points during care and considers informed consent an ongoing process. In their attempt to provide guidance on informed consent to clinicians offering cancer susceptibility testing, Geller et al. (63) cited this "process" model as the ideal for informed consent involving genetic testing in both a clinical and research setting.

Instituting Lidz's process model would be very helpful in improving informed consent as would be freeing informed-consent language from the legalistic constraints that add to its incomprehensibility. However, it is our contention that neither one of these changes is sufficient because they begin with an inadequate underlying model of informed consent. Figure 26.1 presents that model schematically.

Figure 26.1 illustrates an informed-consent encounter that might be considered, from the point of view of bioethical, clinical, and research practice,

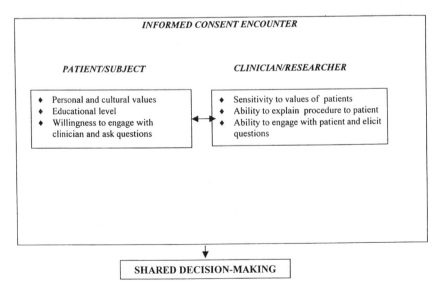

Figure 26.1 Ideal informed-consent encounter from a clinical and bioethical perspective.

an ideal. The shared decision-making process that results is seen as the outcome of an interaction between patient/subject and clinician/researcher that goes on within the informed-consent encounter. As represented here, the patient/subject has personal and cultural values and the clinician is sensitive to them. The patient has a certain educational and cognitive level, and the clinician is attuned to it and able to communicate in language that the patient can comprehend. Questions are asked and answered, and this requires the patient's willingness to ask questions and the clinician's skills in creating an environment that elicits those questions, as well as the appropriate knowledge to answer them. In concert, these things constitute a shared decision-making process. The joint nature of this encounter is shown by the two-sided arrow.

While this is already a great deal to ask, there is an essential fallacy in the view of informed consent represented by Figure 26.1: The informed-consent encounter is shown as a bounded interaction between two parties within a clinical encounter. In reality, however, some of the most important barriers to effective informed consent occur well before the clinician/researcher and patient/subject enter the consultation room, and they derive from the world outside that clinical encounter—a world that is unacknowledged in this view of informed consent. Yet the clinical encounter is not a world apart in which the patient (or potential research subject) may freely choose between alternatives, and has an equal probability of making any particular choice. Neither is it a world in which the clinician/researcher is free from external pressures. Figure 26.2 is a representation of some of the most important of the structural factors that shape the informed-consent encounter well before clinician/researcher or patient/subject step into a room together.

Beginning with the clinician/researcher, confusions resulting from the different role expectations involved in clinical care and in research are little studied. However, there is interesting work by anthropologist Pamela Sankar (64) on this point in which Sankar points out that the social interaction between an individual and a clinician changes dramatically when the clinician is a researcher. Instead of always seeking more time and information from a busy clinician, the prospective research subject now has time and information lavished upon her or him. Far from being the supplicant, the prospective research subject is now the pursued. Although Sankar's work was in the context of ill patients enrolled in trials of experimental treatments, genetics research presents similar problems. In linkage studies, for example, researchers are dependent on finding rare families—namely large families with an unusual burden of disease and with many affected and unaffected living relatives. When such a family is found, they are tremendously valuable, potentially tempting a researcher toward efforts at persuasion. Data presented below will speak to these points in order to demonstrate the complex dynamics that may make informed consent extremely difficult to operationalize in certain

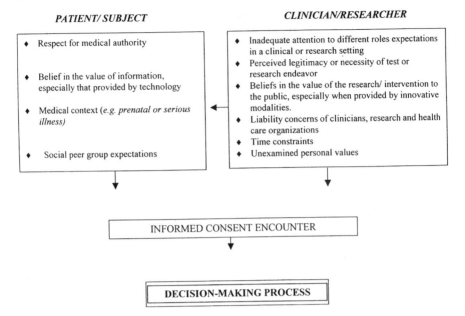

PATIENT/ SUBJECT

- ◆ Respect for medical authority

- ◆ Belief in the value of information, especially that provided by technology

- ◆ Medical context (*e.g. prenatal or serious illness*)

- ◆ Social peer group expectations

CLINICIAN/RESEARCHER

- ◆ Inadequate attention to different roles expectations in a clinical or research setting
- ◆ Perceived legitimacy or necessity of test or research endeavor
- ◆ Beliefs in the value of the research/ intervention to the public, especially when provided by innovative modalities.
- ◆ Liability concerns of clinicians, research and health care organizations
- ◆ Time constraints
- ◆ Unexamined personal values

INFORMED CONSENT ENCOUNTER

DECISION-MAKING PROCESS

Figure 26.2 External factors that shape the informed-consent encounter.

genetics studies. However, in all medical encounters, the depth of respect for medical authority is a factor often underestimated by providers.

The perception of the legitimacy or necessity of the test or research endeavor is itself shaped by a broader belief in the value of information, especially information provided by medical technology. This value, which amounts to an American cultural belief, is, in general, shared by patient/subject and provider/researcher. It might be described by the following propositions: All information is knowledge, knowledge is power; medical information yields increased control of one's world and also leads directly to disease prevention.

In addition, the particular medical context is important as well. For the patient/subject, belief in the importance of the research or the value of the medical information is likely to be especially strong in situations of personal vulnerability—such as the prenatal period or in the context of the risk of a serious and much feared illness, such as cancer, or when there is a belief that research is a key to a cure or that an intervention has an imprimatur of being important for public health. But in the case of serious illness, the provider/researcher has a correlative need to help in some way, which will increase his or her motivational bias.

Liability concerns can exert considerable pressure on clinicians (and researchers) in many situations. However, the case is paradoxical when it comes to informed consent, as it is the ethical need for informing patients that has itself created the potential legal cause for liability and thus has pressured clinicians and researchers into an emphasis on the far more narrow concern of documenting that consent has been obtained.

Finally, some very pragmatic considerations, such as time constraints on clinicians, may have a profound effect on the most sincere intention and desire to inform patients fully and thoughtfully. The issue of time constraints is of particular concern in a clinical setting where time pressures will be much more severe and a thorough informed-consent discussion, especially on a topic filled with both medical and moral complexity, is not a quick procedure.

Patients also may enter the informed-consent encounter having already heard about the test or procedure being offered. In the case of prenatal testing, for example, peer pressure has turned much optional testing into an expected routine of pregnancy; a woman may have to deal not only with her physician but also with her family and peer group if she chooses to forgo certain tests. Similarly, a physician or researcher may have difficulty being nondirective if this individual is not aware of personal biases in favor of or against certain procedures.

Finally, as opposed to the ideal picture of informed consent in Figure 26.1, in which the arrow between provider/researcher and patient/subject is bidirectional, in Figure 26.2 the unidirectional arrow indicates the tendency of these effects to act on the patient, not vice versa.

The points discussed above will be expanded below in the context of four examples. Although certainly not exhaustive, the examples are intended to represent a spectrum of settings in which public health and genetics might meet. The first two examples involve clinical care; the second two concern research endeavors. However, it will be seen that the lines between clinical care and research cannot always be sharply and clearly drawn.

The first example describes the unintended influence of provider attitude and setting on the rates of use of a prenatal test and demonstrates how these structural influences, if unacknowledged, can override even elaborate attempts at informed consent. The second example is a discussion of the history and logic behind the lack of informed consent for newborn screening programs. The third example is drawn from Press' observation of one day in a "gene-hunting" family linkage study that demonstrates some of the familial complexity unique to genetics. The final example examines the dilemmas involved in doing genetic research on stored tissue samples.

Example 1: Prenatal Screening: The Case of Maternal Serum Alpha-Fetoprotein Testing

For women in most times and places, pregnancy is likely to be associated with feelings of vulnerability and the desire to protect their developing baby. For American women, pregnancy is a time of ongoing medical interaction through a recommended schedule of monthly and then weekly prenatal medical visits. Research seeking to isolate what aspects of prenatal care are tied to improved birth outcomes have cited information provision about topics like nutrition and signs and symptoms of pregnancy-related medical problems, rather than any active medical interventions. Thus in pregnancy, virtually all the structural forces referred to in Figure 26.2 are present: Prenatal care is routine and strongly socially sanctioned, and it provides valued and protective information during a vulnerable period in a patient's life. Press and Browner conducted research on how women's decisions about the use of one prenatal screen—maternal serum alpha-fetoprotein (MSAFP)—might be affected by these, and other, structural factors.

Maternal serum alpha-fetoprotein (MSAFP) screening was developed to detect neural tube defects (NTDs) in the fetus. Among the most commonly reported of serious birth defects, NTDs lead to varying degrees of physical and cognitive impairment and, in the case of anencephaly, are incompatible with life. Alpha-fetoprotein is a substance produced by the developing fetus. In the early 1970s research suggested that levels of alpha-fetoprotein in maternal serum could be used as a noninvasive, inexpensive modality of screening for NTDs (65,66). Population-based screening seemed desirable as over 90% of NTDs occur to women at no known risk. The initial research was done in Britain where some of the highest worldwide incidences of NTDs are found (approximately 5 to 6 per 1000 births) (67); researchers in Britain saw this as a public health problem (66,68) and acted quickly to investigate the usefulness of MSAFP as a population screen in actual practice.

The subsequent story of the rapid, and perhaps precipitous, adoption of maternal serum alpha-fetoprotein (MSAFP) screening as a part of routine prenatal care has been chronicled elsewhere (69–71). A significant part of this story in the United States was the Legal Alert (72) from the American College of Obstetricians and Gynecologists to its members, warning of liability jeopardy if MSAFP were not offered to pregnant patients. Clearly this was a structural force of major proportions. California, where Press and Browner (38) conducted their research, is the only state in the U.S. to mandate the offer of MSAFP testing to all pregnant women. Many California physicians interviewed by Press and Browner volunteered that they saw the mandate to offer testing as tantamount in medicolegal terms to a mandate to get their patients to accept testing (38,73).

Press and Browner found that these pressures on physicians translated, for the patient, into an unexplained emphasis on this test by their health care providers. It was found that this, together with the structural forces that enhanced the acceptability of anything offered as part of prenatal care, acted strongly to diminish informed decision making about MSAFP. Specifically, the extent to which pregnant women in the study felt that they had actually made a decision to accept testing was negligible. Almost 85% of those who agreed to testing answered no to the question "Did you have to think much before deciding to be tested?" and the most frequent reasons given for taking the test were: "I don't know, I just took it," "Why not?" and "The more information I have about my baby the better."

Therefore, Press and Browner (38) hypothesized that provider attitude and other structural factors in the medical setting would be the strongest determinants of the rate of uptake of MSAFP in any health care setting. Investigating this proved difficult, however, because most empirical studies have focused on the characteristics of the women who refuse testing (74–80); such a research plan follows logically from the typical assumptions made about informed consent, which focus on free and autonomous decisions rather than on the structural factors that shape and constrain those decisions.

Nevertheless, a close examination of those figures on test use that have been reported support Press and Browner's contention. First, various studies show a very wide range of test use (from as high as 98% to as low as 30%) (66,67,74,75,80–91), and this variation seems to correlate with what is reported in, or can be deduced from, the study about physician attitudes and/or other structural factors.

The first data on uptake came from a UK pilot study to corroborate the usefulness and acceptability to patients and providers of MSAFP as a screen for NTDs. The UK Collaborative Study (67) was a massive project to screen close to 20,000 pregnant women at 19 locations in England, Scotland, and Wales. Test uptake rates of up to 98% suggested that MSAFP screening was clearly an acceptable option; the fact that this was shown through screening of this huge number of pregnancies made the results seem particularly authoritative. In fact, the UK Collaborative Study stands as an example of how a pilot study, done with a public health imprimatur on a large-scale basis, can appear to authorize rather than interrogate the acceptability of a screening procedure.

The next large-scale pilot study was done in Canada. Researchers in charge of this program were also enthusiastic about testing (85), and here again the test uptake rate was well above 90%. However, during this same period, smaller and more local studies were being done on MSAFP screening, and not all the results were equally favorable. For example, Roberts et al. (84) report a much lower rate of test uptake in a study of smaller obstetrics clinics in South Wales, a location comprising patients quite similar to those in the UK Collaborative Study. Roberts and colleagues explained their very different results by citing physicians in their rural area who, they claimed, were reluctant to "interfere" with pregnancies and thus did not refer women early enough in their pregnancy for testing to be feasible.

In the United States, Madlon-Kay et al. (91) studied the attitudes of physicians in rural Minnesota toward MSAFP and found these family practitioners to be generally unenthusiastic about the screening. Only one-third said they would want to be tested if they or their spouse were pregnant, citing anxiety and the possibility of further testing that could jeopardize the pregnancy. Although close to 90% said they offered the screening to their pregnant patients, only 22% reported that more than half their patients were, in fact, being screened. The authors of the study themselves conclude that the physicians' "ambivalence about MSAFP testing appears to be conveyed to their patients" (91).

The importance of broader structural factors, such as logistic ease, is suggested by the work of Gardner et al. (83) in North Carolina where an

MSAFP program was instituted and a specific program goal was to provide support to make offering the screening as convenient as possible for physicians. In reporting the results of this study, investigators compared their MSAFP acceptance rates with rates reported elsewhere in the United States and concluded that their higher rates were linked directly to the organizational structure of their program.

Finally, it is not surprising that it is in California, with its official mandate to offer testing, that rates of MSAFP uptake are the highest in the country (90).

Example 2: Informed Permission for Newborn Screening

It makes little sense to talk about informed consent for the care of young children (92). Traditional notions of informed consent are based on the idea that patients are entitled to make decisions for themselves in light of their own values. This premise is not met when one person is making a decision on behalf of another, as parents do for their young children and as spouses do for their disabled partners. We tend to honor these third-party decisions because they represent the best judgment made by those who care the most for the patient who is unable to decide on one's own, but we refer to this sort of authorization as "permission" to distinguish it from "consent."

All states require that newborns be screened shortly after birth for a variety of disorders, including phenylketonuria (PKU), congenital hypothyroidism, and hemoglobinopathies such as sickle cell anemia (93). Although these programs have unique features, one of the most remarkable is that in all but one or two states, screening is essentially mandatory and parental permission is not sought. Most states do permit parents to refuse screening for at least some religious reasons, exemptions that remain from the time of the Nixon administration when receipt of federal funds was conditioned on honoring religious objections. The religious exemptions, however, do not significantly affect the mandatory nature of newborn screening; for the most part, parents are not informed that they can refuse or even that their children are being screened. The mandatory nature of these programs is all the more remarkable in light of the fact that a committee of the National Academy of Sciences declared in 1975 that informed consent was necessary for newborn screening (94). Why has this recommendation not been heeded? The main argument for making screening mandatory, and the one that holds sway to this day, goes like this: The benefits of newborn screening to the affected children who are detected and given prompt treatment are obvious. No reasonable parent would refuse newborn screening. (A subset of this assertion is that refusal of newborn screening is tantamount to medical neglect that would warrant state intervention.) It is difficult and hence costly to talk with parents about newborn screening, and some argue that giving parents such information would only alarm them. As a result, it is an unwarranted expenditure of money and effort to seek parental permission.

Many of the elements of this argument are flawed, and many important issues are ignored. Although the overwhelming majority of parents would, if asked, accept newborn screening, refusal of screening is not unreasonable and certainly is not evidence of actionable medical neglect. Most of the diseases sought in newborn screening programs have been quite rare. For example, PKU affects approximately 1 in 10,000 infants, whereas maple syrup urine disease (MSUD) affects about 1 in 300,000 (95). As a result, the likelihood is very low that any particular child whose parent refuses screening is actually affected. Put another way, most children who are not tested in fact will do fine. Moreover, screening itself has adverse consequences, which have not been adequately taken into account. As high as 90% or even more of abnormal newborn screening results actually turn out to be false-positives—that is, the babies who get these abnormal results do not actually have the disease that is being sought. Determining which children are truly affected and which are not requires further testing, additional costs, and physician visits, all in the first few and often chaotic months of babies' lives. The most distressing consequence of the inevitability of false-positive test results is that, although most parents whose children ultimately are shown not to be affected are reassured and go on to enjoy their healthy babies, this is not always the case. A small percentage of parents continue to worry that their babies actually do have the condition associated with the initial abnormal result, or some other disease, and so view their newborns as sickly and vulnerable.

New technologies, such as tandem mass spectrometry and genetic testing, will soon make it possible to expand dramatically the number of disorders that can be detected in the newborn period; it will also be possible to include less rare disorders in a constantly expanding panel of tests (96). Unfortunately, for many of these disorders, the benefits of early detection and intervention will be neither clear nor quite so dramatic as what can be achieved by early intervention for PKU. When there is a lack of clarity about the need for or efficacy of early treatment, the benefits of screening become much less clear. In addition, testing may contain risks—for example, the identification of healthy carriers in addition to affected children. Such information could be deleterious on a familial and psychological level and pose risks of discrimination and stigmatization. As the benefit-to-risk ratio becomes less favorable, the moral necessity of seeking parental permission for screening increases as does the reasonableness of parental decisions to refuse.

The problem with the argument that it costs too much to seek parental permission when parents are likely to agree anyway is that it goes too far. Following this reasoning to its logical conclusion would mean that clinicians who care for children would rarely have to seek parental permission because parents usually do at least part of what their children's physicians recommend. The absurdity of this result demonstrates that the primary justification for seeking permission is not to permit parents to refuse interventions, although that is certainly one purpose. The real reasons for talking with parents and seeking their permission are far more complex.

Whether one relies for justification on ethical, religious, or legal notions of the role of the family, or on the practical reality that children are with parents much of the time, the fact is that parents are the primary caretakers and decision-makers for children. Acknowledging and honoring this role is an important reason for including parents in decision making. A more utilitarian argument is that parents are more likely to follow the clinician's recommendations when they believe their concerns have been heard and when they have a role in deciding what to do for their children. Parents need to be involved in making choices because they can function better if they know what is going on and because they bear the consequences most directly when something adverse happens to their children. Although clinicians typically do not think about these arguments in any detail, these are some of the many reasons why clinicians understand that parental permission must be sought before diagnostic and therapeutic interventions can be undertaken unless there is a really valid reason not to do so.

One could hypothesize that the reason why most state-run newborn screening programs do not require parental permission is that legislators, regulators, and laboratory personnel understandably focus on the potential benefits of screening. Because these actors are removed from the clinical situation, they do not automatically think about the centrality of communication to patient care or about the adverse consequences of screening that occur in practice. They are not in the habit of talking with parents on a routine basis to try to build a collaborative relationship based on trust and respect, and they do not have to look parents in the eye when a test has unintended consequences for both child and family members. If legislators and regulators did have these experiences, many would endorse the need for educating and seeking permission from parents for newborn screening.

Example 3: Gene Hunting at a Family Picnic

Another important setting in which public health and genetics are likely to interact is epidemiological research to establish the penetrance of specific alleles in a gene linked to disease and to investigate gene–gene and gene–environment interactions in the expressivity of that disease. This research raises many of the ethical issues discussed above (e.g., the possibility of this information being used in a discriminatory fashion; psychological morbidity; possibilities of family disruption; and privacy concerns when DNA samples cannot be made anonymous without compromising the goals of the investigation) and requires careful informed-consent protocols. Yet such research presents some strikingly new challenges.

For example, as multiple members of a family are enrolled, participation may lead to a social redefinition or realignment of a family unit, exacerbating tensions and/or strengthening familial bonds (24,97,98). This heightened sense of family may become a powerful motivation for research participation, increasing coercion on uninterested family members. The hope of older members of the family to be able to do something for the younger and future members may also make it particularly difficult to keep the line between research and clinical care from blurring. An entirely unexamined issue, however, is how the inclusion of entire families, whom the research encourages to coalesce as social units, may present the researcher with unanticipated difficulties and ones that challenge informed consent. The data below—representing the investigator's ethnographic observations—illustrate some of these novel challenges for informed consent in the context of familial genetics research. They come from a family study looking for new mutations in susceptibility genes for breast/ovarian cancer. This sort of "gene-hunting" is a standard first step in demonstrating the association of a gene and a disease and will continue to be a necessary part of genetic research in the future.

The family in this example became involved in the research when the proband was diagnosed with breast cancer at the age of 37. She quickly became a quasi-member of the research team, calling her relatives and encouraging them to be part of the study and to give permission for obtaining their medical records. This role transformation can be seen as the mirror image of the transformation Sankar talks about in the role of the clinician from "doctor" to "researcher." Ethnographic observation suggested that this unacknowledged role change in the proband, and ultimately her family, led to confusion and difficulty for the researcher and for the possibility of informed consent.

When the family's pedigree was complete and medical records had confirmed diagnoses of breast cancer in numerous relatives, it became necessary to obtain DNA samples from a large number of individuals. Following a model used by other "gene-hunters," and before them by public health researchers investigating disease outbreaks in populations, it was decided that the researchers would go to a location convenient for the entire family rather than asking individual family members to come to the university.

Research-team preparations for the day focused on the logistics of collecting, marking, and storing blood samples, and getting consent forms signed by all family members. Little attention was paid to the interpersonal political aspects of the encounter of the research team with the family unit. However, evidence of a shift in the balance of power seemed obvious from the moment it was discovered that the Principal Investigator's (PI) preference for a private event in a family home had been ignored. Instead, the community hospital was chosen by the family, with placards in the entryway announcing the arrival of the researchers, and the family's local oncologist and the hospital administrator in attendance. This implicit struggle for the ownership of the event would continue throughout the day as family members sought to meet their own needs.

As 40 members of the family assembled and conversed, a frequent theme was concern about "the young people" in the family, suggesting that a significant motivator of participation in the study was the hope that it would help protect the younger generations of the family from the cancer history the older generation had suffered—and that such progress would happen soon. When the blood drawing began, the family was impatient with the length of time it took to get informed consent. They had come ready to give blood and did not want to listen to more explanations of the parameters of the study and its risks. When mothers brought their small children up to give a specimen, it was difficult for the team to persuade them that they did not need the children's blood. Several parents were insistent—if it would help the study they saw no reason not to test the children. The phlebotomists were not prepared to elaborate on the issues involved. Things started to bog down as such incidents occurred and eventually informed-consent forms were quickly signed with little or no further discussion.

Although the PI was a bench scientist and had a clear intention to avoid any clinical interaction with his research subjects, clinical questions quickly arose. In the exchange that had perhaps the highest emotional charge of the day, the proband had an interchange with three of her first cousins. It began when she mentioned that she had already had her ovaries removed. One first cousin responded, saying that she had periodic CA125 testing, to which the proband answered, "But that tells you when you have the disease. Why wait?" Another first cousin countered, "What are you saying, that we should all go have our ovaries taken out?" And the third of the first cousins said, "A Pap smear will detect ovarian cancer, right?" Uncertain of the answer, all turned to the PI who answered that a Pap smear won't detect ovarian cancer. "Well what does detect it?" he was asked. "That's hard," he answered, and began to discuss the problems with various detection modalities. He was quickly interrupted by one of the cousins, who asked, "Well, what should I do?" While the PI stood silent, trying to figure out how to deal with this blatant request for clinical advice, many of the women in the family talked among themselves, repeating bits of information they had gleaned on oophorectomy, surgical menopause, and the possibilities of adoption. Eventually the conversation trailed off, with the PI neither contributing useful medical advice nor clearly still in control of the flow of the day's agenda.

But the greatest problems for the Principal Investigator arose when a family member asked: "When will you be able to tell people who have been tested if they have the gene?" The PI replied apologetically and somewhat confusingly, that results would not be given owing to lack of scientific certainty involved in either a positive or a negative result. He did not, however, explicitly remind the family members that they had all agreed to this in the Consent Form, nor did he use the opportunity to revisit the potential *social, legal, and psychological* risks of this sort of research.

Questions from the family continued, demonstrating variable degrees of sophistication about genetics but a uniform hunger for the results, until finally the PI said: "If we are certain that a family has the gene, we will invite them to participate in a separate results disclosure study. . . . When [this] psychosocial study is funded we will invite you into the disclosure study." This seemed to satisfy the family, and someone asked, "When will that study be funded?" The PI, desperately optimistic, replied, "Eight months to one year." The psychosocial "disclosure study" was never funded.

Example 4: The Use of Stored Tissue Samples and Medical Records for Research

Testing of human biological materials is an integral part of medical care. For the most part, the materials that remain after the completion of testing are discarded, but certain types of individual samples, ranging from surgical pathological specimens to newborn screening blood spots, typically are retained, sometimes for years. Similarly, human biological materials are collected and stored or put into tissue culture in a growing number of research protocols.

In the past few years, the question of whether and when these retained materials can appropriately be used for purposes other than those for which they were originally collected has been raised with increasing intensity (99,100). These uses include quality assurance, test development, and tracking, but the use that has received the most attention is research, particularly genetics research.

The knowledge that can be gained from studying human biological materials depends to a significant degree on the ability to correlate particular samples with clinical information about the individuals from whom they were obtained. One can assess allelic variation by analyzing the DNA of isolated tissue samples and even the prevalence of certain genotypes if one has a population-based sample of tissues, but understanding the relationship of genotype to phenotype requires access to clinical information as well. Thus, the most pressing question is under what conditions retained biological samples and medical records can be linked and used for research.

Several developments have contributed to the current interest in examining the limits of the need to obtain informed consent to use of medical records and tissue samples for research. One is the power of the new tools of genetics, which increasingly can reveal much about the future health of the individual and his or her relatives. Another is the power of information technologies that, by permitting manipulation of large data sets in ways that were simply impossible before, can be used both to improve our understanding of human disease and to invade the individual's privacy. True anonymity is becoming harder and harder to achieve, particularly in studies that link DNA results with clinical information. Another factor is the renewed debate in our highly diverse society about the role of research and the rights and obligations of individuals and communities. Most citizens strongly favor research at least in terms of their willingness to devote public monies to its pursuit, and many individuals actively seek to participate in research, often as a way to obtain innovative therapy (101). Others, however, worry that the results of research will open the door to discrimination and stigmatization (102).

Until recently, however, and despite the apparent requirements of the federal regulations for the protection of human subjects from research risks, medical records and tissue samples collected in the course of clinical practice were often used for research without the knowledge, or any sort of meaningful consent, of patients. (Patients do typically sign very broad waivers embedded in the middle of lengthy forms when they enter a hospital or consent to surgery, but no one would contend seriously that these waivers constitute meaningful consent for research uses.) The situation was more complex for records and samples collected in the course of research. If examination of these materials was contemplated at the outset of the project, these uses typically were disclosed in the initial consent process. Investigators who subsequently thought of new questions they wished to pursue using these materials, however, rarely recontacted subjects to obtain consent for the new research.

Defining the appropriate role for informed consent can be achieved only if considered in the context of all the efforts that should be made to protect the interests of the individuals whose information and materials are being studied. Other protective elements include designing protocols to use the least identifiable data necessary to meet the scientific goal and putting measures in place to protect the security of data. Effective third-party review of protocols should focus on these elements. When these steps are taken, informed consent will be required when the protocol poses more than minimal risk to the person, a condition most likely to occur when the patient will be contacted in the future either to obtain more information or particularly to be given specific research results. More generally, respect for individuals and the growing emphasis on transparency in information policies require that potential uses for research need to be identified, if possible, and disclosed to patients and subjects prior to the collection of medical information and biological samples. The National Action Plan for Breast Cancer has developed documents that can serve as templates for use in the clinical setting. Such disclosures can then afford individuals the opportunity at least to opt out of such uses.

Conclusions and Recommendations

The examples presented here do not pretend to cover comprehensively the arenas in which public health and genetics might come together, either in research or in clinical programs. However, it is hoped they can point to the major issues that need consideration when implementing such programs.

In terms of prenatal genetic screening, the most important issue is that an offer of information about one's developing baby is never neutral. The desire to protect one's child, combined with the trust which contemporary women place in health care providers and the health care system in regard to pregnancy and childbirth, give a profound impetus toward the acceptance of any offer of noninvasive testing; they also make any test that is important enough to be offered appear automatically important enough to be accepted. Thus, it is crucial that the informed-consent process not be pro forma. In fact, an emphasis on obtaining consent can work mainly to *promote* consent unless there is a concomitant emphasis on the real necessity for a decision to be made by the woman or couple.

In our discussion of newborn screening programs, we discussed the usual practice of excluding parents from the decision-making process. Although we believe that informed consent should be the general standard for all aspects of public health and genetics, we recognize that, in certain situations, such as screening of children who are not in a position to make decisions for themselves for disorders where early detection is highly beneficial, a lesser standard may make sense. However, we find flawed the argument that any sort of consent process for newborn screening is always unnecessary and excessively cumbersome, and we advocate strongly for the use of a standard of informed permission for any neonatal genetic screening tests that might be introduced in the future, particularly if the disorders are not well understood, treatments or benefits are of unproven value, and/or the test identifies carriers as well as affected newborns.

The third example cited above highlights ways in which all genetics research inevitably involves families, and how working with families introduces completely new dynamics, needs, and tensions. Once family members are involved, it is very difficult to separate such research from clinical care, either theoretically or pragmatically. In addition, researchers will have to be aware of the needs and strategies of the families themselves. These problems become even more complicated if the families are from small and identifiable minority populations. All of this leads us to suggest strongly that a high level of informed consent be necessary for such research. We consider this to be necessary whether or not individual results will be given back to research participants—although differing strategies will be involved in different situations. Similarly, informed consent is also required for at least some protocols that examine medical records and stored human biological materials. In addition, we counsel that the issue of sharing information on genotype with research participants and with relatives of participants is one of considerable complexity that should be thought through carefully well in advance of beginning any research endeavor.

If all of our examples point to the need for great seriousness in considering and implementing informed consent, what conclusions and guidance can we derive from them about how to "do" informed consent per se? We believe that in designing modes of obtaining informed consent, explicit consideration must be given to the structural forces that may make truly informed consent difficult in each particular situation. For example, the preexisting cultural power of medical authority in contemporary American society may be particularly determinative in prenatal situations, whereas the motivation to assuage guilty concern about having passed on a "bad gene" to a child may motivate participation in certain types of research. Moreover, it must be realized that these structural forces have the potential to increase in importance and impact when coupled with any program that purports to have the public's health at stake.

Finally, we would hope that the message taken from these examples is that as genetics and public health come together, the model of "informed consent" that needs to be developed is one of true collaboration between patient/research participant and health care provider/researcher—a collaboration in which both are encouraged to delve more deeply and explicitly into their own needs, values, and motivations for offering, accepting, or refusing genetic information or research participation in a public health and genetics endeavor.

References

1. Smith JD. Reflections on mental retardation and eugenics, old and new: Mensa and the Human Genome Project. Ment Retard 1994;32:234–238.

2. Ledley FD. Distinguishing genetics and eugenics on the basis of fairness. J Med Ethics 1994;20:157–164.

3. Garver KL, Garver B. The Human Genome Project and eugenic concerns. Am J Hum Genet 1994;54:148–158.

4. Marks J. Historiography of eugenics. Am J Hum Genet 1993;52:650–652.

5. Markel H. The stigma of disease: implications of genetic screening. Am J Med 1992;93:209–215.

6. Faden RR. Human-subjects research today: final report of the Advisory Committee on Human Radiation Experiments. Acad Med 1996;71:482–483.

7. Faden R. The Advisory Committee on Human Radiation Experiments: reflections on a presidential commission. Hastings Cent Rep 1996;26:5–10.

8. Kass NE, Sugarman J, Faden R, Schoch-Spana M. Trust: the fragile foundation of contemporary biomedical research. Hastings Cent Rep 1996;26:25–29.

9. Roy B. The Julius Rosenwald Fund syphilis seroprevalence studies. J Nat Med Associ 1996;88:315–322.

10. Dowd SB, Wilson B. Informed patient consent: a historical perspective. Radiol Technol 1995;67:119–124.

11. Roy B. The Tuskegee syphilis experiment: biotechnology and the administrative state. J Nat Med Assoc 1995;87:56–67.

12. Murray TH. Genetics and the moral mission of health insurance. Hastings Cent Rep 1992;22:12–17.

13. Porkowski R. The genetic testing debate: new technologies present challenges in risk selection. J Insur Med 1988;20:57–61.

14. Hudson KL, Rothenberg KH, Andrews LB, et al. Genetic discrimination and health insurance: an urgent need for reform. Science 1995;270:391–393.

15. Rothenberg KH. Genetic information and health insurance: state legislative approaches. J Law Med Ethics 1995;23:312–319.

16. Alper JS, Geller LN, Barash CI, et al. Genetic discrimination and screening for hemochromatosis. J Public Health Policy 1994;15:345–358.

17. Billings PR, Kohn MA, de Cuevas M, Beckwith J, Alper JS, Natowicz MR. Discrimination as a consequence of genetic testing. Am J Hum Genet. 1992;50:476–482.

18. Draper E, Hubbard R, Henifin MS. Genetic screening of prospective parents and of workers: some scientific and social issues. Int J Health Serv 1985;15:231–251.

19. Rothstein M. Genetic discrimination in employment and the American with Disabilities Act. Houston Law Rev 1992;29:23–85.

20. Rothenberg KH, Fuller B, Rothstein M, et al. Genetic information and the workplace: legislative approaches and policy challenges. Science 1997;275:1755–1757.

21. Grandjean P, Sorsa M. Ethical aspects of genetic predisposition to environmentally-related disease. Sci Total Environ 1996;184:37–43.

22. Pukkala E, Auvinen A, Wahlberg G. Incidence of cancer among Finnish airline cabin attendants. BMJ 1995;311:649–652.

23. Huggins M, Bloch M, Wiggins S, et al. Predictive testing for Huntington disease in Canada: adverse effects and unexpected results in those receiving a decreased risk. Am J Med Genet 1992;42:508–515.

24. Green J, Richards M, Murton F, et al. Family communication and genetic counseling: the case of hereditary breast and ovarian cancer. J Genet Counsel 1997;6:45–60.

25. Grobstein R. Amniocentesis counseling In: Kessler S (ed). Genetic counseling: psychological dimensions. New York: Academic Press, 1979.

26. Glass RM. AAAS conference explores ethical aspects of large pedigree genetic research. JAMA 1992;267:2158.

27. Jonsen AR, Durfy SJ, Burke W, et al. The advent of the "unpatients." Nat Med 1996;2:622–624.

28. Kenen RH, Schmidt RM. Stigmatization of carrier status: social implications of heterozygote genetic screening programs. Am J Public Health 1978;49:116–120.

29. Nelkin D, Tancredi L. Dangerous diagnostics: the social power of biological information. New York: Basic Books, 1990.

30. Juengst ET. The ethics of prediction: genetic risk and the physician–patient relationship. Genome Sci Technol 1995;1:21–36.

31. Green RM, Thomas AM. Whose gene is it? A case discussion about familial conflict over genetic testing for breast cancer. J Genet Counsel 1997;6:245–253.

32. Reilly PR. Panel comment: the impact of the Genetic Privacy Act on medicine. J Law Med Ethics 1995;23:378–381.

33. Byrne DJ, Napier A, Cuschieri A. How informed is signed consent? BMJ Clin Res Ed 1988;296:839–840.

34. Hekkenberg RJ, Irish JC, Rotstein LE, et al. Informed consent in head and neck surgery: how much do patients actually remember? J Otolaryngol 1997;26:155–159.

35. Hopper KD, Azjdel M, Hulse SF, et al. Interactive method of informing patients of the risks of intravenous contrast media. Radiology 1994;192:67–71.

36. Lavelle-Jones C, Byrne DJ, Rice P, et al. Factors affecting quality of informed consent BMJ 1993;306:885–890.

37. Taub HA, Baker MT, Sturr JF. Informed consent for research: effects of readability, patient age, and education. J Am Geriatr Soc 1986;34:601–606.

38. Press NA, Browner CH. "Collective fictions": similarities in reasons for accepting maternal serum alpha-fetoprotein screening among women of diverse ethnic and social class backgrounds. Fetal Diagn Ther 1993;8S1:97–106.

39. McCormack D, Evoy D, Mulcahy D, et al. An evaluation of patient's comprehension of orthopaedic terminology: implications for informed consent. J R Coll Surg Edinb 1997;42:33–35.

40. Little JM. Leeders Logic, hermenuetics and informed consent. Arch Intern Med 1988;148:1385–1389.

41. Lidz CW, Appelbaum PS, Meisel A. Two models of implementing informed consent. Arch Intern Med 1988;148:1385–1389.

42. Andrews LB. Compromised consent: deficiencies in the consent process for genetic testing. J Am Med Womens Assoc 1997;52:39–42.

43. Holtzman NA. Primary-care physicians as providers of frontline genetic services. Fetal Diagn Ther 1993;8(Suppl)1:213–219.

44. Sadler M. Serum screening for Down's syndrome: how much do health professionals know? Br J Obstet Gynaecol 1997;104:176–179.

45. Grossman SA, Piantadosi S, Covahey C. Are informed consent forms that describe clinical oncology research protocols readable by most patients and their families? J Clin Oncol 1995;12:2211–2215.

46. Hopper KD, TenHave TR, Hartzel J. Informed consent forms for clinical and research imaging procedures: how much do patients understand? Am J Roentgenol 1995;164:493–496.

47. Jubelirer SJ, Linton JC, Magnetti SM. Reading versus comprehension: implications for patient education and consent in an outpatient oncology clinic. J Cancer Educ 1994;9:26–29.

48. Meade CD, Wittbrot R. Computerized readability analysis of written materials. Comput Nurs 1988;6:30–36.

49. Philipson SJ, Doyle MA, Gabram SG, et al. Informed consent for research: a study to evaluate readability and processability to effect change. J Investig Med 1995;43:459–467.

50. Rivera R, Reed JS, Menius D. Evaluating the readability of informed consent forms used in contraceptive clinical trials. Int J Gynaecol Obstet 1992;38:227–230.

51. Briguglio J, Cardella JF, Fox PS, et al. Development of a model angiography informed-consent form based on a multi-institutional survey of current forms. J Vasc Interv Radiol 1995;6:971–978.

52. Bernhardt BA, Geller G, Doksum T, et al. Prenatal genetic testing: content of discussions between obstetric providers and pregnant women. Obstet Gynecol 1998;91: 648–655.

53. Hofman KJ, Tambor ES, Chase GA, et al. Physicians' knowledge of genetics and genetic tests. Acad Med 1993;68:625–632.

54. Redelmeier DA, Rozin D, Kahneman D. Understanding patients' decisions: cognitive and emotional perspectives. JAMA 1993;270:72–76.

55. Kahneman D, Tversky A. Variants of uncertainty. Cognition 1982;11:143–157.

56. Tversky A, Kahneman D. The framing of decisions and the psychology of choice. Science 1981;211:453–458.

57. O'Connor AM. Effects of framing and level of probability on patients' preferences for cancer chemotherapy. J Clin Epidemiol 1989;42:119–126.

58. Bursztajin HJ, Chanowitz B, Gutheil TG, et al. Micro-effects of language on risk perception in drug-prescribing behavior. Bull Am Acad Psychiatry Law 1992;20:59–66.

59. Steethman SE, Mileman PA, van't Hof MA, et al. Blind chance? an investigation into the perceived probabilities of phrases used in oral radiology for expressing chance. Dento Maxillo Facial Radiol 1993;22:135–139.

60. White LJ, Jones JS, Felton CW, et al. Informed consent for medical research: common discrepancies and readability. Acad Emerg Med 1996;3:745–750.

61. Feldman-Stewart D, Chammas S, Hayter C, et al. An empirical approach to informed consent in ovarian cancer. J Clin Epidemiol 1996;49:1259–1269.

62. Braddock CH, Fihn SD, Levinson W, et al. How doctors and patients discuss routine clinical decisions: informed decision making in the outpatient setting. J Gen Intern Med 1997;12:339–345.

63. Geller G, Botkin JR, Green MJ, Press N, et al. Genetic testing for susceptibility to adult-onset cancer: the process and content of informed consent. JAMA 1997;277:1467–1474.

64. Sankar P. The ritualization of informed consent to medical research. Invited presentation American Anthropological Association, 95th Annual meetings, San Francisco, November 1996.

65. Brock DHJ, Sutcliffe RG. Lancet 1972;ii:197–199.

66. Brock DHJ, Bolton AE, Monaghan JM. Prenatal diagnosis of anencephaly through maternal serum alpha-fetoprotein measurement. Lancet 1973;ii:923–924.

67. Report of the UK Collaborative Study on alphafetoprotein in relation to neural tube defects. Lancet 1977;1:1323–1333.

68. Ferguson-Smith MA, Rawlinson HA, May HM, et al. Avoidance of anencephalic and spina bifida births by maternal serum alpha-fetoprotein screening. Lancet 1978;24:1330–1333.

69. Holtzman NA. From research to routine: how is the road paved? In: Gastel B, Haddow JE, Fletcher JC, et al. (eds). Maternal serum alpha-fetoprotein: issues in the

prenatal screening and diagnosis of neural tube defects. Proceedings of a conference held by the National Center for Health Care Technology and the Food and Drug Administration, July 28–30, 1980, Washington, DC, pp. 153–158.

70. Press NA, Browner CH. Why women say yes to prenatal diagnosis. Soc Sci Med 1997;45:979–989.

71. Annas GJ. Is a genetic screening test ready when the lawyers say it is? Hastings Cent Rep 1985;15:16–18.

72. American College of Obstetrics and Gynecology. Professional liability implications of AFP tests. May 1985; DPL Alert.

73. Browner CH, Press NA. The production of authoritative knowledge in prenatal care. Med Anthropol Q 1996;10:141–156.

74. Bennet MJ, Gau GS, Gau DW. Women's attitudes to screning for neural tube defects. Br J Obstet Gynaecol 1980;87:370–371.

75. Berne-Frommel K, Josefson G, Kjessler B. Who declines from antenatal serum alpha-fetoprotein screening—and why? Acta Obstet Gynecol 1984;63:687–691.

76. Sikkink J. Patient acceptance of prenatal alpha-fetoprotein screening: a preliminary study. Fam Pract Res J 1990;10:123–131.

77. Dembert ML, Watson RE, Mick SS, et al. Women's attitudes toward the serum alpha-fetoprotein test. Conn Med 1983;47:525–529.

78. Faden RR, Chwalow AJ, Quaid K, et al. Prenatal screening and pregnant women's attitudes toward the abortion of defective fetuses. Am J Public Health 1987;77:288–290.

79. Jorgensen FS. Declining an alpha-fetoprotein test in pregnancy. Why and who? Acta Obstet Gynecol Scand 1995;74:3–11.

80. Tymstra TJ, Bejema C, Beekhus JR, et al. Women's opinions on the offer and use of prenatal diagnosis. Prenat Diagn 1991;11:893–898.

81. Wald NJ, Cuckle HS, Boreham J, et al. Antenatal screening in Oxford for fetal neural tube defects. Br J Obstet Gynaeocol 1979;86:91–100.

82. Macri JN, Haddow JE, Weiss RR. Screening for neural tube defects in the United States: a summary of the Scarborough conference. Am J Obstet Gynecol 1979;133:119–125.

83. Gardner S, Burton B, Johson AM. Maternal serum alpha-fetoprotein screening: a report of the Forsyth County project. Am. J Obstet Gynecol 1981;40:250–253.

84. Roberts CJ, Hibbard EM, Elder GH, et al. The efficiency of a serum screening service for neural tube defects: the South Wales experience. Lancet 1983;2:1315–1318.

85. Doran TA, Valentine GH, Wong PY, et al. Maternal serum alpha-fetoprotein screening: report of a Canadian pilot project. Can Med Assoc J 1987;137:285–293.

86. Kyle D, Cummins C, Evans S. Factors affecting the uptake of screening for neural tube defects. Br J Obstet Gynaecol 1988;95:560–564.

87. Byrne-Essif K, Naber JM, Colmorgen GHC. Acceptance of maternal serum alpha-fetoprotein screening in Wilmington hospital's obstetrical clinic. Del Med J 1988;60:569–571.

88. Sanden ML, Bjurulf P. Pregnant women's attitudes and knowledge in relation to access to serum-alpha-fetoprotein test. Scand J Soc Med 1988;16:197–204.

89. Marteau TM, Johnston M, Shaw RW, et al. Factors influencing the uptake of screening for open neural tube defects and amniocentesis to test for Down's syndrome. Br J Obstet Gynaecol 1989;96:739–748.

90. Deukmejian G, Allenby CL, Kizer KW. A report to the legislature: review of current genetic programs. Sacramento: State of California Health and Welfare Agency, Department of Health Services, Genetic Disease Branch, 1990.

91. Madlon-Kay DJ, Reif C, Mersy DJ, et al. Maternal serum alpha-fetoprotein testing: physician experience and attitudes and their influence on patient acceptance. J Fam Pract 1992;35:395–400.

92. Committee on Bioethics, Informed Consent, Parental Permission, and Child Assent in Pediatric Practice. Pediatrics 1995;95:314–317.

93. Clayton EW. Screening and treatment of newborns. Houston Law Rev 1992;29: 85–148.

94. Committee on Screening for Inborn Errors of Metabolism, Genetic Screening. Programs, principles, and research. Washington, DC: National Academy of Sciences Press, 1975.

95. Scriver CR. The metabolic and molecular bases of inherited disease (7th ed). New York: McGraw-Hill, 1995.

96. Levy HL. Newborn screening by tandem mass spectrometry: a new era. Clin Chem 1998;44:2401–2402.

97. Heimler A, Zanko A. Huntington disease: a case study describing the complexities and nuances of predictive testing of monozygotic twins. J Genet Counsel 1995;4:125–137.

98. Chapple A, May C, Campion P. Lay understanding of genetic disease: a British study of families attending a genetic counseling service. J Genet Counsel 1995;4: 281–300.

99. Clayton EW, Steinberg KK, Khoury MJ, et al. Informed consent for genetic research on stored tissue samples. J Am Med Assoc 1995;274:1786–1792.

100. Clayton EW. Informed consent and genetic research. In: Rothstein MA (ed). Genetic secrets: privacy, confidentiality, and new genetic technology. New Haven, CT: Yale University Press, 1997, pp. 126–136.

101. Thomas A. Public support for medical research—how deep, how enduring? Acad Med 1998;73:178–179.

102. Employers should be barred from accessing genetic information, Americans say in ncgr survey. http://www.ncgr.org/ncgr/news/1998/0304.html.

27

Public health surveillance of genetic information:
Ethical and legal responses to social risk

Scott Burris, Lawrence O. Gostin, and Deborah Tress

The practice of public health begins with effective surveillance of physical characteristics, diseases, behavior, and environmental conditions that significantly influence a population's well-being. As the roles of specific genetic characteristics are better understood, epidemiologists will more often consider adding selected genetic information to the conditions subject to surveillance. Although surveillance of genetic information will significantly advance the public's health, it also entails some real and perceived risks. The social objective is to achieve the public good that comes from genetic information without unreasonable or unethical interference with the civil liberties of individuals. Even when individual interests are well protected by law, however, perceptions of risk to social status, employment, or other relationships can persist and confound useful public health data collection. This chapter explores the problem that such "social risk" poses to public health collection of genetic data, discusses the capacities and limitations of law as an antidote to social risk, and presents ethical principles for understanding and assessing the benefits and risks of population-based genetics. It concludes with recommendations for surveillance policy and research.

Public Health Surveillance for Genetic Information

What Is Public Health Surveillance?
Promoting the public's health and preventing disease and disability will increasingly require the translation of the new genetic vocabulary into practices that improve the health of the public. Public health practitioners will be required to investigate the distribution of genetic variations that are associ-

ated with diseases, assess the prevalence of particular diseases with genetic components, evaluate genetic tests and interventions for preventing diseases on a population basis, and assure the quality of genetic tests (1). Surveillance, defined as the "ongoing, systematic collection, analysis, and interpretation of outcome specific data for use in the planning, implementation, and evaluation of public health practice," (2) will be a valuable tool in this work.

The purposes of public health surveillance are to assess public health status, define public health priorities, evaluate programs, and stimulate research (2). Data collected through surveillance are used to study the prevalence, geographical distribution, and natural history of a disease. Surveillance data can help detect epidemics, define problems, generate hypotheses and stimulate research, evaluate control measures, monitor changes in infectious agents, detect changes in health practices, and facilitate planning. Data are gathered from a variety of sources, and in a variety of ways. Some information and conditions are required by statute or regulation to be reported by physicians, laboratories, and institutions to public health authorities. In addition, biological specimens, vital records, sentinel surveillance, registries, surveys of providers and individuals, administrative data systems, and other sources all provide data for public health uses. In most instances, the data were created or collected originally for purposes other than surveillance.

The data in surveillance systems may be collected with personal identifiers, with coded identifiers, or anonymously. Whether identifiers are needed depends on the subject matter within the data system, the type and source of the data, and the anticipated uses of the data. In many cases, names are collected principally for the purpose of detecting duplicate reporting to enhance the accuracy of the system, or to ensure comprehensive information on a particular case. In other instances, identifiers allow for data to be linked from different systems for epidemiologic research (2) or case investigations. The individual may not be specifically notified about data collection, and is not asked to give informed consent. However, the existence of reporting laws and regulations gives at least constructive knowledge that data systems exist and that individual information will be collected (3–5).

Surveillance for Genetic Information

Nearly every human disease has a genetic component that will eventually be relevant to disease prevention. Surveillance is important to gathering the information needed to study the public health impact of genes on the population; to determine the prevalence, distribution, and frequency of predisposing genetic variation; to track the morbidity and mortality associated with genetically linked diseases; to identify modifiable risk factors for disease and disability; and to evaluate the use and effectiveness of genetic tests and other interventions (1,6,7).

The relative contributions of genes and environmental factors will vary significantly for different diseases, as will the needs and methods of surveillance. Surveillance for diseases and disorders where the presence of the genetic trait equals the presence of the disease, such as Huntington's disease and Tay-Sachs, may be useful for determining the prevalence and distribution of the gene and the disease, to target services, and to evaluate programs. For other conditions, such as phenylketonuria, the genetic trait plus a particular environmental factor creates the disease or condition (8). Some genetic information identifies individuals as carriers who may have a greater or lesser risk of passing on various diseases and conditions to their offspring.

The diseases and conditions of greatest concern from a public health standpoint will probably be found to result from a more complex interaction between single or multiple mutations and factors in the social and physical environment (1,9). For many common chronic diseases, such as heart disease and cancer, the genetic factor may be one of several modifiable or nonmodifiable individual and environmental risk factors. A person's genetic composition is also thought to be a factor in the susceptibility to many infectious diseases including HIV/AIDS. Therefore, the predictive value of the genetic information will vary substantially. Surveillance activities for the particular diseases could include relevant genetic information in addition to other risk factors. In many of these cases, the presence or absence of the genetic trait may be of limited value on its own, but significant in the context of other factors, and for subsequent epidemiologic and clinical investigations.

Surveillance for genetic information is already occurring. Birth defects surveillance systems and registries are an important source of genetic information on a national, state, and local level (2,3,10,11). These systems vary in that some rely on available information, whereas others are the product of active case finding (2). Newborn screening programs collect data that can be used for valuable surveillance on the prevalence and distribution of the underlying disease conditions tested, to assess the effectiveness and need for particular screening tests in various populations, and to evaluate prevention and intervention activities. Many states have established programs to provide otherwise unavailable or inaccessible genetic services to selected populations. Data derived from the provision of such services can be critical to assess the prevalence of various conditions in the state, to evaluate whether the services offered are appropriate and effective, and in planning future health services and prevention programs (12,13).

Defining the Social Risks of Surveillance

Throughout the history of American public health, surveillance has generated occasional opposition, based on fears that the collection of data by the government threatened the civil rights, social status, or economic interests of individuals. Opposition to surveillance has in some instances slowed its implementation, reduced cooperation by both reporters and subjects, and led those at risk to avoid diagnosis and other medical services. Leading examples include tuberculosis reporting (14,15), venereal disease surveillance (16), and named reporting of HIV disease (17,18). Opposition to surveillance typically reflects the deep anxieties and social divisions revealed by a specific health condition, rather than a categorical enmity toward public health data collection: People who object to HIV surveillance do not typically oppose surveillance for measles or malaria (19). In such cases, successful surveillance depends upon the effectiveness of public health agencies in broadly addressing the factors engendering opposition.

Defining Social Risk
Part of the difficulty in assessing the impact of social risk on health-related decisions has been the lack of a generally accepted definition of the phenomenon of social risk itself. One of us has offered this definition: Social risk in health behavior is the danger that an individual will be socially or economically penalized should she become identified with an expensive, disfavored or feared medical condition (18). It has two distinct components: (*1*) "the threat," that is, the attitudes and behavior that cause or threaten social harm; and (*2*) "the perception of risk," namely the attitudes and beliefs about the threat among those who are in some way tied to the trait or disease. Social risk will influence acceptance of surveillance whenever the social construction or economic cost of a disease creates at least the perception of a risk that, alone or in combination with other factors, outweighs the benefits of obtaining diagnostic or therapeutic care.

The threat and the perception of social risk are independent to a considerable degree. This independence has been a notable characteristic of the social risk of public health surveillance, and it may be the most important characteristic of social risk for policymakers to recognize. It explains why, as in the case of HIV, the essentially spotless record of public health in protecting surveillance data, and strong privacy legislation, can fail to quiet opposition to named reporting. It suggests that the current lack of strong legal protection against the social risks of genetic testing will not necessarily lead to widespread opposition to genetic surveillance.

The Potential Social Risks of Genetic Surveillance
The concern that progress in genetics could create social risk is founded on historical experience with other health conditions. For the most part, scholarly treatment of the issue focuses on ethical and legal principles, stimulated by historical analogies and contemporary anecdotes (20–22). There have been only a small number of empirical investigations of the prevalence of threats or perceptions of social risk (23–28). These studies almost uniformly rely on

self-report of the experiences of small, convenience samples. Several focus on attitudes or behavior under hypothetical circumstances. Many studies that touch on issues of social risk do so only tangentially in the course of studying a broader range of factors influencing health care utilization (29,30).

These studies, although useful, can hardly be considered a sufficient empirical basis for the construction of effective policies addressing the social risks of genetics, and some commentators suggest that the risk of genetic discrimination may be overstated (31). Available data do not allow reliable estimation of the prevalence of discrimination, stigma, social hostility, or other manifestations of social risk. As in other areas of prevention, the important and complex question of how perceptions of risk arise and influence individual behavior has been largely ignored. The psychological process of risk assessment has been well studied, but the many insights of this body of work have been slow to permeate the analysis of health behavior (32). Further research on both the threats of social risk and their perceptions should be a high priority.

The experience with HIV has shown the dangers to policy-making of a lack of rigorous empirical investigation of social risk (18). Recent research in the field of HIV/AIDS has undermined the claim that reporting in and of itself inhibits testing rates generally (33), but it has also reinforced the conclusion that the availability of anonymous testing is important to reach people at risk regardless of the reporting rules in place (34). In the absence of sufficient data, we should be very cautious about assuming that social risk will be a problem influencing the willingness of people to be tested under conditions of reporting, or that reporting will increase social risk. We can and should avoid broad claims about the social risks of genetic technology in favor of a more nuanced and contextualized analysis of both the possible threats and the perceptions of risk posed by particular kinds of genetic information.

A first step for further investigation—and for policy-making in the inevitable absence of adequate data—is to define a sufficiently broad universe of potential harms associated with genetic surveillance. It is helpful to consider a range of vulnerability, which can be both economic and psychosocial. Economic harm includes, potentially, losing access to insurance, a decrease in employability, and loss of economic support (as, for example, where genetic information leads to a divorce). Psychosocial vulnerability includes stigma, loss of social status or marriageability, and exposure to social hostility because of one's condition. (Stigma, which is classically defined as a sense of spoiled identity shared by the person with the stigmatizing condition (35), should be distinguished from social hostility, defined as negative social attitudes toward a condition which are not shared by the person with the condition (18).) We should assume that vulnerability will vary from person to person and with the type of genetic information collected (36).

The absolute risk of economic harm *caused by surveillance* is probably quite low, simply because the likelihood of the information being divulged by public health agencies is low (17) and can be further reduced by collecting the data anonymously or with coded identifiers. It does not follow that the perception of risk will also be low. People who are highly averse to the consequences of a breach may overestimate the risks of its occurrence, particularly if they have heard horror stories of lost privacy (37). Similarly, people's attitudes to surveillance may be a function of their attitudes toward government or professional elites generally. They may not understand that the health department is independent of the police department. Fear of government data collection may be based on bad experiences with the data-collection practices of private employers or insurers. Commentators have observed that many African Americans mistrust medical and public health authorities (38) and are dubious of professional claims that new medical technologies will be used for socially just ends or in a fair way (39). We cannot assume that people subject to surveillance know what surveillance is, what conditions are subject to reporting (33), or who has access to the information. Even people who understand that data are being collected by a trustworthy health department may perceive a risk that a future legislature or administration will change the rules and use the data in a harmful way (40).

The risk of psychosocial harm from surveillance may be greater than the risk of more tangible economic losses. Even if no one else learns about a person's genetic information, the subject may experience anxiety about the government possessing personal information. If the subject feels stigma, he or she may suffer the agonies associated with strategies of concealment and selective disclosure (35). The creation of the data makes the subject a potential source of disclosure (41,42), and the harm to an individual's socioeconomic status resulting from a disclosure of genetic information will be no less real because the revelation comes from the individual rather than the government or a health care professional.

Assessing the actual and perceived social risk of genetic surveillance is complicated by the fact that most surveillance information is created outside the public health system for other purposes. Most genetic information will be generated by physicians in the health care system, through screening tests and medical histories. Such health care records currently enjoy much less protection than do public health data, are used for more purposes, and by more actors. The same information that is absolutely protected from disclosure by the health department may be readily available to an employer or an insurer from medical records. Under these circumstances, the marginal increase in psychosocial risk entailed in collecting the data for public health purposes is virtually nil. Ironically, opposition to surveillance may arise in part because public health data collection is perceived as unnecessary (compared to medical care) and preventable (as compared to collection by insurance companies and employers). Conversely, people who are highly conscious of the poor protection accorded to health records may resist surveillance because they do not see a distinction between public health agencies and other collectors of data.

If the perception of a risk from surveillance is a combination of more generalized fears of, and attitudes toward, the use of genetic information, it may often be meaningless to speak of the social risks of surveillance. A perception of high social risk associated with the information being collected by anyone has the potential to influence the acceptability of surveillance at either or both the policy level (Should surveillance be conducted?) and the individual one (Will people carrying the genetic information avoid the data-collection process?). Moreover, individuals may be as much concerned with anticipated psychosocial harms as with economic harms. It follows that promotion of the acceptability of surveillance is dependent upon a broader effort to address the social risks of collecting genetic information, and must consider more aspects of the problem than are necessarily encompassed in terms like breach of privacy and discrimination.

Addressing the Threat of Social Risk: Privacy of Public Health Data

The threat of social risk directly caused by surveillance can be addressed, at least in part, by strict state public health records privacy laws. Virtually all states do, in fact, protect the privacy of public health data (43,44), but the protection is uneven, not simply across the states but within them (45). States generally provide some protection to health data collected for public health purposes, though it is quite common for the level of protection to vary with the type of disease (46,47).

Public health privacy laws generally encompass information gathered by public heath agencies in the course of executing their duties. Disclosure is allowed for public health purposes, such as case investigation, but with an explicit or implicit requirement that release be necessary to achieve a bona fide public health goal. Disclosure is also commonly authorized for research purposes, with conditions that would preclude further dissemination of identifying information about an individual. In addition, many states authorize disclosure pursuant to subpoena or court order—(for example, Arkansas (48), California (49), Hawaii (50)). Other states place disclosure within the discretion of public health officials (e.g., Pennsylvania) (51).

Some states have reformed their laws to protect all information that the government collects, including communicable disease data, under a single statute (52,53). A small number of states have adopted legislation based upon a model statute for protecting and disclosing public health data (53–55). In most states, however, the statutes are decades old and reflect changes neither in disease nor record-keeping technology (45). Responsible public health practices in health departments make flaws in privacy law largely a matter of theoretical concern, but reform of public health privacy laws is nevertheless an important element of an effective response to the social risk of disease.

Having recognized that the greatest risk of breach of privacy probably comes from the original collector of the data, or the insurer or employer who acquires access as payer for health care, we have to address the broader issue of medical records privacy as it applies to genetic information. It is useful to think of a genetic information infrastructure, defined as the basic, underlying framework of collection, storage, use, and transmission of genomic information (including human tissue and extracted DNA) to support all essential functions in genetic research, diagnosis, treatment, and reproductive counseling (56). Despite the technical problems and the cost, several governmental (57,58) and private (59) committees have proposed automation of health data, including genomic information. Several conceptual and technological innovations are likely to accelerate the pace of automation of health records: patient-based longitudinal clinical records that include genetic testing and screening information (60); unique identifiers and the potential to link genomic information to identifiable persons; and genetic databases for clinical, research, and public health purposes. No matter how effective the protection of public health data, the threat of social harm arising from genetic information will depend to a considerable degree on the protection of privacy in nonpublic medical and insurance records.

Few states provide comprehensive protection to health care records (55,61). Several states have passed specific genetic privacy legislation that dramatically restricts disclosure of and access to genetic information without the informed consent of the subject (62–65). The informed-consent requirements generally apply to the conduct of a genetic test in a clinical setting. Some of the statutes further extend the informed-consent requirements to any subsequent release of the information, unless covered by a statutory exception, and so in some cases could be read to prohibit reporting for public health purposes (62,63,66). Some of these laws include a specific prohibition on discriminatory uses of the information (21,67–72). Some include restrictions and requirements on retention, disclosure, and notice (63). Some require destruction of biological samples and test results after a set amount of time, at the completion of a project or at the request of the individual (73). Common exceptions might include the release and retention of data used in anonymous research, genetic testing conducted pursuant to newborn screening requirements, law enforcement, and paternity testing (62,63,74).

Meaningful legal protection of personal health privacy, although a popular concept, has proven difficult to establish as law. The pressure for access arises in large part because of the usefulness of the data to insurers, employers, and other commercial and official actors. Public health, too, benefits from ready access to health records. Surveillance would in many instances be enhanced by the capacity to search computerized medical records. At a minimum, it has traditionally depended upon the ability of physicians freely to report cases to the health department. While protecting medical privacy probably helps reduce the perception of social risk associated with public health data collection, it is important to bear in mind that privacy laws that do not distinguish between public health and individual medical records will place unnecessary and counterproductive burdens on public health efforts. Applying a requirement of individual informed consent to information reported to or shared among health departments would be particularly harmful.

Addressing the Perception of Social Risk from Surveillance

Though the actual risk of social harm directly caused by surveillance is low, perceived risks (and higher actual threats arising in other settings) can create a context in which public health data collection is politically problematic or is resisted by subjects. Public health agencies therefore have a stake in assuring that people are not only protected from the social risks of genetic information they carry but that they are aware of this protection. Law is one important source of protection, but health officials must be conscious of its limitations.

Laws addressing the threat of improper release and discriminatory behavior can help reduce the perception of risk, and can do so even if such laws do not actually reduce the threat. Commentators on genetic issues have extensively discussed protection from discrimination, involuntary testing, and breach of the privacy of medical records (56,75–78). Proposals such as the creation of law-enforcement databases of genetic information have been assessed for their possible impact on the perception of social risk (79). At least half the states have passed legislation limiting genetic discrimination by health insurers, and several have laws prohibiting genetic discrimination in employment (75). The federal Health Insurance Portability and Accountability Act of 1996 (HIPAA) prohibits insurers from considering a genetic trait without the manifestation of disease as a preexisting condition for coverage purposes (80). Both scholars and litigators have explored the applicability of general disability, race, and gender discrimination laws to people who have or are perceived to have gene-based impairments (81–83). The creation of property rights in genetic information is another possible means of increasing the control that individuals have, and perceive themselves to have, over their genetic information (75).

Limits of law as an Antidote to Social Risk

Adequate privacy and antidiscrimination legislation is justifiable from a purely moral perspective, and is the necessary foundation for a practical system of public health surveillance. For all its potential, however, law is subject to several limits to its effectiveness in influencing individual health behavior, and may have some counterproductive influence. Law does not deal directly with many forms of social risk. It does not, for example, protect individuals from current social hostility or stigma that does not take the form of actionable discrimination, though it may reduce overt expression of negative attitudes and even help change attitudes in the long run (84,85). It may not provide protection against discrimination for an action, such as having an abortion, that arises because of genetic information but is itself distinct. Even those threats that are addressed are not always addressed completely. Very small companies, for example, are often covered neither by federal nor state discrimination law. Likewise, it will be impossible even with the strictest confidentiality laws to keep genetic information out of the hands of the insurers who are paying for the testing that creates the information. At least some genetic information will be considered valid underwriting information that insurers will legally be able to collect under our current system of insurance regulation (78). Many commentators regard HIPAA as a failure, because of insurers' ability to use genetic information in setting coverage rates (86).

More broadly, the notion that a law will influence individuals to provide a risky piece of information to a health care provider or the state is deceptively simple. An individual's willingness to rely on the law in making choices about future health behavior is subject to at least three factors whose presence cannot be assumed. To be directly influenced in genetic-related health behavior by law, a person must be aware of the existing legal protection. Knowledge of gene-related legal protection among those who have or may have socially risky genetic information has not been studied, but the available data tell us that individuals are rarely well informed about the law (87) and often do not take legal action when they could reasonably do so (88).

Second, people are unlikely to rely on legal protection in planning their conduct if they do not perceive themselves to be entitled to legal protection. There are many reasons why a person who believes he might carry socially risky genetic information may not believe he is entitled to legal help. Stigmatized people sometimes blame themselves for the social risks they encounter, or regard such risks as inevitable (89,90). Some individuals might mistrust "the system" as a general matter, or believe it to be designed to protect the rights of more powerful people and institutions in the society. Many others will have had purely negative interactions with the system, such as being arrested or harassed by police. These factors can make the law particularly weak in dealing with the social-risk perceptions of marginalized populations.

Finally, a person willing to rely on the law for protection in the event genetic information causes harm must presumably believe that it will be effective in providing the protections it promises, including adequate remedies. For many people, the prospect of a money award some months or years after losing a job or suffering public humiliation may not appear to be a good trade-off for the health benefits secured by running the risk. This factor is particularly important given that the individual can easily choose the almost completely reliable option of not creating the datum in the first place.

The Dangers of "Genetic Exceptionalism"

Laws that treat genetic information as uniquely problematic reflect and strengthen a sense of "genetic exceptionalism," the idea that genetic information is unique and deserving of special protection. Although not all statutes distinguish genetic information from nongenetic medical information (91,92), proposed and existing legislation often treat genetics as uniquely powerful and distinct from the rest of medicine (93). This approach poses several problems.

First, although genetic data can be regarded as distinct in its implications for family members and its rare ability to predict future illness, genetic information is more like, than different from, other health information. One might narrowly define "genetic information" as the product of DNA-related tests, but much genetic disease is diagnosed through direct clinical observation and family history. Broader definitions may expand genetic information to all genetic-related diseases, yet many diseases are known to have a genetic component, and more, if not most, diseases are likely to be found to have genetic links in the future. Even classic infectious diseases such as HIV infection have genetic components. Scientists have shown that some genetic variations inhibit acquisition of infection, and it is likely that the degree to which a person progresses from HIV infection to AIDS will, in part, be genetically determined. It is also difficult to separate genetic from nongenetic information in a medical record. Are sex, eye color, blood type, and nationality genetic or nongenetic data? As we learn more about the role of genetics in disease, attempts to separate genetic information from other types of information will become even more vexing. For these reasons, some commentators have suggested that valid reasons exist to treat genetic information no differently from other medical information (94).

This problem is related to a second one: Providing special protection to genetic information will often be unfair because it treats people facing the same social risks differently based on the biological cause of their otherwise identical health conditions. Why, for example, should a woman who has developed breast cancer of genetic origin (e.g., BRACA1 or -2) be given greater protection than a woman who has developed breast cancer because of environmental or behavioral factors? Even diseases that are solely genetic are not inherently special so as to give rise to unusual claims to legal protection. A debilitating, ultimately fatal condition exposes those who have it to pain, emotional distress, and social risk with substantially equal severity whether it is caused by a gene, like Huntington's, or a virus, like HIV (95). Indeed, it is conceivable that genetic illnesses are less in need of legal protection than sexually transmitted diseases, which often carry a stigma arising from the perception that they are just desserts for voluntary behavior.

On a practical level, we must be cautious that the very people whom policymakers hope to encourage to take advantage of genetic testing may become more reluctant because of the heightened focus on its exceptional nature. Treating genetics as distinct from the rest of medicine may enhance the stigma of genetics testing, even as legislators attempt to remove its stigmatizing effects (96). This can create public fears and misapprehensions about genetics that could discourage individuals from seeking testing and treatment, and thwart future scientific progress. Conversely, by focusing only on genetics information, legislators could convey the perception that the public need not worry about the confidentiality of other kinds of medical information, thus fostering complacency in an area where insufficient protections might exist.

The Public Health Ethics of Surveillance

The discipline of bioethics has become influential in the development of health care policy and medical practice. Public health, although often seen as a quintessentially utilitarian enterprise, likewise raises profound moral questions that can benefit from an ethical analysis. If "public health" is defined as *the process of maximizing, within the bounds of possibility set by the resources allocated, the level and distribution of satisfactory health in a population*, then its pursuit entails an endless series of choices about the definition and determinants of health, and the best means of its just and effective attainment (45). The ethical system that has developed for analyzing health care decisions is of limited use in considering measures aimed at creating the conditions in which the population as a whole can be healthy. Fundamental questions of equality and justice in the distribution of scarce resources and the allocation of the burdens of disease control and prevention require a distinct "ethics" of public health. Such a system of thought has been slowly emerging over the past two decades (97), taking shape in such documents as the Council for International Organizations of Medical Sciences' 1991 International Guidelines for Ethical Review of Epidemiological Studies (98). It was one of the interests of Jonathan Mann, whose untimely death is a loss to this endeavor as to so many others (99). Such a system would recognize the limits of an individualistic orientation in assessing the costs and benefits of population-oriented health measures, by, for example, focusing less on individual relative risk and more on population attributable risk (100). It would place on those who are at low personal risk an obligation to make or accept changes in social behavior necessary to reduce the toll of ill health on others in the community (97). At a minimum, "[s]uch an ethic would ensure that no group or person was arbitrarily excluded from protection and that the burdens of collective action were fairly shouldered by all" (97).

In the absence of a fully developed system of public health ethics, we may still profitably ask three questions that can help us assess whether surveillance for genetic information is a just tool for public health.

1. *Will surveillance enhance the health of the population?* To find a genetic surveillance measure "ethical" in the public health sense, we need to determine that it has a reasonable probability of leading to information that can be used to reduce the incidence of genetic illness or mortality in the society as a whole or in a significant population facing a special threat. If it does not, the measure, however useful to individuals, ought not be an important public health priority, and may not be worthy of significant public-sector resources. By the same token, however, a measure may be compelling in its importance to public health even though it has limited value to any one person in the population.

2. *Is surveillance for particular genetic information a wise and just use of resources?* Rationing in public health is a "moral imperative ... in the face of scarce resources" (101). Ideally, each public health dollar will be spent to achieve the greatest marginal increase in the level and distribution of well-being in the population, and the socioeconomic costs of any intervention—including the social risk—will not fall disproportionately on any group within the population. Public health ethics make explicit the competition for scarce resources that has often proven difficult to address in the patient-centered maze of medical ethics. Measures that are of significant value to some relatively healthy patients might be ethically dubious from a public health perspective if the resources could be used instead to improve the lot of a relatively less healthy group, or to increase by even a small degree the overall health of the population. Similarly, the individual pursuit of low relative risk has no place in the ethical practice of public health when it comes at the expense of reduction in the population attributable risk. Public health measures might entail infringements on individual civil liberties, and more generally upon an individual's status in the society, but only where they can be justified by a compelling necessity (102).

3. *Will surveillance be acceptable to the population being observed?* This principle has roots in both practicality and morality. Public health depends largely on voluntary compliance with its guidelines. Resistance can raise costs enormously, the more as prevalence of the condition rises. Thus, both the success of a public health intervention, and its cost, depend significantly on the degree to which its targets perceive it to be more beneficial than costly.

Genetic information could often be useful to the public's health. Genomic data can help track the incidence, patterns, and trends of genetic carrier states or disease in populations. Carefully planned surveillance or epidemiological activities facilitate rapid identification of health needs. This permits reproductive counseling, testing, health education, and treatment resources to be better targeted, and it points the way for future research. Even the collection of data about low prevalence condition or a small population could have long-term benefits to population health through the advancement of biomedical knowledge. Surveillance typically provides its benefits at a low economic cost, and the marginal cost of adding information to the list of already reportable data is probably slight. The main concern about collecting genetic information is its potential social risk.

We have already suggested that the social risk to individuals remains largely unexplored by empirical research, and may well have been overstated. To assess genetic surveillance properly, we need more information about both the perception and the threat of social risk. Given the potential variability of the phenomenon, it would be most useful to gather this data as specific types of information are proposed for surveillance. Whatever the level of risk, both the threat and the perception may be reduced through such devices as anonymous or coded collection of data, and strong legal guarantees of privacy, nondiscrimination, and access to medical care.

Although we consider surveillance to pose a low social risk to individuals, a more diffuse but equally compelling risk of genetic technology has been identified and may be implicated by surveillance: An ethical public health policy would look at broader social questions arising from how we construct genetic health, in part through surveillance. A new technology providing new forms of information about health and disease can have dramatic effects on how these concepts are understood in society (16). In a society that sometimes seems enamored with the power of genomic information, genomic data are often thought capable of explaining much that is human: personality, intelligence, appearance, behavior, health, and disease (103,104). A widespread belief that health is "in the genes" may have the effect of bolstering a cultural conception of health as individualized and dependent upon medical management. Genetic screening will add yet more "risk factors" to the individual's medical health inventory, and enhance the view that each individual is responsible for his or her own health. While this conception of health has some advantages in disease control, it also can lead to victim-blaming and a neglect of communal provision for health (105).

Genetic concepts of illness might also promote group blame and eugenic ideas in new guises (31,106,107). Susan Wolf has warned of the rise of what she calls "geneticism," which, "like racism and sexism, . . . is a long-standing and deeply entrenched system for disadvantaging some and advantaging others" based on their genetic traits (108). Proponents of surveillance for genetic information will have to recognize and take some responsibility for addressing the social meaning of genetic information.

Recommendations

Our analysis of ethics, law, and social risk suggest the following list of needs. From researchers:

- More research on the social risk of genetic information, focusing on specific kinds of information, and examining both the prevalence of socially harmful behavior and the perception of social risk.
- More research into what extent, and how, individuals rely on law in making health choices.
- Research to determine what measures are effective in reducing perceptions of social risk.

From legislators:

- Effective protection of medical privacy, and separate and even stricter protection of the privacy of public health records.
- Effective protection of all citizens against discrimination based on genetic information. Liberally construed disability laws may be sufficient for this purpose, but it is not yet clear whether the Americans with Disabilities Act (ADA) and state laws will provide this protection. Race and sex discrimination laws might also play a role, wherever conditions are sex linked or associated with racial or ethnic groups.
- Efforts to reform or ameliorate the effects of our current system of health insurance on access to care for people with heightened risks.

From public health agencies:

- Careful attention to the complex relationship between overall genetic social risk and the particular social risks of surveillance.
- Use of appropriate public health ethical criteria for assessing public health uses of data.

In considering new legislation to address concerns about the use and misuse of genetic testing and genetic information, it is important particularly at the state level to distinguish between public health and other uses of genetic data, and to review and consider the existing state framework for public health and medical research. Public health authorities and researchers should be afforded the opportunity to define their needs, including access to information to conduct public health functions. Having a clear understanding of the various programs that may involve genetic testing and information, states can then assess the potential impact of proposed legislation in the areas discussed above. Any potential impact on public health programs and research should be carefully balanced against the underlying goals of the legislation. In some cases the goals of the legislation may be promoted by specifically addressing deficiencies in the public health framework, particularly the legal ability to protect participants or to provide necessary confidentiality protections.

Conclusions

Surveillance (more data) is usually good and poses little risk for people on whom data are collected. The actual risk of surveillance can be minimized by rigorously protecting public health data from being used for other purposes, such as law enforcement, and by promoting social conditions in which people are safe from mistreatment and discrimination based on genetic makeup. No matter how well we succeed in reducing the threat of social risk, surveillance will still often be controversial, because of concerns about the social risks posed by the collection of sensitive data. For surveillance to be ethical from a public health point of view, the data have to efficiently promote the health of the population; their collection should be acceptable to the population, and the data must be protected. To protect public health data, we need effective laws protecting public health records, but we must also bear in mind that legal protection may not always be sufficient to reduce perceptions of social risk, particularly among those who are suspicious of government or alienated from the legal system. Implementing surveillance programs about which there are serious questions of acceptability requires a solid foundation of laws prohibiting arbitrary discrimination based on health status, but also political and other efforts to address perceptions of social risk that cannot be eliminated by law.

References

1. Centers for Disease Control and Prevention. Translating advances in human genetics into public health action—a strategic plan. Atlanta, GA, October 1, 1997.

2. Teutsch SM, Churchill RE. Principles and practice of public health surveillance. New York and Oxford: Oxford University Press, 1994.

3. Mich. Comp. Laws Ann. §333.5721 (1997).

4. Cal. Health & Saf. Code §§103825, 103875 (1997).

5. Ga. Code Ann. §31-12-2(b) (1997).

6. Khoury MJ and the Genetics Working Group. From genes to public health: the applications of genetic technology in disease prevention. Am J Public Health 1996;86: 1717–1722.

7. Holtzman NA, Watson MS (eds). Promoting safe and effective genetic testing in the United States: final report of the task force on genetic testing. Baltimore: Johns Hopkins University Press, 1998.

8. Khoury MJ, Beatty T, Cohen B. Fundamentals of genetic epidemiology. New York and Oxford: Oxford University Press, 1993.

9. Khoury MJ. Genetic epidemiology and the future of disease prevention and public health. Epidemiol Rev 1997;19:175–180.

10. Iowa Code Ann. §136A.4-6 (1997).

11. Ky. Rev. Stat. Ann. §211.665 (1997).

12. Minn. Stat. Ann. §13.385 (1997).

13. Mo. Rev. Stat. §191.323 (1997).

14. Fox DM. Social policy and city politics: tuberculosis reporting in New York, 1889–1900. Bull Hist Med 1975;49:169–194.

15. Rothman S. Seek and hide: public health departments and persons with tuberculosis, 1890–1940. J Law Med Ethics 1993;21:289–295.

16. Brandt AM. No magic bullet: a social history of venereal disease in the United States since 1980. New York and Oxford: Oxford University Press, 1987.

17. Gostin LO, Hodge J Jr. The "names debate": the case for national HIV reporting in the United States. Albany Law Rev 1998;61:679–743.

18. Burris S. Law and the social risk of health care: lessons from HIV testing. Albany Law Rev 1998;61:831–895.

19. Burris S. Public health, "AIDS exceptionalism," and the law. John Marshall Law Rev 1994;27:251–272.

20. Institute of Medicine. Social, legal, and ethical implications of genetic testing in assessing genetic risks: implications for health and social policy. Washington, DC: National Academy Press, 1994.

21. Hudson KL, Rothenberg KH, Andrews LB, Kahn MJE, Collins FS. Genetic discrimination and health insurance: an urgent need for reform. Science 1995;270:391–393.

22. Underwood RH, Cadle RG. Genetics, genetic testing, and the specter of discrimination: a discussion using hypothetical cases. Ky Law J 1996–97;85:665–693.

23. U.S. Congress, Office of Technology Assessment. The role of genetic testing in the prevention of occupational disease. Washington, DC: U.S. Government Printing Office, 1983.

24. U.S. Congress, Office of Technology Assessment. Genetic tests and health insurance: results of a survey. Washington, DC: U.S. Government Printing Office, 1992.

25. Billings PR, Kohn MA, de Cuevas M, Beckwith J, Alper JS, Natowicz MR. Discrimination as a consequence of genetic testing. Am J Hum Genet 1992;50:476–482.

26. Lapham E, Kozma C, Weiss JO. Genetic discrimination: perspectives of consumers. Science 1996;274:621–624.

27. Benkendorf JL, Reutenauer JE, Hughes CA, et al. Patients' attitudes about autonomy and confidentiality in genetic testing for breast–ovarian cancer susceptibility. Am J Med Genet 1997;73:296–303.

28. Botkin JR, McMahon WM, Smith KR, Nash JE. Privacy and confidentiality in the publication of pedigrees: a survey of investigators and biomedical journals. JAMA 1998;279:1808–1812.

29. Lerman C, Seay J, Balshem A, Audrain J. Interest in genetic testing among first-degree relatives of breast cancer patients. Am J Med Genet 1995;57:385–392.

30. Clayton EW, Hannig VL, Pfotenhauer JP, et al. Lack of interest by nonpregnant couples in population-based cystic fibrosis carrier screening. Am J Hum Genet 1996;58:617–627.

31. Wertz DC. Society and the not-so-new genetics: what are we afraid of? Some future predictions from a social scientist. J Contemp Health Law Policy 1997;13: 299–346.

32. Kowalewski MR, Henson KD, Longshore D. Rethinking perceived risk and health behavior: a critical review of HIV prevention research. Health Educ Behav 1997;24:313–325.

33. Nakshima AK, Horsley R, Frey RL, Sweeney PA, Weber JT, Fleming PL. Effect of HIV reporting by name on use of HIV testing in publicly funded counseling and testing programs. JAMA 1998;280:1421–1426.

34. Bindman AB, Osmond D, Hecht FM, et al. Multistate evaluation of anonymous HIV testing and access to medical care. JAMA 1998;280:1416–1420.

35. Goffman E. Stigma: notes on the management of spoiled identity. Englewood Cliffs, NJ: Prentice Hall, 1963.

36. Hall MA. Insurers' use of genetic information. Jurimetrics J 1996;7(Fall):13–22.

37. Tversky A, Kahneman D. Availability: a heuristic for judging frequency and probability. In: Kahneman D, Slovic P, Tversky A (eds), Judgement under uncertainty: heuristics and biases. Cambridge: Cambridge University Press, 1982, pp. 163–178.

38. Allen AL. Genetic testing, nature, and trust. Seton Hall Law Rev 1997;27: 887–892.

39. Roberts DE. The nature of blacks' skepticism about genetic testing. Seton Hall Law Rev 1997;27:971–979.

40. Burris S. Driving the epidemic underground? a new look at law and the social risk of HIV testing. AIDS Public Policy J 1997;12:66–78.

41. Mansergh G, Marks G, Simoni J. Self-disclosure of HIV-infection among men who vary in time since seropositive diagnosis and symptomatic status. AIDS 1995;9:639–644.

42. Lerman C, Peshkin BN, Hughes C, Isaacs C. Family disclosure in genetic testing for cancer susceptibility: determinants and consequences. J Health Care Law Policy 1998;1:353–372.

43. Gostin LO, Lazzarini Z, Neslund VS, Osterholm MT. The public health information infrastructure: a national review of the law on health information privacy. JAMA 1996;275:1921,1923–1925.

44. Gostin LO, Lazzarini Z. Childhood immunization registries: a national review of public health information systems and the protection of privacy. JAMA 1995;274:1793–1799.

45. Gostin LO, Burris SC, Lazzarini Z. The law and the public's health: a study of infectious disease law in the United States (in press).

46. N.Y.C.L.S. Pub. Health §§2306 and 2782 (1994).

47. Cal. Civ. Code §1798.24 (1995).

48. Ark. Stat. Ann. §20-15-904 (1994).

49. Cal. Health & Saf. Code §121070 (1996).

50. Haw. Rev. Stat. §325-101 (1994).

51. Pa. Stat. Ann. tit. 35 §521.15 (1998).

52. Minn Stat. ch. 13 (1996).

53. Mont. Code Ann. §50-16-603 (1994).

54. Rev. Code Wash. §70.02.005 et seq. (1994).

55. Gostin LO. Health information privacy. Cornell Law Rev 1995;80:451–507.

56. Gostin LO. Genetic privacy. J Law Med Ethics 1995;23:320–330.

57. Congressional Office of Technology Assessment. Protecting privacy in computerized medical information. Washington, DC, 1993; OTA-TCT-576.

58. U.S. Department of Health and Human Services. Final report of the task force on the privacy of private-sector health records, Washington, DC, 1995.

59. Donaldson MS, Lohr KN (eds). Health data in the information age: use, disclosure, and privacy. Washington, DC: National Academy Press, 1994.

60. Gostin LO, Turek-Brezina J, Powers M, et al. Privacy and security of personal information in a new health care system. JAMA 1993;270:2487–2493.

61. Confidentiality of Medical Information Act, Cal. Civil Code §§56 to 56.37 (1982 & Supp. 1998).

62. Ga. Code Ann. §§33-54-1 to -8 (1997).

63. N.J. Stat. Ann. §§10:5-43 to -49 (1997).

64. Ill. Comp. Stat. §§513/5-30 (1998).

65. Or. Rev. Stat. §§659.700-659.720 (1997).

66. La. Rev. Stat. Ann. §213.7 (1998).

67. Bornstein RA. Genetic discrimination insurability and legislation: a closing of the legal loopholes. J Law Policy 1996;4:551–610.

68. Rothenberg K, Fuller B, Rothstein M, et al. Genetic information and the workplace: legislative approaches and policy challenges. Science 1997;275:1755–1757.

69. Ind. Code §27-8-26-5 (1998).

70. Kan. Stat. Ann. §40-2259 (1997).

71. Tex. Ins. Code Ann. §21.73 (1997).

72. Cal. Health & Saf. Code §1374.7 (1997).

73. Vernon's Tex. Code Ann., Labor Code, §21.401 to 21.405 (1997).

74. Or. Rev. Stat. §51-659.710 (1997).

75. Yesley MS. Protecting genetic difference. Berkeley Tech Law J 1998;13:653–665.

76. Mehlman MJ, Durchslag MR, Neuhauser D. When do health care decisions discriminate against persons with disabilities? J Health Polit Policy Law 1997;22:1385–1408.

77. Rothstein MR. The law of medical and genetic privacy in the workplace. In: Rothstein M (ed). Genetic secrets: protecting privacy and confidentiality in the genetic era. New Haven, CT: Yale University Press, 1997, pp. 281–288.

78. Kass NE. The implications of genetic testing for health and life insurance. In: Rothstein M (ed). Genetic secrets: protecting privacy and confidentiality in the genetic era. New Haven, CT: Yale University Press, 1997, pp. 299–316.

79. McEwen JE. DNA data banks. In: Rothstein M (ed). Genetic secrets: protecting privacy and confidentiality in the genetic era. New Haven, CT: Yale University Press, 1997, pp. 231–251.

80. Pub, Law 104–191, 104th Cong, 2d Sess. (1996).

81. Blanck PD, Marti MW. Genetic discrimination and the employment provisions of the Americans with Disabilities Act: emerging legal, empirical, and policy implications. Behav Sci Law 1996;14:411–432.

82. Gin BR. Genetic discrimination: Huntington's disease and the Americans with Disabilities Act. Colum Law Rev 1997;97:1406–1434.

83. Norman-Bloodsaw v. Lawrence Berkeley Laboratory, 135 F.3d 1260 (9th Cir. 1998).

84. Lessig L. The regulation of social meaning. U Chicago Law Rev 1995;62:943–1045.

85. Sunstein CR. Social norms and social roles. Colum Law Rev 1996;96:903–968.

86. Cocco M. The right medicine for health care. Newsday, July 14 1998, p. A30.

87. Ellickson R. A critique of economic and sociological theories of social control. J Legal Studies 1987;16:67–99.

88. Weiler PC, Hiatt HH, Newhouse JP, Johnson WG, Brennan TA, Leape L. A measure of malpractice: medical injury, malpractice litigation, and patient compensation. Cambridge, MA: Harvard University Press, 1991.

89. Coates D, Penrod S. Social psychology and the emergence of disputes. Law Society Rev 1980–81;15:655–680.

90. Musheno MC. Legal consciousness on the margins of society: struggles against stigmatization in the AIDS crisis. Identities 1995;2:102–122.

91. Me. Rev. Stat. Ann. tit. 18-A, §9-310 (1996).

92. Ohio Rev. Code Ann. §3729.46 (1997).

93. N.J. Rev. Stat. §2a (1996).

94. NIH-DOE Working group on ethical, legal and social implications of human genome research, genetic information and health insurance, 1993.

95. Rothstein MR. Genetic privacy and confidentiality: why they are so hard to protect. J Law Med Ethics 1998;26:198–204.

96. Markel H. The stigma of disease: implications of genetic screening. Am J Med 1992;93:209–215.

97. Beauchamp DE. Exploring new ethics for public health: developing a fair alcohol policy. J Health Polit Policy Law 1976–77;1:338–354.

98. See various essays collected in Dickens BM, Gostin L, Levine RJ (eds). Research on human populations: national and international ethical guidelines. Law Med Health Care 1991;3–4:157–266.

99. Jonathan M. Mann, medicine and public health, ethics and human rights. Hastings Cent Rep 1997; May–June: 6–13.

100. Northridge M. Public health methods: attributable risk as a link between causality and public health action. Am J Public Health 1995;85:1202–1204.

101. Morrow RH, Bryant JH. Health policy approaches to measuring and valuing human life: conceptual and ethical issues. Am J Public Health 1995;85:1356–1360.

102. Gostin LO, Lazzarini Z. Human rights and public health in the AIDS pandemic. New York and Oxford: Oxford University Press, 1997.

103. Nelkin D. The double-edged helix. NY Times, February 4, 1994, p. A23.

104. Lander ES. Scientific commentary: the scientific foundations and medical and social prospects of the human genome project. J Law Med Ethics 1998;26:184–188.

105. Rose G. Sick individuals and sick populations. Int J Epidemiol 1985;14:32–38.

106. Stone DH, Stewart S. Screening and the new genetics; a public health perspective on the ethical debate. J Public Health Med 1996;18:3–5.

107. Harper P. Genetics and public health. Br Med J 1992;304:721–724

108. Wolf S. Beyond 'genetic discrimination': toward the broader harm of geneticism. J Law Med Ethics 1995;23:345–349.

VI

COMMUNICATION, EDUCATION, AND INFORMATION DISSEMINATION

28

Principles and practices of communication processes for genetics in public health

Celeste M. Condit, Roxanne L. Parrott,
and Beth O'Grady

The Nazis' horrifying abuses of putative information about the hereditary characteristics of human beings constitute essential cautionary lessons for any national effort to disseminate genetic information. For ethical reasons, and to ensure public support in the face of widespread sensitivity to these ethical challenges, public health programs that employ genetic technology must carefully heed these lessons. This chapter describes two basic requirements of the communication processes and outcomes necessary to an ethical and socially responsible use of genetic medicine in a public health framework. The chapter begins by reviewing the reasons that there are exceptional ethical burdens on genetic medicine and then outlines the transactional model of communication and its applications in public health genetics. It concludes by describing research on the effects-based pretesting of the attitudinal effects of public health messages about genetics.

The Legacy of Eugenics

The idea that people's natures could be fundamentally defined by qualities inherited through their "blood" was a key ingredient of Nazi social programs (1). This proto-genetic belief set justified segregation, sterilization, and ultimately extermination of millions of people. While the more democratic political system in the United States prevented the resort to anything like death camps, the eugenic movement in the United States did produce tens of thousands of sterilizations, which subsequent research has demonstrated to have been motivated not by clear medical criteria, but rather by the pragmatic goals and biases of administrators of local mental health institutions (2).

At least three important lessons for the use of genetic information arose from these initial attempts to employ hereditary information on a social scale. First, genetic information is readily employed in a stigmatizing fashion. Second, genetic information should be used for the well-being of individuals, not for the perceived future good of a people or nation. Third, genetically based decisions must be made by individuals, based on their own values and preferences, not on externally imposed criteria, whether or not these criteria are perceived to be true and just by socially sanctioned experts (3). Although these lessons probably do not constitute comprehensive and sufficient criteria for morally acceptable public programs about genetics (4), they are certainly minimally necessary criteria.

The history of public health genetic programs is undeniably one tainted by great evil. The evils remain a continuing danger in large part because genetic perspectives too easily (though not necessarily) bleed into eugenic worldviews (3). This history and these ideological associations make "genetic exceptionalism"—that is, treatment of genetic medicine as a unique form of medicine— a necessity.[1] Whether its technical features are identical with other forms of medicine or not, genetic medicine is exceptional because of its history and its ideological linkages. From the perspective of some social critics, this may mean that any efforts by public health agencies to use or advocate genetic information and technologies is itself evil. However, the possibility remains open that if done with care and respect for the ethical issues involved, public health efforts to utilize genetics might bring great benefit to individuals without producing the harms of eugenics. The processes utilized to communicate genetic information to the public will be crucial in these efforts.

Communication Processes

Public health communication about genetics will necessarily be designed, in part, to convey information about available genetic tests and technologies to the general public. To avoid the evils of eugenics, such communication programs must be designed to achieve these ends (a) by focusing on the well-being of the individuals who are the targets of the messages, (b) while actively protecting the rights of individuals to free choice with regard to application of any genetic technologies to themselves (or to their young children), and (c) without increasing the stigma associated with particular genetic configurations (or even perhaps while decreasing it).

---

[1] It may be desirable to make the procedures applied to genetic medicine the model for most medical programs, and to that extent genetic medicine would no longer be exceptional. However, because public health initiatives must deal with issues of contagion that are dissimilar in significant ways from issues of genetic disease, there will necessarily be some cases where public health initiatives cannot live up to the standards of individual autonomy that should and can inhere in genetic medicine.

To fulfill these goals, the process of communication must be designed on a *transactional* model rather than an *expert* model (5). Expert models of technical communication presume that the communication interaction is directed and controlled by the expert's judgments. The expert initiates communication and provides information to the layperson, who acts as source of information only at the bequest of the expert, and with regard to the information that the expert deems to be of interest. The layperson does not serve as the initiator of the communication, except perhaps to initiate communication to improve her or his health. The layperson is also expected to act in the ways prescribed by the expert; if not, the person can be judged to be "noncompliant." The expert model has been widely challenged in medicine generally (6–11) and overwhelmingly rejected by the informed genetics community in the United States with regard to genetic counseling (12–14). The model is similarly inappropriate to mass communication about genetics, and a transactional model offers a more appropriate approach.

A transactional model of communication posits that the communication interaction should be guided, not by the expert, but by the mutual orientation of all involved parties to each other's perspectives and concerns in an ongoing process of exploration leading to decisions and action (5). In the case of medical genetics, of course, the final decision rests with the affected individual, not with the technical expert. However, unless the decision is guided by an open transactional process, it cannot be said to be a free choice, even if the individual is in putative agreement with the actions chosen (15). The transactional model of communication is appropriate in medical communication because all parties involved in the communication process bring different types of expertise to the interaction. Medical geneticists may bring expert knowledge about inheritance pathways, genetic procedures, and side effects of genetic technologies, but laypersons bring expert knowledge of their personal situation (which determines the actual relevance and outcomes of any application of the technologies), and they convey definitive knowledge of their own values and interests.

Genetic counseling as a discipline and a practice has explored in some detail applications of transactional models under the rubrics of "client centered" or "nondirective" counseling (12–14). Although the use of transactional counseling is under attack for financial (16), institutional (17), and ideological reasons (18,19), it remains a widely agreed-upon goal for interpersonal interactions about genetic health care decision making. Legislation to require that insurance companies provide access to substantive genetic counseling by a genetic counselor certified by the National Society of Genetic Counselors in any case where coverage of genetic testing is provided would be an important step toward maintaining the positive transactional orientation established by the early work in genetic medicine. A similarly transactional set of goals and procedures is necessary for the communication of genetic information in the public arena.

Implementation of a transactional approach requires that public health campaigns about genetic issues should not be unilaterally generated by genetic experts working in public health agencies. Rather, active sustained interaction with potential target audiences and with the general public should be included in the process of designing programs and health communication messages. Several mechanisms can be used for gaining active public participation in the public health communication process. Public opinion surveys can provide some static information about the range of public attitudes about the broad issues under discussion. However, focus groups, audience studies (20), and "town meetings" (21) can afford more dynamic input about particular ideas, at least with particular target audiences. Web-based technologies can also provide access for additional input to proposals and procedures. Any public health agency that is developing public health proposals for use of direct genetic technologies should maintain a web page or similar communication strategies with current goals, options, and proposals, and a mechanism for public debate about those proposals.

Additionally, representatives of target groups and public representatives should be included in development of goals and procedures. This requires a partnership between medical professionals and widely varied groups including general and condition-specific consumer interest groups (e.g., The Alliance of Genetic Support Groups) and organized public interest groups (the Black Women's Health Project, the Women's Health Network, ACT-UP, League of Women Voters, Christian Coalition, Ecumenical Council, and others). There will necessarily be contention about who is included and what positions are most valued. However, the history of genetic programs in the United States suggests that community-based projects that are guided by the input of community representatives—for example, Tay-Sachs (22)—are more effective and less ethically unsatisfactory to the community than are programs that are perceived as imposed from outside—sickle cell testing, for example (23).

Broad participation in the generation of a public health genetics campaign needs to derive from both specific target audiences (potential "consumers" of the offered technology) and the general public. Too often, "consumers" and the "public" are conflated in expert thought. However, one's role as a potential "consumer" of a genetic technology is different from one's role as a member of the general public (24). One's interests as a consumer relate primarily to personal well-being, whereas one's role as a member of the public requires consideration of the broad range of interests and needs of all of the members of one's polity. Because public health projects are done in the "name" of the public, the perspectives of the general public must be fairly incorporated (and not simply dismissed because the expertise of nongeneticists is different from that of technical personnel). Moreover, as public health genetics are provided to preserve the health of the potential consumer, such consumers must also be included in both program and message development.

Transactional communication processes are challenging. It is far easier to imagine oneself as an expert disseminating wisdom than to engage in the contentious debates inevitably engendered by public and consumer involvement. However, the limited success of health campaigns that employ the expert model (25), as well as the ethical dictates of genetic medicine, suggests the need for accepting these challenges. This need is more widely accepted for some public health applications than for others, but it pertains in all cases, if to somewhat different degrees.

Most experts in genetic medicine recognize the need for transactional approaches in reproductive genetics—that is, in the use of prenatal testing and abortion to select among fetuses. There is also a fairly widespread acceptance of the transactional model with regard to adult testing of adult-onset diseases, though there is some continuing disagreement about the ways in which this transactional approach should be implemented and regulated.

For example, the appropriateness of the commercial advertisement of the availability of testing for genotypes associated with above-average risks of breast cancer has been challenged, but any control of communication approaches used by commercial agencies faces constitutional limitations. These issues of freedom of commercial speech, based as they are in individual constitutional rights, do not, however, restrict the choices by public health agencies about what information to disseminate. Thus, given the complexities of genetic testing, it seems to be a general obligation of public health agencies to move forward in a transactional manner, to the extent that they move forward at all. Previous research on Huntington's disease similarly supports the need for transactional approaches in adult testing of adult-onset diseases (26).

The arena in which the transactional model is most likely to be contested is with regard to the application of genetic technologies to children. In these cases, young children are not capable of fully participating in transactional communication processes as equal partners nor of making free and autonomous decisions (though the appropriate cutoff age is disputed, in part because each individual develops these capabilities gradually and at a somewhat different rate). Consequently, the decision-making authority over children's health is held in trust and split between parents and the state. In most issues, parents have a presumptive right to make decisions for their youngsters in matters where choices must be made during childhood. However, in medical, educational, and other basic welfare matters, the state imposes limits on the scope of parental authority. The state insists that children must be free from physical abuse and receive basic education, shelter, clothing, and life-sustaining medical care (even if the parents' deepest religious commitments oppose that care). Parents thus do not enjoy the same breadth of rights of decision for their children as they enjoy for themselves. Based on these recognized restrictions on parental rights, legally mandated genetic screening of newborns has been implemented and defended for medical conditions with immediate and serious clinical manifestations and where treatments are available that are at least partially efficacious (PKU—phenylketonuria—forms the classic example, but not the sole one; see ref. 27). As direct genetic tests become available for such diseases and for others, genetic testing of newborns and older children becomes a potential target of public health programs.

These programs, however, must be limited in scope to those disease conditions that will have an immediate and substantial health effect on the child (28). This means that newborn and childhood genetic testing for predispositions to delayed-onset conditions such as Huntington's chorea, adult-onset diabetes, or cystic fibrosis are not compatible with our system of rights and values, nor is such testing appropriate for conditions that do not threaten health, unless symptomology is present (e.g., Fragile X syndrome). These restrictions arise from the limited authority that both the parents and the state have to make decisions for children's lives owing to the privacy rights of every individual with regard to genetic information.

Parents and the state are authorized to make decisions of fundamental long-term consequences for children only when the children cannot reasonably make such decisions themselves and the decision must be made immediately to safeguard the well-being of the child. With delayed-onset conditions and current medical technologies, there are no pressing reasons to usurp the rights of children to make their own decisions about genetic testing (decisions which the children will be capable of making autonomously at a later time). There is strong evidence and wide consensus that these decisions are highly consequential for an individual's sense of self and therefore fall under the zone of the rights to privacy and autonomy (22). Neither parents nor the state have the right to usurp that privacy and autonomy unless there is immediate and serious medical need to protect the life and health of the child.

Parents have sometimes asserted their right to make these decisions on non-medical grounds (e.g., to make informed financial decisions for the family as a whole). The argument is that knowing about the future financial needs and abilities of a child will enable parents to plan better for all members of the family, for example. However, the same logic would allow parents to contract marriages for their children in advance. Knowing that a child will later marry a millionaire rather than a pauper would certainly help in planning the financial allocations of resources within a family, but our society has ruled out such contract marriages as a violation of personal autonomy.

Rights to make decisions about genetic testing are of the same character, and potentially of the same import, as are rights to make decisions about one's marriage. Neither the parent nor the state has the right to usurp those rights for convenience. Both public health criteria and parental criteria allow intervention and violation of individual autonomy only in cases of immediate exigency. In general, the ethical issues seem similar with regard to genetic testing of those individuals who have been involuntarily institutionalized for mental incapacities, but we believe that greater explicit discussion of the issues with regard to these groups is needed before general policy determinations can be made.

Public health initiatives to apply genetic testing to newborns must thus be limited to a narrow set of disease conditions. However, even, in the cases where governmental agencies may assert an interest on behalf of the child, there are reasons to believe that a transactional (voluntary) approach to the communication between the parents and the agency might be superior to a nonvoluntary approach. Not only is a transactional approach ethically preferable, but some research suggests that it will also be more effective. For example, research on PKU screening has indicated that voluntary programs have actually been more effective than nonvoluntary programs (22). This result confounds the assumptions of the expert-information model of communication, but is in line with the assumptions of a transactional model. When parents are engaged in a transactional manner and voluntarily involve their family in testing, they are more likely to follow through on treatment regimens because they understand and are committed to their value.

Given that the transactional approach is both ethically superior and likely to be equally or more effective, it seems peculiar that any other approach would be employed. However, transactional communication is more difficult for untrained medical personnel and also more expensive, especially in time and stress. Despite these difficulties, any public health agency that chooses mandatory genetic testing in the name of "efficiency" or "necessity" needs to attend closely and seriously to the heavy preference for those values in totalitarian societies (29). In the American case, a failure to achieve the necessary ethical standards could arise from perfectly good intentions. The desire to save a particular child from concrete and specific debilitating mental and physical conditions may seem in the immediate instance to weigh more heavily than concerns about rights and ethics that are abstract and distant. However, the trade-off is not truly between rights and concrete care for children. The trade-off is between financial concerns over "efficiency" and rights/ethics. Although dictating an outcome may seem more desirable in an immediate case, and although it may be more "efficient" in the large scale, it is ultimately less desirable in general, not only because it erodes the fundamental bulwark of individual rights, but also because it may generate lower participation and follow-through by other potentially afflicted individuals.

The erosion of individual rights is particularly of concern because screening for PKU could be taken as a precedent for multiplex genetic screening of newborns for any possible condition. Although newborn screening for PKU (and a few other relatively rare conditions) may be defensible because of the immediate and tangible benefits and the relatively low costs to parents, society, and children, this is likely to be atypical of disease conditions covered in multiplex genetic screening. Testing for cystic fibrosis, for example, offers a tempting candidate for inclusion in newborn or childhood screening. However, population-scale testing for cystic fibrosis is not medically necessary for the potentially afflicted individual. If an individual has no symptoms, there is no need for treatment, and if an individual has symptoms, the diagnosis and treatment may be initiated based on symptomology. Given that genetic testing may reveal recessive genes and that these may have serious implications for personal identity, familial relationships, and reproductive planning, testing that is not motivated by pressing medical needs is pernicious. At most, genetic testing may be medically useful as a back-up to uncertain clinical diagnosis.

On the population scale, cystic fibrosis testing has been advocated for reproductive planning (30), not for individual benefit. Population-scale newborn screening for conditions such as PKU could thus provide a back-door entry for population-based reproductive genetic influence by the government. If these programs are not employed within a transactional process at both the public and personal levels, one may have inadvertently implemented a eugenics program in the vicious sense of that term.

In addition, there is disagreement about whether parents should be able to choose on behalf of their children any testing for delayed-onset conditions (31); our analysis suggests they should not. However, there are certainly no ethically permissible grounds for government agencies to mandate genetic testing of children for delayed-onset conditions. Permitting nonvoluntary testing of children for PKU and the few other conditions in which such testing might be of immediate benefit to the child risks establishing an ethically dangerous precedent. Given that use of voluntary programs is likely to be as effective if not more effective than nonvoluntary programs, the benefits of transactional approaches seem well worth their additional economic costs. If we cannot afford to do genetic testing ethically, we would argue, we cannot afford to do it at all.

We conclude, therefore, that a transactional process is desirable, if not necessary, for all public health genetics. In mass communication campaigns, this process should include active involvement of representatives from target audiences (potential "consumers") and from the broader public in both program design and message design and evaluation. At the level of the individual consumer, it should require transactional, voluntary approaches. While we believe thoroughly in the importance of appropriate processes, we do not believe in their sufficiency. Consequently, adoption of these transactional communication processes needs to be accompanied by direct pretesting of messages to ensure that they do not increase stigma about particular genetic configurations, particularly that they do not increase attitudes that are genetically deterministic and discriminatory.

Testing the Attitudinal Effects of Messages

In the past two decades, backers of public health campaigns have become increasingly sophisticated about the messages they produce (32–34). Pretesting of messages to ensure that they have some positive impact toward achieving their target goals is increasingly recognized as desirable, if not essential. In the case of genetics, however, pretesting of messages should also attend to the socioethical impact of public health messages. A message that succeeds at encouraging people to seek genetic testing, but which simultaneously stigmatizes persons with some genetic configurations, would not be desirable. This section of this chapter reviews ongoing research indicating that (a) different forms of similar messages about genetics can have different attitudinal effects on target audiences, (b) even sophisticated critics are not successful at guessing what the attitudinal impacts of a message will be, and (c) a resort to technical vocabularies does not resolve the problem of negative attitudinal effects. Consequently, the existing research supports the need for pretesting of specific messages with their target and general audiences for stigmatizing effects as a necessary means for ensuring that public health messages do not encourage undesirable attitudes about genetics.

Attitudinal Components of Stigma: Discrimination and Determinism

Past critical and ethical studies have identified at least two major components of genetic stigmatization—genetic determinism and genetic discrimination (for a review of this literature, see ref. 3). *Genetic discrimination* consists of actions taken or attitudes toward a person that are based solely on the person's genetic configuration. Responses to a person based solely on the individual's genetic configuration are discriminatory because in all cases one's characteristics are only partially and probabilistically related to one's genes. Even if genes were the only factors influencing a particular condition, factors of timing and developmental interaction among genes play a vital and important role in the manifestation of particular characteristics—at the very least with regard to their timing and degree. (In the vocabulary of genetics, genes inevitably vary in their penetrance and expressivity.) But most human characteristics of interest are not the result solely of specific genes, but rather of interactions among several genes and various environmental factors including nutrition, toxic substances, culture, social structure, and upbringing. Even the most apparently clear cases of so-called single-gene diseases—such as sickle cell, cystic fibrosis, or Huntington's chorea—vary enormously with regard to severity, range of symptoms, or, in the latter case, time of appearance. To respond to someone's genetic configuration rather than to the clinical or tangible characteristic itself is therefore discriminatory.[2] The gene is not an accurate substitute for the person or for any of the person's characteristics.

Discriminatory attitudes about genetics derive much of their stigmatizing impact from their basis in excessively deterministic attitudes about genetics. *Genetic determinism* identifies genes as the sole relevant causal feature of an individual's characteristics and life courses. From genetically deterministic perspectives, if one's genes are identified as abnormal or insufficient, then one's core identity is thereby identified as insufficient and abnormal as well. Therefore, even in the absence of explicit discriminatory statements, messages that enhance attitudes that are genetically deterministic are socially and ethically undesirable. This does not mean that all statements about the causal or influential role of genes in human characteristics are unacceptable. Positions, attitudes, and statements that recognize the probabilistic nature of genetic systems and that place those genetic configurations within the multiple environmental inputs and developmental processes involved in the production of human characteristics can be unobjectionable. However, when false, unsupported, or tenuously supported claims of genetic absolutism are made, the charge of genetic determinism is appropriately levied. Thus, claims to exclusive genetic impact have been reasonably defended—for example, with regard to the so-called nurturing gene in mice (35), but few cases of human behavioral genetics today meet the test of sufficient support. Such research must include careful manipulation and control of a range of environmental factors to be informative.

Investigators as politically disparate as E. O. Wilson (36) and Alper and Beckwith (37) have emphasized that measures of heritability demonstrate that genes have an impact but they do not directly measure this impact against the relative role of environmental impact. Even twin studies do not generally provide wide variations in environment nor do they control for or even rigorously explore the different components of environment. Hence, studies of the sort that have been performed to date do not show the relative influence of genes over environment on various human characteristics, but only show that genes have some important influences. Statements that over-claim the role of genes or the scientific support for that role in any particular condition might

---

[2] Responding to someone's genetic condition may not be pernicious (hence "discriminatory" in the negative sense) when it is used to justify socially supported voluntary clinical monitoring and the voluntary adoption of services to reduce outcomes associated with specific genetic configurations. In such cases, the genetic configuration is responded to directly solely as a voluntary personal effort to gain additional information of a non-genetic type. In an opposite vein, some responses to persons based on their manifest characteristics may be discriminatory, but these would not constitute *genetic* discrimination and so would be dealt with on other grounds. Where manifest characteristics are mistakenly responded to as though they were genetic characteristics, there is genetic discrimination; such responses are based in false genetic determinism (see below).

rightly be classified as genetically deterministic, whereas statements that merely identify the existence of a substantial role for genes are appropriate, because they are accurately limited to the existing knowledge base.

Most thoughtful people will agree that public health messages that increase genetic stigmatization are likely to be both counterproductive and unethical. Such messages will probably be counterproductive because the threat of being stigmatized is likely to drive individuals away from testing rather than move them toward it. Such messages are unethical because they apply negative judgments to people based on criteria that are not related to merit or even actual characteristics, but only to potential characteristics. It is reasonable to assume that we have a national consensus that our tax dollars should not be spent on stigmatizing ourselves or our fellow citizens. Most ethical and social scholars agree that the key components of such stigma are genetic discrimination and genetic determinism. The question then arises: Can levels of determinism and discrimination be increased or decreased by varying the message form?

Attitudinal Impacts of Different Message Forms
Early research results suggest that variations in the form of genetic messages can result in quite substantial changes in the levels of discriminatory attitudes of message recipients, at least among some key target audiences. In 1997, a study by Condit and Williams (38) explored the impact of two different forms of a genetic "news" report on an important target audience of the new genetics—college students. Audience studies employ the methodology of analyzing the response to specific messages by particular audience segments or "target audiences" for a variety of pragmatic and theoretically grounded reasons.[3] Condit and Williams (1997) analyzed college students because they comprise an important target audiences for public media about the new genetics. College graduates are the group most likely to voluntarily use the next generation of genetic technologies (39,40).

In the study (38), the 137 research participants were asked to read one of two versions of a message about a family with a disease associated with a particular genetic configuration. One version of the message, labeled "voluntary hereditarianism," was assembled from news reports printed between 1970 and 1975. Voluntary hereditarianism is a worldview suggesting that individuals should make choices about their reproduction with regard to the "normality" of their offspring, but that these choices should actively consider genetic selections that will be good for both the society and for future offspring. The key metaphor in this discourse was the reference to one's genetic inheritance as a "lottery"—where heredity was a matter of winning or losing against present

---

[3] Audience studies choose to explore particular segments of audiences rather than to provide representative samples of entire populations so as to avoid submerging distinctive group differences in a general mean. Selection of relevant audience segments is based on a variety of criteria, but use of the target audience of a particular message is obviously one important basis.

odds. We presumed that this message would be perceived as more deterministic and discriminatory than the second version of the message, which was assembled from news reports printed between 1989 and 1992, and which we labeled "medical genetics." Medical genetics discourse presents a worldview suggesting that individuals are in control of their reproduction with regard to the "health" of offspring, but it also raises socioethical questions about the range and appropriateness of these decisions (for more information, see ref. 38). The key metaphor of the "medical genetics" discourse was the reference to one's DNA as constituting a "blueprint" that provided a plan for one's personal characteristics.

After reading one of the two versions of the message, each participant was asked a series of closed questions about the opinions about genetics held by the author of the message. This provided a manipulation check on the success of the construction of the distinctive features of the two messages. Participants were next asked a series of closed questions about their own attitudes about genetics. They were then asked several open-ended questions exploring their interpretations of the lottery and blueprint metaphors cited above.

The manipulation check indicated that the levels of determinism in the two messages were not successfully varied. This failure prevented analysis of differential effects, but it is an instructive failure, because our efforts to vary the message focused on three features that we thought reflected different levels of determinism: (1) the use of absolute terms such as "results in" instead of partial tems such as "predisposes" or "susceptibility"; (2) the inclusion or omission of statements about the role of environment; and (3) the use of the blueprint versus lottery metaphor. These null findings suggested that such audiences might not construct alternative understandings of determinism levels based on these factors. As indicated below, the qualitative study suggested that readers responded to issues of determinism along three dimensions—partiality/totality, probability/absoluteness, and fixity/malleability— and future studies are in the proposal stage to attempt to integrate these dimensions into a scale for measuring determinism.

The manipulation check indicated that the levels of discriminatory or judgmental affect toward those with genetic diseases was successfully varied ($p < 0.001$). This variation in the message had a surprisingly strong impact on the audience member's own stated attitudes with regard to genetic discrimination. The composite mean of seven questions designed to assess discriminatory effect was 26.8 (SD = 6.96) for those who had been exposed to the voluntary hereditarianist discourse, as opposed to 30.7 (SD = 6.72) for those exposed to the medical genetics discourse ($p < 0.001$). The strength of this difference is particularly striking given that the audience members merely read a single one-page message about genetics. This suggests quite clearly that messages about genetic health topics can have dramatically different impacts on public attitudes, depending on the particular components included in the message and the phrasing of the message. Public health advocates therefore have reason to be seriously concerned that any messages they generate be designed such that they do not have the side effect of increasing the levels of discrimination and determinism in public attitudes. This, however, turns out to be a task demanding more than moral intuition or even sustained critical reflection.

The Failure of Critical Predictions

The inability of Condit and Williams to manipulate successfully the perceived level of determinism in the genetics news reports provides one hint that constructing messages with desired attitudinal effects is not a matter that can be taken at face value. Further evidence of the inability of sophisticated critical analysis to predict the impact of particular word choices comes from the open-ended questions in the study. Social critics have generally concurred that the "blueprint" metaphor in genetics is both inherently deterministic and discriminatory in its meanings (3,41). The blueprint metaphor states that genes are like blueprints that lay down the outlines of our future characteristics and life courses. The study by Condit and Williams (38) asked participants to explain what they thought the lottery metaphor meant, what they thought the blueprint metaphor meant, and to compare the two.

The results demonstrated clearly the limits of critical prediction of audience interpretations. Whereas 39 of the 137 participants gave explicitly deterministic interpretations of the blueprint metaphor, a plurality, 58, gave non- or even antideterministic interpretations (others did not provide relevant responses or gave contradictory answers). The basis for these interpretations was that the audience members understood genes and the blueprint metaphor as being partial, probabilistic, and malleable. Hence, they saw blueprints as only part of a final construction, they saw blueprints as only probabilistic, not absolute designs, and they viewed the human building as a malleable product that could be revised either through individual will or through technology (for more detail on these findings, see ref. 42). In contrast, they saw the lottery metaphor as offering two absolute and dichotomous choices that could not be modified: "win" or "lose."

Similarly, only 7 respondents offered explicitly pro-discriminatory interpretations, while 39 offered explicitly antidiscriminatory interpretations of the blueprint metaphor. Thus, in this in-depth qualitative study, audience readings of the blueprint metaphor were far more variable than the critics had suggested, and they tended to lean in the opposite direction to that suggested by the critics. Although this is only one audience segment, it is the segment one would expect to be most deterministic and discriminatory in their worldview, because they are the group demographically positioned most similarly to early eugenicists. The fact that even such audiences as these did not produce readings of these messages that are strongly deterministic and discriminatory constitutes telling evidence that such meanings can hardly be called inherent to these terms.

If social critics who attend closely to discourse cannot predict successfully the impact of a particular message with regard to determinism and discrimination, one alternative might appear to be to stick tightly to technical vocabularies to avoid bias. Some recent evidence suggests that this also is likely to be an unsuccessful approach.

Scientific Terminologies Have Attitudinal Components

When issues of biased word choice are raised, scientists and other technical personnel often seek to resolve the problem by rigorous adherence to technical vocabularies. Unfortunately, such an approach in the case of genetics may be unworkable because public audiences hold meanings for technical vocabularies that include strong affective elements. A recent study by Condit and O'Grady explored the interpretations of the key term "mutation" held by lay and expert audiences. The expert audience consisted of 35 active research scientists in genetics at four universities. Two lay groups were surveyed. One was a group of 107 undergraduates at the University of Georgia. The other was a group of 31 primarily middle-aged, upper-middle-class white women accessed through a tennis directory. The latter group was chosen to provide a population that would be roughly similar to the experts in income, age, and race, while the students provided a third population that was similar, though younger.

After introductory open-ended questions, the readers were asked this question: "If a physician told you that your child or fetus had a genetic mutation but that this mutation did not cause any known harm, how worried would you be for your child's well-being?" The possible answers were (1) Not at all worried, (2) Slightly worried, (3) Moderately worried, or (4) Very worried. The one-way ANOVA indicated a statistically significant difference among the groups [$F(2, 170) = 44.84, p < 0.001$)], with both the tennis group (mean 2.77; SD 0.762) and the student group (mean 2.90; SD 0.800) differing substantially from the expert group (mean 1.49; SD 0.702). This question was designed to explore the impact of the meaning of the word *mutation*, independent of any presumed effects of an actual mutation. However, there are clearly other factors (such as fear of medical or technical communication settings) that might separate lay from expert audiences.

Thus, participants were next asked to check off the meanings they associated with the term "mutation." Chi-square tests between the tennis group and the expert group revealed no statistically significant differences with regard to three potentially associated terms (terms were selected on the basis of a historical study of public discourse by O'Grady, unpublished data). Both groups saw mutations as "variations" but not as "planned" or "intentional." More tennis players saw mutations as "expected" (21/31) than did experts (14/21), but if a 0.05 level of significance is corrected for multiple items, the 0.024 p value is not significant.

A clear difference existed between the two groups on two key terms. The scientists saw mutations as "necessary" (35/35) and "not undesirable" (29/35), whereas the tennis group tended to be significantly less likely to see mutations as "necessary" (14/31; chi square 20.1, $p < 0.000$) or as "not undesirable" (16/31; chi square 7.40; $p < 0.007$). The responses of college students were similar to those of the tennis audience (chi square tests of college students vs. experts and of college students and tennis players combined vs. experts show the same patterns, though they are based on unequal sample sizes). The open-ended questions in the study revealed that the scientists interpreted mutations as necessary because of the scientists' evolutionary worldview, and they interpreted mutations as not undesirable both because of that worldview and because of the utility of mutations in their own labwork. Scientists were more likely to define mutations at the microscopic level, especially in terms of alterations in base-pair sequences, whereas lay audiences associated mutations with physical consequences such as extra digits.

A candidate for an alternative term, "genetic alteration," showed a similar divergence in interpretations. If these groups, who are demographically similar to the scientists, and who differ from them primarily with regard to age and expertise, produce different understandings of these messages, then it seems even more unlikely that groups who are demographically different as well as different in expertise will produce meanings similar to those of the experts. These results therefore suggest that a resort to technical terminologies is not likely to guarantee messages free of biasing and/or stigmatizing effects and also that, due to their special experiences and interests, technical experts are unlikely to be any more reliable than are critics at predicting successful message contents for variable target audiences.

Pretesting Messages for Ethical, Attitudinal Impacts
Initial research indicates that different forms of public health messages about genetics may have strong impacts on attitudes about genetic discrimination and perhaps other factors such as genetic determinism. This research also suggests that neither the judgments of social critics nor those of geneticists provide a reliable source for ensuring that these messages do not carry unintended negative attitudinal impacts. Two courses of action are supported by these conclusions. First, research studies are needed to explore the interpretations that different audience segments have of different terms and components of genetic messages. This will provide further and more solidly based guidelines for construction of public health messages about genetics. Second, even when messages are designed with the results of such research in mind, they need to be pretested with representatives from the target audiences to assess their attitudinal impact on key ethical features. Audience studies

incorporating both qualitative and quantitative information provide one appropriate means of making such assessments.

Conclusions

The effort to incorporate the findings of molecular medical genetics into public health initiatives entails long-term and serious social consequences. If the benefits of these endeavors are to outweigh potential adverse consequences for individuals and for the society at large, the means of communication employed in designing these programs and implementing them need to be carefully constructed. Current socioethical and empirical research indicates the insufficiency of an expert model of communication and the desirability of a transactional model. This will require continued change in the way public health agencies do their jobs, so that target audiences and the public at large continue to become more active agents in program and message design and evaluation.

Additionally, however, direct testing of message effects is desirable to ensure that messages designed to achieve specific health objectives do not have the pernicious side effect of increasing the level of discriminatory and deterministic attitudes among the public. There is also a pressing need for more empirical information about communication processes in genetic medicine. Although substantial research exists on genetic counseling (43–47), mass communication of health campaigns (47), transactional communication processes in general and in health arenas specifically (48–50), and there is a growing literature exploring genetic worldviews (41,51,52), very few studies integrate communication research per se with the genetic context (exceptions include 53–55). Implementation of genetic technologies is not likely to wait upon communication research in this area. But appropriate communication processes are essential in this ethically freighted and socially significant medical arena. This makes additional communication research on genetics a pressing priority.

Acknowledgments

The authors thank Anna Williams, Wylie Burke, and two anonymous reviewers for their helpful readings of earlier versions of this chapter.

References

1. Kevles DJ. In the name of eugenics: genetics and the uses of human heredity. Cambridge, MA: Harvard University Press, 1995.

2. Smith JD, Polloway EA. Institutionalization, involuntary sterilization, and mental retardation: profiles from the history of practice. Ment Retard 1993;31:208–214.

3. Condit CM. The meanings of the gene: determinism, discrimination, and perfectionism in U.S. public discourse. Madison: University of Wisconsin Press, 1999.

4. Paul DB. The politics of heredity: essays on eugenics, biomedicine, and the nature–nurture debate. Albany: State University of New York Press, 1998.

5. Stacks D, Hickson M, Hill, SR. Introduction to communication theory. Fort Worth, TX: Holt, Rinehart, & Winston, 1991.

6. Marshall AA. Whose agenda is it anyway? Training medical residents in patient-centered interviewing techniques. In: Ray EB (ed). Case studies in health communication. Hillsdale, NJ: Lawrence Erlbaum, 1993, pp. 15–30.

7. Stewart M, Roter D. Communicating with medical patients. Newbury Park, CA: Sage, 1989.

8. Davis MS. Variations in patients' compliance with doctors' advice: an empirical analysis of patterns of communication. Am J Public Health 1968;58:274–288.

9. Anderson RJ. Methods of improving patient compliance in chronic disease states. Arch Intern Med 1982;142:1673–1675.

10. Donovan JL, Blake DR. Patient non-compliance: deviance or reasoned decision-making? Soc Sci Med 1992;34:507–513.

11. Parrott R, Kilgore M, Parker R. Negotiating child health care routines through paediatrician–parent conversations. J Lang Soc Psychol 1992;11:35–45.

12. Benkendorf JL, Callanan NP, Bobstein R, Schmerler S, FitzGerald KT. An explication of the National Society of Genetic Counselors (NSGC) code of ethics. J Genet Counsel 1992;1:31–39.

13. Wachbroit R, Wasserman D. Clarifying the goals of nondirective genetic counseling. Philos Public Policy 1995;15:1–6.

14. Rothenberg KH, Thomson EJ. Women and prenatal testing: facing the challenges of genetic technology. Columbus: Ohio State University Press, 1994.

15. Petchesky RP. Abortion and woman's choice: the state, sexuality, and reproductive freedom. Boston: Northeastern University Press, 1985.

16. Mahowlad MB, Verp MS, Anderson RR. Genetic counseling: clinical and ethical challenges. Annu Rev Genet 1998;32:547–559.

17. Bernhardt BA. Empirical evidence that genetic counseling is directive: where do we go from here? Am J Hum Genet 1997;60:17–20.

18. Brunger F, Lippman A. Resistance and adherence to the norms of genetic counseling. J Genet Counsel 1995;4:151–168.

19. Michie S, Bron F, Bobrow M, Marteau TM. Nondirectiveness in genetic counseling: an empirical study. Am J Hum Genet 1997;60:40–47.

20. Morley D. The nationwide audience: structure and decoding. London: British Film Institute, 1980.

21. Garland MJ, Anderson B, Jimison H. The scorecard as consumers see it: focus group results. A policy brief for the Oregon Health Policy Institute. Project: The Oregon Consumer Scorecard, August 1996.

22. Andrews LB, Fullerton JE, Holtzman NA, Motulsky AL (eds). Assessing genetic risks: implications for health and social policy. Washington, DC: National Academy Press, 1994, pp. 42, 43, 261.

23. Duster T. Backdoor to eugenics. New York: Routledge, 1990.

24. Goodnight GT. The personal, technical, and public spheres of argument: a speculative inquiry into the art of public deliberation. Argument Advocacy 1982;18: 214–227.

25. Dervin B. Mass communicating: changing conceptions of the audience. In: Rice RE, Paisley W (eds). Public communication campaigns. Beverly Hills, CA: Sage, 1981, pp. 71–88.

26. Clarke A, Flinter F. The genetic testing of children: a clinical perspective. In: Marteau T, Richards M (eds). The troubled helix: social and psychological implications of the new human genetics. Cambridge: Cambridge University Press, 1996, pp. 164–176.

27. Paul, DB. The history of newborn phenylketonuria screening in the U.S. In: Holtzman NA, Watson MS (eds). Promoting safe and effective genetic testing in the United States: final report of the task force on genetic testing. NIH-DOE Working Group on Ethical, Legal, and Social Implications of Human Genome Research, 1997;137–160.

28. Holtzman NA, Watson MS (eds). Promoting safe and effective genetic testing in the United States: final report of the task force on genetic testing. NIH-DOE Working Group on Ethical, Legal, and Social Implications of Human Genome Research, 1997, p. 10.

29. Hasian MA Jr. The rhetoric of eugenics in Anglo-American thought. Athens: University of Georgia Press, 1996.

30. U.S. Congress, Office of Technology Assessment. Cystic fibrosis and DNA tests: implications of carrier screening. OTA-BA-532. Washington, DC: U.S. Government Printing Office, 1992.

31. The prenatal and childhood testing resolution . . . expert opinions spark debate. Perspect Genet Counsel 1995/1996;17:8–10.

32. Atkin CK, Friemuth V. Formative evaluation research in campaign design. In: Rice RE, Atkin CK (eds). Public communication campaigns (2nd ed). Newbury Park, CA: Sage, 1989, pp. 131–150.

33. Freimuth VS, Van Nevel JP. Reaching the public: the asbestos awareness campaign. J Communic 1981;31:155–167.

34. Freimuth VS, Hammond SL, Edgar TL, Monahan JL. Reaching those at risk: a content-analytic study of AIDS PSAs. Communic Res 1990;17:775–791.

35. Brown JR, Hong Ye, Bronson RT, Diekkes P, Greenberg, ME. A defect in nurturing in mice lacking the immediate early gene fosB. Cell 1996;86:297–309.

36. Wilson, EO. Consilience: the unity of knowledge. New York: Knopf, 1998.

37. Alper JS, Beckwith J. Genetic fatalism and social policy: the implications of behavior genetics research. Yale J Biol Med 1993;66:511–524.

38. Condit CM, Williams M. Audience responses to the discourse of medical genetics: evidence against the critique of medicalization. Health Communic 1997;9:219–236.

39. Beeson D, Golbus M. Decision-making: whether or not to have prenatal diagnosis and abortion for X-linked conditions. Am J Med Genet 1985;20:107–114.

40. Coffman MA, Kinney SK, Shisler JN, Leuthard JL, DePersio SR. Reproductive genetic services in rural Oklahoma. In Reproductive genetic testing: impact upon women, fetal diagnosis and therapy, 1993;8(Suppl. 1):128–141.

41. Nelkin D, Lindee S. The DNA mystique: the gene as cultural icon. New York: W. H. Freeman, 1995.

42. Condit CM. How the public undestands genetics: non-deterministic and non-discriminatory interpretations of the "blueprint" metaphor. Public Understand Sci 1999;8:169–180.

43. Bartels DN, LeRoy BS, Caplan AL (eds). Prescribing our future: ethical challenges in genetic counseling. New York: Aldine de Gruyter, 1992.

44. Kessler S. Psychological aspects of genetic counseling: VI. a critical review of the literature dealing with education and reproduction. Am J Med Genet 1989;34:340–354.

45. Stadler MP, Mulvihill JJ. Cancer risk assessment and genetic counseling in an academic medical center: consultands' satisfaction, knowledge, and behavior in the first year. J Genet Counsel 1998;17:279–298.

46. Wolff G, Jung C. Nondirectiveness and genetic counseling. J Genetic Counsel 1995;4:3–25.

47. Winett LB, Wallack L. Advancing public health goals through the mass media. J Health Communic 1996;1:173–196.

48. Tinker TL. Recommendations to improve health risk communication: lessons learned from the U.S. Public Health Service. J Health Communic 1996;1:197–217.

49. Dervin B. Audience as listener and learner, teacher and confidante: the sense-making approach. In: Rice RE, Atkin CK (eds). Public communication campaigns (2nd ed). Beverly Hills, CA: Sage, 1989, pp. 67–86.

50. Krishnatray PK, Melkote SR. Public communication campaigns in the destigmatization of leprosy: a comparative analysis of diffusion and participatory approaches. A case study in Gwalior, India. J Health Communic 1998;3:327–344.

51. Rosner M, Johnson TR. Telling stories: metaphors of the Human Genome Project. Hypatia 1995;10:104–129.

52. Peters T. Playing God: genetic determinism and human freedom. New York and London: Routledge, 1997.

53. Conrad P. Public eyes and private genes: historical frames, news constructions, and social problems. Social Probl 1997;44:139–154.

54. Conrad P, Weinberg D. Has the gene for alcoholism been discovered three times since 1980?: a news media analysis. Perspec Social Probl 1996;8:3–25.

55. Durant J, Hansen A, Bauer M. Public understanding of the new genetics. In: Marteau T, Richards M (eds). The troubled helix: social and psychological implications of the new human genetics. Cambridge: Cambridge University Press, 1996, pp. 235–248.

29

Training in public health genetics

Susan M. Caumartin, Diane L. Baker,
and Carl F. Marrs

The term *public health genetics* describes the incorporation of the advances in genetics and molecular biology into public health research, education, and practice. Examples of contributions from the field of genetics that will enhance our ability to protect and promote the public's health include the identification of genes that contribute to the maintenance of health and of genetic mutations that result in disease; the investigation of the frequency of alleles in populations, subpopulations, and families, and the risks that mutations impose on these groups; the examination of whether genes act alone or in gene–gene or gene–environment interactions; and the identification and articulation of associated ethical, legal, and social issues.

Paradigm Shift in Public Health

The explosion of research activity in human genetics and the increasing information resulting from the international effort to decipher the human genome make it essential that public health students be educated in the basic principles of human genetics (1). Students of all disciplines—epidemiology, biostatistics, health behavior/health education, environmental/industrial health, and health management/policy—must add to their discipline-specific skills an understanding of the role genetics will play. Students of public health do not need to be geneticists. They should, however, be public health specialists who possess an understanding of how the application of human genetic information and technology is creating a paradigm shift in public health and prevention strategies (2).

Public health has historically viewed genetic disease as rare and unmanageable by traditional public health practice (3). We now understand that, broadly speaking, all disease has a genetic component (4) and that, in most cases, that component is only part of the complete disease equation.

Chronic and infectious diseases are best understood in the context of interactions among environmental, behavioral, and genetic risk factors. Common chronic diseases are now the greatest cause of morbidity and mortality in the United States, with heart disease and cancer most responsible (5,6). Although important environmental and behavioral risk factors have been identified and general population recommendations made, the unraveling of individual susceptibility to cancer and heart disease will allow for more powerful predictive and preventive measures.

Genetic variations in individuals resulting in differential susceptibility also play an important role in understanding infectious diseases. For example, CCR5 and CCR2 chemokine receptor variations in humans can affect susceptibility and disease progression after exposure to HIV (7). Similarly, red blood cell variations such as sickle cell anemia, G6PD (glucose-6-phosphate dehydrogenase) deficiency and thalassemia all provide protection against malarial parasites (8). As genomic information increases, many more examples of disease susceptibility alleles are being found (9).

Public health risk prevention recommendations are typically community- or population-wide, with limited ability to tailor the intervention or message to the high risk individual or family. A more individualized risk assessment, paired with better insight into disease management and immune response, should become possible with the emerging information about genetic mutations. Individual and family susceptibility would thus be combined with known environmental and behavioral risk factors so that more specific and appropriate recommendations can be made. Primary prevention of disease may eventually be defined as the interruption of known risk factors that contribute to the development of a disease in those with an inherited susceptibility (4). The objective is to reduce disease phenotype, not prevent or alter individual genotype (4,10). In other words, based on the identification of an inherited susceptibility (genotype), prevention would mean the alteration of environmental and behavioral risk factors that would reduce the likelihood of disease development and symptom manifestation (phenotype).

With the integration of genetics into public health theory and practice, there must be a concurrent focus on the ethical, legal, and social issues that accompany the development and application of genetic tests, the use and confidentiality of the information derived from those tests, and the privacy and informed consent of the individual being tested. Public health professionals need to be aware of the complexities of genetic testing and the meaning and use of test results. They should anticipate and become sensitive to the possibility of changing social pressures created by the very existence of such genetic testing. One need not look very far into public health history to be reminded of the abuses that have occurred in the name of genetics (11).

Public Health Education

The Institute of Medicine, in its 1988 study of public health, defines the mission of public health as "fulfilling society's interest in assuring conditions in which people can be healthy" (12). To achieve this mission, the competencies of the health professional must evolve with the changing landscape of threats to the community's health and the increasing amount of information resulting from each new era of scientific investigation. Historically, this has been accomplished through new educational programs.

Twenty-eight accredited schools of public health and over 300 universities nationally offer a masters of public health (MPH) degree or other public health graduate degree. It is estimated that about 5000 public health students graduate annually in the United States (13). These professionals are trained as multidisciplinary problem-solvers in one of five major public health disciplines: epidemiology, biostatistics, health behavior/health education, environmental science and health services, and policy administration. Many schools of public health also offer degrees or concentrations in maternal and child health, nutrition, international health, biomedical laboratory science, and public health practice/program management. In this chapter we focus on the need for incorporating an understanding of human genetics as applied to health promotion and disease prevention in schools of public health.

Public Health Genetics Education

Individual departments within schools of public health will choose to incorporate genetic information as appropriate for their specific discipline, ranging from understanding the nature and characteristics of disease, to risk appraisal and intervention strategies designed to deal with health issues resulting from genetic variability.

Epidemiology, Biostatistics

The utility of genetics is obvious in epidemiology, which focuses on the fundamental causes of disease. Epidemiologists and biostatisticians develop efficient and robust designs and analytical methods for examining health concerns that lead to improved understandings of underlying mechanisms. They identify genetic factors that place populations, subpopulations and families at risk. Health-risk appraisals will benefit from this knowledge of genetics by helping to identify individuals with inherited susceptibilities to major diseases, such as heart disease and cancer. At-risk individuals in presymptomatic stages may be offered preventive interventions earlier.

Epidemiology and biostatistics also play critical roles in the assessment of gene frequency, gene–gene interaction, host/pathogen genetics and the specific role of mutations as risk factors in various diseases. Through their analytical models, biostatisticians and epidemiologists will study the long-term effects of genetic differences on disease etiology and severity.

Environmental and Industrial Health

Every human disease, common or rare, chronic or infectious, involves a complex interplay of genetics, environment, and behavior. The public health areas of environmental and industrial health have historically identified the effects of chemical, biological, and physical factors on health and disease. Genetic information provides a blueprint on which to impose these factors. Environmental health specialists can assess gene–environment interactions and identify and test various environmental modifications to reduce adverse outcomes associated with specific genotypes. Given the extraordinary impact that common chronic diseases will have on the world's aging population, it will be critical for epidemiologists and environmental health specialists to apply an understanding of genetic mechanisms to reduce disease risk and disability and develop successful interventions.

Health Behavior and Health Education

Health behavior/health education specialists can assess public demand for genetic information, educate the public on genetic issues and evaluate the psychosocial impact of this information on individuals, families, and populations. Health behaviorists/educators are responsible for developing educational strategies that will communicate the complexities of genetics to the lay public and for developing effective behavior modifications that prevent disease in those with an inherited susceptibility. Education of the public in this area can be conceptualized as a population- or family-based version of traditional genetic counseling. The goal will be to assist the public in making reasoned decisions about their use of genetic testing, understanding test results, and analyzing the impact that test results may have on their lives (14). Health behaviorists might also contribute to an understanding of individual variation in utilization of genetic services. Additionally, behavioral scientists in public health have a key role in defining the ethical and social dimensions and implications of genetic technology.

Health Policy

Genetics adds an important new focus to public health policies and their impact on the delivery of services. Health-policy specialists identify, analyze, and address the ethical, legal, and social issues arising from an ever-expanding body of genetic knowledge and new technologies. These include the public's right to autonomy, privacy, confidentiality, and equity. Issues of privacy and confidentiality are important in light of genetic information about health risks and their potential effects on discrimination in employment and health insurability. Practitioners must ensure that the promise and realization of new knowledge is not compromised by misuse of that knowledge.

Changing Needs of the Workplace

The explosion of information about the role that genetics plays in our understanding of health and disease will alter and enhance our concept of public health practice, research, and education (15). A bewildered public soon will be asking what all these genetic advances mean, and public health professionals should be prepared to respond. Students of public health need to be trained now for the(se) future demands.

With this in mind, schools of public health will want to anticipate the evolving needs of diverse workplace settings. Public health graduates will continue to be employed at federal, state, and local public health agencies, health care provider organizations, research institutes, consulting firms, advocacy organizations, educational institutions, and a variety of industrial settings. Whether they work as scientists, program planners and managers, policy analysts, political advisers, educators, economists, biostatisticians, epidemiologists, lawyers, or health advocates, public health graduates will be challenged to examine the need to address genetic issues.

For genetic education in schools of public health to be relevant to this variety of workplace settings and roles, the curricula need to have breadth to relate to all essential public health disciplines and core functions and to be integrated with courses in all academic departments. Broad-based public health genetics programs are necessary to provide the application of genetic knowledge and technology in the variety of settings where public health is practiced.

Training to Meet the Need

In the same way that all public health students should be aware of the health impact of smoking, diet, exercise, radiation, pollution, and poverty, public health students of every discipline will need to appreciate the impact that genetic information will have on public health theory and practice. Responding to this need, all schools of public health will want to incorporate genetics where appropriate into their courses. Courses as diverse as law, risk management and communication, principles of health behavior, public health ethics, and aging and chronic disease will benefit from the integration of genetic information. Further, some schools of public health may decide to develop masters-level professionals with more detailed knowledge and skills in public health genetics. In the future, the need for more focused expertise and research in public health genetics may become apparent, creating the need for doctoral-level training. Schools of public health will benefit from drawing on the resources of medicine, nursing, law, social work, psychology, and other disciplines to create an interdisciplinary environment wherein the genetics curriculum will be enriched in depth and options.

Genetic principles and applications are important in providing all public health professionals with a more comprehensive understanding of health and disease. To understand the complex role of genetics in health and disease, one must first understand basic genetic principles. Some students arrive with previous training in molecular biology or human genetics, but many students have had little or no biology background when they enter a graduate-degree program in public health. For these students, the school could require mastery of introductory human genetics prior to entry into the program, or an introductory public health genetics course could be provided within the school.

Offering a course that begins with basic cellular biology and moves through DNA, cytogenetics, and modes of inheritance, to recent advances in genetics and molecular biology including the Human Genome Project, gene therapy, and molecular diagnosis of human disease would be appropriate. Applications of genetic advances and diseases relevant to public health practice should be emphasized, while the ethical, legal, and social implications of these advances are highlighted and discussed.

Additional course offerings could include genetic epidemiology, statistical genetics, population genetics, cancer genetics, risk assessment, and principles of health behavior. Perhaps most fundamental, though, to a public-health-based genetics curriculum is a course that focuses on the ethical, legal, and social issues arising from the application of the advances of genetics and molecular biology into public health research, education, and practice.

Issues of privacy and confidentiality, use of genetic information in epidemiological research, sharing of information within and outside families, and the right not to receive genetic information can all be considered. Because genetic testing and screening have become public health interventions, students can consider when and how such programs should be expanded, the extent to which they should be voluntary or mandatory, and the use of the resulting information by insurers and employers. Utilization of genetic information by these parties raises issues not only of balancing the interests of the parties, but also the balancing of public interests with individual rights and freedoms.

Emerging genetic technologies raise the familiar issues of access, quality, and cost. Students need to examine whether genetic testing and screening, genetic diagnosis, and emerging gene therapy should be treated differently from other medical technologies. These issues raise questions about the definition of health and disease—for example, whether a gene-influenced condition represents a disease to be prevented or treated, or is an instance of human variation to be tolerated or even valued.

Students should discuss the historical link between public health and eugenics. They should consider how emerging genetic technologies can be utilized in public health without repeating the stigmatization, harms, and discrimination of past eugenic practices.

A course that educates students in the ethical, legal, and social implications of genetics in public health is not only a necessary component of public health genetics education; it also provides a vehicle for demonstrating how basic science, epidemiology, human behavior, and policy development and implementation are linked in the study and practice of public health.

Future Directions

What are the future directions for training in public health genetics? Based upon the above analysis of the need and current directions, recommendation(s) may be to:

- Incorporate genetic education into the curricula of all schools of public health, either as an elective or special program, or as a component of all departments and an increasing number of courses. This approach to public health genetics education will parallel the approach being taken by the Centers for Disease Control and Prevention, which applies genetics to all major components of public health practice (16).
- Educate the faculty of schools of public health about the implications of genetics for the disciplines in which they teach and carry out research. Workshops, seminars, conferences, and web-based educational materials can support faculty development in this area.
- Assume an increasing role in the genetics education of health professionals, policymakers, and the public at large. This role should be bi-directional, educating the public and eliciting public views as a guide to policy-making.
- Explore collaborations with health professional organizations in the education of current and future practitioners. Pursue the development of continuing education conferences and institutes and participate in local/regional educational programs.
- Establish collaborative relationships with other university units and programs related to genetics (e.g., medicine, nursing, social work, public policy, sociology, biology, law). Genetics is a multifaceted subject area

that can facilitate effective interdisciplinary approaches to teaching and research.

- Encourage public health genetics research by public health faculty. Genetics can become a significant component of a diverse body of research, encompassing basic sciences, social sciences, policy, demonstration projects, and community-based participatory research.

Public health educators must assume a leadership role in preparing future public health professionals who will understand and know how to apply the rapidly expanding knowledge and technology in the genetics area to the practice of public health for the achievement of public health goals. In pursuing this mission, it is vital that schools of public health emphasize not only the science of genetics but also the ethical, legal, and social implications. The field of public health will then ensure that the ethical principles and societal goals on which it is based are reflected in the ways that genetic advances are applied to the protection and promotion of the public's health in the 21st century.

Acknowledgments

We thank Bruce Chin, Ph.D., Toby Citrin, J.D., and Thomas Hickey, Dr.P.H., all from the University of Michigan, School of Public Health, for their time, effort, and contributions in the writing of this chapter. We also thank Carolyn Hogan for her contribution in the preparation of this chapter. Support for the writing of this chapter was provided, in part, by National Institutes of Health grant 1 R25 HG01511-01A1.

References

1. Omenn GS. Comment: genetics and public health. Am J Public Health 1996; 86:1701–1704.

2. Khoury MJ. Relationship between medical genetics and public health: changing the paradigm of disease prevention and the definition of a genetic disease. Am J Med Genet 1997;71:289–291.

3. Schull WJ, Hanis CL. Genetics and public health in the 1990s. Annu Rev Public Health 1990;11:105–125.

4. Khoury MJ. From genes to public health: the applications of genetic technology in disease prevention. Am J Public Health 1996;86:1717–1722.

5. Hickey T, Speers MA, Prohaska TR (eds). Public health and aging. Baltimore: The Johns Hopkins University Press, 1997.

6. McGinnis JM, Foege WH. Actual causes of death in the United States. JAMA 1993;270:2207–2212.

7. Winkler C, Modi W, Smith MW, et al. Genetic restrictions of AIDS pathogenesis by an SDF-1 chemokine gene variant. Science 1998;279:389–393.

8. Roth EF. Red cell polymorphisms and the malaria hypothesis. Diagn Med 1985;8:28–35.

9. Qureshi ST, Skamene E, Malo D. Comparative genomics and host resistance against infectious diseases. Emerg Infect Dis 1999;5:36–47.

10. Juengst ET. "Prevention" and the goals of genetic medicine. Hum Gene Ther 1995;6:1590–1605.

11. Pernick MS. Public health then and now: eugenics and public health in American history. Am J Public Health 1997;87:1767–1772.

12. Institute of Medicine. The future of public health. Washington, DC: National Academy Press, 1988.

13. Katz W. 1996 Annual data report. Washington, DC: Association of Schools of Public Health, 1998.

14. Sorenson JR, Cheuvront B. The Human Genome Project and health behavior and health education research. Health Educ Res: Theory Pract 1993;8:589–593.

15. Collins FS. Shattuck lecture—medical and societal consequences of the Human Genome Project. N Engl J Med 1999;341:28–37.

16. Taskforce on Genetics in Disease Prevention. Translating advances in human genetics into public health action: a strategic plan. Atlanta, GA: Centers for Disease Control and Prevention, 1997. (available at *http://www.cdc.gov/genetics/Strategic.html*)

30

Consumer perspectives on genetic testing:
Lessons learned

Mary E. Davidson, Karey David, Nancy Hsu,
Toni I. Pollin, Joan O. Weiss, Nachama Wilker,
and Mary Ann Wilson

Genetic tests are moving rapidly from the laboratory to the medical clinic and from the detection of rare disorders to risk prediction for more common health problems. As health care consumers, we face an impressive confluence of new technologies—DNA sequencing and genetic testing on the one hand and the construction of massive electronic information systems that centralize personal, medical, and genetic information in rapidly changing health care delivery systems on the other. Ethical, legal, psychological, and social concerns associated with these new diagnostic tools, especially with the development of tests for more common health problems, will color and impact individual and family decision making about the use of genetic testing. In the rush of technological progress, shifts in health care delivery, and consequent policy considerations, the implications of genetic testing for families and communities must not be overlooked.

Ever since its formation in 1986, the Genetic Alliance (formerly Alliance of Genetic Support Groups)—a coalition of consumers, professionals, and support groups concerned with the needs of individuals and families living with genetic conditions—has worked to educate the general public and providers about the subtle, personal, and familial ramifications of genetic testing. Using the firsthand experiences of its consumer members as a powerful educational tool, the Alliance advocates for the development of genetic-testing protocols and dynamic informed-consent standards to ensure autonomous and informed decision making that is founded on current, accurate information at every step of the testing, diagnostic and treatment-management process.

Also published in *Families, Systems a Health* Ms #98.09—"Consumer Perspective on Genetic Testing: Implications for Building Family-Centered Public Policies."

As legislators, researchers, providers, and health care administrators begin to shape genetic testing policies, clinical protocols, and standards, we must listen closely to the experience and wisdom of the generation of consumers of genetic services who came before us. To focus attention on the lessons learned, the Alliance collected personal narratives from consumers with firsthand experience with genetic testing and screening.

The five Alliance members who provided narratives of their genetic testing experiences represent a range of genetic disorders and conditions—Tay-Sachs, neurofibromatosis II, familial adenomatous polyposis, sickle cell anemia, and cystic fibrosis—and diversity of geographic, ethnic, and religious backgrounds and ethical viewpoints. Their experiences demonstrate the impact of genetic testing on real people and underscore the need for broader genetics information, education, and counseling support.

These same issues and concerns will confront the next generation of genetic consumers as genetic technologies move rapidly into the detection and prediction of more common health problems. With advances in genetic research and technology and improved understanding of complex gene disorders, the concept of the consumer is moving from a small to a much larger population and from a rare disease focus to a more universal and common context.

Scientists, ethicists, medical professionals, and other experts routinely play major roles in public policy decision making. The Alliance draws on more than a dozen years of firsthand experience with genetic educational programs for professionals and the public to present consumer perspectives on the policy implications of genetic testing and to demonstrate consumer participation as a value-added component in policy development. This chapter presents a unique window into the personal experiences of five individuals and their families who have had front-line experience with genetic testing.

Personal, Familial, and Societal Implications of Genetic Testing

The experiences of living with a genetic disorder illuminate the issues facing individuals and families who are considering genetic testing. The narrators included here recount their experiences of coming to grips with the heredity of the condition, deliberating over medical options based on predictive but inconclusive test results, facing the issues and extraordinarily difficult choices during pregnancy raised by genetic testing, weighing the benefits and consequences of knowing a diagnosis, and choosing between the advantages of genetic testing and the risks of misuse of genetic information.

The presentation of these personal accounts is not intended as a comprehensive guide to the range of issues involved in testing for each genetic disorder. Each narrator's feelings about genetic testing are influenced in part by the specific condition involved and in part by individual and family attitudes and beliefs. Reactions to genetic testing can vary tremendously from individual to individual, family to family, and community to community; however, the ethical, social, psychological, and legal issues raised by genetic testing—at once complex, profound, and uncharted—largely cut across individual, family, and ethnocultural borders.

In each account, the individual simply tells his or her own story and does not presume to represent everyone living with the condition. Together, however, the experiences convey a range of motivations and personal values that individuals and families bring to the complex process of genetic testing. By listening closely to experienced consumer voices such as these, health professionals can learn about the implications of genetic testing, the crafting of public policies, and the development of clinical standards.

Consumer Involvement in the Development of Genetic Testing Programs

Tay-Sachs Disease

Classical Tay-Sachs is an autosomal recessive, degenerative disorder of the central nervous system that affects infants. Babies appear normal at birth and seem to develop normally for the first few months of life, but by 6 to 9 months, normal development slows. Development soon ceases entirely and regression sets in. By 18 months of age, most children with Tay-Sachs are blind, paralyzed, unresponsive, and suffering from repeated seizures due to an enzyme deficiency that causes the abnormal buildup of a fatty substance in the nerve cells of the brain, gradually crippling the nervous system. The disease progresses relentlessly, resulting in death by 5 years of age.

> *Sedra's infant daughter was diagnosed with Tay-Sachs at 1 year of age. The following is Sedra's personal account of that experience and her involvement, after learning about her infant daughter's condition, in community education about Tay-Sachs and testing programs. Sedra concludes: "Prenatal testing is never a simple experience, regardless of one's perspective, test outcome or decision."*

One day someone looked me in the eye and said, "Your daughter has a rare genetic disease for which there is no cure or treatment. She will deteriorate and die before the age of five. There's nothing you can do."

My daughter was one year old when she was diagnosed. While she was still at home, my efforts focused on finding the energy, time, and skills to care for her and the rest of my family. Then came the awareness that caring for her at home was becoming a 24-hour-a-day activity. I was rapidly coming to the understanding that I didn't possess the training or skills to handle the complex medical problems that were arising day by day. It was becoming clear that some alternative plan had to be considered. We looked, researched, and finally made the decision that hospitalizing her at the Tay-Sachs Unit of Kingsbrook Jewish Medical Center was the best option available to us.

To this day, while I understand intellectually the reasoning that went into that decision, I still feel as if on February 7, 1969, I abandoned my child. That awful sense, along with the huge vacuum created in my life when the challenge of caring for her was gone, left me with an intense drive. Even if there was nothing I could do to save my own child, I had to do *something*, find some way to fight back, or at least to move forward.

In May of 1969, three months after my daughter was hospitalized, I called together a small group of friends and neighbors. We sat around my living room exploring ways in which we could work together. We decided to form a chapter of National Tay-Sachs and Allied Diseases (NTSAD). Our primary thrust at that time (with no screening or treatment available) was simply to *be there* to assist families confronted by the then little known, yet monstrous experience called Tay-Sachs.

Timing is everything. Within a year, scientific breakthroughs concerning Tay-Sachs began popping up. The missing enzyme was discovered. The potential for identifying carriers surfaced and with it the ability for prenatal diagnosis to predict if the developing fetus of a high-risk couple had the disease or was unaffected. With this information in hand, a pediatrician at Johns Hopkins Hospital, Dr. Michael Kaback, conceived a unique strategy to combat this fatal genetic disorder. Dr. Kaback reasoned that if he could educate the community at highest risk for Tay-Sachs, the Ashkenazi Jewish community; provide an accessible, convenient way for members of this community to be tested for carrier status; and link high-risk couples to genetic counseling and follow-up services, the tragedy of Tay-Sachs disease could be prevented. So, in 1970, Dr. Kaback initiated the first community-based mass carrier screening and prevention program.

All of these developments created an incredible momentum for the young Philadelphia Tay-Sachs chapter. Suddenly, there was a simple and practical strategy to prevent the tragedy of Tay-Sachs disease, and all we had to do was tell *everyone* about it and find the means (financial and logistical) to deliver a Tay-Sachs testing program to all those people. And so we did.

In October 1972, we opened the doors of the Tay-Sachs Prevention Program (TSPP) at Thomas Jefferson University. Created and funded by the Philadelphia chapter of NTSAD, it was and continues to be a comprehensive genetic screening and counseling program aimed at preventing the tragedy of Tay-Sachs disease by identifying carriers and providing a full range of services to help high-risk couples have full, healthy families. By the end of 1997, 74,520 people had been tested and some 3,220 carriers identified. We are proud of TSPP's accomplishments; many tragedies have been averted, and many healthy babies have been born to high-risk couples.

Along with that sense of pride has come, for me, a far deeper understanding of the complexity of the carrier screening process. I know that when we began this adventure, it all seemed so clear, so simple. In fact, the most important lesson I've learned, the only thing I remain absolutely certain about, is it's not simple; the more we learn, the more complicated it gets. We developed this program to give people important information that we thought would be well received. Sometimes, it's not. I have found that most people choose to get tested to confirm that they are not carriers. They are generally not happy to find out they are carriers, no matter how much genetic counseling you provide. It's not simple.

Prenatal testing is an integral part of this program and most carrier couples opt to test their unborn babies for Tay-Sachs disease. Prenatal diagnosis is a heavy-duty, stressful experience and, while most of the time couples are given good news, about one in four times a couple is informed that the fetus is affected and that they must make a decision about terminating a wanted pregnancy. So, while one tragedy has been prevented, a significant loss remains. And what happens if a couple decides to undergo testing and prenatal diagnosis and elects not to terminate an affected pregnancy? Will an insurance company cover the care of that child? Will a couple really have the right to choose to bear a child with Tay-Sachs? It is definitely not simple.

Family Choices in Genetic Testing and Research: Discrimination Issues

Although Tay-Sachs causes massive damage and certain death at a young age, other genetic conditions have a less well defined outcome or range of expression. Issues and concerns vary in range and intensity according to the particular genetic disease, age of onset, disease severity, and available medical options. When thinking about genetic screening for other conditions—where impact and prognosis are less predictive—other complex choices unavoidably arise, as well as concerns about unauthorized disclosures of personal genetic information and discrimination.

Neurofibromatosis (NF)

Neurofibromatosis (NF) is an autosomal dominant genetic condition characterized by numerous tumors stemming from the covering of the nerves. Most of the tumors are benign but can become intrusive and cause problems with other body systems. People affected with NF also face an increased risk for malignant tumors.

There are two genetically distinct forms of NF. Neurofibromatosis type 1 (NF1) is characterized by multiple café-au-lait spots on the skin, multiple benign tumors on the peripheral nervous system, and growth abnormalities. It is associated with an increased risk for optic glioma (tumor on the optic nerve), scoliosis, learning disabilities, and cancer. Neurofibromatosis type 2 (NF2) is characterized by tumors (vestibular schwannomas) on both acoustic nerves that cause hearing loss and deafness, cataracts at an early age, brain tumors, and multiple spinal tumors. Symptoms usually appear in the late teens or, in some cases, even earlier. Neurofibromatosis is a heterogeneous condition, requiring affected individuals to be monitored for possible symptoms and changes throughout their lives. For some, in addition to the stress that accompanies any serious medical condition, NF can lead to special psychosocial adjustment problems stemming from its unpredictable course and potential for stigmatizing deformity in physical appearance (1).

> *Donna, whose husband and two of their three children have NF2, discusses her feelings about the use of prenatal genetic testing for NF2. Donna debates the pros and cons of pursuing a genetic diagnosis: the ability to monitor the condition and prevent complications versus the risk of genetic discrimination.*

How and where do I begin to tell you my thoughts on genetic testing? It's a question that leads to many more questions. Genetic testing can be good or bad. It depends a lot on your personal point of view on several issues.

One of the first things that is done once a gene is identified in relation to a hereditary condition is to try to develop a prenatal test. You can hardly mention genetics without the question of babies popping up. The first, and probably most volatile, issue related to genetic testing is whether or not abortion is a moral choice. I don't consider it to be a moral choice, and this colors my feelings about prenatal genetic tests. If someone did a prenatal genetic test and found that my child carries the gene for "our" disorder, would that make my child less worthy of life than a child who didn't have the gene? (My husband has NF2, but we are a team—NF is ours, not just his alone, to deal with.) At the time we were having children, there was no prenatal test for NF2. Our decision was a no-brainer. If there had been a test, knowing before our babies were born that they had NF2 would only have served to make the pregnancies more stressful for us.

We were involved through blood-sample testing in a research program that was seeking to find the NF2 gene. Our testing was hardest on my son, who was very young at the time. It was difficult to watch the children face those needles to give blood, but it was important to us that the gene be found because it might be helpful in developing a treatment. We felt it was also important to their futures to know—if it was possible to know— who had NF and who did not. Anyone who did have the NF2 gene mutation would need special monitoring and would generally fare better with early treatment, particularly to preserve hearing, if a problem did develop.

Our son's perception of NF was a more frightening one than his sister's. At a young age, he saw the pain that it can cause. Knowing that he has the gene was—and I suspect still is—scary for him in more ways than it is for his sister, who also tested positive. I think those fears have calmed as he has watched his father's rapid recoveries from surgeries, but they cannot be discounted or ignored. My son knows that he has tumors and can point them out to you. When his father and sister were in the hospital, he asked several times, "Am I going to have to have a surgery?" We have told him honestly that he probably will have to have one some day, but probably not for a long time. We encourage him to concentrate on eating healthy, playing, learning, and all of the fun things that children are supposed to do and try not to worry about surgeries.

What about other relatives? We knew my husband's father and paternal grandfather had NF2. His brother was examined but refused without explanation to give blood for the genetic test. We don't know whether it was because he simply doesn't like needles, he didn't want to know if he had NF2, or he thought he would have had symptoms by his age and felt it was unnecessary. My husband's uncle was also unwilling to participate in the research beyond answering a few questions, though he has some suspicious symptoms. With genetic testing, there are often people who adamantly want to know whether they have a disorder and people who just as adamantly do not want to know.

What are the pros and cons of knowing whether or not someone has this disorder? Would it always be considered a plus to find out? Knowing that a person has NF2 allows for earlier treatment of vestibular schwannomas, which grow on both auditory nerves and typically cause deafness. Earlier treatment, primarily surgery, can sometimes preserve some or most of the hearing. Waiting until the tumors are large enough to cause a noticeable hearing problem may reduce or ruin the chances of saving any hearing and preserving facial control and balance function. Also, NF2 can cause spinal tumors and scoliosis. These symptoms need monitoring in affected children because spinal tumors can cause loss of mobility, among other things, and scoliosis can cause pain as well as posture and pulmonary problems.

What could happen to health insurance coverage if NF was diagnosed by a genetic test? Well, worst-case scenario, you get the work equivalent of a "pink slip." We knew this was a possibility. My husband's insurance is part of a group policy through his employer, so the probability of their axing him in a major corporation because of a genetic test was slim in our view. The fact that he has a genetic disorder and needs the health coverage for himself and the children has kept him from going into business for himself, a regret that he has learned to live with.

If he changes jobs, what happens? This is something that has always concerned us. It's difficult to prove discrimination of any type, and with all the genetic testing out there, there will eventually be abuses if there aren't already. This is an issue that greets all of us in this time of technological and medical advances. Many employers require physicals which include blood tests when they hire a new employee. It is just a matter of time before those tests are sophisticated enough to detect more and more genetic disorders or predispositions. How will people prove that they were not hired because a blood test showed that they had the gene for some type of cancer, NF, or a host of other genetic conditions? Making this discrimination against the law won't stop it unless the physicals are entirely banned. Even then, there will continue to be people who walk into an interview with an obvious ailment and don't get the job because of it.

Family Choices in Genetic Testing and Research:
Testing Children

Familial Adenomatous Polyposis (FAP)

While the majority of cancer occurs sporadically, inheritable genetic mutations that predispose cancer are being discovered. Most of the discussion of "cancer genes" centers around inheritable mutations that greatly increase the chance that an individual will develop a particular type(s) of cancer but do not guarantee the development of cancer.

Familial adenomatous polyposis (FAP), an autosomal dominant genetic condition that causes approximately 1% of all colon cancer, is an exception. People with this condition develop hundreds to thousands of polyps, or colorectal adenomas, throughout the colon, usually as a teenager to young adult. Polyps are mushroom-like growths found in the gastrointestinal tract, primarily inside the colon. If these polyps are left untreated, they will become cancerous. At present, when polyps become numerous, removal of the colon is the only method available to prevent colon cancer (2).

> *Ann and members of her family have firsthand knowledge of the issues associated with the diagnosis and treatment of an inherited cancer. Ann speaks frankly, from the viewpoint of a mother who, together with her two daughters, is diagnosed with FAP: "Life was not over but it was painted a different color."*

Back in 1984, I found myself acutely ill and learned I had a rare genetic disorder, familial adenomatous polyposis (FAP). My family became involved in research programs shortly after surgery to remove my colon. In late 1992, Johns Hopkins Hospital in Baltimore, Maryland, where the FAP registry is located, asked if we would be interested in participating in a genetic study.

My husband and I looked upon the genetic testing as a welcome opportunity to evaluate the status of our daughters. We could now have confirmation, before actual physical manifestations, of whether or not they too had FAP. The girls, now 12 and 10 years old, had already experienced one distasteful physical examination (sigmoidoscopy) at ages 10 and 8. No polyps had been found in either daughter.

It is really difficult to describe how we felt during this time. I pictured many different scenarios. Would I be strong enough for them? Would they hate me? Would only one of them have the disease? We had now been living with this possibility for approximately 9 years at the time.

We explained, as best you can to children that age, what the testing was, what was expected of us, and why we had decided to participate. We had to meet with the people running the project so they could explain the purpose, take some blood, and answer some questions. The girls also had an opportunity to speak with genetic counselors on the telephone during the waiting period.

The Hopkins staff members were as interested in the family's reaction as we were in obtaining the results. We gave the girls choices: we could obtain the results and not tell the girls, we could all be present when the results were given, or we could not receive the results at all. The third option was never considered.

Originally, the girls were going to be present when the results were disclosed, but the uncooperative winter weather of 1993 forced us to reschedule the disclosure meeting. My husband and I decided not to have the girls present. I guess that given more time to think about it, we weren't sure we could handle our reactions and theirs at the same time.

"Both girls have the FAP gene . . ." I remember not being surprised, but I didn't hear much after that. I was thinking about what their reactions might be and my husband's reaction. When would we be looking at surgery? Is my husband sorry he married me? A tremendous sadness and, of course, fear came over us. Even though the test results were not a surprise, we both wondered, "Did we hear her [the researcher] correctly?"

Now came the time to tell the girls. Some time prior to the scheduled day, we had told them that we were meeting with the researchers. We didn't remind them of the meeting that morning, but when she came home from school, our 12-year-old daughter called me at work and chatted about her day. Just as she was getting ready to hang up, she said, "Did you get the results of the test?" Almost offhandedly it seemed, I said, "Yes, I will talk to you about it when we get home." She asked, "OK, but are we [she and her sister] the same?" I answered, "Yes."

She recently said she did not know how she would have handled having a different test result from her sister. Her younger sister, now 15 years old, claims that was not a factor, now or then, for her.

When I arrived home that day, the girls were both waiting impatiently. I can still see the oldest standing in the dining room, the younger one off in the background. When I told them the news, the oldest sort of shouted, "What am I going to do now? Who is going to take care of me? What about insurance? Who will pay for this? What about my children?"

There was no opportunity to give an answer between questions. I was shocked. We had never discussed costs or insurance. We may have briefly discussed having children, but I was quite surprised that she blurted all of this out. There were no public tears, ever, by either one of them. Eventually, we addressed each of her questions, inadequate as our answers might have been at that time. The questions were overwhelming for us as adults. I can't imagine how a 12-year-old perceived them.

The youngest, then 10 years old, said very little. Her sister said it all, I guess. She did go to school and tell a friend that she had cancer. Fortunately, that friend's mother called me and suggested that I have a talk with her, which we did. Our younger daughter treats much of life, especially awkward and unpleasant situations, with humor, which is beneficial for all of us.

Shortly after we got the genetic test results, at a previously scheduled physical examination, polyps were found in both girls. My husband and I both realized that life will never be the same. I don't mean life is over, but it's just painted a different color. A new agenda was suddenly placed on our table. Work took a back seat. We looked to the future and made some rather drastic changes. We sold the building where we had our law practice and relocated our office to a home addition. We wanted to be available for whatever we would face.

Once the testing was completed and the disease manifested itself, we really did not have daily discussions about it. As the time would draw closer to the annual appointment, we would all be a little on edge and some speculative discussions would arise. I found it interesting that both girls chose FAP as a research project for school.

In November 1995, we were told that our younger daughter needed to start planning for surgery. From the onset, her polyps seemed to be more aggressive in their growth pattern than our older daughter's. In March 1996, she was scheduled for surgery. After investigating all of the surgical options, we decided on a two-stage ileoanal reservoir. This would mean that she would have one surgery to create the internal pouch, which meant she would have a temporary ileostomy. If all went well, she would then be scheduled for her takedown, or reattachment. From the point of the second surgery, adaptation can take 6 months to 1 year. With the exception of a few minor setbacks, our daughter has come through with flying colors.

We were hoping to delay any surgery on our older daughter until she graduated from high school, but we were told in August 1996 that she now had to start thinking of surgery. She had her first surgery in January 1997, and a second stage the following March.

Both girls coped extremely well with the surgery. They are very different, and our preparation for surgery was slightly different for each. We would feed them information a little at a time over a period of months. Although you have very little control with any disease, we attribute part of our daughters' success and ability to bounce back to their normal schedules, to being well prepared and having some control over time frames. Above all, we have managed to get the girls through without a trace of cancer.

Genetic testing is certainly beneficial for FAP families. For those who test negative, it can eliminate the unpleasant and unnecessary testing that accompanies FAP. Testing would further benefit an FAP family who may manifest polyps later in life. That family would have additional time to learn about and understand the disease and make better informed choices with less pressure. This is especially important if the source is a recent mutation, as it was in my case. Approximately 30% of people with FAP were the first person in the family to have the mutation. Testing can provide families with time frames convenient for the family to plan and care for someone undergoing any surgery.

A Family's Experience as Motivation for Advocacy

Sickle Cell Anemia

Sickle cell anemia is an autosomal recessive blood disorder caused by a mutation in the gene for the β-subunit of hemoglobin. Under certain conditions, the sickle mutation results in rigid, sickle-shaped red blood cells that have difficulty moving through capillaries, decreasing the oxygen supply to the body's tissues. Symptoms of sickle cell disease include joint pain and a tendency for infection, fever, stroke, organ enlargement, weakness, heart problems, and growth delay. Sickle cell disease is most common among those of African descent, with a prevalence of approximately 1 in 600 in the African American population and a carrier rate of 1 in 12 (3). It is believed that the high prevalence of sickle cell trait in the African population arose from the mutated gene's ability to protect against malaria (4).

The history of sickle cell disease illustrates the potential for discrimination that arises with genetic testing. The promising discoveries related to sickle cell anemia of the 1970s resulted in gross abuses of genetic test information and tragic injustice for healthy and productive individuals. Many who were healthy carriers of sickle cell trait, or were simply presumed to be affected because they were in a high-risk racial group, lost jobs, health care, homes, families— the very fabric that holds life together. As we learn more about the genetics underlying conditions, it is important to remember the lessons of the sickle cell experience.

> *Larry and Michelle have three children ages 20, 15, and 13. Two children were diagnosed with sickle cell disease at a young age. They talk about living with children diagnosed with serious, chronic genetic conditions, and the difficulties associated with understanding and using test results.*

LARRY: As a young married couple, we had our vision of what the American dream would mean to us. As for so many other couples, children were part of that vision. To be honest, when our first child was born, we had not heard of genetic testing. The choice of genetic testing was not given to us. Michelle's mother had been told that she carried the trait, but this information was not passed on to us.

When our little girl was born in April 1978, she was beautiful and healthy-looking; we had no idea that this vibrant child had a war of cells going on inside her. When she went to the doctor for her 6-month checkup, the doctor informed us that tests showed that she had abnormal cells and he was referring us to a physician at a different hospital who could do more accurate testing. He gave our daughter a kiss on her forehead and said good-bye. His nurse was almost in tears. At the new doctor's office, my wife met a doctor who explained all the possible reasons why the initial test showed abnormalities. He also explained in detail what would need to be done if the genetic test proved our daughter had some form of sickle cell disease. After the tests were completed, our worst fears were realized. It was a blow that would eventually test our faith in God, family, doctors, and each other.

The nightmare began that day and continued to get worse as we realized that our insurance company looked at people with incurable diseases like sickle cell disease as a no-win situation. This issue brought on the additional burden of negotiating payment to the hospital based on portions of our child's bills that were not being paid by our insurance company. Within three years of her birth, we were in such debt that we were forced to file bankruptcy.

We reached a point of no return when our third child was born. Because of the particular trait I carry (β-thalassemia, which was not detectable at that time), the prenatal testing available showed no disease-causing abnormalities, just as with our first son. This time the test was wrong. Our third child—a second son—has been much sicker than our daughter, and his complications have at times been more complex and obviously more expensive.

MICHELLE: Our family's reaction to our children's illness has been varied. My father was very supportive, but he had no idea how to express his sadness for what we were going through. The way that he showed his support was to show up at the hospital and sit with me every once in a while. My mother's reaction was to start joining different sickle cell organizations, but she totally baffled me by paying attention only to our daughter and not to our son. This is still going on. Some of my husband's family members told me that to have this illness happen, I must have been an evil person or that I must have done something wrong to make God so mad at me. To have two sick kids was unheard of in this perfect family of actors, singers, judges, politicians, and an Olympic gold medal winner; how dare I! Others in the family just ignored the situation. No one would come to the hospital, then or now.

LARRY: As parents, we realize that if our children recognize that we have given up, in most instances, so will they. This was a deciding factor in our desire to get Involved the national PR campaign in "Health Security Express: A Call for Universal Health Care." We joined the national fight for the next family who would face these growing health care issues. We were fighting for the people outside our bus, the very people who cursed us and rocked our bus, scaring the children. We realize that we all have genetic flaws and it's only a matter of time before a condition surfaces in one of their family members. Then they, too, become a part of society that feels misunderstood and unwanted.

Larry and Michelle's circumstances illustrate the conflicts that can arise between an individual's right to genetic information and a family member's right to privacy. In not being told their genetic background, the couple was denied some of the choices they otherwise would have had. Had the couple's relatives had the opportunity to address their own emotional reactions to the knowledge that they were carriers, as well as to understand the scientific basis for it, family relationships might have been preserved, and learning their daughter's diagnosis would not have been compounded by the confusion of learning withheld "family secrets."

The experience of this couple also demonstrates an important lesson about genetic testing that is becoming particularly important as new tests continue to be developed. During the years that Larry and Michelle were having children, only the sickle cell mutation, not the β-thalassemia mutation that Larry was later found to carry, could be detected by DNA analysis.

In addition, the family's experience presents another lesson: For testing to be useful to consumers, there must be a more complete understanding about medical utility, the limitations of "positive" and "negative" results, and the impact of new genetic information on extended family relationships. This complicated phenomenon is one of many issues also confronting those who are trying to determine applications for cystic fibrosis testing.

Consumer's Perspectives on the Potential for Misuse of Genetic Testing

Cystic Fibrosis (CF)

Cystic fibrosis (CF) is the most common single-gene disorder affecting Caucasians. The CF gene codes for a protein involved in salt transport, and its symptoms include pulmonary difficulty caused by the presence of thick mucus, pancreatic insufficiency, and decreased fertility. The prevalence of this autosomal recessive disease is approximately 1 in 2500 in the Caucasian population (e.g., approximately 1 in 25 Caucasians is a carrier). Carrier testing by DNA analysis detects only 90% of the mutations in Caucasian carriers, so 10% of the carriers in this population will have false-negative test results. Incidence and detection rates in other populations vary, with test sensitivity comparatively low in some ethnic groups. As with sickle cell disorder and neurofibromatosis, the severity of symptoms is not predictable from the results of the genetic test and can vary significantly, even among those with the same mutation.

> *Suzanne, a successful lawyer, is 35 years old, and has CF. She hopes that genetic research is not diverted by the more immediate and tangible profits available in genetic testing technologies, and that the search for cures and better treatments of genetic disorders continues its current rapid momentum.*

I have always believed in the value of information and the right to know as much as possible about ourselves and our futures; however, the recent recommendation of a panel of experts to offer prenatal genetic screening for cystic fibrosis genes to all pregnant couples has caused me to reevaluate my perspective (5).

Having lived with CF for 35 years, I believe it is a manageable, chronic illness. Cystic fibrosis is a genetic disease that affects the respiratory, digestive, and reproductive systems. The disease is rare and primarily affects Caucasians. An individual must inherit two copies of the mutated gene, one from each parent, to have CF.

I was diagnosed with CF in 1964, at 7 months of age. At the time there were few treatments for CF and little hope for people with the disease. Referring to current medical information, my parents believed that I had a 50% chance to live through kindergarten. When I was old enough to understand these statistics, I had outlived them. I have now graduated from law school.

To treat my symptoms, I take pancreatic enzyme supplements with every meal to aid digestion and antibiotics to fight lung infections. I perform daily chest physical therapy by taking Pulmozyme to loosen the mucus and cough it up, thus reducing my chances of lung infections. I have been hospitalized for an intestinal blockage, appendicitis, and sinus surgeries, but no lung infections. I recently developed insulin-dependent diabetes due to CF. I have also participated in numerous clinical trials, including the Pulmozyme trial.

Despite the growing population of adults with CF who are living quality lives, genetic tests for CF threaten to reduce our value as human beings to our genetic information. Cystic fibrosis is not a uniform condition. Although prenatal tests may accurately detect the genes for CF, they cannot determine which genes will lead to a healthy life, as in my case, or to a lifelong struggle with the disease. I have two identical copies of the main genetic mutation for CF and, were the prenatal CF test available in the 1960s, I may not have been born.

I am not the only person living well with CF. People with CF are living productive lives, attending high school and college, getting married, having careers, and having children of their own. The current life expectancy is about 31 years of age; however, for individuals born with CF today, the life expectancy can be much higher (5). I have many friends with CF. Many are older and are doing quite well. Some are younger and have struggled with their health. A few have received lung transplants. All of us anticipate new drugs to cure the disease.

There are about 23,000 people with CF living in the United States Approximately 35.6% of this population are now adults; about half of this population will be adults by the year 2000. A survey in 1995 reported that 35% of young adults with CF worked full-time, and almost 90% had completed a high school education (5).

New medical treatments have improved the length and quality of our lives. Pulmozyme, the first new drug for CF, thins the mucus in the lungs, thus reducing the chance for lung infections (5). In December 1997, the Food and Drug Administration (FDA) approved TOBI, the first inhaled antibiotic treatment for CF [The Washington Post, December 24, 1997]. New treatment approaches target the genetic cause or causes of CF to correct the cellular defect (5).

I believe we will cure CF in my lifetime. With our knowledge of CF and with research on new treatments rapidly advancing, I believe the decision by the NIH [National Institutes of Health] panel to offer genetic testing for CF to all pregnant couples is inappropriate (5). I believe this widespread use of genetic testing for CF could reduce the number of people living with CF in an inappropriate manner, negatively impact the perception of society toward people with disabilities, and threaten the desire of biotechnology and pharmaceutical companies to pursue treatments and cures for people with CF. For these reasons, I challenge the appropriateness of using prenatal testing for CF for all pregnant couples, especially in the absence of reliable mechanisms to ensure truly informed decision making. Our society should focus on developing new treatments for CF and treating people with disabilities as equals. Given the premium that society places on "perfection" and the absence of adequate social acceptance and support for people who are less than perfect, prenatal CF testing may actually reduce parental choice. I am concerned that testing technol-

ogy will increase peer pressure to eliminate the problem of CF by terminating the children who will have it. We are faced with using a new technology to eliminate certain genetic diseases and people with those diseases.
Just because we can eliminate disease in this way does not mean that we
should. We must continue to protect the most frail in our society.

It is essential that testing coercion does not occur. Suzanne, who is concerned about the effects of actively offering CF carrier testing to all pregnant
couples and couples planning pregnancies, warns against sending "a message
to potential parents of children with certain genetic traits that they are irre-
sponsible in not using prenatal tests to terminate an affected baby."

Informed consent and freedom of choice need to be carefully protected for
the genetics consumer. It is equally crucial that individual decisions regarding
testing be supported in cases not involving a pregnancy, such as those surrounding testing for adult-onset disorders such as breast cancer or
Huntington's disease. Suzanne emphasizes an important point:

> I must also stress that genetic testing must remain an option that individ-
> uals may choose to forgo. The decision to forgo testing must remain just
> as much a voluntary option as the decision to take the test. Furthermore,
> it is also an individual's decision to use the information from the test in a
> way that best suits his or her life. My hope is that some individuals will
> decide to continue pregnancies despite the knowledge that the outcome
> will be children with CF. However, I fully recognize that this is an indi-
> vidual decision. Once made, it must be supported by medical profes-
> sionals, health insurers, and society.

It should be noted that Suzanne's personal view regarding the availability
of testing does not necessarily represent all individuals with CF. Some individuals believe that, whereas their lives are worthwhile, it is important that
others have the opportunity to choose to avoid having a child with CF and the
associated emotional, physical, and financial challenges that accrue from this
decision.

Policy Implications of Genetic Testing:
The Role of Consumers

The five contributors to this chapter speak passionately about what genetic
testing means to them and their families. Their stories bring to life the range
of experiences and issues associated with the testing experience—the personal, ethical, and family challenges; the complicated medical options; and the
fears surrounding genetic discrimination.

For many individuals and families, the impact of receiving genetic testing
results is powerful beyond imagination. Test results can indicate future risk

probabilities or even early death. They can reveal secrets about the past, confirm personal identities, or suggest shared family destinies. They can also give rise to adverse family reactions.

By sharing their stories with us, these five consumers highlight a number of important common themes regarding genetic testing:

- Consumers must be guaranteed the right to make voluntary, informed choices about genetic testing.
- Consumers must have access to accurate information and supportive counseling to make informed decisions about genetic testing and to use the information it provides appropriately.
- As with any medical diagnosis, the identification of a genetic condition has the potential to impact dramatically on the health and psychosocial adjustment of the individual.
- Health professionals offering genetic testing must have a thorough understanding of the benefits and limitations of such testing and the needs of the individuals and families who seek their care.
- Concerted and systematic efforts must succeed in preventing the social, legal, and institutional stigmatization of individuals with genetic disorders and in guaranteeing their right to voluntary, informed choices about genetic testing.
- Genetic services must include a broad range of testing, clinical, and support services, including counseling prior to genetic testing or screening, while awaiting test results and after receiving test information.
- The implications of genetic testing and diagnosis reach beyond the individual being tested, to the individual's family and extended family circle. Test results can indicate that others in the family are at risk for the same disorder or suggest that unsuspecting family members might be carriers of a genetic condition.
- The implications of genetic testing also reach out to the larger community of individuals who may have no interest or desire to know their genetic makeup and may be concerned that information about the genetic characteristics of their community might be used as fuel for discrimination and stigmatization.
- As the number of genes known to cause or increase susceptibility to diseases—particularly common diseases—grows, the number of individuals and families affected by and making decisions about genetic testing will grow exponentially.

Consumer Recommendations

The number of genetic conditions for which tests are available is multiplying rapidly. The identification of a large number of genetic conditions and traits will eventually become a simple and quick procedure. However, genetic tests have arrived before the public fully understands how to use them to get the answers they need without jeopardizing their rights; before many health care professionals are prepared to use them to maximize quality patient care; and before policymakers are sufficiently literate in the science and ethics of genetics to shape appropriate public policies. Genetic-testing technologies cannot live up to their full potential until public and professional genetic literacy becomes a reality.

Geneticists, genetic counselors, and health care professionals with genetics training can work appropriately with individuals and their families, balancing genetic concerns with sensitivity, respect, and unconditional regard. To protect the privacy of genetic information and to prevent discrimination in health and life insurance, employment, and other life opportunities, these same concerns must be addressed at state and national levels where regulatory policies, standards of care, and genetics legislation are being crafted. Comprehensive genetics public policies are needed to guarantee that consumers have access to accurate information, education, counseling support, privacy, and nondiscrimination. Broad-based public education programs are needed for the general public to become informed genetics consumers, familiar with the basic terminology of genetics, risk probability, and susceptibility. With these safeguards in place, individuals will be equipped to evaluate the benefits and risks of genetic testing for themselves and their families and better prepared to live with their decisions.

Ultimately, both the appropriateness and the utility of genetic testing depend on the extent to which individuals are supported in their decisions. Until protective federal legislation has been enacted, decision making about genetic services will necessarily involve weighing the advantages of a genetic diagnosis against the risks of misuse of genetic-test results and genetic discrimination. Supportive education and counseling services that are sensitive to an individual's personal and family values facilitate the decision making process. Consumers considering genetic testing deserve the opportunity to ask questions and be given answers from skilled health care providers knowledgeable about genetics.

Conclusions

The consumer narratives shared earlier underscore the necessity for developing genetic-testing policies reflective of real human needs and responsive to consumers need for access to affordable, sensitive, and quality genetic services. The lessons learned by those with firsthand experience of genetic testing and screening are invaluable resources for building public policy that is respectful of individual, family and community needs and values.

For decision making about genetic testing to be truly optional and autonomous and for legislative policy to develop meaningfully, the input and insight of every segment of the genetics community, the public at large, and consumers from every ethnocultural community must be taken into account. There are growing numbers of opportunities for consumers to become active voices in public policy discussions including institutional review boards, grant-review committees, public health panels, conference planning committees, managed-care appeals boards, state legislative committees, state and federal commissions, federal agency advisory committees, and others.

In this new era of genetic-testing technology, as growing numbers of genetic conditions and traits are identified and genetics becomes mainstream medicine, there is the potential that every member of the general public will be identified with a genetic condition or predisposition. Through active consumer involvement in provider education and public-policy decision making we can look forward to the fulfillment of the promises of genetic testing and genetics research for individuals, families, and the swelling community of genetics consumers.

Appendix A   Alliance Educational Programs Build on Consumer Experience

Helpline and Information Resource Center (IRC): The Genetic Alliance (formerly Alliance of Genetic Support Groups) maintains a direct link to consumers of genetic services and the general public through a toll-free helpline service, 1-800-336-GENE. Helpline callers receive referrals to national support organizations, genetic counseling services, and other sources of information and assistance. These direct and daily contacts uniquely allow the Alliance to gauge the changing pulse of the consumer community and the general public, identifying concerns and unmet needs as they arise and translating these into policy initiatives.

Frequent questions received through the helpline include: "Will insurance cover genetic testing?" and "Can I get all my bad genes tested?" It is not uncommon to hear from an individual who has a genetic condition, or a family member with a genetic condition, yet still has many unanswered questions about the condition, its inheritance pattern, and the testing options available. Some consumers express apprehension about genetic discrimination and the possible misuse of genetic information; others falsely cling to assumptions about doctor–patient privacy rights or assume that the confidentiality of genetic testing results is protected by existing federal and state laws.

Interactions through the helpline graphically demonstrate the inadequacy of current public genetic literacy regarding the ethical, legal, and social implications of genetic testing and screening. From the perspective of its 12 years of helpline experience, the Alliance is convinced that proactive educational programs targeting providers and allied health professionals can create knowledgeable and skilled providers and consumers of health care services.

Consumer Voices Network (CVN): By making consumers full and equal partners in the policy-formulation process from start to finish, the promises of genetics research can be integrated effectively, appropriately, and ethically into health care services, health care systems, and genetic public policies. The Consumer Voices Network (CVN) articulates the common concerns of consumers and works to enlarge consumer participation in discussions that shape and define public policies that will meaningfully impact their lives.

To foster consumer voices and to promote public awareness of genetics and genetics services and policies, the CVN is expanding focus on policy in its *Alert* newsletter, new website resources, and legislative links E-mail broadcasts. The membership conference in September 1998, "Forging Genetic Partnerships: Researchers, Policymakers and Consumers," trained consumers to be effective advocates with news media, policymakers, and health care providers. The 1999 conference, "Genetics in the New Millennium: Meeting the Challenges," will set the stage for increased consumer participation in public-policy issues and forums.

Alliance consumer opportunities include working with news media to promote understanding of the consumer experience, increasing consumer involvement in the development of public policies reflective of their needs, and developing partnerships with other stakeholders in the genetics community. In the coming years, consumers with expertise in public health, newborn screening, clinical research, privacy and confidentiality, informed consent, and other issues will be recruited and matched with national and local conferences on specific public-policy topics.

Human Genome Education Model Project (HuGEM): The HuGEM Project is a joint educational initiative of the Georgetown University Child Development Center and the Genetic Alliance. The program draws from both consumer and professional resources and focuses on the ethical, legal, and psychosocial issues associated with genetic technologies, services, and research to enhance health care professional awareness.

A survey taken in 1994 of 332 Alliance consumer members validated consumer consensus that voluntary, face-to-face, and written informed-consent procedures, as well as genetic counseling, should be available to everyone undergoing genetic testing or screening. Survey results also suggested that consumers perceived a connection between the existence of a genetic disorder and actual and anticipated genetic discrimination (6). Fearing genetic discrimination, 9% of the respondents (or members of their families) refused to be tested for genetic conditions, 18% did not reveal genetic information to insurers, and 17% did not give genetic information to employers (7).

HuGEM II has launched a national educational initiative to bring genetics and associated ethical issues to the attention of seven health care professional associations: the American Dietetic Association (ADA); the American Occupational Therapy Association (AOTA); the American Psychological Association (APA); the American Physical Therapy Association (APTA); the American Speech-Language-Hearing Association (ASHA); the National Association of Social Workers (NASW); and the Council of Social Work Education (CSWE). The graduate curricula of these health care professionals characteristically do not include scientific, clinical, or policy courses relevant to problems and issues facing individuals diagnosed with genetic conditions. Working from a "train the trainer" approach, HuGEM staff and consumer volunteers travel to the national conferences of these professional organizations to present workshops on genetics and the ethical, legal, and psychosocial issues raised by cutting-edge genetic research and genetic tests that are increasingly faced by their clients.

Partnership for Genetic Services Pilot Program: By developing strong partnerships among consumers, medical geneticists, genetic counselors, and primary-care providers, the Alliance's Partnership for Genetic Services Pilot Program is working to address the need for scientific, educational, and social resources to provide complete and compassionate health care in the 21st century. The program promotes a quality of care that integrates the genetic information explosion, medical technology, and psychosocial implications into the context of our changing health care system.

By introducing families and individuals living with genetic disorders and their unique needs and resources to second-year medical students and primary-care providers in managed-care organizations, the Partnership Program aims to enhance quality genetics services. The Partnership Program will develop the capacity of managed-care sites to identify individuals who can benefit from genetics services and assist pilot sites in delivering quality genetics services to consumers in a family-centered and culturally appropriate manner. Primary-care providers will have the opportunity to gain awareness of the implications of genetic testing and conditions for routine patient management. The Partnership will introduce valuable consumer-oriented resources that are available within the support group community and that can be used to supplement medical management.

References

1. Gutmann DH, Aylsworth A, Carey JC, et al. The diagnostic evaluation and multidisciplinary management of neurofibromatosis 1 and neurofibromatosis 2. JAMA 1997;278:51–57.

2. Giardiello FM, Brensinger JD, Peterson GM, et al. The use and interpretation of commercial APC gene testing for familial adenomatous polyposis. N Engl J Med 1997;336:823–827.

3. Reid JH. Common problems in sickle cell disease. Am Fam Physician 1994;49:1477–1486.

4. Makgoba MW. Molecular basis of resistance and susceptibility to malaria. Lancet 1997;350:678–679.

5. U.S. Dept of Health and Human Services, National Institutes of Health. Consensus development conference statement: genetic testing for cystic fibrosis. Bethesda, MD: 1997.

6. Kozma C, Lapham EV, Weiss JO. Genetic discrimination: perspectives of consumers. Science 1996;274:621–624.

7. Kozma C, Lapham EV, Weiss JO Whom would you trust with your genetic information? (abstracts). Am J Hum Genet 61:1997;4:A24.

Appendix B   Useful Educational Materials

Books and Articles

Andrews, Lori B.; Fullarton, Jane E., et al. (eds.). *Assessing Genetic Risks: Implications for Health and Social Policy*. Washington, DC: National Academy Press, 1994.

Baker, Catherine. *Your Genes, Your Choices: Exploring the Issues Raised by Genetic Research*. American Association for the Advancement of Science, Directorate for Education and Human resources Programs, 1200 New York Ave., NW, Washington, DC 20005: 1997. *http://ehr.aaas.org/ehr/books/index.html*. Video available.

Biesecker, Leslie G. "Orphan Tests." *Cambridge Quarterly of Healthcare Ethics*. Cambridge: Cambridge University Press, 1996, pp. 300–306.

Cowley, Geoffrey. "Flunk the Gene Test and Lose Your Insurance." *Newsweek*. December 23, 1996.

Drlica, Karl A. *Double-edged Sword. The Promises and Risks of the Genetic Revolution.* Reading, MA: Addison-Wesley, 1996.

Findlay, Steven. "Genetic Testing Poses Questions of Privacy." *USA Today*, 1996.

Genetic Testing. Mary Ann Liebert, Inc., 2 Madison Ave., Larchmont, NY 10538-1962.

"Genetic Discrimination: A Prejudice Is Born." *Science News*, 150, October 26, 1996.

Gutmann, Monika. "Is Cancer in Your Genes?" *USA Weekend*, February 7–9, 1997.

Holtzman, Neil A.; and Watson, Michael S. *Promoting Safe and Effective Genetic Testing in the United States*. Final Report of the Task Force on Genetic Testing. September 1997.

Hudson, K.L.; Rothenberg, K.H.; Andrews, L.B., et al. "Genetic Discrimination and Health Insurance: An Urgent Need for Reform." *Science* 1995;270:391.

Johannes, Laura. "Study on Inherited Diseases Finds Bias." *The Wall Street Journal*, October 25, 1996.

Lapham, E.V.; Kozma, C.; and Weiss, J.O. "Genetic Discrimination: Perspectives of Consumers." *Science* 274:621–624.

Mittman, I.S.; Penchaszadeh, V.B.; Secundy, M.G., et al. "The National Dialogue on Genetics." *Community Genetics* 1998;1:111–202.

Pear, Robert. "States Pass Laws to Regulate Use of Genetic Testing." *New York Times*. October 18, 1997.

Rothenberg, K.; Fuller, B.; Rothstein, M.; et al. "Genetic Information and the Workplace: Legislative Approaches and Policy Challenges." *Science* 1997;275: 1755–1757.

Smolowe, Jill. "Genetic Testing's Growing Ability to Predict Disease Makes It Vital to Soften the Shock of Seeing the Future." *Time*, 1997.

Teichler-Zallen, Doris. *Does It Run in the Family? A Consumer's Guide to DNA Testing for Genetic Disorders*. Rutgers, NJ: Rutgers University Press, 1997.

Weiss, J.O.; Allen, L.; Marche-Escola S.; et al. "Consumer Perspectives on Genetic Testing, Research and Services for Ethnoculturally Diverse Populations." *Community Genetics* 1998;1:118–123.

Wexler, Alice. *Mapping Fate: A Memoir of Family, Risk, and Genetic Research*. Berkeley, CA: University of California Press, 1996.

"What You Need to Know About Genetic Testing Now." *UC Berkeley Wellness Letter*, December 1996.

Booklets

"Chromosome Rearrangements Discovered Through Prenatal Diagnosis." (1998) Pacific Northwest Regional Genetics Group.

"Gene Testing and Gene Therapy: What They Mean to You and Your Family." March of Dimes Birth Defect Foundation, 1275 Mamaroneck Ave., White Plains, NY 10605.

"Gene Testing for Cystic Fibrosis." National Institutes of Health Consensus Development Conference Statement, Office of Medical Applications For Research. Bethesda, MD, April 14–16, 1997.

"Gene Testing for Huntington's Disease." Huntington's Disease Society of America. 140 West 22nd St., 6th Floor, New York, NY 10011.

"The Human Genome Project: From Maps to Medicine." National Institutes of Health. Bethesda, MD. Publication No. 95-3897.

"Informed Consent: Participation in Genetic Research Studies." Alliance of Genetic Support Groups. 4301 Connecticut Ave. NW, 404, Washington, DC 20008.

"It's Your Choice" [Cystic Fibrosis]. Division of Genetics, University of Rochester Medical Center. Rochester, NY 14642.

"Understanding Genetic Testing." National Cancer Institute. Bethesda, MD. Publication No. 96-3905, January 1997.

"What Are Clinical Trials All About? A Booklet for Patients with Cancer." National Cancer Institute, 1997. NIH Publication No. 97-2706.

"Why Do DNA Testing or Banking? A Fact Sheet for Families." Pacific Northwest Regional Genetics Group, Oregon Health Sciences University. CDRD Clinical Services Building, 901 E. 18th Ave., Eugene, OR 97403-5254.

Videos

"A Question of Genes: Inherited Risks" (an Educator's Guide). Oregon Public Broadcasting. 7140 SW Macadam Ave., Portland, OR 97219-3099. September 1997.

"The Ethical Question (Fragile X Syndrome)." Division of Continuing Medical Education, American Medical Association, 515 No. State St., Chicago, IL 60610.

"Genetic Testing for Breast Cancer Risks: It's Your Choice." National Action Plan on Breast Cancer, HHS-PHS, Office on Women's Health, 200 Independence Ave. SW, Room 718F, Washington, DC 20201.

"Is There a Place for Me?" Neurofibromatosis, Inc. 8855 Annapolis Road, 110, Lanham, MD 20706-2924.

"Optimizing Genetic Services: Consumers and Providers Speak Out." The Eunice Kennedy Shriver Center, Funded by the New England Regional Genetics Group, P.O. Box 542, Mount Desert, ME 04660; (207) 288–2704.

"Our Genetic Heritage." March of Dimes Birth Defects Foundation, 1275 Mamaroneck Ave., White Plains, NY 10605; (914) 428–7100.

"Predictive Testing: Presentations by Patients," Michael Hayden, M.D. Ph.D. Dept. of Medical Genetics, University of British Columbia, (604) 875-3535, *mrh@ulam. generes.ca.*

"The Same Inside." March of Dimes Birth Defects Foundation, P.O. Box 1657, Wilkes-Barre, PA 18703, 1983. Educator's Guide with Lesson Plans Included. Closed captioned for the hearing impaired.

"The HuGEM Project: An Overview of the Human Genome Project and Its Ethical, Legal and Social Issues." HuGEM Project, Georgetown University Child Development Center, 3307 M St. NW, 401, Washington, DC 20007-3935.

"The HuGEM Project: Opportunities and Challenges of the Human Genome Project." HuGEM Project, Georgetown University Child Development Center, 3307 M Street NW, 401, Washington, DC 20007-3935.

"The HuGEM Project: Issues of Genetic Privacy and Discrimination." HuGEM Project, Georgetown University Child Development Center, 3307 M Street NW, 401, Washington, DC 20007-3935.

"The HuGEM Project: Genetic Testing Across the Lifespan." HuGEM Project, Georgetown University Child Development Center, 3307 M Street NW, 401, Washington, DC 20007-3935.

"The HuGEM Project: Working Together to Improve Genetic Services." HuGEM Project, Georgetown University Child Development Center, 3307 M Street NW, 401, Washington, DC 20007-3935.

"The Human Genome Project." National Human Genome Research Institute. Bethesda, MD 20892; (301) 402-0911; *http://www.nhgri.nih.gov.*

"The HuGEM Project: Genetic Testing Across the Lifespan." HuGEM Project, Georgetown University Child Development Center, 3307 M Street NW, 401, Washington, DC 20007-3935.

Websites

Alphabet Soup
   http://www.acadia.net/nergg/soup.html
Blazing a Genetic Trail: A Report from the Howard Hughes Medical Institute
   http://www.hhmi.org/genetictrail/
Council of Regional Networks for Genetic Services
   http://www.cc.emory.edu/PEDIATRICS/corn/corn.htm
Cystic Fibrosis Consensus Statement
   odp.od.nih.gov/consensus/statements/cdc/106/106_stmt.html
Directory of Genetic Support Groups
   http://members.aol.com/dnacutter/sgroup.htm
Family Village
   http://familyvillage.wisc.edu/index.htmlx
Gene Almanac
   http://vector.cshl.org/index1.html
The Gene Letter
   http://www.geneletter.org/
Genetic Alliance
   http://www.geneticalliance.org
Genetics Education Center: University of Kansas Medical Center
   http://www.kumc.edu/gec/

Genetics Resource Center
  http://www.pitt.edu/~edugene/resource
Genetics Webliography
  http://www.dml.georgetown.edu/~davidsol
Genetic Testing Task Force
  www.nhgri.nih.gov/Policy_and_public_affairs/Elsi/tf_gentest.html
Human Genome Education Model Project
  www.dml/georgetown.edu/hugem
March of Dimes
  http://www.modimes.org
The National Human Genome Research Institute
  http://www.nhgri.nih.gov/
National Organization for Rare Disorders
  http://www.rarediseases.org/
National Society of Genetic Counselors
  http://www.nsgc.org/index.html
Office of Genetics and Disease Prevention
  http://www.cdc.gov/genetics/
Office of Rare Diseases
  http://cancernet.nci.nih.gov/ord/
TheTech
  http://www.thetech.org/exhibits_events/online/genome/overview.html
The UMDNJ and Coriell Research Library. The New Genetics: A Resource for
Teachers and Students
  http://arginine.umdnj.edu/~swartz/teachgen.html
Woodbine House Book Publishers: Publishers of the Special-Needs Collection
  http://www.woodbinehouse.com

31

Using the Internet to disseminate genetics information for public health

Leslie A. O'Leary and Debra L. Collins

As a result of the Human Genome Project, most, if not all, of our genes will be mapped and sequenced by the year 2003 (1). Already, genes are being discovered at an incredible pace. Although most of the genes that have been identified are associated with rare genetic disorders, genes that confer susceptibility to common diseases such as cancer, heart disease, and diabetes are also being discovered. As these "susceptibility" genes are identified, clinical and epidemiologic data regarding their association with specific diseases will become available. This information will have tremendous impact on public health, particularly in terms of disease prevention and health promotion. Therefore, it is crucial that the information be distributed both accurately and rapidly.

The traditional method of disseminating scientific information to the medical and public health community has been primarily through publication of peer-reviewed manuscripts in scientific journals. Unfortunately, this process often delays the release of important information for several months to years. As data from the Human Genome Project accumulate rapidly, a new approach for disseminating this information is crucial. The Internet is an avenue by which information can be distributed inexpensively to millions of people both rapidly and accurately. This chapter will focus on the use of the Internet as a method of disseminating genetic information for public health.

History of the Internet

Although many people believe the Internet is a recent development, its origin dates back to the 1960s when the Advanced Research Projects Agency (ARPA), a research and development agency of the United States

Department of Defense, developed a computer communication network that became known as ARPANET. The ARPANET revolutionized the world of communications and provided the foundation for the Internet (2).

The objective of ARPANET was to link computers located at various scientific laboratories across the country so that computer resources could be shared among researchers. In 1969, the first four computers, located at the University of California at Los Angeles, the Stanford Research Institute, the University of California at Santa Barbara, and the University of Utah, were linked (2). Before long, computers from other areas (e.g., Harvard University, Carnegie Mellon University) were added, and ARPANET began to grow.

The first public demonstration of ARPANET was held in October 1972, at the First International Conference on Computer Communication in Washington, DC (2). Soon after, other countries began developing their own networks, but ARPANET remained the largest and most sophisticated. However, during the 1980s, other networks such as CSNET, BITNET, and NSFNET were being developed, and by the end of 1989, ARPANET had been dissolved; sites were removed from ARPANET and put on NSFNET (2). The NSFNET was faster and easier to connect to than ARPANET, and it became the backbone for what is now called the Internet.

During the 1980s, the Internet was used primarily by academic, governmental, and private research organizations. However, Internet usage exploded in the early 1990s when individual access to the Internet became available via commercial providers. In 1981, there were approximately 230 computers on the Internet (3); by the end of 1999, more than 100 million Americans will be on the Internet, according to Jupiter Communications, a New York research firm (4). Currently, the Internet is not only being used by academic, governmental, and private research organizations, but it is also being used commercially to advertise and sell products. Approximately two million Web pages are added daily in the U.S. alone (5). Because of its capability to distribute information rapidly, accurately, and inexpensively, the Internet has become one of the most popular methods of disseminating information.

Internet Services

The most fascinating features of the Internet are the services and information it provides. The most commonly used services include *electronic mail* (E-mail), the *file transfer protocol* (FTP), and the *World Wide Web* (WWW). Electronic mail, defined as messages sent and received electronically, is the most frequently used feature of the Internet and is the primary reason for its heavy use. Originating in the 1960s, E-mail has become one of the most effective means of communication. It is fast, reliable, and inexpensive and allows people to communicate with each other regardless of geographic boundaries. An E-mail address consists of two parts, the *username* and the *hostname*, which are separated by the symbol "@". A type of E-mail that has become increasingly popular is mail distributed through *mailing lists*. Mailing lists allow people to send a message to an E-mail address where the message is copied and then sent to all members who subscribe to the mailing list, thus enabling a person to communicate simultaneously with multiple people worldwide. Most mailing lists focus on a specific subject. For example, the *genetics mailing list* (genetics@listserv.cdc.gov), which is moderated by the Office of ,Genetics and Disease Prevention at the Centers for Disease Control and Prevention, focuses on information related to genetics and public health.

Another commonly used Internet service is the *file transfer protocol* (FTP), which makes possible the transfer of files between computers on the Internet. Using FTP and the Internet, individuals can distribute software or documents rapidly and inexpensively. For example, public health researchers worldwide can transfer information to each other within a matter of a few seconds, as well as access documents such as the Centers for Disease Control and Prevention's *Morbidity and Mortality Weekly Report* (6).

When most people talk about the Internet, they are usually referring to the *World Wide Web* (WWW). The WWW, which is a multimedia branch of the Internet, was developed in 1990 by researchers at the European Laboratory for Particle Physics (CERN) as a method of sharing information among physicists (2,7). The WWW is a network of documents, called web pages, linked together by a coding system that can electronically describe data, called hypertext language. Information from one web document (web page) to another can be accessed by clicking on highlighted hypertext in one document with a mouse. The documents can contain information in the form of text, graphics, video clips, or sound. Currently, the WWW is the predominant mechanism by which people access the Internet.

Search Engines and Finding Information on the Internet

New WWW resources are added or updated frequently in response to new technology, including improvements in hardware and Internet browsers. With the plethora of WWW information available, *search engines* are invaluable. Many (e.g., AltaVista, HotBot, Northern Light, Lycos, Infoseek) use keyword searches; however, each search engine produces different search results because of the differences in indexing systems used. Metasearch sites use several search engines simultaneously and rank the results.

Search engines use software, referred to as *spiders*, *robots*, or *worms*, to index a database of downloaded documents and resources (with titles, *URLs*, *headers*, *full text*, and other information) from various hosts linked to the Internet. A few thousand to more than a million web sites or pages may be included, depending on the search engine's database and the quality of the indexing.

All search engines provide a link to the sites retrieved in the results displayed, usually in order of relevance. The ranking of the information sought will depend on the keywords used, the way the search was requested, and the way the information on the page is indexed by a search engine. Some sites are also available in multiple languages and are accessible for the visually impaired through speech-translation programs.

Each search tool provides instructions for its use. The Frequently Asked Questions (FAQ) section is updated regularly and describes new features. There is no single comprehensive search tool for the WWW (web), and more than one search engine may be needed to find information. Some tips for using search engines are provided below:

- Use the most unique or unusual word associated with the topic.
- Use quotation marks around phrases; otherwise, the terms are searched individually.
- Note spelling errors and variations (e.g., color/colour).
- Use Boolean operators (AND, OR, NOT, or other operators) to keep a search from yielding too much, or too little, information.
- Use advance search features such as adjacency, proximity, or truncation (to find words near each other, or containing the same prefix or stem).
- Use specific field searches (such as URL or title), date, media type, and/or location.
- Some search engines allow "plain-English" word order, phrase, case-sensitive, and field-based searching.
- Some search engines specifically search the web, FTP sites, newsgroup articles, telnet sites, E-mail addresses, and/or electronic-news headlines.
- Some search engines allow searches in languages other than English.
- New locations of established sites are often announced prominently in clinical journals. One can also find relocated sites with searching tools by using keywords specific for the resource. Medical center librarians may be helpful as well.

Using the Internet to Educate Public Health Professionals in Genetics

Progress in the Human Genome Project has led to an explosion of genetic information. Genes are being discovered on a weekly basis, with more than 10,000 genes identified by the end of 1999 (8). In addition, genetic tests are being developed and marketed to the general public at an incredible pace. Currently, more than 700 genetics tests are available for medical practice (9). Because of the plethora of genetic information that is forthcoming, Sikorski and Peters (10) predict that most of the up-to-date information necessary to practice genomic medicine will be found on the Internet. Because of the potential impact this information may have on society in terms of disease prevention and health promotion, it is essential that public health professionals are educated in the field of medical genetics.

The Internet is also changing the way people learn. Traditionally, individuals were educated via lectures and books in a classroom setting. Nowadays, much of the material that was previously presented in classroom format can now be found on the Internet. As an example, the Global Health Network (11) has developed an Internet-based course in epidemiology to educate medical students and those in other health-related professions worldwide. The objectives of the course, referred to as the *Supercourse: Epidemiology, the Internet and Global Health* (12), are to provide an overview of (*1*) epidemiology using case examples, (*2*) the Internet using the interactive medium, and (*3*) the integration of epidemiology/public health and the Internet. It is likely that similar courses related to genetics and public health will also soon be available on the Internet.

Several WWW sites that contain educational information on genetics are now accessible on the Internet. The information contained on these websites varies in both level and content, ranging from material suitable for the general public to information geared toward health professionals and researchers. The Information for Genetic Professionals website (13) at the University of Kansas Medical Center provides links to clinical, research, and educational resources for genetic counselors and medical geneticists. Information on training programs in genetics is also available on the Internet. The University of Pittsburgh's Graduate School of Public Health, which offers a degree program in human genetics (14), and the University of Michigan, which offers an interdepartmental program in public health genetics (15), have websites that provide information on their training programs. Information on other training programs in genetics or public health are available on the Internet and can be obtained by using search engines or by visiting a university's website.

Public Health and the Internet

The goals of public health are to reduce disease, premature death, and disability in human populations. These goals are accomplished in a variety of ways through a multidisciplinary approach consisting of science, programs, and services. However, a critical component to improving the health of the public is information exchange and communication. Because the Internet has no geographic boundaries, it is an excellent mechanism for disseminating public health information. Already many of the medical and scientific journals (e.g., *British Medical Journal* [16], *American Journal of Human Genetics* [17], *American Journal of Public Health* [18]) can be accessed on-line (some with a paid subscription).

As the Internet gained popularity in the 1990s, its potential as a mechanism of disseminating information to improve public health worldwide became recognized (19). Today, use of the Internet in public health is expanding. Most state health departments (e.g., New York State Department of Health [20]), as well as federal (e.g., Centers for Disease Control and Prevention [21]) and international health organizations (e.g., World Health Organizations [22]) have developed sites on the WWW. Most of these sites have contact information to assist people who have questions or need further information.

With the plethora of genetics information that is forthcoming as a result of the Human Genome Project, it is not surprising that many public health professionals are turning to the Internet for genetic information. Data on gene variants, laboratories that do genetic testing, policy statements, and patient support organizations are all available on the WWW. For example, if a public health researcher needs information on gene variants associated with cystic fibrosis this individual can access such information from an on-line genetic database such as the Online Mendelian Inheritance In Man (OMIM™) (23). Similarly, if information is requested on laboratories that do genetic testing for cystic fibrosis one could access the GeneTests™ (9) website, which is an on-line directory of laboratories providing testing for genetic disorders. Although these resources may not currently be available for all diseases, it is likely that as the information becomes available for other disorders it will be put on the Internet.

Public health organizations are not only turning to the Internet to obtain information, but many are also designing websites that are specific to their own genetics program. For example, many state health departments, as well as federal and international agencies, have developed websites that are specific to their genetics programs (e.g., California Department of Health Services Genetic Disease Branch [24]). The Office of Genetics and Disease Prevention at the Centers for Disease Control and Prevention (CDC) maintains a website providing access to current information about the impact of human genetic research on public health and disease prevention (25). Included on this website are links to other sites (e.g., genetic databases, regional and state genetics programs) that contain pertinent information on genetics and public health.

A website that is currently being developed that will be useful to both public health officials and to researchers and policymakers is the Human Genome Epidemiology Network (HuGE Net) website (26). This site contains the cumulative (and often changing) information on epidemiologic aspects of human genes, ranging from the prevalence of gene variants in various populations to the evaluation of genetic test and services. Other features of the site will include (1) updated medical literature searches for specific genes; (2) links to Internet sites and databases with population-based information on specific genes; (*3*) commentaries, editorials, and opinion pieces; (*4*) announcements of conferences, workshops, and training opportunities in human genome epidemiology; (*5*) funding opportunities in human genome epidemiology; and (*6*) a forum for communication and dialogue. Public health professionals will be able to use this information to develop both prevention and intervention strategies.

Genetic Resources on the Internet

Already there is an enormous amount of genetics information available on the Internet, and more is added every day. The resources available range from highly technical reports geared toward geneticists and health-related professionals to information on support groups and organizations for consumers. Most of this information is free and can be viewed by anyone with Internet access. For resources that are not free (e.g., software programs) many provide demonstration files on-line for preview prior to purchase. Below are some examples of resources that might be useful to both public health professionals and consumers. Additional WWW resources on genetics are listed in the Appendix.

Medical Genetic Databases

Online Mendelian Inheritance in Man (OMIM™) (8), the Internet version of *Mendelian Inheritance in Man*, 12th edition (27), is a resource first published by Victor A. McKusick, M.D., in 1966. OMIM is maintained by the National Center for Biotechnology Information (NCBI) and is continually updated with information from peer-reviewed journals in genetics, molecular biology, and related disciplines. *Mendelian Inheritance in Man*/OMIM is considered the most authoritative reference for information on inherited traits. The printed version of McKusick's catalogue focuses on single-gene traits (e.g., cystic fibrosis), whereas the on-line version also includes chromosomal conditions (e.g., cri-du-chat syndrome), as well as multifactorial traits (e.g., Alzheimer disease) (8,27).

OMIM provides a comprehensive description and overview of more than 10,000 genetic conditions. Each listing describes the condition, including clinical features, mode of inheritance, molecular and cytogenetic findings, diagnostic criteria, clinical management, and references. Each OMIM entry is given a unique six-digit number, a McKusick number, whose first digit indicates the mode of inheritance. The presence or absence of an asterisk (*) or number symbol (#) before an entry number provides information about the locus/phenotype/gene relationship. The numbering system also designates allelic variants. If prenatal diagnosis is available for a condition, it is probably mentioned in the molecular genetics or diagnosis section. If there is no information specifically given, this does not mean that prenatal diagnosis is not available, as there may be implied capability of prenatal diagnosis if the DNA mutation is identified or there is known linkage.

GeneClinics (28) is an on-line resource that contains comprehensive clinical descriptions, diagnostic criteria, management and counseling issues, molecular laboratories, and genetic support group links for specific genetic conditions. It is maintained by certified genetics professionals affiliated with the University of Washington. The disease profiles are written by experts and are peer-reviewed. By July 2000, some 250 disease profiles will be included. GeneClinics (28) complements GeneTests™ (9), which is a directory of medical genetics laboratories.

Genetic Testing Laboratories

GeneTests™ (9) is an on-line international directory of clinical and research genetic laboratories and is a valuable resource for locating laboratories offering genetic testing. This database maintains up-to-date information on genetic testing for more than 650 conditions from over 400 laboratories. Access is through user registration. GeneTests (9) is overseen by board-certified clinical geneticists and genetic counselors at the University of Washington, with support from the National Library of Medicine. GeneTests (9) can be searched by gene, laboratory, laboratory director, or OMIM catalogue number. The website will expand in the future to contain educational material aimed at non-genetics health care providers. This material will include a glossary and sections on the benefits of genetic testing, general uses of genetic testing, indications for referral for a genetics consultation, a genetics clinic directory, components of genetic counseling, and instructions on how to order a genetic test.

Genetic Support Groups

Numerous Internet sites provide information on specific genetic conditions for patients, health care professionals, policymakers, and the general public. Information varies between organizations regarding basic genetics, clinical features, management, treatment, medical advances, references, and community resources. Support groups frequently provide the full-published text of their brochures on their websites. Some sites focus on specific categories of genetic conditions, such as cancer (Cancer Family Alliance) or deafness (The Heredity Hearing Impairment Resource Registry—NIDCD HHIRR). The Alliance of Genetic Support Groups (29) maintains a database of current information on support groups for more than 300 genetic and rare conditions. The Alliance's website is regularly updated to provide accurate addresses, phone numbers, and other valuable information. The Genetic and Rare Conditions Information (30) website provides links to genetic support groups, educational materials, and research resources. Included are local, national, and international not-for-profit and private support groups.

Professional Genetic Organizations

All the professional genetic organizations have websites with information about public-policy statements and other pertinent topics. The website entitled "A World of Genetic Societies" (31) contains an overall list of professional genetic organizations. Membership directories are also accessible from this site, as well as information on genetic centers, education programs, and resources. A listing of professional organizations can also be found on the CDC's Office of Genetics and Disease Prevention website (25).

Information for Genetic Professionals (13) is a website overseen by a board-certified genetic counselor at the University of Kansas Medical Center. This site is updated continuously with input from international genetic resources. Included are resources for patient care, research, and education. Links are provided to clinical genetic centers, genome centers, and sites that focus on ethical and legal issues associated with genetics. Updated information about WWW resources in this chapter is available at that site.

Quality of Internet-Based Genetics Information

Although the Internet provides an excellent mechanism of disseminating information, one must be aware that the quality of information on the Internet varies widely, ranging from highly technical professional articles to anecdotal information on a personal home page, newsgroup site, or other public area. Internet information may or may not adhere to the established guidelines, peer-review, indexing, and cataloguing standards of published medical literature. However, the quality of genetic information on the Internet continues to improve as governmental agencies, educational institutions, research centers, and clinics add informative materials.

Numerous organizations have published criteria for assessing the quality, reliability, and validity of health information on the Internet (32,33). Criteria include (*1*) evaluating the credibility and conflicts of interests (qualifications of the medical advisors or scientific advisory board, website owner or sponsor, website author and credentials) and (*2*) evaluating the structure and content of the website (site-review process, frequency with which the site is updated, attribution of sources, comprehensiveness, accuracy, readability, and dating material). A website is more useful if it is easy to find and easy to navigate. The number of other websites that link to the site is also a means of estimating the value of the site. Moreover, indications of site utilization can be helpful, but misleading, as web site access statistics are not standardized and often difficult to interpret. Repeated visits to a page by the same individual may not be distinguishable from repeated visits from several individuals. Therefore, the number of visits to a web site cannot be equated with the number of visitors.

A set of principles and ethical guidelines for medical and health information on the WWW are set forth by the Health on the Net Code of Conduct (HONcode) (34). The HONcode is displayed on sites that clearly indicate that they (*1*) provide information about the medical health professional or author, (*2*) respect medical information privacy, (*3*) display the last modification date, (*4*) provide bibliographic references and updated links to other sources, (*5*) provide scientific references for health treatments and benefits, (*6*) display the E-mail address of the website manager, and (*7*) provide statements regarding site sponsorship and funding.

Summary

Few technological advances have had as much of an impact on communication and information dissemination as the Internet. Once used primarily by academic, government, and private research organizations, the Internet is now used by most businesses and schools, and is found in many households. Its ability to distribute current information rapidly, accurately, and inexpensively makes it the ideal mechanism for disseminating the vast amount of information being generated as a result of the Human Genome Project. In an effort to stay informed and up-to-date, public health professionals are likely to depend on the Internet as a repository for genetics information. The Internet will undoubtedly play a crucial role in disseminating genetics information to public health professionals and to individuals in the new millennium.

References

1. Collins FS, Patrinos A, Jordan E, et al. New goals for the U.S. Human Genome Project: 1998–2003. Science 1998;282:682–689.

2. Hafner K, Lyon M. Where wizards stay up late. New York: Simon & Schuster, 1996.

3. Glowniak J. History, structure and function of the Internet. Semin Nucl Med 1998;28:135–144.

4. Petersen A. The web's explosive growth poses a challenge for users: how to make the most of it. Wall Street Journal. December 6, 1999, p. R6.

5. Rout L. Editor's Note. Wall Street Journal. December 6, 1999, p. R4.

6. Centers for Disease Control and Prevention. Morbidity and Mortality Weekly Report. World Wide Web URL: *http://www2.cdc.gov/mmwr/*.

7. Doyle DJ, Ruskin KJ, Engel TP. Symposium: a clinician's guide to the Internet. The Internet and medicine: past, present, and future. Yale J Biol Med 1996;69:429–437.

8. Online Mendelian Inheritance in Man, OMIM (TM). Center for Medical Genetics, Johns Hopkins University (Baltimore, MD) and National Center for Biotechnology Information, National Library of Medicine (Bethesda, MD), 1999. World Wide Web URL:*http://www.ncbi.nlm.nih.gov/omim/*.

9. GeneTests™ World Wide Web URL: *http://www.genetests.org.*

10. Sikorski R, Peters R. Genomic medicine. Internet resources for medical genetics. JAMA 1997;278:1212–1213.

11. The Global Health Network. World Wide Web URL:*http://www.pitt.edu/HOME/GHNet/GHNet.html.*

12. Supercourse: Epidemiology, the Internet and global health. World Wide Web URL: *http://www.pitt.edu/~super1/.*

13. Information for Genetic Professionals. World Wide Web URL: *http://www.kumc.edu/gec/geneinfo.html.*

14. University of Pittsburgh Graduate School of Public Health Human Genetics Program. World Wide Web URL: *http://info.pitt.edu/~gsphhome/hgen/oldindex.htm.*

15. University of Michigan Public Health Genetics. World Wide Web URL: *http://www.sph.umich.edu/genetics/.*

16. British Medical Journal. World Wide Web URL: *http://www.bmj.com/index.shtml.*

17. American Journal of Human Genetics. World Wide Web URL: *http://www.journals.uchicago.edu/AJHG/.*

18. American Journal of Public Health. World Wide Web URL: *http://www.apha.org/journal/AJPH2.htm.*

19. LaPorte RE, Akazawa S, Hellmonds P, et al. Global public health and the information superhighway. BMJ 1994;308:1651–1652.

20. New York State Department of Health. Wadsworth Center. World Wide Web URL: *http://www.wadsworth.org/.*

21. Centers for Disease Control and Prevention. World Wide Web URL: *http://www.cdc.gov/.*

22. World Health Organization. World Wide Web URL: *http://www.who.int/.*

23. Online Mendelian Inheritance in Man, OMIM (TM). Johns Hopkins University, Baltimore, MD. MIM Number: *602421: Date last edited: 5/20/1999, World Wide Web URL: *http://www.ncbi.nlm.nih.gov/omim/.*

24. California Department of Health Services Genetic Disease Branch. World Wide Web URL: *http://www.dhs.cahwnet.gov/org/pcfh/GDB/gdbindex.htm.*

25. Centers for Disease Control and Prevention. Office of Genetics and Disease Prevention. World Wide Web URL: *http://www.cdc.gov/genetics/default.htm.*

26. Centers for Disease Control and Prevention. Human Genome Epidemiology Network (HuGE Net). World Wide Web URL: *http://www.cdc.gov/genetics/hugenet.*

27. McKusick VA. Mendelian inheritance in man: catalogs of human genes and genetic disorders (12th ed.). Baltimore, MD: Johns Hopkins University Press, 1998.

28. GeneClinics. World Wide Web URL: *http://www.geneclinics.org/.*

29. Alliance of Genetic Support Groups. World Wide Web URL: *http://www.geneticalliance.org/.*

30. Genetic Conditions and Rare Conditions Information. World Wide Web URL: *http://www.kumc.edu/gec/support/.*

31. A World of Genetic Societies. World Wide Web URL: *http://www.faseb.org/genetics/.*

32. Kim P, Eng TR, Deering MJ, et al. Published criteria for evaluating health-related web sites: review. BMJ 199;318:647–649.

33. Wyatt JC. Commentary: measuring quality and impact of the World Wide Web. BMJ 1997;314:1879–1881.

34. Boyer C, Selby M, Scherrer JR, et al. The health on the net code of conduct for medical and health web sites. Comput Biol Med 1998;28:603–610. World Wide Web URL: *http://www.hon.ch/HONcode/Conduct.html.*

Appendix

Selected On-line Genetic Resources
Alliance of Genetic Support Groups: Contains current information on support groups for more than 300 genetic and rare conditions. Includes accurate addresses, phone numbers, a printed brochure, a list of addresses, and phone numbers. Web site: *http://www.geneticalliance.org/*

Chromosomal Variation in Man: A Catalogue of Chromosomal Variants and Anomalies: Consists of a systematic collection of important citations from the world's literature reporting on all common and rare chromosomal alterations, phenotypes, and abnormalities in humans. Web site: *http://www.wiley.com/products/subject/life/borgaonkar/online.htm.*

Department of Energy Human Genome Program: Focuses on reaching the goals of the U.S. Human Genome Project in cooperation with the extramural division of the National Human Genome Research Institute of the National Institutes of Health. Web site: *http://www.er.doe.gov/production/ober/hug_top.html.*

GeneClinics (formerly Genline): Contains comprehensive clinical descriptions, diagnostic criteria, management and counseling issues, molecular laboratories, and genetic support group links for specific genetic conditions. Web site: *http://www.geneclinics.org*

GeneTests^{TM} (formerly Helix): An on-line international directory of clinical and research genetic laboratories that provide genetic testing. Web site: *http://www.genetests.org*

Genetic Conditions and Rare Conditions Information: Links users to support groups, and to educational and research resources. Web site: *http://www.kumc.edu/gec/support/*

Genetic Professional Organizations: Provides addresses of, and information on, international genetics groups. Web site: *http://www.kumc.edu/gec/prof/soclist.html*; Web site: *http://www.faseb.org/genetics*

The Human Genome Epidemiology Network (HuGE Net): Contains information on the epidemiologic aspects of human genes. Web site: *http://www.cdc.gov/genetics/hugenet/*

Human Cytogenetics Database: Includes cytogenetic data on more than 1000 chromosome aneuploidies. Web site: *http://www.oup.co.uk/isbn/0-19-268206-7*

Information for Genetic Professionals: Provides links to clinical, research, and educational resources for genetic counselors, clinical geneticists, and medical geneticists, as well as information on training programs in genetics. Web site: *http://www.kumc.edu/gec/geneinfo.html*

London Dysmorphology Database (LDDB): Includes a clinical description of more than 3000 nonchromosomal, multiple congenital anomaly syndromes. Web site: *http://www.oup.co.uk/isbn/0-19-268796-4*

March of Dimes: Offers information on specific birth defects or infant health problems, pre-pregnancy, pregnancy, teen pregnancy, newborn care, effect of exposure to drugs and environmental hazards during pregnancy (teratogens), support groups, and genetics. Web site: *http://www.modimes.org*

National Human Genome Research Institute (NHGRI): Heads the Human Genome Project for the National Institutes of Health. Web site: *http://www.nhgri.nih.gov/*

NORD (National Organization for Rare Disorders, Inc.): Provides education, advocacy, research, and service for voluntary health organizations serving people with rare disorders and disabilities. Web site: *http://www.rarediseases.org/*

Office of Genetics and Disease Prevention (OGDP): Provides access to current information about the impact of human genetic research on public health and disease prevention. Web site: *http://www.cdc.gov/genetics/default.htm*

Office of Rare Diseases (ORD): Disseminates information on more than 6000 rare diseases, including research, scientific and medical publications, as well as patient support groups. Web site: *http://rarediseases.info.nih.gov/ord/*

OMIM^{TM} (Online Mendelian Inheritance in Man): Catalogue of human genes and genetic disorders. Web site: *http://www3.ncbi.nlm.nih.gov/Omim/*

POSSUM (Pictures of Standard Syndromes and Undiagnosed Malformations): Lists descriptions of more than 2500 single-gene, chromosomal, skeletal, and complex genetic syndromes from the medical literature, as well as from the Genetics Clinic at the Murdoch Institute, Victoria, Australia. Web site: *http://www.possum.net.au*

The National Library of Medicine's search service provides access to over 10 million citations in MEDLINE, and other related databases and online journals. Web site: *http://www.ncbi.nlm.nih.gov/entrez/query.fcgi/*

Note: Because of the dynamic nature of the WWW, some URLs may have changed since this list was compiled.

Index